Oncology: Clinical Research

Oncology: Clinical Research

Edited by Georgia Cassidy

hayle
medical

New York

Hayle Medical,
750 Third Avenue, 9th Floor,
New York, NY 10017, USA

Visit us on the World Wide Web at:
www.haylemedical.com

ISBN: 978-1-63241-892-0

Trademark Notice: Registered trademark of products or corporate names are used only for explanation and identification without intent to infringe.

Cataloging-in-Publication Data

Oncology : clinical research / edited by Georgia Cassidy.
    p. cm.
Includes bibliographical references and index.
ISBN 978-1-63241-892-0
1. Oncology. 2. Tumors. 3. Cancer. 4. Tumors--Treatment. 5. Cancer--Treatment.
I. Cassidy, Georgia.
RC254 .O53 2020
616.994--dc23

Table of Contents

Preface

It is often said that books are a boon to mankind. They document every progress and pass on the knowledge from one generation to the other. They play a crucial role in our lives. Thus I was both excited and nervous while editing this book. I was pleased by the thought of being able to make a mark but I was also nervous to do it right because the future of students depends upon it. Hence, I took a few months to research further into the discipline, revise my knowledge and also explore some more aspects. Post this process, I begun with the editing of this book.

Oncology is a branch of medicine concerned with the prevention, diagnosis and treatment of cancer. Cancer is a disease, which involves abnormal growth of a cell. These cells have the potential to invade or spread to other parts of the body. There are different forms of cancer such as esophageal cancer, blood cancer, cervical cancer, lung cancer, stomach cancer, etc. Consumption of tobacco or alcohol, obesity and advanced age are some of the common factors that increase the risk of cancer. Common diagnostic tests used in this domain include computed tomography, biopsy, ultrasonography, magnetic resonance imaging, etc. Treatment methods include radiation, chemotherapy surgery, surgery, targeted therapy and hormonal therapy. This book studies, analyses and upholds the pillars of oncology and its utmost significance in modern times. A number of latest researches have been included to keep the readers up-to-date with the global concepts in this area of study. It is a resource guide for experts as well as students.

I thank my publisher with all my heart for considering me worthy of this unparalleled opportunity and for showing unwavering faith in my skills. I would also like to thank the editorial team who worked closely with me at every step and contributed immensely towards the successful completion of this book. Last but not the least, I wish to thank my friends and colleagues for their support.

Editor

Human papillomavirus genotypes associated with cervical precancerous lesions and cancer in the highest area of cervical cancer mortality, Longnan, China

Jin Zhao[1*†], Zhong Guo[1†], Qiang Wang[2], Tianbin Si[3], Shuyan Pei[1], Chenjing Wang[1], Hongmei Qu[1], Jianbin Zhong[1], Ying Ma[1], Cong Nie[1] and Dan Zhang[1]

Abstract

Background: The mortality of cervical cancer in Longnan is as high as 39/10 million, ranking first in China.

Methods: Between 2012 to 2016, 329 samples with cervicitis, cervical intraepithelial neoplasia grade 1 to 3 (CINI to III), and invasive squamous cell carcinoma (SCC) were collected. HPV genotypes were examined with a validated kit for 23 different HPV subtypes.

Results: Compared to cervicitis, the HPV positivity is significantly higher in CINI, CIN II/III, and SCC (38.60%, 74.60%, 87.50% and 89.05%, $P < 0.001$) and the positivity is also higher in SCC compared to CINI ($P < 0.01$). The most frequently detected genotypes were HPV16 in cervicitis, HPV16, 58 and 52 in CINI and CIN II/III, and HPV16, 58 and 18 in SCC groups. HPV16 positivity in cervicitis, CINI, CIN II/III, and SCC patients were 45.46%, 46.81%, 60.32% and 78.69%, respectively. Compared to cervicitis and CINI, the odds ratios (OR) for SCC in HPV16 positive patients were 2.96 (95% confidence interval [CI]: 1.09–8.00, $P < 0.05$) and 4.20 (95% confidence interval [CI]: 2.05–8.61, $P < 0.001$), respectively. In addition, the multiple infections in cervicitis, CINI, CINII/III and SCC group are 9.09%, 27.66%, 26.98% and 25.41% and HPV16 + 58 was the most common combinations.

Conclusion: These findings highlight the key role of HPV16, 58, 52 and 18 in the development of CIN and SCC in Longnan women and a fully aware of regional differences in HPV genotype distribution are tasks for cervical cancer control and prevention.

Keywords: Human papillomaviruses, Cervicitis, Cervical intraepithelial neoplasia grade I to III, Invasive squamous cell carcinoma

Background

Human papillomaviruses (HPV), double-stranded and non-enveloped DNA viruses (7 ~ 8 kb long), are a group of remarkably diverse DNA viruses from the Papillomaviridae family, which are causally involved in the etiology of various benign and malignant neoplastic lesions of mucosal and skin epithelium [1, 2]. Currently, more than 200 different HPV genotypes have been identified.

Genotypes HPV16, 18, 31, 33, 35, 39, 45, 51, 52, 56, 58 and 59 are regarded as high risk types (hr-HPV) because they are identified in high-grade squamous intraepithelial lesions (HSIL) and invasive cervical cancer tissues [3–5]. On the other hand, the genotypes HPV6 and 11 are considered as low-risk types [4, 6].

Cervical cancer (CC) is a major fatal malignancy among women, causing about 265,700 deaths annually world-wide. Nearly 90% of cervical cancer deaths occur in developing countries, such as China [7]. The cervical cancer incidence in China is high, with 132,300 new cases each year, yielding a rate of 27 per 100,000 women [8]. Epidemiological studies and experimental data verify

* Correspondence: gz6768@163.com
†Equal contributors
[1]Medical College of Northwest University for Nationalities, Lanzhou 730030, People's Republic of China
Full list of author information is available at the end of the article

that persistent HPV infection is considered to play a key role in the development of CC [9]. Cervical intraepithelial neoplasia (CIN) reflects a continuous and progressive CC process, and high grade squamous intraepithelial lesions (HSIL) with HPV infection, can develop and progress to CC over a period of 8 to 12 years [10].

The prevalence of HPV infection and the reported type-specific distribution varies greatly by geographic region and ethnicity. For example, HPV16 is slightly more prevalent in Europe and North America, HPV 31 is more prevalent in South/Central America, HPV 33 and 45 are more prevalent in Africa, and HPV 52 and 58 are more prevalent in Asia [9, 11–17]. Furthermore, the data from mainland China indicated that HPV16, 18, 33, and 58 were the most common types in women with CC in Henan, central China [18], whereas HPV16, 58, 18 and 33 were the most prevalent types in CIN2+ (high-grade cervical lesions, including CINII/III, and CC) in women in Liaoning, northeast China [19], and HPV16 and 58 were the most common types in CC and high-grade precancerous lesions in Chengdu, southwestern China [20].

Longnan of Gansu Province, located in the remote areas of Northwest of China, is the high incidence areas of cervical cancer and cervical cancer mortality as high as 39/10 million, ranking first in China [21]. This study aims to investigate the prevalence and distribution of HPV oncogenic genotypes in patients with cervicitis, CINI, CINII/III, or invasive squamous cell carcinoma (SCC) in Longnan. The results will help to establish more cost-effective follow up and guiding significance for cervical cancer prevention.

Methods
Study subjects
A total of 329 Longnan patients aged 17 ~ 79 years samples were initially included in the present study between January 1, 2012, and January 30, 2016: 57 in the cervicitis group, 63 in the CINI group, 72 in the CINII/III group, and 137 in the SCC group. All the samples were obtained from patients who underwent biopsies with colposcopy or advanced operations. In all of samples, 305 were obtained at the No.1 Hospital of Longnan City as well as 24 samples from Gansu Provincial Cancer Hospital. All patients gave written informed consent for their participation. This study has been approved by the Ethics Committees of Northwest University for Nationalities prior to its start. All the samples were formalin-fixed and paraffin-embedded. All specimens were evaluated by at least 2 experienced pathologists in their respective hospital's pathology department. Cervicitis, CINI, CINII/III and squamous cervical cancer (SCC) were diagnosed according to the standard criteria [22].

HPV genotype screening using the human papillomavirus genotyping kit
The Human Papillomavirus Genotyping kit for 23 Types was produced by Yaneng Bioscience co., LTD (Shen Zhen, China), and the kit was applied for with permit number 3400994 in 2008 by the Fresh Armed State Drug Administration, China. The kit was used to perform Polymerase chain reaction (PCR) to amplify the L1 gene in conjunction with reverse dot blot (RDB) analysis to identify the HPV subtypes. This method offers a simple testing strategy involving a membrane chip that can detect infections from multiple HPV subtypes, including 18 high-risk types (HPV16, 18, 31, 33, 35, 39, 45, 51, 52, 53, 56, 58, 59, 66, 68, 73, 83 and MM4) and 5 low-risk types (HPV 6, 11, 42, 43 and 44). This method had a sensitivity of 103 copies/ml and a specificity of 99%; β-globin was used as an internal positive control [23].

DNA extraction and polymerase chain reaction (PCR) conditions
DNA was extracted from 4–5 serial sections (4 μm thick) by hot dehiscing using the Human Papillomavirus Genotyping kit for 23 Types, according to the manufacturer's instructions. The tissues prepared for extraction included representative tumor tissues and the adjacent normal tissue. The quality of the extracted DNA was verified using a spectrophotometer (260/280 nm ultraviolet light). The extracted DNA was concentrated by high-speed centrifugation at 4 °C. For each PCR reaction, 5 μL extracted concentrated DNA was used in a final reaction volume of 25 μL. The PCR amplification conditions were as follows: preheating at 95 °C for 10 min, followed by 40 cycles of denaturation at 94 °C for 30 s, annealing at 42 °C for 90 s, and extension at 72 °C for 30 s, with a final extension at 72 °C for 5 min. The amplification were then denatured and subjected to hybridization.

To test the quality of the DNA, the kit was also used to amplify the housekeeping gene β-globin within the same reactions as an internal positive control. We also used a verified HPV multiple infection cervical intraepithelial neoplasia sample as a positive control and distilled water as a negative control; all control samples were subject to the same treatments and processed at the same time as the experimental samples. To ensure the samples were not contaminated within the lab, every test was carried out with fresh wash buffer and all samples were independently tested in two isolated labs by blind assignment.

HPV detection and typing
We use the reverse dot blot (RDB) method for HPV detection and typing. The 25 μL reaction volumes containing the amplified fragments were hybridized to

the dot blot membrane in 6 mL hybridization solution ($2 \times$ SSC, 0.1%SDS) at 51 °C for 2 h. After a stringent wash, the hybridized membrane was probed by adding a streptavidin-horseradish peroxidase conjugate (which binds to the biotinylated PCR products) and a substrate (3,3′,5,5′-Tetramethylbenzidine) to generate a blue precipitate at the site of the probe dot. The results were inspected by macroscopic observation, and the results were deemed reliable when the PC (positive control) dot appeared as a clear round blue dot. A clear round blue dot was scored as positive for the corresponding HPV subtype, a dilute blue dot was scored as weakly positive, and the absence of a dot was scored as negative.

Statistical analysis

Statistical analysis was performed using SPSS version 19.0 (SPSS, Chicago, IL). Differences between groups were examined using the χ^2, or Fisher's exact probability test according to the characteristics of the data distribution. The odds ratio (OR) and relative 95% confidence interval (CI) were calculated. The significance level α was set at 0.05.

Results

Genotypes detected in Cervicitis, CINI, CINII / III and SCC

We identified 329 eligible patients with a mean age of 43.5 years (range, 17 ~ 79) from the medical records. Of these patients, 57 were confirmed as cervicitis, 63 were CINI, 72 were CINIИIII, and 137 cases were SCC. The HPV positive rates in the cervicitis, CINI, CINIИIII and SCC were 38.60% (22/57), 74.60% (47/63), 87.50% (63/72) and 89.05% (122/137), respectively; the HPV positive rate was significantly higher in CINI, CINIИIII and SCC than that in cervicitis ($P < 0.001$). and the positivity is also higher in SCC compared to CINI ($P < 0.01$. Fig. 1).

The distribution of HPV genotypes according to cervical lesions is shown in Fig 2. HPV16 was the most common genotype in cervicitis, accounting for 45.46% (10/22). In the CINI group, HPV16 was the most common genotype, accounting for 46.81% (22/47), followed by HPV58 (21.28%, 10/47), HPV52 (17.02%, 8/47), HPV33 (12.77%, 6/47), HPV 51 (6.38%, 3/47) and 59 (6.38%, 3/47). For the CIN IИIII group, HPV16 was also the most common genotype, accounting for 60.32% (38/63), followed by HPV58 (25.40%, 16/63), HPV52 (12.70%, 8/63), HPV31 (6.35%, 4/63) and 33 (6.35%, 4/63). The 5 most common genotypes in patients with SCC were HPV16 (78.69%, 96/122), HPV58 (20.49%, 25/122), HPV18 (6.56%, 8/122), HPV59 (4.92%, 6/122) and 52 (4.10%, 5/122), in descending order. None genotype of the differences between groups were significant except

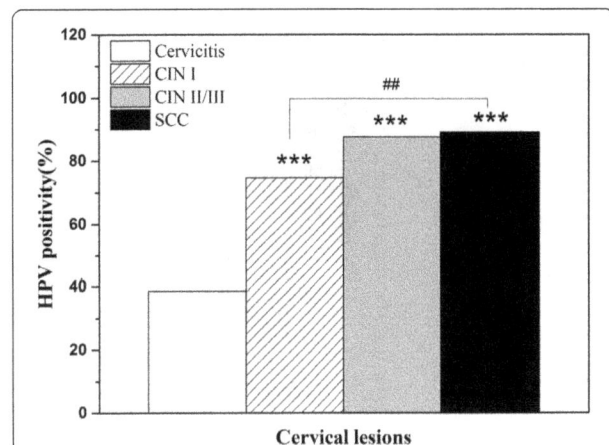

Fig. 1 Prevalence of HPV infection in the study groups. *** $P < 0.001$ CINI, CINII/III, SCC vs. cervicitis; ## $P < 0.01$ SCC vs. CINI. Percentages for co-infections with two or more HPV strains were calculated separately for each one. Abbreviations: HPV, human papillomavirus; CIN, cervical intraepithelial neoplasia; SCC, squamous cell carcinoma

HPV16 infection in SCC compared to cervicitis, CINI and CINIИIII ($P < 0.001$, $P < 0.01$. Fig. 2).

OR for HPV16 infection

Because HPV16 was significantly higher in invasive SCC, logistic regression analysis was used to calculate the odds ratios (OR) and 95% confident intervals (95%CI) of such infections. Compared to cervicitis and CINI, the odds ratios (OR) for SCC in HPV16 positive patients were 2.96 (95% confidence interval [CI]: 1.09–8.00, $P < 0.05$) and 4.20 (95% confidence interval [CI]: 2.05–8.61, $P < 0.001$, respectively (Table 1).

HPV genotypes of multiple infections in Cervicitis, CINI, CINII / III and SCC

Some women were infected with 2 or 3 types of HPV simultaneously (Table 2). Compared to cervicitis (9.09%, 2/22), more patients with CINI, CIN IИIII and SCC had multiple HPV infections, however, as the cervical lesion grade increased, the prevalence of multiple HPV infections gradually deceased (27.66%, 13/47; 26.98%, 17/63 and 25.41%, 31/122, respectively). Double infections accounted for the majority of multiple infections, 4.55%(1/22), 21.28%(10/47), 20.64%(13/63) and 21.31%(26/122) for cervicitis, CINI, CIN IИIII and SCC respectively. Of those, HPV16 + 58 was the most common combinations, and HPV52 + 33 in CINI subgroup, HPV16 + 33 and HPV16 + 52 in CIN IИIII subgroup were also common genotypes combination. In the cervicitis, CINI, CIN IИIII and SCC subgroups, 4.5%(1/22), 6.38%(3/47), 6.35%(4/63), 4.10% (5/122) of patients had triple HPV infections. The combinations and prevalence of the HPV genotypes in multiple infections for each cervical lesion group and subgroup are specified in Table 3.

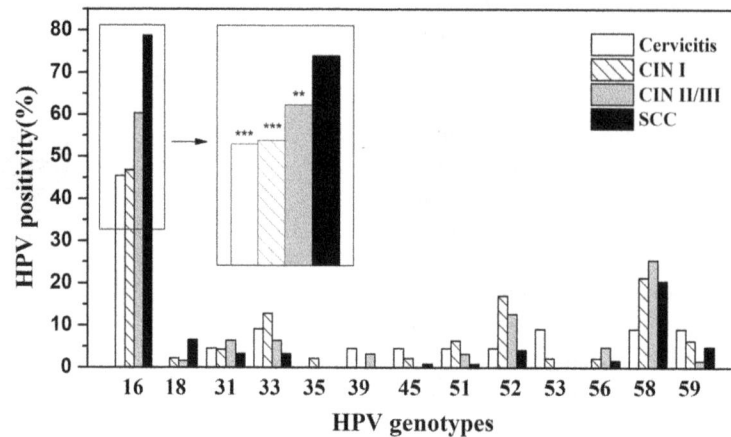

Fig. 2 Distribution of HPV infection in the study groups. ** $P < 0.01$ vs. SCC; *** $P < 0.001$ vs. SCC. Percentages for co-infections with two or more HPV strains were calculated separately for each one. Abbreviations: HPV, human papillomavirus; CIN, cervical intraepithelial neoplasia; SCC, squamous cell carcinoma

Discussion

Our data showed that 38.60% of patients with cervicitis, 74.60% with CINI, 87.50% with CINIИII, and 89.05% with SCC were positive for HPV DNA. HPV infection rates were significantly higher in CINI, CINIИII, and invasive SCC than in cervicitis patients, but they never reached 100%. In addition, in our population, HPV 16 was the dominant genotype and HPV 33, 53, 58 and 59 were the second dominant genotypes for cervicitis. HPV genotypes 16, 58, and 52 were the dominant high-risk HPV in patients with CINI and CINIИII, however for invasive SCC, the dominant high-risk HPV were 16, 58 and 18. Besides of the genotypes suggested above, HPV 6, 11, 31, 33, 51, 56 and 59 also were detected. In some reports in which HPV16, 18, and 45, HPV16, 18 and 33 or 16, 18 and 58 were most commonly detected in cervicitis [11, 24–26], CINI, CINIИII and SCC patients. Despite the small sample size of our subgroup, the dominant genotypes remained stable across the cervicitis, CINI, CINIИII and SCC groups, which supported the credibility of our data. In addition, HPV16 was significantly associated with SCC, the ORs were 2.96 (CI: 1.09–8.00) and 4.20 (CI: 2.05–8.61, respectively, when compared to cervicitis and CINI. The absence of a similar significant association between other genotypes may have been due to the small size of study groups.

In our group of CINI, CINIИII and SCC patients, the positivity for HPV DNA are consistent with those in most other studies [11, 24–30]. For example, the reports

Table 1 ORs of HPV16 for SCC

OR	95% CI	P
2.96 (Compared to cervicitis)	1.09 – 8.00	< 0.05
4.20 (Compared to CIN I)	2.05 – 8.61	< 0.001

Abbreviations: *HPV* human papillomavirus, *CIN* cervical intraepithelial neoplasia, *SCC* squamous cell carcinoma, *OR* odds ratio, *CI* confidence interval

from Shanghai of 239 patients with CINI and USA of 411 patients with CINIИII, in which the rates of HPV DNA positivity were 74.9% and 82.0–92.0%. For the regions of worldwide, the rate of HPV DNA positivity in SCC was 87.0–90.9%. In addition, the positivity of HPV16 infection in CINI, CINIИII and SCC patients is 46.81%, 60.32% and 78.69% respectively, which is also consistent with the most reports [11, 24, 31, 32]. These evidences further suggested that the performance of HPV detection kit is credible and our data likely reflect the real association pattern between HPV infection and cervical cancer or precancerous lesions in local area.

The distribution of dominant HPV genotypes showed obvious regional differences [33]. HPV18 is reported to be one of the two most carcinogenic HPV genotypes (HPV16 and 18), accounting for $10 \sim 15\%$ of cervical cancers [11, 24, 32]. In our population, the prevalence of HPV18 in patients with cervicitis, CIN I, CIN II/III and invasive SCC were 0%, 2.13%, 1.59% and 6.56%, respectively. The overall prevalence rate of HPV18 is very lower, but consistent with a recent Korea report, where only 6 (2.5%) out of the 243 high-risk HPV positive subjects showed HPV18 infection [34]. HPV52 is also considered as a high-risk genotype and is especially frequent in Northern America, Africa, and Asia [35, 36]. In our population, the prevalence of HPV52 in patients with cervicitis, CIN I, CIN II/III and invasive SCC were 4.55%, 17.02%, 12.70% and 4.10%, respectively and was largely higher than in other reports, in which HPV52 prevalent rates ranged up to 2.4% in women with normal cytological findings, 5.1% in women with CIN II/III and were 2.5% in women with SCC [36]. In present study, HPV 58 is a dominant high-risk genotype and the prevalence of HPV58 in patients with cervicitis, CIN I, CIN II/III and invasive SCC was 9.09%, 21.28%, 25.40 and 20.49%, respectively. Although the overall prevalence

Table 2 Simple and multiple of HPV infections in the study groups

Genotype	Simple infections	Multiple infections		
		Double	Triple	Total
cervicitis	90.91% (20/22)	4.55% (1/22)	4.5% (1/22)	9.09% (2/22)
CIN I	72.34% (34/47)	21.28% (10/47)	6.38% (3/47)	27.66% (13/47)
CIN II/III	73.02% (46/63)	20.64% (13/63)	6.35% (4/63)	26.98% (17/63)
SCC	74.59% (91/122)	21.31% (26/122)	4.10% (5/122)	25.41% (31/122)

Abbreviations: *HPV* human papillomavirus, *CIN* cervical intraepithelial neoplasia, *SCC* squamous cell carcinoma

rate of HPV58 in our research is very higher than the reports of Japanese and world, in which HPV58 prevalence rates are 7.0% in patients with CIN II/III and 3.3% ~ 13.3% in patients with SCC [10, 37], our result is consistent with some recent Chinese reports [33, 38], where 16.4%, 20.1%, 23.5% and 31.4% patients with cervicitis, CIN I, CIN II/III and invasive SCC and 29.1% and 24.3% patients with CIN II/III and invasive SCC showed HPV58 infection.

Our data suggested that more patients with CINI, CIN IИII and SCC had multiple HPV infections compared to cervicitis, however, the rates of multiple HPV infections in CIN I, CIN II/III and SCC patients showed a slightly decreasing trend with severity of lesions. Although this

Table 3 Combinations of HPV types in multiple infection in the study groups

Genotype	Cervicitis	CIN I	CIN II/III	SCC
Conbinations of HPV types in double infections				
HPV16+18				1.64% (2/122)
HPV16+33			4.76% (3/63)	1.64% (2/122)
HPV16+52			4.76% (3/63)	
HPV16+58		4.26% (2/47)	6.35% (4/63)	9.84% (12/122)
HPV16+other types		6.38% (3/47)	1.59% (1/63)	5.74% (7/122)
HPV51+11		2.13% (1/47)		
HPV52+31		2.13% (1/47)		
HPV52+56				0.82% (1/122)
HPV52+33		4.26% (2/47)		
HPV58+53	4.5% (1/22)			
HPV58+56			1.59% (1/63)	
HPV58+59				0.82% (1/122)
HPV58+other types			1.59% (1/63)	0.82% (1/122)
Combinations of HPV types in triple infections				
HPV16+18+33				0.82% (1/122)
HPV16+18+59				0.82% (1/122)
HPV16+31+33			1.59% (1/63)	
HPV16+56+81				0.82% (1/122)
HPV16+58+31				0.82% (1/122)
HPV16+58+33		2.13% (1/47)		
HPV16+58+43			1.59% (1/63)	
HPV16+59+43				0.82% (1/122)
HPV18+33+35		2.13% (1/47)		
HPV18+58+31			1.59% (1/63)	
HPV45+53+59	4.5% (1/22)			
HPV58+31+42			1.59% (1/63)	

Abbreviations: *HPV* human papillomavirus, *CIN* cervical intraepithelial neoplasia, *SCC* squamous cell carcinoma

finding is partially consistent with the results of previous studies, in which Francois et al. and Meizhu Xiao et al. found that the rates of multiple hr-HPV infections in CINII, CINIII, and CC patients declined gradually [38, 39], the rates of multiple HPV infections of our survey was significantly lower than in these reports. This difference may occur because the prevalence of HPV-positive status also vary varies among geographic locations and populations. Moreover, the small size of group in our study may be one of the reason of lower positivity of multiple HPV infections. However, in a worldwide pooled analysis of 167 adenocarcinoma of the cervix patients, the multiple-infection rate was 8.9%, obviously lower than the simple infection prevalence of 91.1% [18]. Thus, our data which reflected Multiple HPV infections might be indeed be associated with the development of cervical lesions, or women with multiple HPV infections might be more susceptible to cervical carcinogenesis, or multiple HPV infections might produce conditions that confer immunological protection against persistent infection [40].

Our data indicated that the combination of HPV16 + 58 plays a dominant role in all cervical lesion groups, contrary to findings in the Jewish Israeli population and in Austrians, but in agreement with findings in women in Beijing, China [41–43]. Thus, the results of this study strongly support the key role of HPV16 and 58 in the development of CC and CIN in women in LongNan, China.

Conclusions
Overall, as demonstrated in our study population, genotypes 16, 58, 52 and 18 are among the predominant HPV and HPV infection increased with cervical lesion, regional differences in HPV genotype distribution and the real carcinogenic HPV revealing need to be mindful in the HPV control and prevention.

Funding
This study was supported by the National Natural Science Foundation of China (31060127. 81260442. 81560508 and 31560254) and Program for Leading Talent of SEAC ([2016] 57).

Authors' contribution
JZ and ZG conceived and designed the study. CN and DZ collected the clinical data. All specimens were evaluated by QW and TBS in their respective hospital's pathology department. SYP and CJW performed all the molecular biology assays for HPV genotyping. HMQ, JBZ and YM analyzed the data and drafted the manuscript. All authors read and approved the final manuscript.

Competing interest
The authors declare that they have no competing interests.

Author details
[1]Medical College of Northwest University for Nationalities, Lanzhou 730030, People's Republic of China. [2]No.1 Hospital of Longnan City, Longnan 746000, People's Republic of China. [3]Gansu Provincial Cancer Hospital, Lanzhou 730050, People's Republic of China.

References
1. Poljak M, Kocjan BJ. Commercially available assays for multiplex detection of alpha human papillomaviruses. Expert Rev Anti Infect Ther. 2010;8(5):1139–62.
2. Nobre RJ, Herráez-Hernández E, Fei JW, Langbein L, Kaden S, Gröne HJ, de Villiers EM. E7 oncoprotein of novel human papillomavirus type 108 lacking the E6 gene induces dysplasia in organotypic keratinocyte cultures. J Virol. 2009;83(7):2907–16.
3. Pillai MR, Lakshmi S, Sreekala S, Devi TG, Jayaprakash PG, Rajalakshmi TN, Devi CG, Nair MK, Nair MB. High-risk human papillomavirus infection and E6 protein expression in lesions of the uterine cervix. Pathobiology. 1998;66(5):240–6.
4. Tornesello ML, Duraturo ML, Botti G, Greggi S, Piccoli R, De Palo G, Montella M, Buonaguro L. Buonaguro FM; Italian HPV working group: prevalence of α-papillomavirus genotypes in cervical intraepithelial neoplasia and cervical cancer in the Italian population. J Med Virol. 2006;78(12):1663–72.
5. Arbyn M, Tommasino M, Depuydt C, Dillner J. Are 20 human papillomavirus types causing cervical cancer? J Pathol. 2014;234(4):431–5.
6. Halec G, Alemany L, Lloveras B, Schmitt M, Alejo M, Bosch FX, Tous S, Klaustermeier JE, Guimerà N, Grabe N, Lahrmann B, Gissmann L, Quint W, Bosch FX, de Sanjose S, Pawlita M. Retrospective international survey and HPV time trends study group; retrospective international survey and HPV time trends study group. Pathogenic role of the eight probably/possibly carcinogenic HPV types 26, 53, 66, 67, 68, 70, 73 and 82 in cervical cancer. J Pathol. 2014;234(4):441–51.
7. Torre LA, Bray F, Siegel RL, Ferlay J, Lortet-Tieulent J, Jemal A. Global cancer statistics, 2012. CA Cancer J Clin. 2015;65(2):87–108.
8. Kim K, Zang R, Choi SC, Ryu SY, Kim JW. Current status of gynecological cancer in China. J Gynecol Oncol. 2009;20(2):72–6.
9. Bosch FX, Manos MM, Muñoz N, Sherman M, Jansen AM, Peto J, Schiffman MH, Moreno V, Kurman R, Shah KV. Prevalence of human papillomavirus in cervical cancer: a worldwide perspective. International biological study on cervical cancer (IBSCC) Study Group. J Natl Cancer Inst. 1995;87(11):796–802.
10. Bosch FX, Burchell AN, Schiffman M, Giuliano AR, de Sanjose S, Bruni L, Tortolero-Luna G, Kjaer SK, Muñoz N. Epidemiology and natural history of human papillomavirus infections and type-specific implications in cervical neoplasia. Vaccine. 2008;26S:K1–16.
11. de Sanjose S, Wim GVQ, Laia A, et al. Human papillomavirus genotype attribution in invasive cervical cancer: a retrospective cross-sectional worldwide study. Lancet Oncol. 2010;11(11):1048–56.
12. Wright Jr TC, Stoler MH, Behrens CM, Apple R, Derion T, Wright TL. The ATHENA human papillomavirus study: design, methods, and baseline results. Am J Obstet Gynecol. 2012;206(1):46e1–11.
13. Diaz M, Kim JJ, Albero G, de Sanjosé S, Clifford G, Bosch FX, Goldie SJ. Health and economic impact of HPV 16 and 18 vaccination and cervical cancer screening in India. Br J Cancer. 2008;99(2):230–8.
14. Kjaer SK, Breugelmans G, Munk C, Junge J, Watson M, Iftner T. Population-based prevalence, type- and age- specific distribution of HPV in women before introduction of an HPV-vaccination program in Denmark. Int J Cancer. 2008; 123(8):1864–70.
15. Castellsagué X, Díaz M, de Sanjosé S, Muñoz N, Herrero R, Franceschi S, Peeling RW, Ashley R, Smith JS, Snijders PJ, Meijer CJ, Bosch FX, et al. Worldwide human papillomavirus etiology of cervical adenocarcinoma and its cofactors: implications for screening and prevention. J Natl Cancer Inst. 2006;98(5):303–15.
16. Schwartz SM, Daling JR, Shera KA, Madeleine MM, McKnight B, Galloway DA, Porter PL, McDougall JK. Human papillomavirus and prognosis of invasive cervical cancer: a population-based study. J Clin Oncol. 2001;19(7):1906–15.
17. Bao YP, Li N, Smith JS, Qiao YL. ACCPAB members. Human papillomavirus type distribution in women from Asia: a meta-analysis. Int J Gynecol Cancer. 2008;18(1):71–9.
18. Shen Y, Gong JM, Li YQ, Gong YM, Lei DM, Cheng GM, Li XF. Epidemiology and genotype distribution of human papillomavirus (HPV) in women of Henan Province. China Clinica Chimica Acta. 2013;415:297–301.
19. Liu X, Zhang S, Ruan Q, Ji Y, Ma L, Zhang Y. Prevalence and type distribution of human papillomavirus in women with cervical lesions in Liaoning Province. China Int J Gynecol Cancer. 2010;20(1):147–53.
20. Jinke L, Dan Z, Yi Z, et al. Prevalence and genotype distribution of human papillomavirus in women with cervical cancer or highgrade precancerous lesions in Chengdu, western China. Int J Gynecol Obstet. 2011;112(2):131–4.

21. Yang L, Huangpu X-m, Zhang S-w, et al. Changes of mortality rate for cervical cancer during 1970's and 1990's periods in china. Acta Academiae Medicinae Sinicae. 2003;25(4):386–90.

22. Kurman RJ, Ellenson LH, Ronnett BM. Blaustein's pathology of the female genital tract. 5th ed. New York: Springer; 2002.

23. Zhi YF, Cha XX, Li XF, Qiu C, Rong SH. Prevalence and genotype distribution of human papillomavirus in women in the Henan Province. Genet Mol Res. 2015;14(2):5452–61.

24. Muñoz N, Bosch FX, de Sanjosé S, Herrero R, Castellsagué X, Shah KV, Snijders PJ, Meijer CJ. International agency for research on cancer multicenter cervical cancer study group. Epidemiologic classification of human papillomavirus types associated with cervical cancer. N Engl J Med. 2003;348(6):518–27.

25. Clifford GM, Rana RK, Franceschi S, Smith JS, Gough G, Pimenta JM. Human papillomavirus genotype distribution in low-grade cervical lesions: comparison by geographic region and with cervical cancer. Cancer Epidemiol Biomarkers Prev. 2005;14(5):1157–64.

26. Wheeler CM, Hunt WC, Joste NE, Key CR, Quint WG, Castle PE. Human papillomavirus genotype distributions: implications for vaccination and cancer screening in the United States. J Natl Cancer Inst. 2009;101(7):475–87.

27. Liang H, Griffith CC, Ma L, Ling B, Feng D, Li Z, Zhao C. The sensitivity of Pap cytology and HPV testing to detect incident cervical cancer: Prior testing results in 178 patients with invasive cervical cancer at a large general hospital in China. J American Soc Cyto. 2015;4(6):S33–4.

28. Zheng B, Li Z, Griffith CC, Yan S, Chen C, Ding X, Liang X, Yang H, Zhao C. Prior high-risk HPV testing and Pap test results for 427 invasive cervical cancers in China's largest CAP-certified laboratory. Cancer Cytopathol. 2015;123(7):428–34.

29. Bhatla N, Lal N, Bao YP, Ng T, Qiao YL. A meta-analysis of human papillomavirus type-distribution in women from South Asia: implications for vaccination. Vaccine. 2008;26(23):2811–7.

30. Li N, Franceschi S, Howell-Jones R, Snijders PJ, Clifford GM. Human papillomavirus type distribution in 30,848 invasive cervical cancers worldwide: Variation by geographical region, histological type and year of publication. Int J Cancer. 2011;128(4):927–35.

31. Dillner J, Rebolj M, Birembaut P, Petry KU, Szarewski A, Munk C, de Sanjose S, Naucler P, Lloveras B, Kjaer S, Cuzick J, van Ballegooijen M, Clavel C, Iftner T. JointEuropean Cohort Study. Long term predictive values of cytology and human papillomavirus testing in cervical cancer screening: joint European cohort study. BMJ. 2008;337:a1754.

32. Walboomers JM, Jacobs MV, Manos MM, Bosch FX, Kummer JA, Shah KV, Snijders PJ, Peto J, Meijer CJ, Muñoz N. Human papillomavirus is a necessary cause of invasive cervical cancer worldwide. J Pathol. 1999;189(1):12–9.

33. Gu Y, Ma C, Zou J, Zhu Y, Yang R, Xu Y, Zhang Y. Prevalence characteristics of high-risk human papillomaviruses in women living in Shanghai with cervical precancerous lesions and cancer. Oncotarget. 2016;7(17):24656–63.

34. Choi JW, Kim Y, Lee JH, Kim YS. The clinical performance of primary HPV screening, primary HPV screening plus cytology cotesting, and cytology alone at a tertiary care hospital. Cancer Cyto. 2016;124(2):144–52.

35. Bosch FX, Lorincz A, Muñoz N, Meijer CJ, Shah KV. The causal relation between human papillomavirus and cervical cancer. J Clin Pathol. 2002;55(4):244–65.

36. Bruni L, Diaz M, Castellsagué X, Ferrer E, Bosch FX, de Sanjosé S. Cervical human papillomavirus prevalence in 5 continents: meta-analysis of 1 million women with normal cytological findings. J Infect Dis. 2010;202(12):1789–99.

37. Watari H, Michimata R, Yasuda M, Ishizu A, Tomaru U, Xiong Y, Hassan MK, Sakuragi N. High prevalence of multiple human papillomavirus infection in Japanese patients with invasive uterine cervical cancer. Pathobiology. 2011;78(4):220–6.

38. Xiao M, Xu Q, Li H, Gao H, Bie Y, Zhang Z. Prevalence of human papillomavirus genotypes among women with high-grade cervical lesions in Beijing. China Med (Baltimore). 2016;95(3), e2555.

39. Francois C, Samuel R, Agnihotram VR, et al. Distribution of human papillomavirus genotypes in cervical intraepithelial neoplasia and invasive cervical cancer in Canada. J Med Virol. 2011;83(6):1034–41.

40. Sang Ah L, Daehee K, Sang SS, et al. Multiple HPV infection in cervical cancer screened by HPV DNA Chip. Cancer Lett. 2003;198(2):187–92.

41. Laskov I, Grisaru D, Efrat G, et al. Are the human papillomavirus genotypes different in cervical cancer and intraepithelial neoplasia in Jewish Israeli women, a low-risk population? Int J Gynecol Cancer. 2013;23(4):730–4.

42. Lucia R, Olaf R, Reinhard H, et al. Human papillomavirus in highgrade cervical lesions Austrian data of a European multicentre study. Wien Klin Wochenschr. 2013;125(19–20):591–9.

43. Ren H, Caiyan X, Songwen Z, et al. Distribution of human papillomavirus genotype and cervical neoplasia among women with abnormal cytology in Beijing. China Int J Gynaecol Obstet. 2012;119(3):257–61.

2

Synchronous bilateral tonsil carcinoma

M-N. Theodoraki*, J. A. Veit, T. K. Hoffmann and J. Greve

Abstract

Background: The incidence of synchronous bilateral tonsil carcinoma seems to be underreported. For adequate oncologic treatment, it is mandatory to remove all primaries to prevent recurrence or metachronic disease. The purpose of this manuscript is to provide a comprehensive review on this topic and to emphasize the need of bilateral tonsillectomy in cases of cancer of unknown primary (CUP) as well as in the case of a unilateral tonsillar carcinoma.

Material and methods: A systematic review of the literature was performed for "bilateral tonsillar neoplasm", "synchronous cancer of the oropharynx" and "cancer of unknown primary in head and neck".

Results: We present a clinical case with bilateral tonsillar carcinoma in initially suggested cancer of unknown primary. Clinically, both tonsillar sites were unsuspicious, but in PET/CT an ipsilateral enhancement of the tonsil area was detected. The pathological work up of bilateral tonsillectomy specimens revealed bilateral squamous cell carcinoma with HPV-type 16 positivity. The review of the literature revealed 29 cases of bilateral tonsil cancer.

Conclusion: The handling of tonsillar tissue in the frame of panendoscopy in the case of CUP is still controversial. We recommend a bilateral tonsillectomy as a routine procedure for cancer of unknown primary as well as unilateral tonsillar carcinoma. Herewith the detrimental consequences of occult metachronous contralateral tonsillar carcinoma can be prevented.

Keywords: Bilateral tonsillar carcinoma, Cancer of unknown primary, Head and neck malignancy, Squamous cell carcinoma, Bilateral tonsillectomy

Background

The detection and treatment of the primary neoplasm in cancer of unknown primary (CUP) of the head and neck (H&N) presents a challenge for the clinician. Currently, the recommended procedure involves imaging techniques as well as panendoscopy with systematic biopsies of localizations with high incidence of occult primary side including an ipsilateral tonsillectomy or at least a biopsy of the ipsilateral tonsil. At first sight, up to 10% of H&N malignancies present as a CUP [1] and the primary tumor can be identified in approximately 21, 5–75% of these cases. As in all H&N malignancies, squamous cell carcinoma presents the most common entity, with the

tonsil being the most frequent localization for an occult primary. Patients with a CUP disease have a decreased overall survival rate compared to other head and neck squamous cell carcinoma (HNSCC) patients [2].

Primary tonsillar carcinoma is the third most common malignancy in H&N area, after thyroid and larynx carcinoma [3]. About 50% of patients are diagnosed with lymphatic metastazation, occurring on the contralateral cervical side in 10–15% [4]. Tonsillar malignancy is likely to be diagnosed in advanced stages with indolent neck mass due to frequent submucosal presentation or deep formations in the crypts with few local clinical symptoms (Fig. 1).

The presence of synchronous malignant tumors in the H&N is not uncommon and is the leading long-term cause of mortality [5]. Within five years, 15% of patients

---

* Correspondence: marie-nicole.theodoraki@gmail.com
Department of Oto-Rhino-Laryngology, Head and Neck Surgery, University Medical Center, Frauensteige 12, 89070 Ulm, Germany

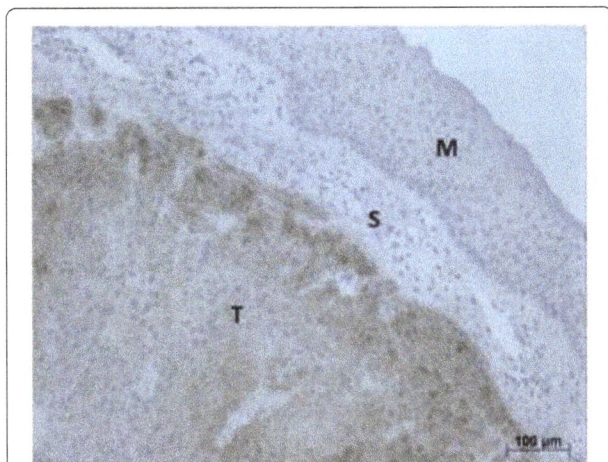

Fig. 1 Immunhistochemical staining of cancer-testis-antigen MAGEA3/A4 with submucosal presentation of a tonsillar carcinoma. Figure of our unpublished data. T = tumor, S = stroma, M = mucosa

with a tonsillar carcinoma present a secondary tumor localized in the H&N [6]. The risk of a secondary malignant tumor in the H&N area is linked by the degree of symmetric chronic exposure to carcinogenic factors of the upper aerodigestive tract. In more recent investigations a strong association of oropharyngeal cancer and -in a lesser extend- CUP-syndromes with human papilloma viruses (HPV) is visible, with significantly better clinical outcome [7].

However, synchronous bilateral tonsil carcinoma is uncommon and only a few cases are reported in literature with the first report in 1971 [8]. The true incidence is likely to be underreported.

The high frequency of tonsillar primaries, as mentioned above, leads to frequent recommendation of unilateral diagnostic tonsillectomy in the context of CUP-panendoscopy [9]. If a tonsillar carcinoma is suspected, a panendoscopy with biopsy or tonsillectomy of the suspected (ipsilateral) tonsil follows. The recommendation for a bilateral tonsillectomy is frequently seen in literature [10] but without consistent performance in clinical practice or integration in corresponding guidelines.

We present a case of a synchronous bilateral tonsil carcinoma with subsequent review of the current literature. This article intends to raise the question of whether a bilateral tonsillectomy should be established as a standard procedure, with the aim of a homogenous approach in cases of cervical CUP-syndrome and/or unilateral tonsillar cancer.

Main text
Materials and methods
A systematic review of the literature was performed via MEDLINE using the terms "bilateral tonsillar neoplasm",

"cancer of unknown primary in head and neck" as well as "synchronous cancer of the oropharynx" from the years 1971 until 2016. All abstracts were reviewed and all publications mentioning a bilateral tonsillar carcinoma were included. The references in the relevant papers were also reviewed. We declare that we have read the Helsinki Declaration and have followed the guidelines in this investigation.

Results
We identified 18 manuscripts describing 29 cases of synchronous bilateral tonsil carcinoma with one case presenting an additional contralateral carcinoma in situ and four cases of contralateral metachronous tonsillar carcinoma. The principal recommendations of these papers are shown in Table 1 [1, 3, 4, 7–21].

Furthermore, we describe a case of a bilateral tonsillar carcinoma confirmed by histopathological analysis following bilateral tonsillectomy in the context of panendoscopy for diagnosis of an occult primary.

Case
A 52-year-old, male patient presented with an eight-week history of a right-sided cervical mass. No further complaints were mentioned. The patient did not consume alcohol nor did he smoke. The oropharyngeal and laryngeal examination revealed just a slight enlargement of the right tonsil compared to the left without induration of the tonsils, ulceration or other abnormalities. An ultrasound of the neck revealed a highly suspect lymph node formation on the right side (TNM: cN2a). A lymph node extirpation followed and indicated a lymph node metastasis of a low-grade keratinizing squamous cell carcinoma. At this point, no HPV diagnostic of the lymph node material was performed. A PET-CT scan performed two weeks after revealed a highly increased metabolism of the right tonsil with highly increased contrast medium uptake and the suspected diagnosis of a tonsillar carcinoma of the right side (Fig. 2). A panendoscopy with bilateral tonsillectomy and systematic biopsies -including a bilateral deep biopsy of the base of tongue- was performed as a standard procedure for CUP staging/diagnostics. Intraoperatively, an induration of the right tonsil was palpated. Neither the contralateral side, nor the base of tongue showed any abnormalities. However, the pathohistological examination showed a synchronous *bilateral* T1 tonsil squamous cell carcinoma with a HPV-16 positivity in the DNA-PCR analysis of tumor tissue. The patient underwent a bilateral tumor resection with a modified radical neck dissection, level I-V of the right side and a left-sided selective neck dissection, level II-V. The TNM-stage was bilateral pT1 pN2a cM0.

Table 1 Literature with previously reported cases of bilateral tonsillar carcinoma

Authors	Year	Country	synchr.	metachr.	Recommendation	HPV-16-status	Primary diagnosis
Patel	2015	USA	3	1	Cases in context of dysphagie after bilateral transoral resection	positive	3× CUP, 1× unilateral carcinoma
Bakkal	2014	Turkey	1		Case in context of primary chemoradiotherapy treatment	n.p.	Bilateral carcinoma
Nakahara	2014	Japan	1		Bilateral tonsillectomy or biopsy if HPV positivity	positive	CUP
Joseph	2014	USA	3	1	Bilateral tonsillectomy	positive	Unilateral carcinoma
Moualed	2011	UK	3		Bilateral tonsillectomy by suspected or proven tonsillar carcinoma	n.p.	Unilateral carcinoma
Mannina	2011	USA	1		Role of PET/CT staging for diagnosis of CUP	positive	CUP
Roeser (poster)	2011	USA	1		Bilateral tonsillectomy if bilateral tonsillar metastasation	positive	CUP
Smith (poster)	2011	USA	1	3	Bilateral tonsillectomy by CUP or unialteral tonsil carcinoma	n.p.	1× CUP, 3× unilateral carcinoma
Monsted	2010	Danemark	1		No recommendation in abstract, article in Danish	unknown	Unilateral carcinoma
Chianchetti	2009	USA	1		Unilateral (or less often) bilateral tonsillectomy by diagnosis of CUP	n.p.	CUP
McGovern	2009	USA	1		Bilateral tonsillectomy if both tonsills enlarged + positive PET-CT scan	positive	CUP
Kothari	2008	UK	5		Bilateral tonsillectomy by diagnosis of CUP	n.p.	CUP
Kozakiewicz	2007	Poland	1		Bilateral tonsillectomy by bilateral cervikal metastasation	unknown	Unilateral carcinoma
Price	2006	UK	1		Role of FDG-PET in diagnosis of CUP, search for primary side	n.p.	CUP
Kazak	2003	Germany	1		Bilateral tonsillectomy by diagnosis of CUP	n.p.	CUP
Koch	2001	USA	2[a]		Bilateral tonsillectomy by diagnosis of CUP	n.p.	CUP
Rajendekumar	1999	UK	1		Search for further head and neck primary	n.p.	Unilateral carcinoma
Schöndorf	1971	Germany		1	Bilateral tonsillectomy by diagnosis of unilateral tonsil carcinoma	n.p.	Unilateral carcinoma

Synchr. synchronous manifestation of bilateral tonsillar carcinoma, *metachr.* metachronous tonsillar carcinoma of the contralateral side; The numbers in the rows synchronous and metachronous demonstrate the number of reported cases in the according publications; [a]1× contralateral carcinoma in situ; *n.p.* not performed

Adjuvant radiotherapy followed in the absence of extracapsular spread.

Discussion

The presence of a bilateral tonsillar carcinoma is rare and only 29 cases are reported in literature. Although many published articles on this topic exist and there is a general consensus that a panendoscopy with representative biopsies should be performed, diverse opinions persist for the handling of the palatine tonsils. An unanimity exists for ipsilateral tonsillectomy but a bilateral procedure is discussed controversially [1].

Although the morbidity of an extended radiation field due to a bilateral primary is increased, the oncologic outcome of missing the second primary by surgery and radiation might be fatal [22]. Due to our clinical experience and the cases reported in literature we provide evidence for bilateral tonsillectomy in cases of CUP-syndrome and unilateral tonsillar cancer with and without HPV-positivity.

A tonsillar carcinoma is more likely to be missed by biopsies than by bilateral tonsillectomy

Simo et al. also described a case of a CUP-syndrome with the detection of primary tumor in a tonsillar remnant by status post tonsillectomy in childhood [23]. Through biopsies, risk of false negative results can arise if the tumor is localized in the submucosa or in deep crypts [24] necessitating another attempt to obtain a representative sample.

The standard therapeutic procedure for unilateral tonsillar carcinoma with T-classification T3 or higher is an adjuvant radiation of the contralateral neck even in an N0 stadium since the risk for contralateral lymph node metastasis is approximately 21% [25]. The contralateral tonsil is usually excluded from the irradiation field to avoid the higher morbidity and oropharyngeal complications. Therefore, a bilateral tonsillectomy seems to be justified. This procedure can prevent the consequences of a late diagnosis as well as improved patient outcome compared to a late diagnosis of metachronous tumor [18]. Another advantage is the resulting symmetric

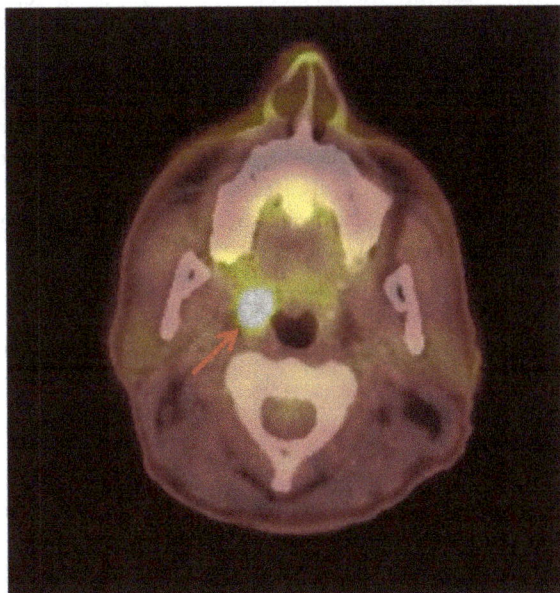

Fig. 2 Axial PET-CT scan. An asymmetric contrast medium enhancement of the *right* tonsil is visible (*arrow*). No enhancement of the *left* tonsil

appearance of the palate arches, which allows for improved oncologic surveillance. In this case a recurrence or a secondary tumor can be more easily detected by means of the disturbance of the symmetry.

Questions of pathogenesis

It is well known that synchronous or metachronous oropharyngeal carcinomas can occur by field cancerization due to symmetrical exposure to noxa [26]. Additionally, recent reports have revealed that Human papilloma viruses (especially subtype 16) increase the risk for developing tonsillar carcinoma [27]. Furthermore, reports exist with speculations of HPV-related oropharyngeal field cancerization and of HPV-related bilateral tonsillar [28]. As we see in Table 1, 6 publications reveal a HPV-positivity in the detected carcinoma in cases with primary diagnosis of CUP-syndrome as well as unilateral tonsillar carcinoma. As it is visible, HPV testing was performed in the more recent publications, demonstrating the relatively new knowledge about the influence of HPV in oral cancer. We present here another case of HPV-positive bilateral tonsillar carcinoma.

In our case, a HPV examination of the metastatic lymph node was not performed and a PET-CT followed to locate a primary tumor. Because of the fact, that the primary tumor in HPV-positive cancers is often occult, a HPV detection in the metastatic lymph node would be helpful for identifying the primary location since 80–90% of HPV positive tumors can be found in the oropharynx (palatine tonsils, base of tongue, lingual tonsils) [1, 29, 30]. Consequently, a HPV positivity in

the resected lymph node could be an additional hint and could facilitate the decision of performing a PET-CT or not. This additional examination is not yet a standardized procedure in our clinic but it is in the process of establishment.

Another relevant question in this context would be if it is justified to perform an additional ablation of the base of tongue in HPV-related CUP to minimize the risk of overseeing the primary tumor. Since risk of complications is higher after this procedure and primary tumors are found more common in the palatine tonsils, literature suggests a bilateral base of tongue resection if the palatine tonsils have already been removed [31]. Hence, an ablation of the base of tongue should be discussed if the case of a HPV positive CUP with bilateral tumor-negative tonsils occurs, which would increase the risk of tumor-localization in the base of tongue. This further option has to be taken in consideration and the risk-benefit ratio has to be discussed with the patient since the procedure is painful and is accompanied with increased bleeding risk.

However, a bilateral tonsillectomy with pathological examination of the whole tissue, like in our case performed, is an important procedure in diagnosis and therapeutic management of HPV positive *and* negative tumors, since tonsillar carcinoma often appear in an early stage with manifestation in the deep crypts, not only in HPV positive but also in HPV negative tumors [4].

Questions of diagnosis

In our case, PET-CT imaging raised the question of an ipsilateral tonsillar carcinoma as a primary tumor for the existing lymph node metastasis. After bilateral tonsillectomy, a synchronous bilateral carcinoma was histologically detected. A unilateral tonsillectomy would have overlooked the contralateral lesion resulting in a late diagnosis of the contralateral tonsillar carcinoma. PET-CT imaging has proved to be useful in detecting primary sites and distant metastasis in patients with solitary lymph node metastasis. Success rates are reported between 25 and 73%, but a false positive rate is stated between 20 and 46%, which could be explained though increased FDG uptake by chronically inflamed tissue or reactive lymph nodes [32]. False negative results can be caused by early lesions or carcinoma in situ [33]. However, the higher sensitivity of PET-CT makes it more useful for finding the primary tumor site than either PET or CT alone. Nevertheless, in our case described above no reliance on the imaging technique was given. In conclusion, an imaging technique, particularly PET-CT, is necessary for reasons described above and can assist in work-up and diagnosis of CUP-syndrome [18], but a bilateral tonsillectomy with histopathological tissue examination, is more reliable for detection of a tonsillar primary [3] and should not be replaced.

Questions of therapy

Bilateral tonsillectomy is recommended as a routine diagnostic tool in 10% of the relevant publications (Table 1). The NCCN 2014 guidelines recommend a tonsillectomy without specifying unilateral or bilateral. Support is growing for the recommendation of bilateral tonsillectomy, but reports can be found with a restrained opinion [1, 24]. For example, Kothari et al. recommend a bilateral tonsillectomy in CUP patients if the PET-CT scan does not reveal any primary [4]. However, this practice can be risky if a false positive result occurs during PET-CT diagnosis, like in our case described. The recommendation of a bilateral tonsillectomy is supported by Moualed et al. who describe two cases of bilateral tonsillar carcinoma with a primary diagnosis of CUP-syndrome and one of bilateral tonsillar carcinoma with a primary diagnosis of being unilateral. They recommend a bilateral tonsillectomy in patients with suspected unilateral tonsillar carcinoma as well as in patients with a cancer of unknown primary [8]. In our clinic we perfom, and therefore we suggest, a bilateral tonsillectomy in non-CUP-cases with a single sided tonsillar carcinoma as well as in all CUP cases regardless HPV status.

An investigation recently published through Fakhry et al. shows a retrospective analysis of the incidence of oropharyngeal cancer after tonsillectomy. The Danish Cancer Registry was analyzed to determine if previous tonsillectomy reduces the future risk for oropharyngeal cancer. They report that remotely performed tonsillectomy resulted in a decreased risk of developing tonsillar cancer [34]. Nevertheless, a prophylactic tonsillectomy can not be recommended and more biomarkers must be developed for the identification of high-risk-persons [35], even more since Zevallos et al. demonstrated an increased risk for base of tongue cancer after previously performed tonsillectomy [36].

Arguments against the contralateral tonsillectomy include the potentially increased morbidity associated with rare but severe complications of a post-tonsillectomy bleeding [24]. The new German guidelines recommend a unilateral tonsillectomy in the case of a unilateral peritonsillar abscess except for patients with a positive history of recurrent acute tonsillitis, where a bilateral tonsillectomy could be justified. However, the morbidity of a bilateral tonsillectomy does not seem to be significantly greater [3, 10]. Anatomical reasons can be the normal architecture of the contralateral tonsil, compared to the increased vascularization of a pathologically changed tonsil. Nevertheless, clinical trials are necessary with

primary endpoint the bleeding risk for reaching representative results. However, extensive tonsillectomy in the context of a very progressive unilateral tonsillar carcinoma can be the cause of an impaired blood supply of the palate and palatal arch with severe consequences in case of a planned reconstruction with a free lap (a.e. m. radialis-transplantation). If a reconstructive procedure is foreseen, this complication has to be considered before a bilateral tonsillectomy is fulfilled.

The patient's perspective

Regarding all steps of diagnosis and therapy, the patient's point of view is not highlighted. After diagnosis, a fast procedure through the above-mentioned examinations is of great importance as the patient's focus is in first line a treatment of the disease in a timely manner. Whether a surgical treatment or a therapy through radiation and chemotherapy is needed, depends in most cases on the TNM stadium. In the case that tumor tonsillectomy with or without neck dissection presents the best option, an additional tonsillectomy of the other side with eventually further reconstructions might be a further stress factor for the patient and accompanied with higher risk of complications like dehiscence or necrosis of the transplanted lap, difficulties in swallowing and in food intake. Nevertheless, if this procedure presents the best option to cure the current cancer disease and to prevent/decrease the risk of secondary carcinomas of the opposite side, which will be discussed prior to intervention with the patient, the proposed procedure will be easier accepted.

Conclusion

It is possible that metachronous tumors of the contralateral tonsil are actually synchronous bilateral tonsil carcinomas, which had not originally been diagnosed. A bilateral tonsillectomy as a diagnostic and partial therapeutic procedure in patients with diagnosis of CUP or confirmed unilateral tonsillar carcinoma should be established as a standard procedure regardless HPV-status. In doing so, the therapy and prognosis can be crucially influenced and the risk for secondary metachronous tumors of the contralateral side can be reduced. The examination of the lymph node metastasis to HPV positivity can give additional hints to an oropharyngeal origin of the primary tumor and should therefore be established in the cascade of CUP-diagnosis. A PET-CT imaging should serve as an indicative investigation and as a supportive diagnostic procedure, but it should not displace panendoscopy with methodical biopsies in combination with a bilateral tonsillectomy. In cases of further soft tissue reconstructions, the possible complication of an alteration of the palatal vasculature has to be considered and an individualized plan needs to be justified.

Abbreviations

CUP: Cancer of unknown primary; FDG: Fluordesoxyglucose; H&N: Head and neck; HNSCC: Head and neck squamous cell carcinoma; PET-CT: Positron Emission Tomography – Computed Tomography

Acknowledgments

None. The results of this manuscript were presented in the German ENT Symposium 2015 in Berlin.

Funding

No funding sources to declare.

Authors' contributions

M-NT data acquisition, analysis and interpretation, drafting the article. JV critical revision of the article. TH critical revision of the article, data interpretation. JG design of work, data analysis and interpretation, critical revision of the article final approval of the version to be published. All authors read and approved the final manuscript.

Competing interests

The authors declare that they have no competing interests.

References

1. Cianchetti M, Mancuso AA, Amdur RJ, Werning JW, Kirwan J, Morris CG, et al. Diagnostic evaluation of squamous cell carcinoma metastatic to cervical lymph nodes from an unknown head and neck primary site. Laryngoscope. 2009;119(12):2348–54. doi:10.1002/lary.20638.

2. Lanzer M, Bachna-Rotter S, Graupp M, Bredell M, Rucker M, Huber G, et al. Unknown primary of the head and neck: A long-term follow-up. J Craniomaxillofac Surg. 2015;43(4):574–9. doi:10.1016/j.jcms.2015.03.004.

3. Moualed D, Qayyum A, Price T, Sharma A, Mahendran S. Bilateral synchronous tonsillar carcinoma: a case series and review of the literature. Eur Arch Otorhinolaryngol. 2012;269(1):255–9. doi:10.1007/s00405-011-1586-y.

4. Kothari P, Randhawa PS, Farrell R. Role of tonsillectomy in the search for a squamous cell carcinoma from an unknown primary in the head and neck. Br J Oral Maxillofac Surg. 2008;46(4):283–7. doi:10.1016/j.bjoms.2007.11.017.

5. Jones AS, Morar P, Phillips DE, Field JK, Husband D, Helliwell TR. Second primary tumors in patients with head and neck squamous cell carcinoma. Cancer. 1995;75(6):1343–53.

6. Schwartz LH, Ozsahin M, Zhang GN, Touboul E, De Vataire F, Andolenko P, et al. Synchronous and metachronous head and neck carcinomas. Cancer. 1994;74(7):1933–8.

7. Joseph AW, Ogawa T, Bishop JA, Lyford-Pike S, Chang X, Phelps TH, et al. Molecular etiology of second primary tumors in contralateral tonsils of human papillomavirus-associated index tonsillar carcinomas. Oral Oncol. 2013;49(4):244–8. doi:10.1016/j.oraloncology.2012.09.009.

8. Schondorf J, Scherer J. Bilateral tonsillar carcinoma. HNO. 1971;19(11):338–40.

9. Mannina EM, Pejavar SM, Glastonbury CM, van Zante A, Wang SJ, Yom SS. Diagnosis of Bilateral Tonsil Cancers via Staging PET/CT: Case Report and Review. Int J Otolaryngol. 2011;2011:928240. doi:10.1155/2011/928240.

10. Koch WM, Bhatti N, Williams MF, Eisele DW. Oncologic rationale for bilateral tonsillectomy in head and neck squamous cell carcinoma of unknown primary source. Otolaryngol Head Neck Surg. 2001;124(3):331–3. doi:10.1067/mhn.2001.114309.

11. Patel AB, Hinni ML, Pollei TR, Hayden RE, Moore EJ. Severe prolonged dysphagia following transoral resection of bilateral synchronous tonsillar carcinoma. Eur Arch Otorhinolaryngol. 2015; doi:10.1007/s00405-015-3540-x.

12. Bakkal BH, Ugur MB, Bahadir B. Bilateral synchronous squamous cell tonsil carcinoma treated with chemoradiotherapy. JPMA J Pak Med Assoc. 2014; 64(4):468–70.

13. Nakahara S, Yasui T, Takenaka Y, Yamamoto Y, Yoshii T, Morii E, et al. Synchronous bilateral tonsillar carcinomas associated with human papillomavirus. Auris Nasus Larynx. 2014;41(1):109–12. doi:10.1016/j.anl.2013.05.006.

14. Smith RO, Pokala K, Medina JE, Krempl GA. Tonsillar carcinoma in the contralateral tonsil. Laryngoscope. 2010;120(Suppl 4):S176. doi:10.1002/lary.21640.

15. Monsted JE. Bilateral squamous cell carcinoma of the tonsils. Ugeskr Laeger. 2010;172(49):3417–8.

16. Roeser MM, Alon EE, Olsen KD, Moore EJ, Manduch M, Wismayer DJ. Synchronous bilateral tonsil squamous cell carcinoma. Laryngoscope. 2010; 120(Suppl 4):S181. doi:10.1002/lary.21645.

17. Kozakiewicz J, Dec M, Miszczyk L, Urbanczyk H. The rare case of simultaneous bilateral cancer of tonsilla palatina with large metastases to lymphoid glands of the neck. Otolaryngol Pol. 2007;61(4):501–4.

18. Kazak I, Haisch A, Jovanovic S. Bilateral synchronous tonsillar carcinoma in cervical cancer of unknown primary site (CUPS). Eur Arch Otorhinolaryngol. 2003;260(9):490–3. doi:10.1007/s00405-003-0590-2.

19. Rajenderkumar D, Chan KK, Hayward KA, McRae RD. Bilateral synchronous tonsillar carcinoma. J Laryngol Otol. 1999;113(3):255–7.

20. Pajor A, Niebudek-Bogusz E, Kaczmarczyk D. Second primary malignant neoplasms in patients treated in the Otolaryngology Clinic AM of Lodz in the years 1981–1989. Otolaryngol Pol. 1995;49(Suppl 20):53–7.

21. Price T, Pickles J. Synchronous bilateral tonsillar carcinoma: role of fluoro-deoxyglucose positron emission tomography scanning in detecting occult primary tumours in metastatic nodal disease of the head and neck. J Laryngol Otol. 2006;120(4):334–7. doi:10.1017/s0022215106000260.

22. Reddy AN, Eisele DW, Forastiere AA, Lee DJ, Westra WH, Califano JA. Neck dissection followed by radiotherapy or chemoradiotherapy for small primary oropharynx carcinoma with cervical metastasis. Laryngoscope. 2005;115(7): 1196–200. doi:10.1097/01.mlg.0000162643.91849.79.

23. Simo R, O'Connell M. Metastatic squamous cell carcinoma of occult primary: beware the tonsillar remnant. J Laryngol Otol. 2008;122(6):641–3. doi:10.1017/s0022215107008341.

24. Tanzler ED, Amdur RJ, Morris CG, Werning JW, Mendenhall WM. Challenging the need for random directed biopsies of the nasopharynx, pyriform sinus, and contralateral tonsil in the work up of unknown primary squamous cell carcinoma of the head and neck. Head Neck. 2014; doi:10.1002/hed.23931.

25. Lim YC, Lee SY, Lim JY, Shin HA, Lee JS, Koo BS, et al. Management of contralateral N0 neck in tonsillar squamous cell carcinoma. Laryngoscope. 2005;115(9):1672–5. doi:10.1097/01.mlg.0000184791.68804.0b.

26. Slaughter DP, Southwick HW, Smejkal W. Field cancerization in oral stratified squamous epithelium; clinical implications of multicentric origin. Cancer. 1953;6(5):963–8.

27. D'Souza G, Kreimer AR, Viscidi R, Pawlita M, Fakhry C, Koch WM, et al. Case-control study of human papillomavirus and oropharyngeal cancer. N Engl J Med. 2007;356(19):1944–56. doi:10.1056/NEJMoa065497.

28. Chepeha D, Eisbruch A. Commentary: clinical nodal staging of human papillomavirus-related oropharyngeal cancer. Cancer J (Sudbury, Mass). 2010;16(3):283. doi:10.1097/PPO.0b013e3181defda7.

29. Begum S, Gillison ML, Ansari-Lari MA, Shah K, Westra WH. Detection of human papillomavirus in cervical lymph nodes: a highly effective strategy for localizing site of tumor origin. Clin Cancer Res. 2003;9(17):6469–75.

30. Chernock RD, Lewis JS. Approach to metastatic carcinoma of unknown primary in the head and neck: squamous cell carcinoma and beyond. Head Neck Pathol. 2015;9(1):6–15. doi:10.1007/s12105-015-0616-2.

31. Byrd JK, Smith KJ, de Almeida JR, Albergotti WG, Davis KS, Kim SW, et al. Transoral Robotic Surgery and the Unknown Primary: A Cost-Effectiveness Analysis. Otolaryngol Head Neck Surg. 2014;150(6):976–82. doi:10.1177/0194599814525746.

32. Calabrese L, Jereczek-Fossa BA, Jassem J, Rocca A, Bruschini R, Orecchia R, et al. Diagnosis and management of neck metastases from an unknown primary. Acta Otorhinolaryngolog Ital. 2005;25(1):2–12.

33. Shintani SA, Foote RL, Lowe VJ, Brown PD, Garces YI, Kasperbauer JL. Utility of PET/CT imaging performed early after surgical resection in the adjuvant treatment planning for head and neck cancer. Int J Radiat Oncol Biol Phys. 2008;70(2):322–9. doi:10.1016/j.ijrobp.2007.06.038.

34. Fakhry C, Andersen KK, Christensen J, Agrawal N, Eisele DW. The Impact of Tonsillectomy upon the Risk of Oropharyngeal Carcinoma Diagnosis and Prognosis in the Danish Cancer Registry. Cancer Prev Res (Philadelphia, Pa). 2015;8(7):583–9. doi:10.1158/1940-6207.capr-15-0101.

35. Misiukiewicz K, Posner M. Role of Prophylactic Bilateral Tonsillectomy as a Cancer Preventive Strategy. Cancer Prev Res (Philadelphia, Pa). 2015;8(7): 580–2. doi:10.1158/1940-6207.capr-15-0153.

36. Zevallos JP, Mazul AL, Rodriguez N, Weissler MC, Brennan P, Anantharaman D, et al. Previous tonsillectomy modifies odds of tonsil and base of tongue cancer. Br J Cancer. 2016;114(7):832–8. doi:10.1038/bjc.2016.63.

3

Predominance and association risk of *Blastocystis hominis* subtype I in colorectal cancer

Amr Mohamed Mohamed[1,2*], Mona Abdelfattah Ahmed[3,4], Sabah Abdelghany Ahmed[4],
Sherif Ahmed Al-Semany[5,6], Saad Saed Alghamdi[1] and Dina Abdulla Zaglool[7,8]

Abstract

Background: *Blastocystis*, a genetically diverse intestinal parasite with controversial pathogenic potential, has increasingly been incriminated for diarrheal illness in immunocompromised individuals including colorectal cancer (CRC) patients. The aim of the current study was to assess the possible association between *Blastocystis* infection and CRC condition in Makkah, Saudi Arabia (KSA).

Methods: Stool samples were collected from 80 non-cancer (NC) and 138 cancer subjects including 74 CRC patients and 64 patients with other cancers outside gastrointestinal tract (COGT). Molecularly confirmed *Blastocystis* isolates were genetically grouped and subtyped using multiplex polymerase chain reaction with restriction fragment length polymorphism (PCR-RFLP) and sequence-tagged site primers-based PCR (PCR-STS), respectively.

Results: *Blastocystis hominis* were confirmed in 29.7, 25 and 15% among CRC, COGT and NC patients, respectively. Obtained *Blastocystis* isolates were initially categorized into 2 groups (A and C), which were subsequently subtyped into 3 different subtypes; subtype-I (38%), subtype-II (44%) and subtype-V (22%). Interestingly, subtype-I was the most predominantly detected subtype (54.5%) among CRC patients with a significant association risk (COR 7.548; 95% CI: 1.629–34.987; $P = 0.004$).

Conclusion: To the best of our knowledge, the current study is the first to provide genetic insights on the prevalence of *Blastocystis hominis* among CRC patients in Makkah, KSA. Moreover, the study suggests for a possible association between subtype-I of *Blastocystis hominis* and CRC, which could indicate a potential influence of Blastocystis on CRC condition. Further studies are required to confirm this association risk and to investigate the possible underlying mechanism of postulated carcinogenic influence of *Blastocystis hominis* subtype-I.

Keywords: *Blastocystis hominis*, CRC, Genetic diversity, Subtypes-I, Association risk

Background

Blastocystis species remains one of the most common intestinal parasites in humans with a prevalence of up to 10% in developed countries, rising to 50–60% in developing countries [1, 2]. It is considered one of the most commonly encountered non-fungal eukaryotic organisms in human fecal samples [3]. Blastocystis is an enteric protozoon found in the intestinal tract of humans and a wide range of animal hosts [4]. Morphologically, *Blastocystis* is a highly polymorphic organism that takes several different forms during its life cycle including vacuolar, cystic, amoeboid, granular, multivacuolar, and avacuolar forms [1, 5].

The pathogenicity of these protozoa is still controversial and inconclusive with non-specific symptoms such as abdominal pain, nausea, vomiting, anorexia, flatulence, weight loss, and acute or chronic diarrhea [6, 7]. Similar to other intestinal parasitism and chronic gastrointestinal illnesses such as irritable bowel syndrome (IBS), *Blastocystis* infection is usually associated with alternate episodes of diarrhea, normal defecation or even constipation.

* Correspondence: amrmohamed2004@yahoo.com
[1]Laboratory Medicine, Faculty of Applied Medical Sciences, Umm Al-Qura University, Makkah 7607, Saudi Arabia
[2]Clinical Laboratory Diagnosis, Department of Animal Medicine, Faculty of Veterinary Medicine, Assiut University, Assiut, Egypt
Full list of author information is available at the end of the article

Symptomatic *Blastocystis* infection has been encountered more commonly among patients of IBS as well as other immunocompromised patients [3, 6, 8].

Molecular studies revealed that the parasite is characterized by an extensive genetic diversity in both humans and animals with a worldwide distribution [9–15]. At least 10 subtypes (ST), ST1 to ST10, have been recognized based on the small subunit ribosomal RNA (SSU rRNA) gene sequence [16]. In addition, three novel subtypes (ST11–ST13) have been identified from captive animals in the zoo [17]. At present, only ST1 to ST9 are considered to colonize in humans [7, 17]. This genetic diversity has supported the hypothesis that the variability in symptoms in patients positive for *Blastocystis* could be due to different pathogenic potential among the subtypes [18–21].

Prevalence studies of *Blastocystis* in immunocompromised individuals have been confined to HIV/AIDS patients and there is general lack of information on the prevalence of the organism in other immunocompromised individuals such as colorectal cancer patients. Therefore the current study aimed to assess the possible relationship between *Blastocystis* infection and malignancy with special reference to CRC. The frequency of *Blastocystis* infection among CRC patients in comparison with other cancer and non-cancer patients were investigated. In addition, the study also aimed to assess the association potential of genetically identified subtype(s) of encountered *Blastocystis* infection with CRC in Makkah, KSA. This represents the first study to explore the genetic diversity of encountered *Blastocystis* isolates and to assess their association significance with colorectal cancer in Makkah, KSA.

Methods
Study subjects
This was a prospective case control study. A total of 218 stool samples were collected from recruited participants attending King Abdulla Medical city (KAMC), Makkah, KSA during the period extended from April 2013 to March 2015. Recruited participants belonged to two main groups. The first group included recently diagnosed patients with malignancy (138) and referred to as cancer patients (CP) while the second group composed of normal subjects visiting the hospital for routine checkup (80) and referred to as non-cancer patients (NC). The cancer patients were categorized into two subgroups; colorectal cancer group (CRC), which included 74 subject and cancers outside gastrointestinal tract group (COGT), which included 64 patients (14 non hogken lymphoma; 11 malignant neoplasm of bladder; 15 malignant neoplasm of uterine adnexa; 9 malignant neoplasm of larynx and 15 malignant neoplasm of breast). Exclusion criteria included any suspected patient started anti-cancer treatment regime and/or receiving any anti-parasitic medication. Ethical

approval for the study was obtained in accordance with the declaration of Helsinki from the Ethics Committee of the Faculty of Applied Medical Sciences, Umm Al-Qura University (AMSEC 10-18-2-2013) and Biomedical Research Ethics committee of King Abdullah Medical City. All investigated patients signed acknowledgment consents to declare their participation agreement.

Isolation and conventional identification of *Blastocystis*
Blastocystis parasites were isolated from suspected stool samples by in vitro cultivation at 37 °C using Jones' medium supplemented with 10% horse serum for 72 h. [22]. Suspected cultures were then sub-cultured in duplicate using Jones' medium at 37 °C for 3 additional days. Afterwards, for each suspected isolate, one culture medium was subjected to microscopic examination for conventional identification of suspected *Blastocystis*, while the second culture medium was kept at -20 °C for further molecular studies.

Molecular identification of isolated Blastocystis
Genomic DNA was isolated from cultures of conventionally identified *Blastocystis* as previously described with few modifications [23]. Briefly, frozen culture media were thawed at room temperature and the suspected *Blastocystis* were harvested by centrifugation at $500 \times g$ for 5 min and washed with sterile phosphate- buffered saline (PBS) (pH 7.4) for 5 times. Obtained cell pellets were then lysed using lysis buffer (20 mM Tris–HCl buffer, pH 8.0, 100 mM NaCl, 25 mM EDTA, pH 8.0) containing 1% SDS and 0.5 mg Proteinase K/ml (Fermentas, USA) and incubated at 55 °C overnight. Genomic DNA was then extracted with phenol/chloroform/ isoamyl alcohol. Extracted DNA was then precipitated in 2 vol of ice-cold ethanol containing 0.3 M sodium acetate (pH 5.2). Obtained DNA pellets were first washed in 70% ice-cold ethanol, and then was resuspended in 50 μl Tris–EDTA (TE) buffer (10 mM Tris, 1 mM EDTA, pH 8.0). DNA concentration of each sample was determined using the BioSpec-nano (Shimadzu Corporation, Japan) and its quality and integrity was tested using the A260/A280 ratio.

Identification of *Blastocystis* isolates was confirmed by molecular amplification of the conserved 1.1 Kbp. Target of SSU rRNA gene using previously described primers Blas-F: (GGA GGT AGT GAC AAT AAA TC) and Blas-R: (ACT AGG AAT TCC TCG TTC ATG) [24]. Amplification protocol was carried out as previously described with some modification [25]. Briefly, 5 μl of template DNA (10 ng/ μl) were used in a total reaction volume of 50 μl. The reaction mix included PCR buffer (20 mmol Tris-HCL (pH 8.4) and 50 mmol KCl), 0.1 mmol each of dNTP (deoxyribonucleotide triphosphate), 1.5 mmol of MgCl2, 50 pmol of each primer, and 1.5 U of HotStar HiFidelity Polymerase (Qiagen). PCR condition consisted of an initial denaturation step at 95 °C for 10 min followed by 35 cycles of denaturation at 95 °C for 1 min, annealing at 53 °C for 30 s, and extension at 72 °C for 1 min.

Grouping and subtyping of Blastocystis by PCR-RFLP and PCR-STS analysis

Grouping of *Blastocystis* isolates was performed by RFLP analysis of the amplified 1.1 kbp. target of SSU rRNA gene using *SpeI* restriction enzyme (New England BioLabs Inc., MA, USA). *Blastocystis* isolates were grouped according to size of obtained digestion products as previously described [26]. Grouped *Blastocystis* isolates were then subjected to subtyping analysis. For this purpose, seven pairs of sequence-tagged site (STS) previously described primers [9] were used for conducting PCR-STS analysis. Primer sets names and sequences as well as predicted product size are shown in Table 1. PCR-STS protocol was conducted as previously described with little modification [9, 23]. Briefly, 5 µl of template DNA (10 ng/ µl) were used in a total reaction volume of 50 µl. The reaction mix included PCR buffer (20 mmol Tris-HCL (pH 8.4) and 50 mmol KCl), 0.1 mmol each of dNTP (deoxyribonucleotide triphosphate), 1.5 mmol of $MgCl_2$, 25 pmol of each primer, and 1.5 U of HotStar HiFidelity Polymerase (Qiagen). The PCR amplification started with an initial denaturation step at 95 °C for 10 min, followed by 35 cycles including denaturation at 95 °C for 1 min, an annealing at 56 °C for 30 s, and an extension step at 72 °C for 1 min. All PCR amplifications were carried out using Applied Biosystems Veriti Thermal Cycler (ThermoFisher Scientific Inc.) After PCR, 10 µl of the PCR product was mixed with 5 µl dye mixture (0.25% bromophenol blue and 0.25% xylene cyanol in 15% Ficoll type 400) and electrophoresed in 1 µl Tris-acetate-EDTA

buffer through a 2% agarose gel containing ethidium bromide (0.5 µg/mL). Bands of the appropriate size were visualized using a Molecular Imager® Gel Doc™ XR System (Bio-Rad Laboratories) according to the manufacturer's instructions and identified by comparison with a 100-bp DNA ladder (DNA molecular weight marker Promega) using Image Lab version 5 (Bio-Rad Laboratories).

Statistical analysis

Statistical analysis of the results was performed using SPSS version 16 (SPSS, Chicago, IL). The frequencies of *Blastocystis* infection and/or its subtypes among different groups of investigated patients were assessed using cross-tabulation followed by Chi square ($X2$) test or Fischer's exact test. A crude odds ratio (COR) with 95% confidence interval (CI) was calculated for frequency analysis as appropriate for assessment of possible association risk. All tests performed were two-sided and P value < 0.05 was considered significant.

Results

Detection and identification of *Blastocystis* isolates

Blastocystis was initially identified conventionally by microscopic visualization of *Blastocystis* stages in culture media. Identification was then confirmed genetically by PCR amplification of the conserved Blastocystis hominis-specific 1.1 Kbp. target of the SSU rRNA gene (Fig. 1). Out of a total of 218 fecal samples from suspected patients with gastrointestinal illnesses, *Blastocystis hominis* were identified in 50 (22.9%) samples. This included 22 (29.7%) of CRC patients, 16 (25%) of COGT patients and 12 (15%) of NC patients (Table 2). A significant difference ($P < 0.05$) of *Blastocystis* infection frequency was evident between CP group and NC groups as well as between CRC and NC groups. However, no significant difference ($P > 0.05$) was evident between COGT and NC groups (Table 2).

Table 1 Different STS primer sets used for differential identification of Blastocystis subtypes along with expected amplified product sizes

STS primer set	GenBank accession no.	Sequences	Product size	Subtype
SB83	AF166086	F-GAAGGACTCTCTGACGATGA R-GTCCAAATGAAAGGCAGC	351	I
SB155	AF166087	F-ATCAGCCTACAATCTCCTC R-ATCGCCACTTCTCCAAT	650	II
SB227	AF166088	F-ATCAGCCTACAATCTCCTC R-ATCGCCACTTCTCCAAT	526	III
SB332	AF166091	FGCATCCAGACTACTATCAACATT R-CCATTTTCAGACAACCACTTA	338	IV
SB340	AY048752	F-TGTTCTTGTGTCTTCTCAGCTC R-TTCTTTCACACTCCCGTCAT	704	V
SB336	AY048751	F-GTGGGTAGAGGAAGGAAAACA R-AGAACAAGTCGATGAAGTGAGAT	317	VI
SB337	AY048750	F-GTCTTTCCCTGTCTATTCTGCA R-AATTCGGTCTGCTTCTTCTG	487	VII

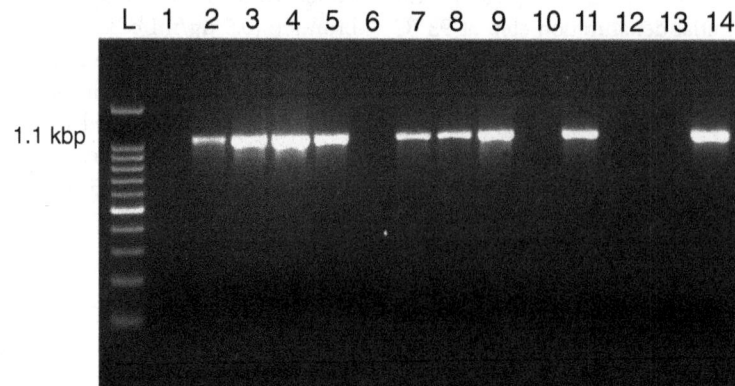

Fig. 1 Representative 1% agarose gel showing the amplification of the *Blastocystis*-specific 1.1 kbp target of the SSU of rRNA gene. (Lane L) shows 100 bp DNA ladder; (Lane 1) represents negative control; (Lanes 2,3,4,5,7,8,9,11and 14) represent positive results for *Blastocystis*; (Lanes 6,10,12 and 13) represent negative results for *Blastocystis*

Moreover, results revealed an associated risk (COR 2.153; 95% CI: 1.053-4.417; $P = 0.044$) between *Blastocystis* infection and cancer condition with a higher risk of association (COR 2.397; 95% CI: 1.087 − 5.286; $P = 0.033$) in CRC group but not in the COGT group.

Genetic grouping and subtyping of *Blastocystis* isolates
Based on RFLP analysis of the amplified 1.1 Kbp target of the SSU rRNA gene, 2 *Blastocystis* groups were reported; group A (230 bp., 430 bp. and 450 bp.) and group C (470 bp. and 650 bp.) (Fig. 2). Accordingly, 39 isolates of obtained *Blastocystis hominis* from suspected patients were categorized as group A while the rest 11 isolates were categorized as group C. further genotypic analysis of recovered *Blastocystis hominis* based on the predicted size of obtained amplicons after PCR-STS assay resulted in subtyping of group A isolates into 2 different subtypes (I and II) and that of group C as only one subtype (V) (Fig. 3). Overall, 40% of recovered *Blastocystis hominis* were identified as subtype II, 38% as subtype I, and 22% were identified as subtype V. In relation to type of patients, subtype I was predominant

(44.7%) in cancer patients while subtype II was predominant (58.3%) among non-cancer patients. Among cancer patients, subtype I was the predominant subtype (54.5%) among CRC patients, while subtype II was predominant (43.7%) among COGT patients (Table 3). Subtype I showed significant higher frequency ($P < 0.05$) in CRC group as compared to other recovered subtypes in the same group. With regard to frequency significance among different groups, subtype I showed significant higher frequency ($P < 0.05$) in CP as compared to NC group. On the other hand, frequency variation between different cancer patients groups revealed significant higher frequency ($P < 0.05$) of subtype I in CRC as compared to COGT group (Table 3). Interestingly, an association risk between *Blastocystis* subtype-I and cancer condition was evident (COR 5.479; 95% CI: 1.232-24.374; $P = 0.013$) with

Table 2 Frequency of Blastocystis infection among CP including CRC and COGT groups as well as NC group of investigated patients

Investigated groups (no.)		Blastocystis infection			
		Positive cases no. (%)		Negative cases no. (%)	
CP (138)	CRC (74)	38 (27.5)[a]	22 (29.7)[b]	100 (72.5)	52 (70.3)
	COGT (64)		16 (25)		48 (75)
NC (80)		12 (15)		68 (85)	
Total (218)		50 (22.9)		168 (77.1)	

Cancer patients (CP); Colorectal cancer (CRC); COGT (Cancer outside gastrointestinal tract); Non cancer (NC)
[a]Blastocystis infection in overall cancer group as compared to NC group ($P = 0.044$)
[b]Blastocystis infection in CRC group as compared to NC group ($P = 0.033$)

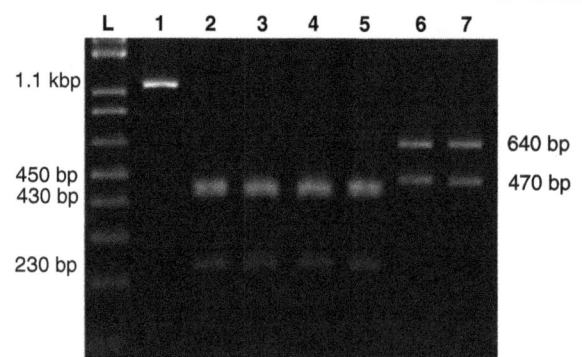

Fig. 2 Representative 1% agarose gel showing *Blastocystis* grouping based on RFLP-PCR of the *Blastocystis*-specific 1.1 kbp target of the SSU of rRNA gene. (Lane L) shows 1 Kbp. DNA ladder; (Lane 1) shows undigested 1.1 kbp target of *Blastocystis*. (Lanes 2–5) show 230 bp, 430 bp and 450 bp digestion products corresponding to *Blastocystis* group A. (Lanes 6 and 7) show 470 bp and 640 bp digestion products corresponding to *Blastocystis* group C

Table 3 Frequency of different *Blastocystis* subtypes isolated from CP including CRC and COGT groups and NC group of investigated patients

Investigated groups (n)		Recovered subtypes of Blastocystis no. (%)					
		I		II		V	
CP (38)	CRC (22)	17 (44.7)[a]	12 (54.5)[b, c, d, e]	13 (34.2)	6 (27.3)	8 (21.1)	4 (18.2)
	COGT (16)		5 (31.3)		7 (43.7)		4 (25)
NC (12)		2 (16.7)		7 (58.3)		3 (25)	
Total (50)		19 (38)		20 (40)		11 (22)	

Cancer patients (CP); Colorectal cancer (CRC); COGT (Cancer outside gastrointestinal tract); Non cancer (NC)
[a]subtype I in CP group against subtype I in NC group ($P = 0.013$)
[b]subtype I in CRC group against subtype I in NC group ($P = 0.004$)
[c]subtype I in CRC group against subtype I in COGT group ($P = 0.024$)
[d]subtype I in CRC group against subtype II in the same group ($P = 0.019$)
[e]subtype I in CRC group against subtype V in the same group ($P = 0.018$)

a greater risk of association (COR 7.548; 95% CI: 1.629 – 34.987; $P = 0.004$) in CRC group.

All raw data of the current work were made available as an additional file (Additional file 1).

Discussion

After dietary factors and tobacco smoke, infectious diseases represent the third leading cause of cancer worldwide. The International Agency on Research of Cancer (IARC) has estimated that 16% of cancer worldwide is initiated by infectious agents including parasites [27]. With regard to relation between parasitic infection and cancerous conditions, few studies investigated the association between *Blastocystis hominis* infection and colorectal cancer. The recently postulated potential carcinogenic effect of *Blastocystis hominis* infection in human host especially in colorectal cancer patients [28, 29] signifies the need for screening of colorectal cancer patients for *Blastocystis hominis* infection. Therefore the current study aimed to investigate the association risk of *Blastocystis hominis* infection and

its subtypes in relation to CRC patients of Makkah region, KSA.

The over all rate of *Blastocystis* infection as revealed in the current study was 22.9%. The current finding is comparable to previously reported frequencies in several countries including Saudi Arabia (17.5%) [30], Malaysia (25.7%) [31], Jordan (25%) [32], Egypt (31%) [33], 25.78% in Venezuela [34] and 22.9% in Argentina [35]. On the other hand, significantly lower infection rates ranged between 9 and 12% were recently reported in Saudi Arabia [36, 37]. The currently recorded higher infection rate could be attributed to the type of targeted patients in the comparable studies where the patients were predominantly immune-competent. Interestingly, the currently recorded rate of *Blastocystis hominis* infection among cancer patients is apparently higher than figures (7.7–13%) previously recorded among other cancer patients [23, 38, 39]. With regard to type of patients, current study revealed significant higher frequency ($P = 0.044$) of *Blastocystis* infection in CP group as compared to NC group. This finding might support the association risk of the parasite with

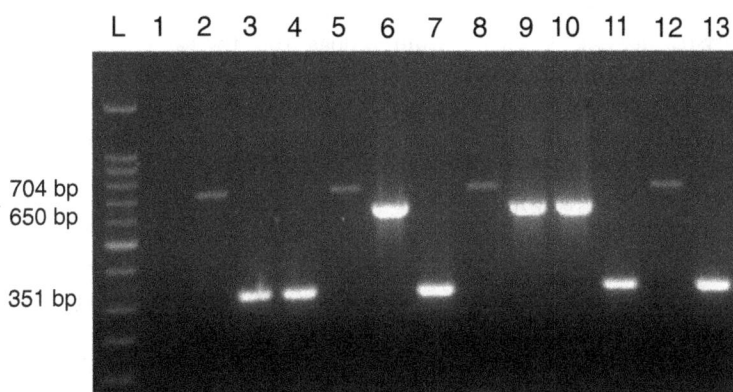

Fig. 3 Representative 1% agarose gel showing *Blastocystis* subtyping based on PCR-STS analysis. (Lane L) shows 100 bp DNA ladder; (Lane 1) represents negative control. (Lanes 2,5,8 and 12) show 704 bp PCR products and represent *Blastocystis* subtype-V. (Lanes 3,4,7,11 and 13) show 351 bp PCR products and represent *Blastocystis* subtype-I. (Lanes 6,9 and 10) show 650 bp PCR products and represent *Blastocystis* subtype-II

immunocompromised condition [23] and denotes that *Blastocystis* infection is not rare and should be looked for routinely in immunocompromised patients. However, with regard to type of cancer, the current study revealed significant ($P = 0.033$) higher frequency of *Blastocystis* infection only in CRC and not COGT group as compared to NC group. These findings contradict the notion of association between *Blastocystis* infection and immunocompromised conditions, yet denote that *Blastocystis* infection is more likely associated with those immunocompromised conditions with gastrointestinal affections as CRC. This likely association was statistically validated in the current study (COR 2.397; 95% CI: 1.087–5.286; $P = 0.033$).

Genetic diversity of *Blastocystis hominis* and its worldwide distribution has been evidenced [9–13]. Genotyping of the parasite has received great attention lately in a trial to link the different pathogenic behaviors of the parasite to its different subtypes. Based on the RFLP analysis of the small subunit ribosomal RNA gene, *Blastocystis hominis* are classified into four groups as previously described [26]. In the current study PCR-RFLP analysis revealed that most of the obtained isolates from suspected patients with gastrointestinal symptoms belonged to group A (78%) while the rest of the isolates were found belonging to group C (22%). Further subtyping of obtained isolates was carried out using PCR-STS assay as previously described [9]. Dissimilar to previous studies, which usually reveal the predominance of one subtype among investigated local population [22, 24, 40], the current study revealed the presence of 3 different subtypes (I, II and V) among investigated patients. The detection of multiple subtypes could be due to the exceptional setting of the study. Makkah, where the current study was conducted, is a unique place in Saudi Arabia and the entire world. Annually, it receives more than three million pilgrims during the pilgrimage season in addition to several other million visitors during the whole year from allover the world [41, 42]. This could have contributed to the acquisition of different *Blastocystis hominis* subtypes from different worldwide settings. In disagreement with previous studies, which had shown the predominance of subtype III among patients with chronic gastrointestinal illness in Malaysia [22], Singapore [24], Egypt [43], Turkey [44], USA [45] and Iran [46], interestingly, the current study have showed the predominance of subtype I and II (38 and 40%, respectively) among targeted patients in Makkah. However, the current finding was in agreement with a previous study in central Thailand, where two subtypes (ST1 and ST2) were found predominant among schoolchildren of a rural community [47]. In the current study subtype II, most likely the one that is non-pathogenic [19], was the most predominantly detected subtype among investigated patients. On the other hand, subtype I, the second most predominately detected subtype among investigated patients, is believed to be one of the known pathogenic subtypes that were implicated in several human diseases and believed to be of animal origin with a zoonotic potential [9, 13]. Evaluation of current study results revealed significant predominance ($P = 0.019$ and $P = 0.018$, respectively) of subtype I as compared to other recovered subtypes (II and V, respectively) in CRC patients. Interestingly, the significant predominance of subtype I among CP group as compared to NC patients included highly significant predominance ($P = 0.004$) in CRC group and not COGT group. Moreover, a strong association risk (COR 7.548; 95% CI: 1.629–34.987; $P = 0.004$) was evident between *Blastocystis hominis* subtype-I infection and CRC condition. This interesting finding supports the postulated carcinogenic effect of certain *Blastocystis hominis* subtypes and their possible influence on colorectal cancer. Recently, in vitro studies documented the ability of *Blastocystis hominis* to induce the growth of colorectal cancer cell lines via inhibiting the apoptotic effect of colon cancer cells. Furthermore, isolated antigens of *Blastocystis hominis* isolates were shown to promote the proliferation of cancer cells via down-regulation of host immune cellular responses [28, 29].

Growing data has evidenced the zoonotic potential of *Blastocystis* spp., where comparable genetic sequences were documented in a number of studies between different *Blastocystis* spp. isolated from both human and animals [48–50]. Moreover, some specific *Blastocystis hominis* subtypes were identified in both humans and animals. Subtype I is a common subtypes that had been identified in both human and a wide range of animal species including pigs, horses, monkeys, cattle, rodents, chickens, quails, and pheasants [10, 50, 51]. Other subtypes were also implicated in both human and animal infections with a potential zoonotic ability like subtype V, the least predominant subtype encountered in the current study, which was reported in both human and dogs from the same sitting in Thailand [49]. In general, it was reported that population closely associated with animals has a higher prevalence of blastocystosis when compared with those not associated with animals [52]. With regard to the current study, the association risk between investigated suspected patients and animals was not inspected. However, it worth mentioning that many residents at Makkah region have some sort of association with animals particularly sheep, goat and camels. Moreover, drinking unpasteurized or even raw milk from dairy animals, a trend that is widely practiced in the region is a potential risk factor for disease transmission from animals to human [3]. Nevertheless, further epidemiologic studies need to be conducted to provide additional evidences to confirm the postulated role of zoonotic transmission of the disease to human population in Makkah, KSA.

Conclusions

The current study is the first to provide genetic insights on the prevalence of *Blastocystis hominis* among CRC patients in Makkah, KSA. Interestingly, the current results suggested a possible association between *Blastocystis hominis* subtype-I and CRC condition, which postulate a potential influence of this pathogen on carcinogenesis of CRC. In deed, these findings need to be confirmed via further controlled epidemiologic and topographic investigations to confirm the proposed association risk and to reveal other possible risk factors that could contribute to the condition. In addition, further studies are required to explore the underlying mechanism of the postulated carcinogenic influence of this pathogen.

Acknowledgements
The authors would like to thank Mr. Mohammed E. Naeem, King Abdullah Medical City, Makkah, KSA and Mr. Ahmed A. Althagafi, Faculty of Applied Medical Sciences, Umm Al-Qura university for their valuable contribution in collection, handling and archiving of related stool specimens.

Funding
The current study was supported by a research grant # 43409023 from the Institute if Scientific Research (ISRRIH), Umm Al-Qura University, Saudi Arabia.

Authors' contributions
AMM, has made substantial contributions to the conception and design of the study, analysis and interpretation of data, drafting and critically revising the manuscript. MAA, contributed in the collection and examination of samples, analysis and interpretation of data. SAA, contributed in the design of the study, analysis and interpretation of data. ShAA, was responsible for recruitment and classification of included cancer patients. SSA, contributed in analysis and interpretation of data and drafting and revising of the manuscript: DAZ, contributed in the collection and examination of samples. All authors gave final approval of the version to be published, and agree to be accountable for all aspects of the work.

Competing interests
The authors declare that they have no competing interests.

Author details
[1]Laboratory Medicine, Faculty of Applied Medical Sciences, Umm Al-Qura University, Makkah 7607, Saudi Arabia. [2]Clinical Laboratory Diagnosis, Department of Animal Medicine, Faculty of Veterinary Medicine, Assiut University, Assiut, Egypt. [3]Medical Parasitology, King Abdullah Medical City, Makkah, Saudi Arabia. [4]Parasitology Department, Faculty of Medicine, Ain-Shams University, Cairo, Egypt. [5]Oncology, King Abdullah Medical City, Makkah, Saudi Arabia. [6]Department of Internal Medicine, Medical Oncology, Mansoura University, Mansoura, Egypt. [7]Medical Parasitology, Al-Noor Specialist Hospital, Makkah, Saudi Arabia. [8]Parasitology Department, Faculty of Medicine, Assiut University, Assiut, Egypt.

References
1. Stenzel DJ, Boreham PF. Blastocystis hominis revisited. Clin Microbiol Rev. 1996;9(4):563–84.
2. Tan KS. Blastocystis in humans and animals: new insights using modern methodologies. Vet Parasitol. 2004;126(1-2):121–44. doi:10.1016/j.vetpar.2004.09.017.
3. Stensvold CR, Lewis HC, Hammerum AM, Porsbo LJ, Nielsen SS, Olsen KE, et al. Blastocystis: unravelling potential risk factors and clinical significance of a common but neglected parasite. Epidemiol Infect. 2009;137(11):1655–63. doi:10.1017/S0950268809002672.
4. Menounos PG, Spanakos G, Tegos N, Vassalos CM, Papadopoulou C, Vakalis NC. Direct detection of Blastocystis sp. in human faecal samples and subtype assignment using single strand conformational polymorphism and sequencing. Mol Cell Probes. 2008;22(1):24–9. doi:10.1016/j.mcp.2007.06.007.
5. Yoshikawa H, Abe N, Iwasawa M, Kitano S, Nagano I, Wu Z, et al. Genomic analysis of Blastocystis hominis strains isolated from two long-term health care facilities. J Clin Microbiol. 2000;38(4):1324–30.
6. Ok Uz, Cirit M, Uner A, Ok E Akcochicek F Basci A and Ozcel MA. Cryptosporidiosis and blastocystosis in renal transplant recipient. Nephron. 1997;75:171-74.
7. Rene BA, Stensvold CR, Badsberg JH, Nielsen HV. Subtype analysis of Blastocystis isolates from Blastocystis cyst excreting patients. Am J Trop Med Hyg. 2009;80(4):588–92.
8. Yakoob J, Jafri W, Beg MA, Abbas Z, Naz S, Islam M, et al. Irritable bowel syndrome: is it associated with genotypes of Blastocystis hominis. Parasitol Res. 2010;106(5):1033–8. doi:10.1007/s00436-010-1761-x.
9. Yoshikawa H, Wu Z, Kimata I, Iseki M, Ali IK, Hossain MB, et al. Polymerase chain reaction-based genotype classification among human Blastocystis hominis populations isolated from different countries. Parasitol Res. 2004; 92(1):22–9. doi:10.1007/s00436-003-0995-2.
10. Noel C, Dufernez F, Gerbod D, Edgcomb VP, Delgado-Viscogliosi P, Ho LC, et al. Molecular phylogenies of Blastocystis isolates from different hosts: implications for genetic diversity, identification of species, and zoonosis. J Clin Microbiol. 2005;43(1):348–55. doi:10.1128/JCM.43.1.348-355.2005.
11. Abe N. Molecular and phylogenetic analysis of Blastocystis isolates from various hosts. Vet Parasitol. 2004;120(3):235–42. doi:10.1016/j.vetpar.2004.01.003.
12. Bohm-Gloning B, Knobloch J, Walderich B. Five subgroups of Blastocystis hominis from symptomatic and asymptomatic patients revealed by restriction site analysis of PCR-amplified 16S-like rDNA. Trop Med Int Health. 1997;2(8):771–8.
13. Yan Y, Su S, Lai R, Liao H, Ye J, Li X, et al. Genetic variability of Blastocystis hominis isolates in China. Parasitol Res. 2006;99(5):597–601. doi:10.1007/s00436-006-0186-z.
14. Souppart L, Sanciu G, Cian A, Wawrzyniak I, Delbac F, Capron M, et al. Molecular epidemiology of human Blastocystis isolates in France. Parasitol Res. 2009;105(2):413–21. doi:10.1007/s00436-009-1398-9.
15. Li LH, Zhang XP, Lv S, Zhang L, Yoshikawa H, Wu Z, et al. Cross-sectional surveys and subtype classification of human Blastocystis isolates from four epidemiological settings in China. Parasitol Res. 2007;102(1):83–90. doi:10.1007/s00436-007-0727-0.
16. Stensvold CR, Alfellani MA, Norskov-Lauritsen S, Prip K, Victory EL, Maddox C, et al. Subtype distribution of Blastocystis isolates from synanthropic and zoo animals and identification of a new subtype. Int J Parasitol. 2009;39(4):473–9. doi:10.1016/j.ijpara.2008.07.006.
17. Parkar U, Traub RJ, Vitali S, Elliot A, Levecke B, Robertson I, et al. Molecular characterization of Blastocystis isolates from zoo animals and their animal-keepers. Vet Parasitol. 2010;169(1-2):8–17. doi:10.1016/j.vetpar.2009.12.032.
18. Souppart L, Moussa H, Cian A, Sanciu G, Poirier P, El Alaoui H, et al. Subtype analysis of Blastocystis isolates from symptomatic patients in Egypt. Parasitol Res. 2010;106(2):505–11. doi:10.1007/s00436-009-1693-5.
19. Dogruman-Al F, Dagci H, Yoshikawa H, Kurt O, Demirel M. A possible link between subtype 2 and asymptomatic infections of Blastocystis hominis. Parasitol Res. 2008;103(3):685–9. doi:10.1007/s00436-008-1031-3.
20. Dominguez-Marquez MV, Guna R, Munoz C, Gomez-Munoz MT, Borras R. High prevalence of subtype 4 among isolates of Blastocystis hominis from symptomatic patients of a health district of Valencia (Spain). Parasitol Res. 2009;105(4):949–55. doi:10.1007/s00436-009-1485-y.
21. Stensvold CR, Christiansen DB, Olsen KE, Nielsen HV. Blastocystis sp. subtype 4 is common in Danish Blastocystis-positive patients presenting with acute diarrhea. Am J Trop Med Hyg. 2011;84(6):883–5. doi:10.4269/ajtmh.2011.11-0005.

22. Tan TC, Suresh KG, Smith HV. Phenotypic and genotypic characterisation of Blastocystis hominis isolates implicates subtype 3 as a subtype with pathogenic potential. Parasitol Res. 2008;104(1):85–93. doi:10.1007/s00436-008-1163-5.

23. Tan TC, Ong SC, Suresh KG. Genetic variability of Blastocystis sp. isolates obtained from cancer and HIV/AIDS patients. Parasitol Res. 2009;105(5):1283–6. doi:10.1007/s00436-009-1551-5.

24. Wong KH, Ng GC, Lin RT, Yoshikawa H, Taylor MB, Tan KS. Predominance of subtype 3 among Blastocystis isolates from a major hospital in Singapore. Parasitol Res. 2008;102(4):663–70. doi:10.1007/s00436-007-0808-0.

25. Jantermtor S, Pinlaor P, Sawadpanich K, Pinlaor S, Sangka A, Wilailuckana C, et al. Subtype identification of Blastocystis spp. isolated from patients in a major hospital in northeastern Thailand. Parasitol Res. 2013;112(4):1781–6. doi:10.1007/s00436-012-3218-x.

26. Yoshikawa H, Dogruman-Al F, Turk S, Kustimur S, Balaban N, Sultan N. Evaluation of DNA extraction kits for molecular diagnosis of human Blastocystis subtypes from fecal samples. Parasitol Res. 2011;109(4):1045–50. doi:10.1007/s00436-011-2342-3.

27. Parkin DM. The global health burden of infection-associated cancers in the year 2002. Int J Cancer. 2006;118(12):3030–44. doi:10.1002/ijc.21731.

28. Chan KH, Chandramathi S, Suresh K, Chua KH, Kuppusamy UR. Effects of symptomatic and asymptomatic isolates of Blastocystis hominis on colorectal cancer cell line, HCT116. Parasitol Res. 2012;110(6):2475–80. doi:10.1007/s00436-011-2788-3.

29. Chandramathi S, Suresh K, Kuppusamy UR. Solubilized antigen of Blastocystis hominis facilitates the growth of human colorectal cancer cells, HCT116. Parasitol Res. 2010;106(4):941–5. doi:10.1007/s00436-010-1764-7.

30. Qadri SM, Al-Okaili GA, Al-Dayel F. Clinical significance of Blastocystis hominis. J Clin Microbiol. 1989;27(11):2407–9.

31. Abdulsalam AM, Ithoi I, Al-Mekhlafi HM, Ahmed A, Surin J, Mak JW. Drinking water is a significant predictor of Blastocystis infection among rural Malaysian primary schoolchildren. Parasitology. 2012;139(8):1014–20. doi:10.1017/S0031182012000340.

32. Nimri LF. Evidence of an epidemic of Blastocystis hominis infections in preschool children in northern Jordan. J Clin Microbiol. 1993;31(10):2706–8.

33. El Masry NA, Bassily S, Farid Z, Aziz AG. Potential clinical significance of Blastocystis hominis in Egypt. Trans R Soc Trop Med Hyg. 1990;84(5):695.

34. Requena I, Hernandez Y, Ramsay M, Salazar C, Devera R. Prevalence of Blastocystis hominis among food handlers from Caroni municipality, Bolivar State, Venezuela. Cad Saude Publica. 2003;19(6):1721–7.

35. Minvielle MC, Pezzani BC, Cordoba MA, De Luca MM, Apezteguia MC, Basualdo JA. Epidemiological survey of Giardia spp. and Blastocystis hominis in an Argentinian rural community. Korean J Parasitol. 2004;42(3):121–7.

36. Al-Braiken FA. Is intestinal parasitic infection still a public health concern among Saudi children? Saudi Med J. 2008;29(11):1630–5.

37. Hawash YA, Dorgham L, el AM A, Sharaf OF. Prevalence of Intestinal Protozoa among Saudi Patients with Chronic Renal Failure: A Case-Control Study. J Trop Med. 2015;2015:563478. doi:10.1155/2015/563478.

38. Koltas S, Ozcan K, Tannverdi S, Paydas S, Baslamish F. The prevalence of Blastocystis hominis in immunosuppressed patients. Ann Med Sci. 1999;8:117–9.

39. Taşova Y, Sahin B, Koltaş S, Paydaş S. Clinical significance and frequency of Blastocystis hominis in Turkish patients with hematological malignancy. Acta Med Okayama. 2000;54:133–6.

40. Katsarou-Katsari A, Vassalos CM, Tzanetou K, Spanakos G, Papadopoulou C, Vakalis N. Acute urticaria associated with amoeboid forms of Blastocystis sp. subtype 3. Acta Derm Venereol. 2008;88(1):80–1. doi:10.2340/00015555-0338.

41. Al-Jasser FS, Kabbash IA, Almazroa MA, Memish ZA. Patterns of diseases and preventive measures among domestic hajjis from Central, Saudi Arabia. Saudi Med J. 2012;33(8):879–86.

42. Shujaa A, Alhamid S. Health response to Hajj mass gathering from emergency perspective, narrative review. Turk J Emerg Med. 2015;15(4):172–6. doi:10.1016/j.tjem.2015.02.001.

43. Hussein EM, Hussein AM, Eida MM, Atwa MM. Pathophysiological variability of different genotypes of human Blastocystis hominis Egyptian isolates in experimentally infected rats. Parasitol Res. 2008;102(5):853–60. doi:10.1007/s00436-007-0833-z.

44. Ozyurt M, Kurt O, Mølbak K, Nielsen HV, Haznedaroglu T, Stensvold CR. Molecular epidemiology of Blastocystis infections in Turkey. Parasitol Int. 2008;57:300–6.

45. Jones MS, Whipps CM, Ganac RD, Hudson NR, Boorom K. Association of Blastocystis subtype 3 and 1 with patients from an Oregon community presenting with chronic gastrointestinal illness. Parasitol Res. 2009;104(2):341–5. doi:10.1007/s00436-008-1198-7.

46. Moosavi A, Haghighi A, Mojarad EN, Zayeri F, Alebouyeh M, Khazan H, et al. Genetic variability of Blastocystis sp. isolated from symptomatic and asymptomatic individuals in Iran. Parasitol Res. 2012;111(6):2311–5. doi:10.1007/s00436-012-3085-5.

47. Leelayoova S, Siripattanapipong S, Thathaisong U, Naaglor T, Taamasri P, Piyaraj P, et al. Drinking water: a possible source of Blastocystis spp. subtype 1 infection in schoolchildren of a rural community in central Thailand. Am J Trop Med Hyg. 2008;79(3):401–6.

48. Noel C, Peyronnet C, Gerbod D, Edgcomb VP, Delgado-Viscogliosi P, Sogin ML, et al. Phylogenetic analysis of Blastocystis isolates from different hosts based on the comparison of small-subunit rRNA gene sequences. Mol Biochem Parasitol. 2003;126(1):119–23.

49. Parkar U, Traub RJ, Kumar S, Mungthin M, Vitali S, Leelayoova S, et al. Direct characterization of Blastocystis from faeces by PCR and evidence of zoonotic potential. Parasitology. 2007;134(Pt 3):359–67. doi:10.1017/S0031182006001582.

50. Yoshikawa H, Abe N, Wu Z. PCR-based identification of zoonotic isolates of Blastocystis from mammals and birds. Microbiol. 2004;150:1147–51.

51. Thathaisong U, Worapong J, Mungthin M, Tan-Ariya P, Viputtigul K, Sudatis A, et al. Blastocystis isolates from a pig and a horse are closely related to Blastocystis hominis. J Clin Microbiol. 2003;41(3):967–75.

52. Rajah Salim H, Suresh Kumar G, Vellayan S, Mak JW, Khairul Anuar A, Init I, et al. Blastocystis in animal handlers. Parasitol Res. 1999;85(12):1032–3.

4

Mouse mammary tumour virus (MMTV) and human breast cancer with neuroendocrine differentiation

Lawson JS[1][*], Ngan CC[1], Glenn WK[1] and Tran DD[1,2]

Abstract

Background: Mouse mammary tumour viruses (MMTVs) may have a role in a subset of human breast cancers. MMTV positive human breast cancers have similar histological characteristics to neuroendocrine breast cancers and to MMTV positive mouse mammary tumours. The purpose of this study was to investigate the expression of neuroendocrine biomarkers – synaptophysin and chromogranin, to determine if these histological characteristics and biomarker expression were due to the influences of MMTV.

Methods: Immunohistochemistry analyses to identify synaptophysin and chromogranin were conducted on a series of human breast cancers in which (i) MMTV had been previously identified and had similar histological characteristics to MMTV positive mouse mammary tumours and (ii) MMTV positive mouse mammary tumours.

Results: The expression of synaptophysin and chromogranin in MMTV positive mouse mammary tumors were all positive (7 of 7 specimens – 100% positive). The expression of synaptophysin and chromogranin in MMTV positive human breast cancers was much less prevalent (3 of 22 – 14%). There was no expression of synaptophysin and chromogranin in the normal breast tissue control specimens.

Discussion: It is not possible to draw any firm conclusions from these observations. However, despite the small numbers of MMTV positive mouse mammary tumours in this study, the universal expression in these specimens of synaptophysin and chromogranin proteins is striking. This pattern of synaptophysin and chromogranin expression is very different from their expression in MMTV positive human breast cancers. The reason for these differences is not known.

Conclusions: The high prevalence of positive expression of synaptophysin and chromogranin in MMTV positive mouse mammary tumours and low expression of synaptophysin and chromogranin in MMTV positive human breast cancers indicates that MMTV is not usually associated with neuroendocrine human breast cancers.

Keywords: Breast cancer, Mouse mammary tumours, Mouse mammary tumour virus, Neuroendocrine breast cancer, Synaptophysin, Chromogranin

Background

There is substantial, but not conclusive, evidence that MMTVs may have a role in a subset of human breast cancers. This evidence is as follows: (i) identification of MMTV–like gene sequences in breast cancer tissues is associated with a 15 fold increase in breast cancer [1], (ii) MMTV-like *env* gene sequences have been identified in 38% of US and Australian human breast tumours but rarely in normal breast tissue controls [2, 3], (iii) MMTV sequences identified in human breast tissues are 95 to 98% homologous with MMTV in mouse mammary tumours [4, 5], (iv) MMTV viral proteins have been identified in human breast cancer [6, 7], (v) Wnt-1 oncogene expression is significantly higher in MMTV-like positive compared to MMTV-like negative breast cancer specimens, which parallels high Wnt-1 expression in MMTV positive mouse mammary tumours [8], (vi) MMTV can infect human cells and randomly integrate its genomic

* Correspondence: james.lawson@unsw.edu.au
[1]School of Biotechnology and Biomolecular Sciences, University of New South Wales, Sydney, Australia
Full list of author information is available at the end of the article

information [9–11], (vii) there is increased prevalence of MMTV-like viral sequences in healthy breast tissues (nil), healthy tissue adjacent to breast cancer (19%), breast hyperplasia (27%), ductal carcinoma in situ (82%) [12], (viii) MMTV–like sequences have been identified in milk from healthy lactating women and three fold increased positivity in milk from women at high risk for breast cancer [13, 14], (ix) MMTV-like sequences have been identified in the saliva of 27% of healthy children, 11% of healthy adults and 57% of adults with breast cancer, which is suggestive of a human to human viral transmission [15], (xi) MMTV-like viral sequences have been identified in breast cancers which developed in a father, mother and daughter of the same family which is suggestive of an infectious condition [16] and MMTV sequences have been identified in benign human breast tissues before the development of MMTV associated breast cancer in the same women [17]. Overall this evidence is consistent with MMTV having similar influences in both human breast cancer and mouse mammary tumours.

We have previously observed that the histological characteristics of MMTV positive human breast cancers are similar to MMTV associated mouse mammary tumours [18]. Many of these MMTV positive human breast cancers also have similar histology to neuroendocrine human breast cancers. Neuroendocrine breast cancer is diagnosed by both histological characteristics and the expression of either synaptophysin or chromogranin proteins [19]. Initially, the World Health Organisation(WHO) classified breast cancers with neuroendocrine features as those breast tumours with over 50% of positive synaptophysin or chromogranin cancer cells. This has since been modified to include breast cancers with any number of synaptophysin or chromogranin positive cancer cells. The WHO classsification now refers to such breast tumours as invasive breast carcinomas with neuroendocrine differentiation [20]. Synaptophysin and chromogranin are proteins secreted by endocrine (hormone producing) cells located in many organs of the body in response to a 'neural' (brain or nervous system) stimulus. While synaptophysin and chromogranin proteins may be secreted by both normal and cancer endocrine cells, their expression is usually higher in malignant cells. This phenomena can be used for diagnostic purposes [21].

In a preliminary investigation we observed that synaptophysin or chromogranin were highly expressed in MMTV associated mouse mammary tumours. As synaptophysin and chromogranin proteins are expressed in human breast cancers which have similar histological characteristics to MMTV positive mouse mammary tumours, we hypothesised that MMTV may be the underlying causal factor.

To explore this hypothesis we investigated by immunohistochemistry, the expression of synaptophysin and chromogranin in a series of MMTV positive human breast cancers and MMTV positive mouse mammary tumours.

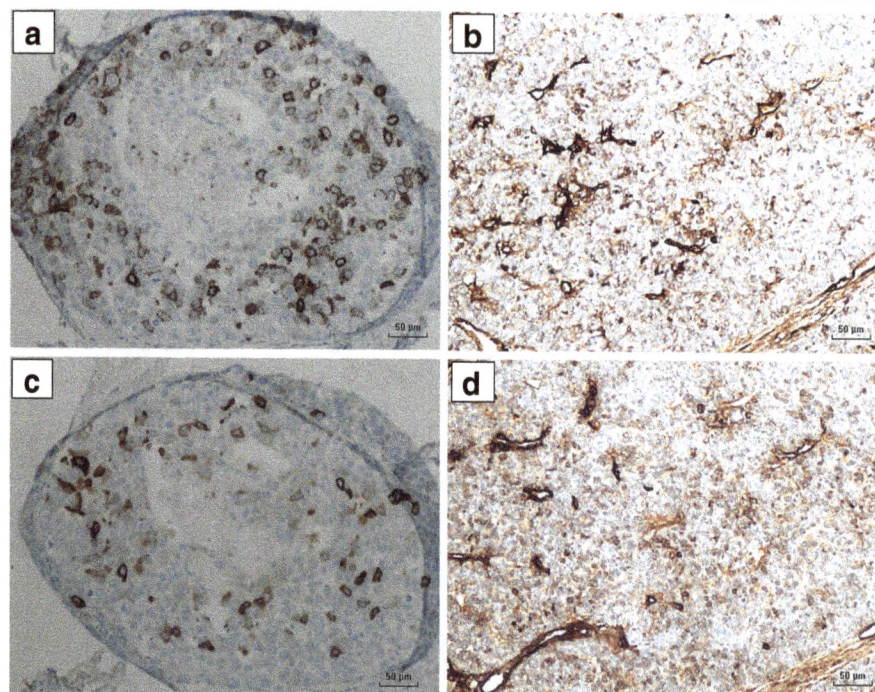

Fig. 1 Synaptophysin & Chromogranin protein expression in MMTV positive human breast cancer & MMTV positive mouse mammary tumour. **a**. Human synaptophysin expression. **b**. Mouse synaptophysin expression. **c**. Human chromogranin expression. **d**. Mouse chromogranin expression

Table 1 Synaptophysin and chromogranin protein expression in MMTV positive mouse mammary tumors, MMTV positive human breast cancers and normal human breast controls

Specimens	MMTV	Synaptophysin	Chromogranin
Mouse mammary tumour	7/7 (100%)	7/7 (100%)	7/7 (100%)
Human breast cancer (selected for MMTV positivity)	22/22 (100%)	2/22 (9%)	2/22 (9%)
Normal human breast controls	0/39 (0%)	0/39 (0%)	0/39 (0%)

We have not been able to identify any prior investigations into the expression of synaptophysin and chromogranin in MMTV positive human breast cancers or MMTV positive mouse mammary tumours.

Here we show that the expression of synaptophysin and chromogranin in MMTV positive breast cancers is not usually associated with human neuroendocrine breast cancers.

Methods
Ethics
This project was approved by the Human Research Ethics Committee of the University of New South Wales, Sydney, Australia (HC11421).

Human breast specimens
Twenty breast cancer archival formalin fixed breast cancer specimens were selected because in previous studies MMTV envelope gene sequences had been identified in these specimens [3]. The MMTV sequences had been identified by PCR techniques following the methods of Wang et al. [2]. In addition each of these breast cancer specimens were selected because their histological

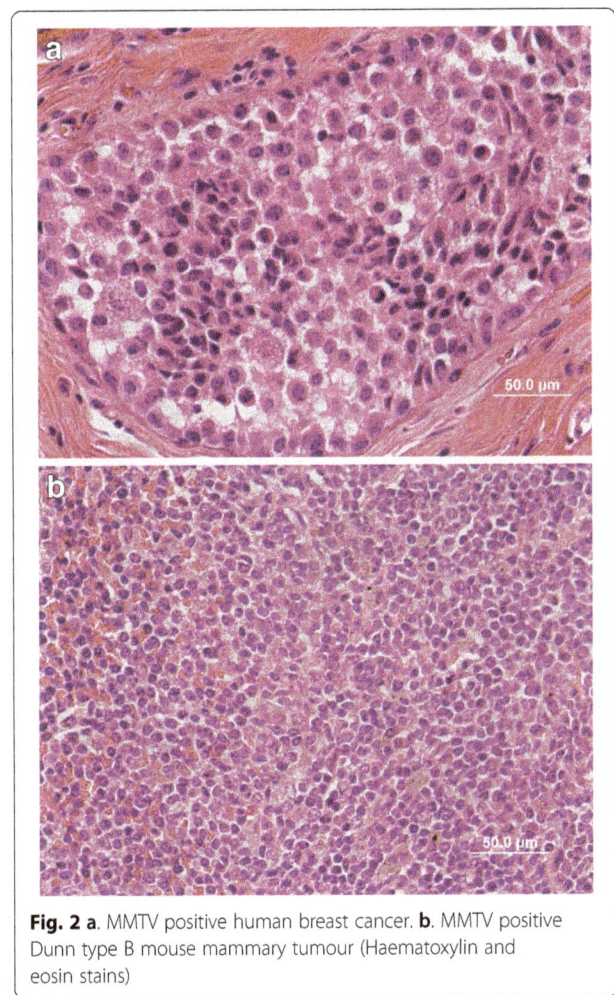

Fig. 2 a. MMTV positive human breast cancer. **b**. MMTV positive Dunn type B mouse mammary tumour (Haematoxylin and eosin stains)

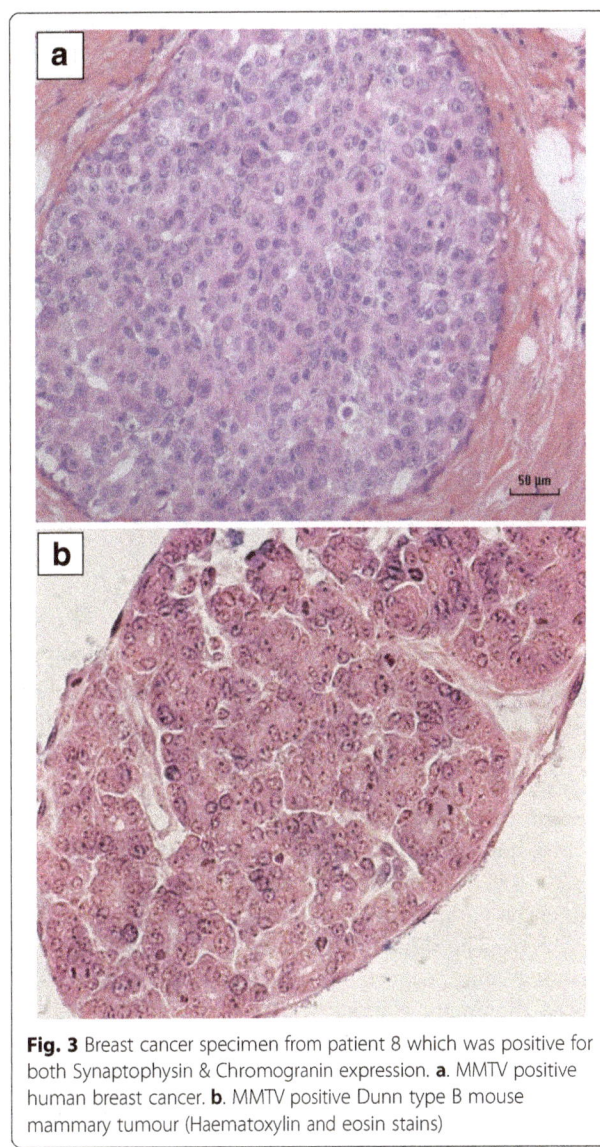

Fig. 3 Breast cancer specimen from patient 8 which was positive for both Synaptophysin & Chromogranin expression. **a**. MMTV positive human breast cancer. **b**. MMTV positive Dunn type B mouse mammary tumour (Haematoxylin and eosin stains)

characteristics were similar to MMTV positive mouse mammary tumours.

Thirty eight normal breast specimens from breast reduction surgery were used as controls. The donors of these specimens were on average younger than the breast cancer patients and therefore should be considered as a comparison group and not age matched controls.

Mouse mammary tumour specimens
Seven mouse mammary tumours in which MMTV envelope gene sequences had previously been identified were used for comparative purposes [22].

Immunohistochemistry
The automated Tissue-Tek Prisma system were used for haematoxylin and eosin staining and Ventana Bench-Mark Ultra were used for the identification of synaptophysin and Chromogranin A proteins. Synaptophysin (Novocastra catalogue number NCL-L-SYNAP-299) and chromogranin A (Dako catalogue number M0869) antibodies were used on formalin fixed paraffin embedded specimens. Both synaptophysin and chromogranin A proteins stain the cell membranes and cytoplasm of the target cells. Pancreatic tissues were used as positive controls for each specimen. Omission of the antibodies was used as negative controls.

Statistics
The non-parametric Kolmogorov-Smirnov test was used to test the significance between the human breast cancer and mouse mammary tumour synaptophysin and chromogranin positivity.

Results
Synaptophysin and chromogranin expression
The outcomes are presented in Table 1 and Additional file 1: Table S1, Additional file 2: Table S2 and Additional file 3: Table S3. The expression of synaptophysin and chromogranin in MMTV positive mouse mammary tumours were all positive (7 of 7 specimens – 100% positive). The expression of synaptophysin and chromogranin in MMTV positive human breast cancers was much less prevalent (3 of 22 – 14%). There was no expression of synaptophysin and chromogranin in the normal breast tissue control specimens. The different positivity for synaptophysin and chromogranin between the human breast cancer and mouse mammary tumour was p = 0.001 and 0.001 respectively, that is highly significant.

The expression of synaptophysin and chromogranin in MMTV positive mouse mammary tumours and MMTV positive human breast cancers are shown in Fig. 1.

Histology
The similar histological characteristics of MMTV positive and neuroendocrine marker positive human breast cancers and MMTV neuroendocrine positive mouse mammary tumours are shown in Fig. 2. Mouse mammary tumour cells are smaller in diameter than human breast cancer cells but have very similar characteristics. However it must be emphasised that the histological characteristics of MMTV positive and synaptophysin and chromogranin *negative* human breast cancers are also similar to MMTV positive mouse mammary tumours. The synaptophysin and chromogranin positive MMTV positive human breast cancers are characterised by intensely stained nuclei which occupy most of the cell, the cells are mostly round and regular in size and are clumped together without glandular acini or lumen. MMTV negative human breast cancers are not similar to MMTV positive mouse mammary tumours.

One human breast cancer specimen was positive for both Synaptophysin and Chromogranin. As shown in Fig. 3 the histological characteristics of this specimen were similar to MMTV positive mouse mammary tumours.

Discussion
We have demonstrated that (i) MMTV positive mouse mammary tumours are all synaptophysin and chromogranin positive (7 of 7 specimens – 100% positive), (ii) in MMTV positive human breast cancers only 3 of 22 (14%) are synaptophysin or chromogranin positive, (iii) there was no expression of synaptophysin and chromogranin in the comparative normal breast specimens and (iv) MMTV positive (and either synaptophysin and chromogranin positive or negative) human breast cancers have similar histological characteristics to neuroendocrine human breast cancers and to MMTV positive mouse mammary tumours.

The expression of synaptophysin and chromogranin proteins in MMTV positive human breast cancers was much less prevalent than in MMTV positive mouse mammary tumours.

These are confusing observations and it is not possible to draw any firm conclusions. However, despite the small numbers of mouse mammary tumours in this study, the universal expression in these specimens of synaptophysin and chromogranin proteins is striking. This pattern of synaptophysin and chromogranin expression is very different from the MMTV human breast cancers. The reason is not known.

The expression or secretion of synaptophysin and chromogranin proteins by endocrine (hormone) producing cells is presumably in response to a neurological or other external stimulus. However, the substantial differences in the expression of synaptophysin and chromogranin in MMTV positive human breast cancer and MMTV positive mouse mammary tumours indicate that MMTV is not usually associated with neuroendocrine human breast cancers.

It has been suggested by Wiedenmann et al. [21] and later by Maeda et al. [23] that the identification of synaptophysin may be useful for the diagnosis of breast cancers. The findings in this current study do not support that suggestion.

Conclusions

The high prevalence of positive expression of synaptophysin and chromogranin in MMTV positive mouse mammary tumours and low expression of synaptophysin and chromogranin in MMTV positive human breast cancers indicates that MMTV is not usually associated with neuroendocrine human breast cancers.

Abbreviation
MMTV: Mouse mammary tumor virus

Acknowledgements
Specimens were provided by Douglass Hanly Moir Pathology. Technical assistance was provided by Benafsha Josufi.

Funding
There was no external funding for this project.

Authors' contributions
JL- initial concepts, identification and collection of specimens, histological assessments, data analyses, preparation of the manuscript. CN – laboratory analyses, preparation of the manuscript. WK - laboratory analyses, preparation of the manuscript. DT- laboratory analyses, preparation of the manuscript. All authors read and approved of the final manuscript.

Competing interests
No author has any competing financial or other competing interests.

Author details
[1]School of Biotechnology and Biomolecular Sciences, University of New South Wales, Sydney, Australia. [2]Douglass Hanly Moir Pathology, Sydney, Australia.

References
1. Wang F, Hou J, Shen Q, Yue Y, Xie F, Wang X, et al. Mouse mammary tumor virus-like virus infection and the risk of human breast cancer: a meta-analysis. Am J Transl Res. 2014;6:248–66.
2. Wang Y, Holland JF, Bleiweiss IJ, Melana S, Liu X, Pelisson I, et al. Detection of mammary tumor virus env gene-like sequences in human breast cancer. Cancer Res. 1995;55:5173–9.
3. Ford CE, Tran D, Deng Y, Ta VT, Rawlinson WD, Lawson JS. Mouse mammary tumor virus-like gene sequences in breast tumors of Australian and Vietnamese women. Clin Cancer Res. 2003;9(3):1118–20.
4. Liu B, Wang Y, Melana SM, Pelisson I, Najfeld V, Holland JF, et al. Identification of a proviral structure in human breast cancer. Cancer Res. 2001;61:1754–9.
5. Melana SM, Holland JF, Pogo BG. Search for mouse mammary tumor virus-like env sequences in cancer and normal breast from the same individuals. Clin Cancer Res. 2001;7:283–4.
6. Bar-Sinai A, Bassa N, Fischette M, Gottesman MM, Love DC, Hanover JA, Hochman J. Mouse mammary tumor virus Env-derived peptide associates with nucleolar targets in lymphoma, mammary carcinoma, and human breast cancer. Cancer Res. 2005;65:7223–30.
7. Melana SM, Nepomnaschy I, Hasa J, Djougarian A, Djougarian A, Holland JF, et al. Detection of human mammary tumor virus proteins in human breast cancer cells. J Virol Methods. 2010;163:157–61.
8. Lawson JS, Glenn WK, Salmons B, Ye Y, Heng B, Moody P, et al. Mouse mammary tumor virus-like sequences in human breast cancer. Cancer Res. 2010;70:3576–85.
9. Indik S, Günzburg WH, Salmons B, Rouault F. Mouse mammary tumor virus infects human cells. Cancer Res. 2005;65:6651–9.
10. Faschinger A, Rouault F, Sollner J, Lukas A, Salmons B, Günzburg WH, et al. Mouse mammary tumor virus integration site selection in human and mouse genomes. J Virol. 2008;82:13.
11. Konstantoulas C, Indik S. C₃H strain of mouse mammary tumor viruses like GR strain infects human mammary epithelial cells albeit less efficiently than murine mammary epithelial cells. J Gen Virol. 2015;96:650–62.
12. Mazzanti CM, Al Hamad M, Fanelli G, Scatena C, Zammarchi F, Zavaglia K, et al. A mouse mammary tumor virus env-like exogenous sequence is strictly related to progression of human sporadic breast carcinoma. Am J Pathol. 2011;179:2083–90.
13. Johal H, Ford CE, Glenn WK, Heads J, Lawson JS, Rawlinson WD. Mouse mammary tumor like virus (MMTV) sequences in breast milk from healthy lactating women. Breast Cancer Res Treat. 2011;129:149–55.
14. Nartey T, Moran H, Marin T, Arcaro KF, Anderton DL, Etkind P, et al. Human Mammary Tumor Virus (HMTV) sequences in human milk. Infect Agent Cancer. 2014;9:20.
15. Mazzanti CM, Lessi F, Armogida I, Zavaglia K, Franceschi S, Al Hamad M, et al. Human saliva as route of inter-human infection for mouse mammary tumor virus. Oncotarget. 2015;6:18355–63.
16. Etkind PR, Stewart AF, Wiernik PH. Mouse mammary tumor virus (MMTV)-like DNA sequences in the breast tumors of father, mother, and daughter. Infect Agent Cancer. 2008;3:2.
17. Nartey T, Mazzanti CM, Melana S, Glenn WK, Bevilacqua G, Holland JF, et al. Mouse mammary tumor-like virus (MMTV) is present in human breast tissue before development of virally associated breast cancer. Infect Agent Cancer. 2017;12:1.
18. Lawson JS, Tran DD, Carpenter E, Ford CE, Rawlinson WD, Whitaker NJ, Delprado W. Presence of mouse mammary tumour-like virus gene sequences may be associated with morphology of specific human breast cancer. J Clin Pathol. 2006;59:1287–92.
19. Adegbola T, Connolly CE, Mortimer G. Small cell neuroendocrine carcinoma of the breast: a report of three cases and review of the literature. J Clin Pathol. 2005;58:775–8.
20. Bussolati G, Badve S. Carcinomas with neuroendocrine features. In: Lakhani et al., editors. WHO Classification of tumours of the breast. Lyon, France: IARC Press; 2012.

21. Wiedenmann B, Huttner WB. Synaptophysin and chromogranins/
    secretogranins–widespread constituents of distinct types of neuroendocrine
    vesicles and new tools in tumor diagnosis. Virchows Arch B Cell Pathol Incl
    Mol Pathol. 1989;58:95–121.

22. Glenn WK, Lawson JS, Whitaker NJ. Mouse mammary tumour-like virus
    gene sequences and specific breast cancer morphology. J Clin Pathol.
    2007;60:1071.

23. Maeda I, Tajima S, Ariizumi Y, Doi M, Endo A, Naruki S, Hoshikawa M,
    Koizumi H, Kanemaki Y, Ueno T, Tsugawa K, Takagi M. Can synaptophysin
    be used as a marker of breast cancer diagnosed by core-needle biopsy in
    epithelial proliferative diseases of the breast? Pathol Int. 2016;66:369–75.

5

Prevalence and risk factors associated with sexually transmitted infections (STIs) among women of reproductive age in Swaziland

Themba G. Ginindza[1*], Cristina D. Stefan[2], Joyce M. Tsoka-Gwegweni[1], Xolisile Dlamini[3], Pauline E. Jolly[4], Elisabete Weiderpass[5,6,7,8], Nathalie Broutet[9] and Benn Sartorius[1]

Abstract

Background: Sexually transmitted infections (STIs) remain an important public health problem with approximately half a billion new cases annually among persons aged 15–49 years. Epidemiological data on STIs among women of reproductive age in Swaziland are limited. The availability of epidemiological data on STIs and associated risk factors in this population is essential for the development of successful prevention, diagnosis and management strategies in the country. The study aimed to determine the prevalence and risk factors associated with STIs.

Methods: A total of 655 women aged 15–49 years were systematically enrolled from five health facilities using a cross-sectional study design. Cervical specimen were tested using GeneXpert CT/NG Assays for *Chlamydia trachomatis (CT)* and *Neisseria gonorrhoeae (NG)*, GeneXpertTV Assay for *Trichomonas vaginalis (TV)*, and GeneXpert HPV Assays for hr-HPV. Blood samples were tested using Alere Determine HIV-1/2Ag/Ab Combo and Trinity Biotech Uni-Gold Recombigen HIV test for confirmation for HIV, and Rapid Plasma Reagin and TPHA test for confirmation for *Treponema pallidum* (syphilis). Genital warts were assessed prior to specimen collection. Survey weighted analyses were done to estimate the population burden of STIs.

Results: The four most common curable STIs: CT, NG, TV, *Treponema pallidum* (syphilis), as well as genital warts were considered in this study. The overall weighted prevalence of any of these five STIs was 19.4% (95% CI: 14.9–24.8), corresponding to 72 990 women with STIs in Swaziland. The estimated prevalences were 7.0% (95% CI: 4.1–11.2) for CT, 6. 0% (95% CI: 3.8–8.8) for NG, 8.4% (95% CI: 5.4–12.8) for TV, 1.4% (95% CI: 1.1–10.2) for syphilis and 2.0% (95% CI: 1.0–11.4) for genital warts. The overall weighted HIV prevalence was 42.7% (95%CI: 35.7–46.2). Among hr-HPV positive women, 18. 8% (95% CI: 13.1–26.3) had one STI, while 6.3% (95% CI: 3.3–11.7) had multiple STIs. Risk factors associated with STIs were being employed (OR = 2.2, 95% CI: 1.0–4.7), self-employed (OR = 2.8, 95% CI: 1.5–5.5) and being hr-HPV positive (OR = 2.0, 95% CI: 1.3–3.1). Age (0.9, 95% CI: 0.8–0.9), being married (OR = 0.4, 95% CI: 0.3–0.7) and not using condoms with regular partners (OR = 0.5, 95% CI: 0.3–0.9) were inversely associated with STIs.

Conclusion: STIs are highly prevalent among women of reproductive age in Swaziland. Thus, a comprehensive STIs screening, surveillance and treatment programme would be justified and could potentially lower the burden of STIs in the country.

Keywords: Sexually transmitted infections, HIV, HPV, Risk factors, Mbabane, Swaziland, Epidemiology, Women, Cross sectional study, Africa

* Correspondence: Ginindza@ukzn.ac.za
[1]Discipline of Public Health, School of Nursing and Public Health, University of KwaZulu-Natal, 2nd Floor George Campbell Building, Mazisi Kunene Road, 4041 Durban, South Africa
Full list of author information is available at the end of the article

Background

Globally, sexually transmitted infections (STIs) remain a significant public health problem mainly in low-income countries [1, 2]. Currently, approximately half a billion new cases occur worldwide each year [3], and more than one million STIs are acquired per day [4]. Of the estimated total of 357 million incident cases of the curable STIs world-wide, 131 million are from *Chlamydia trachomatis* (CT), 78 million are from *Neisseria gonorrhea* (NG), 5.6 million are from syphilis and 143 million are from *Trichomonas vaginalis* (TV) cases [3, 4]. The World Health Organization (WHO) further estimated that 8.3, 21.1 and 59.7 million new cases of CT, NG and TV infections respectively, occur in sub-Saharan Africa (SSA), with the majority of new STIs occurring among the population aged 15 to 49 years [5].

Depending on which STI and the population, in low-income countries largely in SSA, NG, CT, TV, Human papillomavirus (HPV), herpes, and syphilis increase the risk of HIV acquisition and transmission between two to eight fold [4, 6–9]. Furthermore, the inflammation resulting from viral and non-viral STIs increases viral shedding of HIV-1 in the genital tract [10–12] and also increases the risk of HIV-1 transmission to the sex partners [13, 14]. It is estimated that the probability of HIV transmission per sexual contact is 6% if either partner has another STI other than HIV [15] as compared to 0.2% in the absence of STIs [16]. The impact of co-infection of HPV with HIV in the SSA has increased the burden of cervical diseases (such as cervical lesions and cancer), since HIV infected women have a higher prevalence of hr-HPV [17]. Furthermore, STIs such as NG and CT are the major causes of pelvic inflammatory disease (PID) and infertility in women [4]. In low-income countries, impairments associated with STIs are a major cause of mother and child mortality and morbidity in adolescence and also during pregnancy [18, 19].

Factors affecting the spread of STIs, including HIV, have been documented in many epidemiological studies across different populations [20–24]. STIs and HIV share the same behavioral, socioeconomic and demographic risk factors [20, 25], including age at first sexual intercourse, inconsistent condom use, having multiple sexual partners, female sex, being single and the partner's sexual behaviour, location and culture. Furthermore, HIV infection increases the of other STIs [20, 24–28].

There is limited information on the prevalence and risk factors associated with STIs at population level in Swaziland, the country which has the highest prevalence of HIV infection worldwide. The availability of epidemiological data on STIs and associated risk factors in this population is essential for the development of successful prevention, diagnosis and management strategies in the country [29]. This study was therefore, conducted to determine the prevalence and risk factors associated with STIs among women of reproductive age in Swaziland.

Methods

Study setting and population

The study participants were women aged 15–49 years attending five healthcare facilities for routine healthcare and related services such as family planning, vaccination etc., from June to July 2015. This cross-sectional study included all women of reproductive age with a history of or who are currently sexually active and who provided written informed consent. The health care facilities (Mbabane Government hospital, Realign Fitkin Memorial (RFM) hospital, Hlatsikhulu hospital, Sithobela hospital and Siteki Public Health Unit) were located within the four political regions of Swaziland as shown in Table 1. The selection of the sites was based on the criteria of having fully functioning cervical cancer screening services, such as visual inspection with acetic acid (VIA) and cryotherapy. The purpose of including all fully functioning cervical cancer screening units was to achieve the goal of the 'see and treat' approach. All health facilities were using the "see and treat" approach as at the time of the study. VIA was performed, and all those who were VIA-positive were treated with cryotherapy and followed for 12 months. However, these results are not reported in this article.

Sample size

The sample size determination was based on the main research project aim, namely of establishing the burden of HPV infection and HPV-related conditions among women of reproductive age in Swaziland, where the value of the parameter(s) were not known in Swaziland. The prevalence of STIs investigated in the study was a secondary objective. Hence, the use of 50%, which assumes maximum variability and the largest possible sample size, given the predefined precision of ±5% and 95% confidence (5% type I error). Based on this a, sample size of 384 subjects was required to be used. The sample was further increased by a margin of 10% to

Table 1 Study sites per region and number of participants per site

Regions	Study site Code	Sites	Participants per-site
Hhohho	H01	Mbabane government hospital	182
Manzini	H02	RFM hospital	196
Lubombo	H03	Siteki Public Health Unit (PHU)	69
	H04	Sithobela Hospital	69
Shiselweni	H05	Hlathikhulu Hospital	139
Total		5	655

account for potential non-response and multiplied by a design effect (D) of 1.5. The final calculated sample size of the study was 650 women. However, a total of 655 women participated to the study.

Sampling strategy

The recruitment of participants was done in two sampling stages. Firstly, women were stratified by age (seven age-groups) and then sampled in each site using systematic random sampling (every third woman of each age), using the lottery method. The participants were selected from each site until the calculated sample size was achieved per site.

Data collection

Prior to questionnaire administration, willing participants were given all the necessary information about the study, their potential contribution, and their risks and benefits before they signed the informed consent form. Furthermore, all necessary information was included in the study information sheet and informed consent documents. A structured standardized questionnaire was administered by trained nurses to obtain detailed data on socio-demographic characteristics, and sexual, reproductive and gynaecologic histories. Thereafter, the nurse midwife inspected the perineal, vulvar, vaginal and cervical regions of each woman for evidence of genital warts, ulcers, discharge, inflammation or tenderness, and recorded all abnormalities according to the study protocol. Lastly, the specimen collection for each of the tests was performed (see details below). All participants found to be exhibiting genital warts were treated with the WHO-recommended 0.5% podophyllin tincture. Additionally, all participants presenting with STIs on syndromic diagnosis or/and who tested positive for STIs, were treatment as per WHO STIs management guidelines [4], which have been adopted by the Ministry of Health. Thereafter, the participants were invited to return in 1 week for review purposes as recommended by the guidelines. Participants were also requested to communicate with their sexual partners their need to visit the clinic or seek treatment, using the provided tracing slip with a suspected STI code of treatment.

Data were entered using EpiData 3.02 for Windows (The Epi Data Association Odense, Denmark). Each participant was assigned a unique study identity number that was used to link the questionnaire and the biological specimens. Personal information was blinded from the researcher and was kept on site for feedback of the results to the women, and validation of data.

Biological specimen collection and testing

After visual inspection of the vulva, a non-lubricated sterile disposable speculum was inserted and cervical cells were collected using the Xpert CT/NG/TV Endocervical swab (CT/NG/TV SWAB-50) (Cepheid, Sunnyvale, CA, 2014). After HIV pre-counselling, two 4 mL samples of blood (for HIV and syphilis testing) were collected in a vacutainer tube from participants consenting to HIV testing. All specimens were collected and transported daily to the National Referral Laboratory (NRL).

Specimen testing

All specimens testing were tested at the NRL, Mbabane, Swaziland. Since this work is part of the HPV/Cervical cancer study, only overall weighted HPV and HIV prevalence results are presented in this paper, for a purpose of assessing the association between the curable STIs and HPV and HIV.

CT/NG and TV testing

Cepheid Xpert CT/NG assay was used to detect *Chlamydia trachomatis* (CT) and *Neisseria gonorrhea* (NG) infection, and the Cepheid Xpert TV Assay was used to detect *Trichomonas vaginalis* (TV) (Cepheid, Sunnyvale, CA, 2014) [30, 31]. All tests were performed according to the manufacturers' instructions. These are real-time polymerase chain reaction (PCR)-based assays for the simultaneous detection of CT/NG and TV from endocervical specimens.

Treponema pallidum (syphilis)

Treponema pallidum (Syphilis) testing was routinely conducted on all participants who consented to HIV testing using a commercially available standard Rapid Plasma Reagin (RPR) test (Atlas Medical, Cambridge, UK) [32], following the manufacturer's instructions. All reactive specimens were confirmed by *Treponema pallidum* Hemagglutination Assay (TPHA) (Omega Diagnostic, Scotland, UK) [33].

HPV testing

The HPV-DNA testing was done using the GeneXpert HPV assay (Xpert HPV Assay) (Cepheid, Sunnyvale, CA, 2014) [34] according to the manufacture's protocol. The Xpert HPV test gives results from six separate channels: (i) sample adequacy control (SAC), (ii) P1-HPV16, (iii) P2-HPV18/45, (iv) P3-HPV 31/33/35/52/58, (v) P4-HPV51/59 and (vi) P5-HPV39/68/56/66. An individual specimen can be positive for more than one probe.

HIV testing

The Alere Determine HIV-1/2 Ag/Ab Combo test was used to detect both HIV-1/2 antibodies and free HIV-1 p24 antigen [35]. Reactive specimens were confirmed by Trinity Biotech Uni-Gold Recombigen HIV Test [36]. All participants who tested HIV positive were post-counselled and referred to health units offering the necessary HIV treatment, care and support services.

Data and statistical analysis

Data were processed and analysed using Stata 13.0SE (Stata corp. College station, Texas, USA). Data were checked for possible errors and missing values prior to analysis. Age and region-weighted analyses were done to estimate the overall STIs' prevalence and coinfection with HIV and hr-HPV.

Survey weighted analysis was done to adjust the sample characteristic to match the target population (15–49) that they were selected to represent. It is applied to bring the proportion of women in the sample in alignment with the portion of women in the target population. Therefore, all results are reported as weighted. Survey weighted prevalence and 95% confidence intervals (CI) were calculated. In addition, assuming that our study subjects were representative of the female population of the same age strata, we used survey weights to extrapolate sample proportions to population totals (age-region weighted) to estimate burden counts, based on the 2007–2030 population projections aligned to the estimated 2014 population of 377 169 women aged 15–49 years [37]. Differences in prevalence by categorical variables such as site, age, HIV and hr-HPV were assessed using the survey weighted chi-square (χ^2) test. Odds ratios (unadjusted and adjusted) and 95% CIs for potential risk factors associated with STIs were estimated using survey weighted logistic regression models. Variables that were significant at a cut-off of 0.2 in the bivariate regression analyses were selected for inclusion into the final multivariable model. An adjusted p-value of <0.05 was deemed statistically significant.

Results

Characteristics of the study population

A total of 655 women were enrolled in the study within the period of June - July 2015. All the participants had sufficient specimens for the four non-viral STIs testing and only 11 had sufficient specimen for hr-HPV. Table 2 summarizes the key characteristics of the study population. The mean ages (± standard deviation [SD]) for enrolled women was 32.2 (±8.7) years. Their mean age at menarche was 14.4 (±1.7) years, at first intercourse was 17.9 (±2.9) years, and at first pregnancy was 19.4 (±3.9) years. Of the 655 participants, 571 (88.7%) had been pregnant previously, 542 (84.2%) had a history of contraceptive use, 272 (42.6%) had a history of STIs, 116 (18.0%) had STIs that had been treated in the past 12 months, 345 (53.6%) were married or cohabiting, 227 (35.3%) had not completed secondary/high school education, 340 (53.0%) were unemployed and 513 (79.7%) reported one lifetime sexual partner.

Prevalence of STIs

Table 3 shows the weighted prevalence of selected STIs in the samples of women aged 15–49 years. The overall STIs' weighted prevalence (excluding HIV and HPV) was 19.4%, (95% CI: 14.9–24.8) and individual prevalence for *Trichomonas vaginalis* (TV), *Neisseria gonorrhoeae* (NG), *Chlamydia trachomatis* (CT), *Treponema pallidum* (syphilis) and genital warts (GW) was 8.46.0, 7.0, 1.4 and 2.0%, respectively. The overall weighted hr-HPV prevalence and HIV prevalence was 46.2% (95% CI: 42.8–49.5), and 42.7% (95% CI: 35.7–46.2) respectively, (Table 3) (detailed data shown in a previously published article [38]). About 4.0% (95% CI: 2.3–6.0) had two or more STIs (multiple infections) and 6.0% (95% CI: 4.3–8.5) had triple infection (at least one STI, HIV and hr-HPV infection) (Table 3). Among women with hr-HPV, 18.9% (95% CI: 13.1–26.3) had a single STI and 6.3% (95% CI: 3.3–11.7) had multiple STIs. Among HIV positive women, 17.7% (95% CI: 11.5–26.9) had one STI, while 4.2% (95% CI: 1.5–11.3) had multiple STIs (Table 4). About 6.3% (95% CI: 4.4–8.9) women had STIs, HPV and HIV combined coinfections.

Population burden estimates

Tables 3 and 4 show the population burden estimates. Population burden estimates to extrapolate absolute burden counts of the different STIs were made based on the 2007–2030 population projections aligned to the 2014 population estimates of women aged 15–49 years. The overall population burden was estimated at 72 990 (95% CI: 51 111–94 871) as depicted on Table 3. When stratified by each STI, 30 132 (95% CI: 16 633–43 631) were estimated to have TV, 22 055 (95% CI: 11 986–32 124) have NG, 25 024 (95% CI: 11 251–38 797) have CT, 5 072 (95% CI: 1 822–8 322) have *Treponema pallidum* (syphilis), and 6111 (95% CI: 470–12692) have GW. Multiple STIs estimates were 13995 (95% CI: 7 092–20 898) and triple STIs were 23 310 (95% CI: 14 193–32 427). Among HIV positive women, the population burden counts for single STIs were 32 158 (95% CI: 20 200–44 115) and for multiple infection 10 798 (95% CI: 4 032–17 564). Among hr-HPV positive women the population burden counts for single and multiple infection were 27 163 (95% CI: 14 941–39 386) and 6 367 (95% CI: 159–12 893), respectively) (Table 4).

Prevalence of STIs by selected socio-demographic characteristics of the women

Table 5 shows the prevalence of STIs by selected socio-demographic characteristics of the women, and the risk factors associated with STIs (univariable and multivariable logistic regressions). The prevalence of STIs decreased with increasing age, with the highest burden among the 15–19 and 24–29 age groups (29.2 and 27.0%

Table 2 Socio-demographic characteristics of the study population (N = 655)

Demographics	n (%)
Age: n (%)	
Mean ± SD (range)	32 .2 ± 8.7
15–19	39 (6.1)
20–24	111 (17.2)
25–29	131 (20.3)
30–34	116 (18.0)
35–39	103 (16.0)
40–44	80 (12.4)
45–49	75 (11.6)
Marital status: n (%)	
Single	266 (41.3)
Cohabiting	38 (5.9)
Married	307 (47.7)
Divorced/separated	22 (3.4)
Widow	11 (1.7)
Education: n (%)	
Never been to school	24 (3.7)
Primary	130 (20.2)
Secondary/High	373 (57.9)
Tertiary	117 (18.2)
Occupation: n (%)	
Unemployed	340 (53.0)
Employed	255 (39.8)
Self-employed	46 (7.2)
Ever pregnant : n (%)	
Yes	571 (88.7)
No	64 (9.9)
Missing	9 (1.4)
Age at first pregnancy: Mean age (SD)	19.4 (3.9)
No. pregnancies: n (%)	
0	6 (1.0)
1	139 (24.3)
2	127 (22.2)
3+	297 (46.1)
Age Menarche: Mean (SD)	14.39 (1.7)
Age at first intercourse: Mean age (SD)	17.90 (2.9)
Number of Sexual life partner: n (%)	
0	33 (5.1)
1	513 (79.7)
2	61 (9.5)
3+	43 (6.7)
Currently using contraceptives: n (%)	
Yes	542 (84.2)

Table 2 Socio-demographic characteristics of the study population (N = 655) (Continued)

No	95 (14.8)
Missing	7 (1.1)
Ever had STI: n (%)	
Yes	272 (42.6)
No	337 (52.7)
Don't remember	30 (4.7)
STIs treated in the past 12 months: n (%)	
Yes	116 (18.0)
No	520 (80.9)
Don't know	7 (1.1)

respectively) (Table 5). There was no statistically significant difference between age-group observed for all or individual STIs, although the prevalence of CT was slightly higher among women aged 15–19 years (12.1%, 95% CI: 3.4–35.5, $p = 0.32$), NG was higher among 20–24 years old (12.1%, 95% CI: 5.4–25.1, $p = 0.41$) while TV was higher among 25–29 years old (13.9%, 95% CI: 10.6–18.1, $p = 0.15$) as compared to all ages (data not shown).

The prevalence of STIs was significantly higher among single women (26.4%) as compared to married women (11.2%) ($p = 0.001$). Women with secondary/high school education had a prevalence of 22.2% as compared to women who had never been to school (9.1%). Unemployed and self-employed women had a prevalence of 21.6, and 21.8% respectively as compared to employed women (14.7%). There was no statistically significant difference between women who reported being pregnant before as compared to women who had never been pregnant (25.2% vs 18.3%, $p = 0.323$).

Based on the univariate analysis: the mean age, being married, increasing number of pregnancies and not using condoms with ones' regular partner were inversely associated with STIs' risk. Significant differences in proportions regarding those married ($p < 0.001$), the number of sexual partners ($p < 0.001$) and contraceptive use by age group ($p < 0.001$) was observed. Having two and three sexual life-time partners was associated with an increased risk OR = 5.1 (95% CI: 1.2–21.5) and OR = 8.4, (95% CI: 1.3–54.2) respectively for STIs. Being hr-HPV positive was significantly associated with increased risk of STIs (OR = 2.1, 95% CI: 1.3–3.6). In the final logistic regression model (multivariate analysis), factors independently associated with increased risk of STIs were: being employed (OR = 2.2, 95% CI: 1.0–4.7), self-employed (OR = 2.8, 95% CI: 1.5–5.5) and hr-HPV positive status (OR = 2.0, 95% CI: 1.3–3.1). Being married, mean age and not using a condom one's with regular partner were found to be inversely associated in the final model (OR = 0.4, 95% CI: 0.3–0.7, OR = 0.92, 95% CI:

Table 3 The prevalence of sexually transmitted infections (STIs) among women aged 15–49 in Swaziland (n = 655)

STIs	Positive (n)	Crude Prevalence (%)	Survey weighted prevalence % (95% CI)	Population burden[a]	95% CI
Overall	114	17.4	19.4 (14.9–24.8)	72990	51111–94871
TV	51	4.7	8.4 (5.4–12.8)	30132	16633–43631
NG	35	5.2	6.0 (3.8–9.4)	22055	11986–32124
CT	38	5.8	7.0 (4.1–11.2)	25024	11251–38797
Treponema pallidum (syphilis)	9	1.2	1.4 (1.1–10.2)	5072	1822–8322
Genital warts	6	1.0	2.0 (1.0–11.4)	6111	470–12692
HIV	276	42.1	42.7 (35.7–46.2)	153276	127336–179216
Hr-HPV (n = 644)	273	42.1	46.2 (42.8–49.5)	174046	153294–194797
Multiple STIs[b]	20	3.1	4.0 (2.3–6.0)	13995	7092–20898
[c]Triple STIs (n = 644)[d]	38	5.9	6.3 (4.4–8.9)	23310	14193–32427

[a]Population burden estimates extrapolated (using sample statistics) based on the 2007–2030 population projections aligned to the 2014 population estimates
[b]Multiple STIs – having two or more of the screened 5 STIs
[c]Triple infection: at least one other STI including HIV and hr-HPV infection
[d]A total of 11 women had insufficient specimen for hr-HPV testing therefore for the analysis for Triple STIs done on N = 644

0.89–0.95, and OR = 0.5, 95% CI: 0.3–0.9) respectively, as compared to not having a sexual life partner.

Individual STI association with HIV and hr-HPV was assessed. There was a significant inverse association between HIV and CT ($p = 0.001$) but there was a significant positive association between HIV and syphilis ($p = 0.001$). There was a significant positive association between hr-HPV and NG and CT ($p = 0.020$ and $p = 0.001$). A significant association with TV and hr-HPV ($p = 0.058$) was observed (results not shown).

Discussion

The current study in Swaziland shows a high prevalence of STIs (19.4%), corresponding to 72 990 women of reproductive age with STIs. Our data suggests that TV was the most prevalent curable STI (8.4%) among those examined in this study. Furthermore, the prevalence of HIV remains significantly high (42.7%) in this population. The prevalence of the STIs decreased with increasing age however, differences by age groups were not statistically significant. A high percentage of women infected with hr-HPV had one STI (18.8%), while 6.3% had multiple STIs. Single women were at higher risk of being infected with STIs compared to married women (26.4% vs 11.2%, $p = 0.001$). A proportion of the women had triple co-infection (6.3%), interact either directly with one another or indirectly via the host's resources or immune system. Studies have demonstrated that, as compared to infections of single pathogen species, these interactions within coinfected hosts can alter the transmission, clinical progression and control of multiple infectious diseases [39, 40]. In the final logistic regression model, being employed, self-employed and hr-HPV infection status were risk factors positively associated with STIs.

In this study, we collected primary data and biological specimens using a standardized methodology. This is the first study evaluating the prevalence of STIs among women of reproductive age not attending antenatal care in Swaziland. We were able to extrapolate our results on the prevalence of STIs as well as genital warts to the female population in the same age groups of 15–49 years-old using the 2007–2030 population projections aligned to the 2014 population estimates [37]. Another strength of our study is that STIs such as NG, TV and CT were detected using the Gene Xpert PCR (Xpert CT/NG and Xpert TV) which, is a highly sensitive laboratory method for detecting genital infection. An important limitation of the study is the lack of generalizability of the results to the general Swazi female population beyond the age groups studied (15–49 years). In addition, since the study subjects were recruited from heath care facilities, it is arguable that they may not be truly representative of the general population. This could have introduced a selection bias. However, weighting was applied when reporting the summary results for the whole study sample. Lastly, the study participants were required to recall past events, which could result in compromising the accuracy of information provided, due to recall bias. Finally, due to limited resources for our study we did not genotype or test for LR-HPVs.

The high prevalence of STIs (19.4%) in this population indicates that STIs are a serious public health problem in Swaziland. Our findings were consistent with previous studies from similar populations across the Southern African Development Community region (SADC) and other sub-Saharan regions [13, 15, 41–43]. The prevalence of each of the STIs detected among the study population was less than 10% (7.0% for CT, 6.0% for NG, 8.4% for TV and 1.4% for syphilis), but this is still high, which compared to global estimates, where the

Table 4 The weighted prevalence and estimated population burden of other STIs and hr-HPV/HIV co-infection among women of reproductive age in Swaziland

Characteristic	hr-HPV status(N = 644)[a]			HIV status(N = 654)[b]		
	Negative (%, 95% CI)	Positive (%, 95% CI)	Total	Negative (%, 95% CI)	positive (%, 95% CI)	Total
STIs status						
Negative	86.3 (79.4–91.1)	74.8 (67.3–81.1)	81.1(75.6–85.4)	82.2 (72.8–92.8)	78.1 (66.5–90.0)	80.6 (72.1–89.7)
Single	12.1 (7.4–19.1)	18.9 (13.1–26.3)	15.2 (11.8–19.4)	14.4 (9.7–22.6)	17.7 (11.5–26.9)	15.7 (11.2–22.6)
Multiple	1.6 (0.7–3.4)	6.3 (3.3–11.7)	3.7 (2.3–6.1)	3.4 (2.0–5.7)	4.2 (1.5–11.3)	3.7 (2.3–6.0)
Total	100	100	100	100	100	100
	p-value = 0.025			p-value = 0.370		
Population Burden						
STIs status	Negative (%, 95% CI)	Positive n(95% CI)	Total	Negative (%, 95% CI)	Positive n(95% CI)	Total
Negative	171725 (145875–197575)	127553 (110677–144428)	299278 (265003–333552)	183121 (148333–217908)	119746 (90801–148690)	302867 (39415–348608)
Single	24073 (11482–36665)	32158 (20200–44115)	56231 (39657–72806)	31832 (16847–46490)	27163 (14941–39386)	58996 (35732–82259)
Multiple	3197 (671–5723)	10798 (4032–17564)	13995 (7092–20898)	7628 (3919–11336)	6367 (−159–12893)	13995 (7092–20898)
Total	198996 (169168–228822)	170508 (154052–186965)	369504	222581 (190953–254208)	153276 (127336–179216)	357857
	p-value = 0.025			p-value = 0.370		

other STIs (CT, NG, TV, syphilis, Genital warts)
Single STI: one of the 5 STIs screened or observed
Multiple STIs: two or more of the 5 STIs screened or observed
[a] N = 644 : A total of 11 women had insufficient specimen for hr-HPV testing
[b] N = 654 : one with unknown/missing HIV status

Table 5 Risk factors associated with STIs among women aged 15–49 years in Swaziland (N = 655)

Risk factors	STIs (Weighted Prevalence)		Unadjusted (Univariate)		Adjusted (Multivariable)	
	Number + ve/Total	(%, 95% CI)	OR (95% CI)	P-value	ORª (95% CI)	P-value
Overall	114/655	19.3 (14.9–24.8)				
Age						
Mean ± SD (range)	114/655	27 .1 (25.9–28.2)	**0.9 (0.8–0.9)**	**0.001**	**0.9 (0.8–0.9)**	**<0.001**
15–19	13/45	29.2 (14.3–59.4)	**1 (ref)**			
20–24	26/110	22.7 (13.1–37.4)	0.7 (0.2–2.1)	0.520	….	….
24–29	34/127	27.0 (19.0–38.1)	0.9 (0.4–2.1)	0.797	……	….
30–34	20/143	13.0 (6.0–3161)	0.4 (0.1–1.1)	0.081	….	….
35–39	14/94	14.5 (7.7–28.8)	0.4 (0.1–1.2)	0.110	….	….
40–44	6/78	6.9 (1.5–29.9)	0.2 (0.03–1.1)	0.067	….	….
45–49	1/58	1.0 (0.1–8.7)	0.03 (0–0.3)	0.004	….	….
Marital status						
Single	66/271	26.4 (18.5–37.4)	**1 (ref)**			
Living with partner/Cohabiting	9/38	24.2 (9.8–62.3)	0.89 (0.3–2.5)	0.819		
Married	36/313	11.2 (6.7–18.9)	**0.35 (0.2–0.6)**	**0.001**	**0.4 (0.3–0.7)**	**0.001**
Divorced/separated	3/22	15.1 (4.9–38.3)	0.5 (0.13–1.9)	0.289	….	….
widow	0/11	0	—	—	….	….
Education:						
Never been to school	2/24	9.4 (19.0–36.0	**1 (ref)**			
Primary	23/133	21.4 (10.5–47.8)	2.6 (0.4–16.9)	0.299	….	….
Secondary/High	78/380	22.2 (15.4–31.3)	2.7 (0.5–15.4)	0.243	….	…
Tertiary	11/118	7.3 (3.5–16.9)	0.8 (0.1–5.4)	0.777	….	….
Occupation:						
Unemployed	67/346	21.6 (14.2–32.9)	**1 (ref)**		1 (ref)	
Employed	39/258	14.7 (9.8–22.0)	0.63 (0.34–1.16)	0.129	**2.2 (1.0–4.7)**	**0.045**
Self-employed	8/48	21.8 (8.0–47.4)	1.01 (0.32–3.19)	0.982	**2.8(1.5–5.5)**	**0.002**
Pregnant before						
Yes	99/582	18.3 (13.5–24.4)	**1 (ref)**			
No	13/64	25.2 (12.6–48.9)	1.51 (0.65–3.46)	0.323	….	….
No. of pregnancies (Mean)	114/655	2.2 (1.9–2.5)	**0.8 (0.7–0.9)**	**0.008**	….	…
Age Menarche (Mean age)	114/655	13.97 (13.5–14.4)	0.9 (0.7–1.1)	0.166	….	..
Age at first sex (mean age)	114/655	17.2 (16.5–17.9)	0.96 (0.9–1.1)	0.370	…..	…..
Number of sexual partners		2.0 (0.6–3.4)	**1.3 (1. 4–1.5)**	**<0.001**	1.2 (0.9–1.5)	0.197
0	3/33	6.2 (14.2–23.6)	**1 (ref)**		….	…
1	84/522	18.4 (14.2–23.6)	3.4 (1.0–12.3)	0.056	….	….
2	16/62	25.1 (11.3–46.8)	**5.1 (1.1–21.5)**	**0.028**	….	….
3+	11/37	35.6 (15.7–53.3)	**8.4 (1.3–54.2)**	**0.027**	….	….
Condom use with regular partner						
Yes	93/457	21.6 (14.8–31.2)	1 (ref)		1 (ref)	
No	20/194	13.1 (5.7–29.1)	**0.5 (0.28–0.9)**	**0.022**	**0.5 (0.3–0.9)**	**0.034**
Ever had STI						
Yes	41/278	16.2 (10.9–23.4)	**1 (ref)**			
No	63/342	19.8 (15.2–25.3)	1.28 (0.8–2.0)	0.246	….	….
Don't remember	7/30	31.8 (12.0–61.3)	2.42 (0.7–7.8)	0.136	….	….

Table 5 Risk factors associated with STIs among women aged 15–49 years in Swaziland ($N = 655$) (Continued)

STIs treated in the past 12 months						
Yes	24/118	22.6 (13.5–35.5)	**1 (ref)**			
No	89/529	18.7 (14.7–23.6	0.8 (0.5–1.4)	0.376	....	.....
Don't know	1/7	13.9 (12.6–67.3)	0.6 (0.4–8.1)	0.654	....	....
HIV Status:						
Negative	55/373	17.7 (13.4–23.0)	**1 (ref)**			
Positive	59/281	21.9 (15.2–30.4)	1.3 (0.9–2.0)	0.204	.....	....
hr-HPV status:						
Negative	46/371	13.7 (8.9–20.6)	1 (ref)		1 (ref)	
Positive	64/273	25.2 (19.0–32.7)	**2.1 (1.3–3.6)**	**0.007**	**2.0 (1.3–3.1)**	**0.002**

The Bolded data shows the signficant results

[a]Adj. OR: Adjusted Odds Ratio for age, marital status, level of education, occupation, history of pregnancy, age at first sex, history of STIs, STIs treated in the past 12 months, HIV status

prevalence for CT among women range from 2.4 to 6.9%, NG from 0.3% to 1.2, TV from 1.9 to 7.8% and syphilis from 0.2 to 1.3 [44]. Results from the first and second STI sentinel surveillance surveys conducted in 2003 and 2005 respectively in Swaziland, showed that the prevalence of STIs, such as CT, NG, TV and syphilis, and other reproductive tract infections, such as bacterial vaginosis and candidiasis, continue to be among the highest in the country [45, 46]. However, a decline in syphilis has been noted in recent years. According to the 11th Sentinel Surveillance report 2008, recent syphilis infection was tested using *Treponema pallidum* haemagglutination (TPHA), and the prevalence was 1.9% while 4.7% showed a history of syphilis infection by RPR results [47]. A comparison between the 2008 report and recent syphilis infection shows a decreasing trend (1.9%) compared to current study findings (1.4%). The high prevalence of the curable STIs in this population might be linked to the limitation of syndromic STI management, which does not give specific aetiological diagnosis; therefore, most infections are missed by this approach [48, 49]. Although syndromic management has proven to be cost-effective in resource limited settings, our findings demonstrate the evidence for the need of a strong national STIs' surveillance system.

HIV remains one of the major public health challenges in Swaziland, with the highest prevalence among women of reproductive age [50, 51]. This high prevalence reported in our study was consistent with other studies. However, our results were slightly higher as compared to Bicego et al's study on recent patterns in population–based HIV among women age 18–49 years (42.7% vs. 39%) [50]. In a country that has the highest HIV prevalence in the world, the challenge remains to assist uninfected individuals in gaining access to high quality prevention services, including early detection and treatment of curable STIs.

The observed high prevalence of STIs in the younger age groups as compared to the older age groups in our study is consistent with other studies [41, 52, 53]. The decreasing STIs prevalence with increasing age observed in our study, might be the results of the high susceptibility of younger women, lack of protective immune response development, and more risky behavior, such as an earlier age at first intercourse, a high number of sexual partners, and unprotected sex [52].

In this current study, single women and women living with partners (but not married) had the highest prevalence of STIs. Similar evidence has been found in other studies [54, 55]. In our multivariate analysis, married women were 60% less likely to be at risk of STIs as compared to single women (OR = 0.4). A similar outcome was found in others studies showing being married is a protective factor [48, 56].

As far as education is concerned, our findings have shown that women with a lower level of education are most likely to have an STI. Studies have shown that women with less education have an increased risk of STIs [13, 57, 58]. Kakaire et al. highlighted that women with lower education tend to lack formal employment and may be completely dependent on the male sexual partner and unable to negotiate safer sex. They are less likely to access STI preventative information and healthcare services [13]. According to Muula, unemployment may leave women with limited alternatives where they may resort to engaging in high risk behavior such as becoming sex workers or to engaging in transactional sex in which they provide sex in exchange for money and material resources from a partner [59]. However, our study found that employed and self-employed women were at high risk of STIs (OR: 2.2 and OR: 2.8 respectively) as compared to unemployed women. The types of employment might explain the high risk of STIs among employed and self-employed women in our study and the in which businesses they are involved. There is evidence suggesting that women working in high-risk occupation such bars, food facilities, guesthouses and similar facilities are at high risk of STI infection [48].

In this study, the risk associated with STIs among women with two or more sexual life-time partners was five to eight times higher as compared to women with no sexual partners in the univariate analysis. Our findings were consistent with other studies which reported that sexual activity with many partners increases the odds of STIs [53, 54]. However, the association was not statistically significant in our study following adjustment for all possible confounding factors (age, marital status, level of education, occupation, history of pregnancy, age at first sex, history of STIs, STIs treated in the past 12 months, and HIV status), which negatively confounded this relationship. There was a very high collinearity between the number of sexual partners and some of the confounding factors, which may have further affected the coefficients in the stepwise multivariable regression. Though evidence from studies done in South Africa [41, 42], Zambia [60], and Tanzania [48] has demonstrated that having more than one or concurrent lifetime sexual partners was among the risk factors associated with STIs.

Inconsistent condom use as a risk factor for STIs in women has been demonstrated in other studies [61, 62]. In contrast to our study, not using condoms with regular partners was inversely associated with STIs. The possible plausible explanation of our findings might be that, women who reported not using condoms with regular partners had one faithful partner or they had been treated for STIs prior to data collection. However, this will require further investigation. Moreover, condoms remain a critical part in a comprehensive and practical approach to the prevention of STIs [63].

HIV positive status was not associated with STIs in both analyses but when assessed by individual STIs, a significant inverse association between HIV and CT, and significant positive association between HIV and syphilis were observed. No statistically significant association between HIV and NG or TV was observed in the current study. However, studies have indicated that depending on the STI involved and the population, NG, CT, TV, HPV and syphilis increase the risk of HIV acquisition and transmission from two to eight times or more [4, 6, 7]. Furthermore, biological findings support the mechanisms for STIs increasing HIV acquisition and transmission through direct mucosal disruption, recruitment of HIV target cells to the genital tract, and by increased HIV load in plasma and genital secretions [10]. High levels of untreated STIs in sub-Saharan countries are linked to high HIV transmission rates and have been postulated to have contributed to the high prevalence of HIV in the region [16].

A vital clinical and public health consequence of our findings is that hr-HPV was the most significant risk factor associated with STIs infection in both univariate and multivariate analysis (unadj-OR = 2.1 and Adj-OR = 2.0). When assessing the association between hr-HPV and individual STIs, there was a significant positive association between hr-HPV and NG and CT. The strong association between HPV infection and STIs has been demonstrated in previous studies, where infection with hr-HPV types, was a risk factor for CT and NG infection [64–66]. These findings are significantly of high importance for policy and prevention programmes to include HPV infection in the existing STIs prevention programmes in the country.

The curable STIs (CT, NG, TV, and syphilis), and HIV and HPV are sexually transmitted infections, which share the same transmission route and behavioural risk factors. If the curable STIs are not treated, they can lead to a variety of different health risks and greatly increase HIV/HPV transmission risk with further chronic health implications. Collectively, our data have shown the significantly high prevalence of and association between STIs and HIV/HPV coinfection, which tends to subscribe to the new concept in which HIV and HPV infections may be bi-directional, each increasing the risk of the other [67–69] STIs increase the risk of HIV/HPV co-infection. The high hr-HPV/HIV coinfection with the curable STIs and resultant high population burden has implications for both cervical cancer and also for the United Nations (UN) sustainable development goal 3, target 3.3 (SDG 3) [70] (goal 3 aims to reduce new HIV infection through ensuring health and well-being for all, at every stage of life). The STIs are positively increasing the risk of HIV/HPV acquisition, which will make it impossible for countries like Swaziland to achieve SDG 3 target 3.3. Therefore, STIs' control and HPV vaccination, combined with periodic HIV screening and referral to early treatment is needed to end the HIV epidemic in Swaziland.

Conclusion

In conclusion, although STIs may be treated and are curable, they remain a major public health challenge in Swaziland where HIV infection is highly prevalent. Our study indicates that there is a need for a comprehensive STI screening, surveillance and treatment programme in the country.

Abbreviations

CT: Chlamydia trachomatis; HIV: Human immunodeficiency virus; Hr-HPV: High-risk human papillomavirus; NG: Neisseria gonorrhoeae; NRL: National referral laboratory; RFM: Realign Fitkin Memorial Hospital; SDG: United Nations Sustainable Development Goal; STIs: Sexually transmitted infections; TPHA: Treponema pallidum Hemagglutination Assay; TV: Trichomonas vaginalis; VIA: Visual inspection with acetic acid

Prevalence and risk factors associated with sexually transmitted infections (STIs) among women...

39

Acknowledgements

We thank the Kingdom of Swaziland Ministry of Health for allowing us to implement the study, and the support from International Agency for Research on cancer (IARC), WHO- Swaziland local office, Ministry of Health Epidemiology Unit and Sexually Reproductive Health Unit (SRH) and University of Alabama at Birmingham (Minority Health International Research Training (MHIRT) grant). We are so thankful for the laboratory support and capacity building from Cepheid Europe and South Africa.

Funding

The study was funded by the University of KwaZulu-Natal College of Health Sciences Doctoral Research Scholarship grant and another part funding from Health and Welfare Sector Education and Training Authority (HWSETA). The funder had no role in the study design, data collection and analysis, decision to publish.

Authors' contributions

TG designed the study, data collection, carried out the analyses, and wrote the paper. BS analysed data and supervised writing up of manuscript: DX, PEJ, EW, NB, CDS, JMT supervised the study, and analyses, wrote the paper, reviewed and modified with their contributions to the original manuscript. All authors have read and approved of the final version of the manuscript.

Competing interests

The authors declare that they have no competing interests.

Author details

[1]Discipline of Public Health, School of Nursing and Public Health, University of KwaZulu-Natal, 2nd Floor George Campbell Building, Mazisi Kunene Road, 4041 Durban, South Africa. [2]Walter Sisulu University, Umtata, South Africa. [3]Epidemiology Unit, Ministry of Health and Social Welfare, Mbabane, Swaziland. [4]Department of Epidemiology, University of Alabama, Birmingham, USA. [5]Department of Medical Epidemiology and Biostatistics, Karolinska Institutet, Stockholm, Sweden. [6]Department of Research, Cancer Registry of Norway, Institute of Population-Based Cancer Research, Oslo, Norway. [7]Department of Community Medicine, Faculty of Health Sciences, University of Tromsø, The Arctic University of Norway, Tromsø, Norway. [8]Genetic Epidemiology Group, Folkhälsan Research Center, Helsinki, Finland. [9]World Health Organization; Department of Reproductive Health and Research, Geneva, Switzerland.

References

1. Genuis SJ, Genuis SK. Managing the sexually transmitted disease pandemic: a time for reevaluation. Am J Obstet Gynecol. 2004;191(4):1103–12.
2. Menendez C, Castellsague X, Renom M, Sacarlal J, Quinto L, Lloveras B, Klaustermeier J, Kornegay JR, Sigauque B, Bosch FX et al.: Prevalence and risk factors of sexually transmitted infections and cervical neoplasia in women from a rural area of southern Mozambique. Infect Dis Obstet Gynecol. 2010;2010:9. doi: 10.1155/2010/609315. https://www.hindawi.com/journals/idog/2010/609315/.
3. World Health Organisation. Report on global sexually transmitted infection surveillance 2013. Geneva: WHO; 2014.
4. World Health Organisation. Sexually transmitted infections (STIs), fact sheet N°110. Geneva: WHO; 2015.
5. World Health Organisation. Global prevalence and incidence of selected curable sexually transmitted infections. 2012.
6. Boily MC, Baggaley RF, Wang L, Masse B, White RG, Hayes RJ, Alary M. Heterosexual risk of HIV-1 infection per sexual act: systematic review and meta-analysis of observational studies. Lancet Infect Dis. 2009;9(2):118–29.
7. Jin F, Prestage GP, Imrie J, Kippax SC, Donovan B, Templeton DJ, Cunningham A, Mindel A, Cunningham PH, Kaldor JM, et al. Anal sexually transmitted infections and risk of HIV infection in homosexual men. J Acquir Immune Defic Syndr. 2010;53(1):144–9.
8. Grosskurth H, Gray R, Hayes R, Mabey D, Wawer M. Control of sexually transmitted diseases for HIV-1 prevention: understanding the implications of the Mwanza and Rakai trials. Lancet. 2000;355(9219):1981–7.
9. Kaul P, Gupta I, Sehgal R, Malla N. Trichomonas vaginalis: random amplified polymorphic DNA analysis of isolates from symptomatic and asymptomatic women in India. Parasitol Int. 2004;53(3):255–62.
10. Ward HRM. Contribution of sexually transmitted infections to the sexual transmission of HIV. Curr Opin HIV AIDS. 2010;4:305–10.
11. Chaturvedi AK, Madeleine MM, Biggar RJ, Engels EA. Risk of human papillomavirus-associated cancers among persons with AIDS. J Natl Cancer Inst. 2009;101(16):1120–30.
12. Johnson LF, Lewis DA. The effect of genital tract infections on HIV-1 shedding in the genital tract: a systematic review and meta-analysis. Sex Transm Dis. 2008;35(11):946–59.
13. Kakaire O, Byamugisha JK, Tumwesigye NM, Gamzell-Danielsson K. Prevalence and factors associated with sexually transmitted infections among HIV positive women opting for intrauterine contraception. PLoS One. 2015;10(4):e0122400.
14. Sweet T, Welles SL. Associations of sexual identity or same-sex behaviors with history of childhood sexual abuse and HIV/STI risk in the United States. J Acquir Immune Defic Syndr. 2012;59(4):400–8.
15. Basera T, Takuva S, Muloongo K, Tshuma N, Nyasulu P. Prevalence and Risk Factors for Self-reported Sexually Transmitted Infections among Adults in the Diepsloot Informal Settlement, Johannesburg, South Africa. J AIDS Clin Res. 2016;7(1):1-5. https://www.omicsonline.org/open-access/prevalence-and-risk-factors-for-selfreported-sexually-transmittedinfections-among-adults-in-the-diepsloot-informal-settlementjohan-2155-6113-1000539.pdf.
16. Johnson LF, Dorrington RE, Bradshaw D, Coetzee DJ. The role of sexually transmitted infections in the evolution of the South African HIV epidemic. Trop Med Int Health. 2012;17(2):161–8.
17. Clifford G, Franceschi S, Diaz M, Munoz N, Villa LL. Chapter 3: HPV type-distribution in women with and without cervical neoplastic diseases. Vaccine. 2006;24 Suppl 3:S3/26–34.
18. Lindstrand A, Bergstrom S, Bugalho A, Zanconato G, Helgesson AM, Hederstedt B. Prevalence of syphilis infection in Mozambican women with second trimester miscarriage and women attending antenatal care in second trimester. Genitourin Med. 1993;69(6):431–3.
19. Moodley P, Sturm AW. Sexually transmitted infections, adverse pregnancy outcome and neonatal infection. Semin Neonatol. 2000;5(3):255–69.
20. Almonte M, Albero G, Molano M, Carcamo C, Garcia PJ, Perez G. Risk factors for human papillomavirus exposure and co-factors for cervical cancer in Latin America and the Caribbean. Vaccine. 2008;26 Suppl 11:L16–36.
21. Appleby P, Beral V, Berrington de Gonzalez A, Colin D, Franceschi S, Goodhill A, Green J, Peto J, Plummer M, Sweetland S. Cervical cancer and hormonal contraceptives: collaborative reanalysis of individual data for 16,573 women with cervical cancer and 35,509 women without cervical cancer from 24 epidemiological studies. Lancet. 2007;370:1609–21.
22. Laumann EO, Youm Y. Racial/ethnic group differences in the prevalence of sexually transmitted diseases in the United States: a network explanation. Sex Transm Dis. 1999;26(5):250–61.
23. Gindi RM, Erbelding EJ, Page KR. Sexually transmitted infection prevalence and behavioral risk factors among Latino and non-Latino patients attending the Baltimore City STD clinics. Sex Transm Dis. 2010;37(3):191–6.
24. Niyazi M, Husaiyin S, Han L, Mamat H, Husaiyin K, Wang L. Prevalence of and risk factors for high-risk human papillomavirus infection: a population-based study from Hetian, Xinjiang, China. Bosn J Basic Med Sci. 2016;16(1):46–51.
25. Ragin CC, Watt A, Markovic N, Bunker CH, Edwards RP, Eckstein S, Fletcher H, Garwood D, Gollin SM, Jackson M, et al. Comparisons of high-risk cervical HPV infections in Caribbean and US populations. Infect Agent Cancer. 2009;4 Suppl 1:S9.
26. Chadambuka A, Chimusoro A, Maradzika JC, Tshimanga M, Gombe NT, Shambira G. Factors associated with contracting sexually transmitted infections among patients in Zvishavane urban, Zimbabwe; 2007. Afr Health Sci. 2011;11(4):535–42.
27. Cordova D, Huang S, Lally M, Estrada Y, Prado G. Do parent-adolescent discrepancies in family functioning increase the risk of Hispanic adolescent HIV risk behaviors? Fam Process. 2014;53(2):348–63.
28. Ragnarsson A, Ekstrom AM, Carter J, Ilako F, Lukhwaro A, Marrone G, Thorson A. Sexual risk taking among patients on antiretroviral therapy in an urban informal settlement in Kenya: a cross-sectional survey. J Int AIDS Soc. 2011;14:20.
29. UNAIDS. HIV and AIDS estimates (2015): Swaziland. Geneva: UNAIDS; 2015.

30. Cepheid. GeneXpert. Xpert® CT/NG, vol. GXCT/NG-CE-10. GXCT/NG-CE-120. Sunnyvale: Cepheid; 2014.

31. Cepheid. GeneXpert. Xpert® TV, vol. GXTV-CE-10. Sunnyvale: Cepheid; 2014.

32. Atlas Medical. RPR SYPHILIS CARD TEST. Cambridge: Atlas Medical; 2014.

33. Omega Diagnostic. Treponema Pallidum Haemagglutination (TPHA) Test Cells, vol. MSDS 0043. Scotland: Omega Diagnostic; 2004.

34. Cepheid. GeneXpert. Xpert® HPV. GXHPV-CE-10th ed. Sunnyvale: Cepheid; 2014.

35. Alere Determine™ HIV-1/2 Ag/Ab Combo [http://www.alere.com/en/home/product-details/determine-1-2-ag-ab-combo.html]. Accessed 2 Dec 2015.

36. Trinity Biotech PLC. Uni-Gold™ Recombigen®HIV. Bray: Trinity Biotech PLC; 2014.

37. The Kingdom of Swaziland Gorvernment and UNFPA. Swaziland Population Projections 2007–2030. In. Edited by Office CS; 2007

38. Ginindza TG, Dlamini X, Almonte M, Herrero R, Jolly PE, Tsoka-Gwegweni JM, Weiderpass E, Broutet N, Sartorius B. Prevalence of and associated risk factors for high risk human papillomavirus among sexually active women, Swaziland. PloS one. 2017;12(1):e0170189.

39. Sternberg ED, Lefevre T, Rawstern AH, de Roode JC. A virulent parasite can provide protection against a lethal parasitoid. Infect Genet Evol. 2011;11(2):399–406.

40. Pedersen AB, Fenton A. Emphasizing the ecology in parasite community ecology. Trends Ecol Evol. 2007;22(3):133–9.

41. Abbai NS, Wand H, Ramjee G. Sexually transmitted infections in women participating in a biomedical intervention trial in Durban: prevalence, coinfections, and risk factors. J Sex Transm Dis. 2013;2013:358402.

42. Naidoo S, Wand H, Abbai NS, Ramjee G. High prevalence and incidence of sexually transmitted infections among women living in Kwazulu-Natal, South Africa. AIDS Res Ther. 2014;11:31.

43. Tyndall MW, Kidula N, Sande J, Ombette J, Temmerman M. Predicting Neisseria gonorrhoeae and Chlamydia trachomatis infection using risk scores, physical examination, microscopy, and leukocyte esterase urine dipsticks among asymptomatic women attending a family planning clinic in Kenya. Sex Transm Dis. 1999;26(8):476–82.

44. Newman L, Rowley J, Vander Hoorn S, Wijesooriya NS, Unemo M, Low N, Stevens G, Gottlieb S, Kiarie J, Temmerman M. Global estimates of the prevalence and incidence of four curable sexually transmitted infections in 2012 based on systematic review and global reporting. PLoS One. 2015;10(12):e0143304.

45. The Kingdom of Swaziland, Ministry of Health. The National HIV sero-surveillance. Mbabane: Swaziland National AIDS Programme; 2004.

46. The Kingdom of Swaziland, Ministry of Health. National HIV Sero-surveillance. Mbabane: Swaziland National AIDS Programme; 2003.

47. The Kindom of Swaziland, Ministry of Health. 11th Sentinel Surveillance. Mbabane: Swaziland National AIDS Programme; 2008.

48. Francis SC, Ao TT, Vanobberghen FM, Chilongani J, Hashim R, Andreasen A, Watson-Jones D, Changalucha J, Kapiga S, Hayes RJ. Epidemiology of curable sexually transmitted infections among women at increased risk for HIV in northwestern Tanzania: inadequacy of syndromic management. PLoS One. 2014;9(7):e101221.

49. Vuylsteke B. Current status of syndromic management of sexually transmitted infections in developing countries. Sex Transm Infect. 2004;80(5):333–4.

50. Bicego GT, Nkambule R, Peterson I, Reed J, Donnell D, Ginindza H, Duong YT, Patel H, Bock N, Philip N, et al. Recent patterns in population-based HIV prevalence in Swaziland. PLoS One. 2013;8(10):e77101.

51. The Kingdom of Swaziland, Ministry of Health. The 12th round of national HIV sero-surveillance in Swaziland. Mbabane: Swaziland National AIDS Programme; 2010.

52. Oliveira FA, Pfleger V, Lang K, Heukelbach J, Miralles I, Fraga F, Sousa AQ, Stoffler-Meilicke M, Ignatius R, Kerr LF, et al. Sexually transmitted infections, bacterial vaginosis, and candidiasis in women of reproductive age in rural Northeast Brazil: a population-based study. Mem Inst Oswaldo Cruz. 2007;102(6):751–6.

53. N WC, A S. Associated risk factors of STIs and multiple sexual relationships among youths in Malawi. PLoS One. 2015;10(8):e0134286.

54. de Lima YA, Turchi MD, Fonseca ZC, Garcia FL, Cardoso FA DBe, da Guarda Reis MN, de Britto Guimaraes EM, Alves RR, Carvalho NR, de Fatima Costa Alves M. Sexually transmitted bacterial infections among young women in central Western Brazil. Int J Infect Dis. 2014;25:16–21.

55. Nyarko C, Unson C, Koduah M, Nyarko P, Galley J. Risk Factors Of Sexually-Transmitted Infections (Stis) Among Men And Women In A Mining Community In Western Ghana: A Study Of Lifetime Occurrence. Int J Of Scie & Tech Res. 2014 3(12):1-10.

56. de Lima SV, de Mesquita AM, Cavalcante FG, Silva ZP, Hora V, Diedrich T, de Carvalho SP, de Melo PG, Dacal AR, de Carvalho EM, et al. Sexually transmitted infections in a female population in rural north-east Brazil: prevalence, morbidity and risk factors. Trop Med Int Health. 2003;8(7):595–603.

57. Arbabi M, Fakhrieh Z, Delavari M, Abdoli A. Prevalence of Trichomonas vaginalis infection in Kashan city, Iran (2012–2013). Iran J Reprod Med. 2014;12(7):507–12.

58. Singa B, Glick SN, Bock N, Walson J, Chaba L, Odek J, McClelland RS, Djomand G, Gao H, John-Stewart G. Sexually transmitted infections among HIV-infected adults in HIV care programs in Kenya: a national sample of HIV clinics. Sex Transm Dis. 2013;40(2):148–53.

59. Muula AS. HIV infection and AIDS among young women in South Africa. Croat Med J. 2008;49(3):423–35.

60. Crucitti T, Jespers V, Mulenga C, Khondowe S, Vandepitte J, Buve A. Non-sexual transmission of Trichomonas vaginalis in adolescent girls attending school in Ndola, Zambia. PloS one. 2011;6(1):e16310.

61. Ramjee G, Daniels B. Women and HIV in Sub-Saharan Africa. AIDS Res Ther. 2013;10(1):30.

62. Ahmed S, Lutalo T, Wawer M, Serwadda D, Sewankambo NK, Nalugoda F, Makumbi F, Wabwire-Mangen F, Kiwanuka N, Kigozi G, et al. HIV incidence and sexually transmitted disease prevalence associated with condom use: a population study in Rakai, Uganda. AIDS (London, England). 2001;15(16):2171–9.

63. Ali Abdulai M, Baiden F, Afari-Asiedu S, Gyabaa-Febir L, Adjei KK, Mahama E, Tawiah-Agyemang C, Newton SK, Asante KP, Owusu-Agyei S. The risk of sexually transmitted infection and its influence on condom use among pregnant women in the Kintampo North municipality of Ghana. J Sex Transm Dis. 2017;2017:8642685.

64. Samarawickrema NA, Tabrizi SN, Young E, Gunawardena P, Garland SM. Prevalence of trichomonas vaginalis, Chlamydia trachomatis, neisseria gonorrhoeae and human papillomavirus in a sexual health clinic setting in urban Sri Lanka. Int J STD AIDS. 2015;26(10):733–9.

65. Vielot N, Hudgens MG, Mugo N, Chitwa M, Kimani J, Smith J. The role of Chlamydia trachomatis in high-risk human papillomavirus persistence among female Sex workers in Nairobi, Kenya. Sex Transm Dis. 2015;42(6):305–11.

66. Wohlmeister D, Vianna DR, Helfer VE, Gimenes F, Consolaro ME, Barcellos RB, Rossetti ML, Calil LN, Buffon A, Pilger DA. Association of human papillomavirus and Chlamydia trachomatis with intraepithelial alterations in cervix samples. Mem Inst Oswaldo Cruz. 2016;111(2):106–13.

67. Giuliano AR, Botha MH, Zeier M, Abrahamsen ME, Glashoff RH, van der Laan LE, Papenfuss M, Engelbrecht S, van der Loeff MF S, Sudenga SL, et al. High HIV, HPV, and STI prevalence among young Western Cape, South African women: EVRI HIV prevention preparedness trial. J Acquir Immune Defic Syndr. 2015;68(2):227–35.

68. Lissouba P, Van de Perre P, Auvert B. Association of genital human papillomavirus infection with HIV acquisition: a systematic review and meta-analysis. Sex Transm Infect. 2013;89(5):350–6.

69. Rositch AF, Gravitt PE, Smith JS. Growing evidence that HPV infection is associated with an increase in HIV acquisition: exploring the issue of HPV vaccination. Sex Transm Infect. 2013;89(5):357.

70. United Nation GA. Transforming our world: the 2030 agenda for sustainable development, vol. A/RES/70/1. New York: United Nation GA; 2015.

71. The Kingdom of Swaziland, Ministry of Health. National guidelines for HIV testing and counseling. Mbabane: The Kingdom of Swaziland, Ministry of Health; 2014.

6

Hepatitis C virus seroprevalence in the general female population of 9 countries in Europe, Asia and Africa

Gary M. Clifford[1*], Tim Waterboer[2], Bolormaa Dondog[2], You Lin Qiao[3], Dimitri Kordzaia[4], Doudja Hammouda[5], Namory Keita[6], Nahid Khodakarami[7], Syed Ahsan Raza[8,9], Ang Tshering Sherpa[10], Witold Zatonski[11], Michael Pawlita[2], Martyn Plummer[1] and Silvia Franceschi[1]

Abstract

Background: New oral treatments with very high cure rates have the potential to revolutionize global management of hepatitis C virus (HCV), but population-based data on HCV infection are missing in many low and middle-income countries (LMIC).

Methods: Between 2004 and 2009, dried blood spots were collected from age-stratified female population samples of 9 countries: China, Mongolia, Poland, Guinea, Nepal, Pakistan, Algeria, Georgia and Iran. HCV antibodies were detected by a multiplex serology assay using bead-based technology.

Results: Crude HCV prevalence ranged from 17.4% in Mongolia to 0.0% in Iran. In a pooled model adjusted by age and country, in which associations with risk factors were not statistically heterogeneous across countries, the only significant determinants of HCV positivity were age (prevalence ratio for ≥45 versus <35 years = 2.84, 95%CI 2.18-3.71) and parity (parous versus nulliparous = 1.73, 95%CI 1.02-2.93). Statistically significant increases in HCV positivity by age, but not parity, were seen in each of the three countries with the highest number of HCV infections: Mongolia, Pakistan, China. There were no associations with sexual partners nor HPV infection. HCV prevalence in women aged ≥45 years correlated well with recent estimates of female HCV-related liver cancer incidence, with the slight exception of Pakistan, which showed a higher HCV prevalence (5.2%) than expected.

Conclusions: HCV prevalence varies enormously in women worldwide. Medical interventions/hospitalizations linked to childbirth may have represented a route of HCV transmission, but not sexual intercourse. Combining dried blood spot collection with high-throughput HCV assays can facilitate seroepidemiological studies in LMIC where data is otherwise scarce.

Keywords: Hepatitis C virus, Epidemiology, Serology, Liver cancer

Background

About 180 million people, some 3% of the world's population, are estimated to have been exposed to hepatitis C virus (HCV) [1–3]. Of these, 130–150 million (~80%) are chronically HCV infected and at risk for development of hepatitis-C related liver cirrhosis or cancer, which kill approximately 700,000 people each year [4]. Although new HCV treatments offering very high cure rates with short durations and few side effects have the potential to drastically reduce HCV-related mortality, access to diagnosis and expensive treatment remain low, so that the number of people living with HCV is actually reported to be increasing [1].

In 2016, the World Health Assembly adopted a strategy to eliminate viral hepatitis as a major public health threat by 2030, noting that national data on hepatitis virus infection are often lacking [5]. In addition, available HCV surveys often over-represent low-risk groups, particularly younger low-risk persons (e.g. pregnant women and blood donors), whereas HCV prevalence is known

* Correspondence: clifford@iarc.fr
[1]International Agency for Research on Cancer, 150 cours Albert Thomas, 69372 Lyon Cedex 08, France
Full list of author information is available at the end of the article

to increase steadily with age owing to the combination of accumulating risk of exposure and a high probability of infection becoming chronic [6].

Common routes of HCV infection are unsafe injections, inadequate sterilization of medical equipment, and the transfusion of unscreened blood and blood products that have been common in high-income countries till the 1980s and also more recently in low- and medium-income countries (LMIC). Because these practices are largely specific to a given country's medical system, HCV prevalence and the timing of infection spread may differ between bordering countries [2], and national level data on HCV infection is required to inform public health decisions.

Hence, we exploited a series of standardized seroepidemiological surveys in order to describe HCV prevalence and risk factors among the general female population of a heterogeneous range of countries around the world. HCV seropositivity was determined using a high throughput assay that has been shown to provide an accurate and cost-effective tool for assessment of HCV antibodies in large epidemiologic studies [7], and we went on to compare country-specific HCV prevalence with recently generated country-specific estimates of HCV-related liver cancer incidence.

Methods
Population
Between 2004 and 2009, studies were undertaken in 11 areas in 9 countries with the primary aim to estimate the prevalence of genital human papillomavirus virus (HPV) infection, according to a similar protocol developed and co-ordinated by the International Agency for Research on Cancer (IARC). Population sampling methods have been previously described for the individual study centres: Shanxi, China [8]; Shenyang, China [9]; Shenzhen, China [10]; Ulaanbaatar, Mongolia [11]; Warsaw, Poland [12]; Conakry, Guinea [13]; Bharatpur, Nepal [14]; Karachi, Pakistan [15]; Zeralda, Algeria [16]; Tbilisi, Georgia [17]; and Tehran, Iran [18]. In each area, an attempt was made to obtain an age-stratified population-based sample that included at least 100 women in each 5-year age group, from 15-19 up to 65 years and older. The number of included women is sometimes higher than that in the original reports due to relaxing of selection criteria for adequacy of genital specimens. Data from Mongolia have been previously reported in validation studies of the present HCV serological assay [7, 19]. Trained interviewers administered a face-to-face questionnaire that included information on sociodemographic characteristics, sexual behaviour, reproductive and contraceptive history, and smoking habits. All participants signed informed consent forms according to the recommendations of the IARC Ethics

Committee, and of the local ethical review committees in each of the participating countries, which also approved each of the original studies.

Specimen collection
Each participant had a blood sample collected by venopuncture. In Mongolia, this sample was drawn from the cubital fossa into vacuum containers without anticoagulant [19], whereas in all other areas, samples were obtained by fingerstick. In both instances, full blood was then immediately applied to DBS (dried blood spot) filter paper card (Whatman 903 Protein Saver Blood Collection Cards; Schleicher & Schuell) to entirely fill five 14.5 mm diameter circles. DBS cards were dried at room temperature, placed in separate plastic paper zip lock envelopes containing a silica desiccant, and shipped at ambient temperature to the German Cancer Research Center (DKFZ) in Heidelberg, Germany, and stored at -20°C until serological analysis.

Study participants were also invited for a pelvic examination (although a subset, particularly self-reported virgins, declined) and collection of cervical exfoliated cells for HPV DNA testing, performed in the Department of Pathology, VU University Medical Center, Amsterdam, the Netherlands, according to a general primer GP5+/6 + –mediated PCR [20].

HCV serology
Antibodies were eluted from DBS cards according to a previously reported protocol that has been shown to result in high agreement (>96% for HCV antigens) of seropositivity in paired DBS and serum results [19]. In brief, one punch of 6 mm diameter from each DBS was eluted in one well of a 96-well plate in 100 µL PBS at 4°C overnight, and 16 µl of eluate subsequently mixed with 80 µL DBS preincubation buffer.

A multiplex serology assay [19] including antigens to HCV (strain H77, subtype 1a) Core and NS3 proteins was performed as previously described [7]. In brief, full-length coding sequences of Core and NS3 were expressed as double fusion proteins with an N-terminal-GST and a C-terminal tag epitope derived from the large T-antigen of SV40 in E. coli. Fusion proteins were loaded and affinity-purified on glutathione-casein coupled spectrally distinct fluorescence-labeled polystyrene beads (SeroMap; Luminex). DBS eluates were incubated with pooled antigen loaded bead sets. Bound antibodies were quantified with biotinylated goat anti-human IgA, IgM, IgG (Dianova), and R-phycoerythrin–labeled streptavidin in a Luminex 100 analyzer as the median R-phycoerythrin fluorescence intensity (MFI) from at least 100 beads of the same bead set. Antigen-specific MFI values were calculated as previously described [21].

DBS-specific cut-off values for HCV Core (MFI ≥ 967) and NS3 (MFI ≥ 310) were defined as the mean MFI plus three SDs from 235 reference sera that tested negative by a commercial HCV antibody screening assay [19]. Women that were positive for both Core and NS3 proteins were defined as being HCV-positive. In an evaluation against a set of 432 reference sera, this cut-off has been proven to perform similarly, in a single step, to a commercial HCV antibody screening assay (MEIA) followed by RNA confirmation (98% sensitivity, 99% specificity) [7].

When a subset of 2,988 DBS samples from 8 study areas were re-tested on a second occasion to evaluate assay reproducibility, 2,982 (99.8%) were concordantly classified (2,940 HCV-negative, 42 HCV-positive).

Statistical analyses

HPV prevalence was standardized by age using the world standard population (in 5-year age groups from 15-19 to 60-65 years) as a reference [22]. Prevalence ratios (PR) for HCV seropositivity and corresponding 95% confidence intervals (CI) were calculated using unconditional logistic regression adjusted for age (5-year groups) and study area. Heterogeneity of PRs between study areas was tested by calculating the difference between the log likelihood of the model that considered the interaction term between the areas and risk factor of interest and the log likelihood of the model that included the exposure only, and comparing it to the chi-squared distribution with degrees of freedom equal to the number of areas minus one.

Country-specific estimates of HCV-related liver cancer incidence in women were extracted from Plummer et al, Lancet Global Health, 2016 [23], derived by combining country-specific estimates of HCV attributable fraction in liver cancer with Globocan 2012 [24] estimates of female liver cancer incidence.

Results

HCV serology results were obtained for a total of 12,204 women, with study-specific sample sizes varying from 1,516 for Shenzhen, China, down to 892 for Iran (Table 1). Overall median age was 34 years, varying from 30 to 38 years by study center (Table 1). A total of 274 women (2.2%) were HCV-positive. Crude HCV prevalence ranged from 17.4% in Mongolia down to 0.0% in Iran (Table 1). Age-standardization reduced HCV prevalence estimates (by increasing the relative weight of younger age groups, who were less often HCV-positive), but did not change relative differences in HCV positivity between centers.

Table 2 shows the relationship of selected characteristics of study women with HCV positivity. In a model adjusted by age and study area, as appropriate, the only significant determinants of HCV positivity were age group (PR for ≥45 versus <35 years = 2.84, 95% CI 2.18-3.71) and parity (PR for parous versus nulliparous =1.73, 95% CI 1.02-2.93). However, no risk trend was found by number of births. Associations of HCV positivity with risk factors were not statistically heterogeneous across study areas (p values for heterogeneity = 0.17, 0.88, 0.59 and 0.25 for age, sexual partners, parity and induced abortion, respectively).

Findings by age group and parity are also shown separately for Mongolia, Pakistan and China (the three countries with the highest number of HCV-positive women) in Table 3. Statistically significant increases in HCV positivity by age were seen in each of the three

Table 1 HCV prevalence by study center

Geographical area	Median age	N tested	N pos	Crude %	Crude 95% CI	Age-standardized[a] %	Age-standardized[a] 95% CI
Mongolia, Ulaanbaatar	35	1,075	187	17.4	15.2-19.2	10.9	3.3-18.6
Pakistan, Karachi	35	963	31	3.2	2.2-4.5	1.7	0.5-2.9
Georgia, Tbilisi	33	1,431	17	1.2	0.7-1.9	0.7	0.0-1.4
Guinea, Conakry	30	1,253	11	0.9	0.4-1.6	0.5	0.0-1.4
Poland, Warsaw	37	909	7	0.8	0.3-1.6	0.3	0.0-0.9
China, Shenyang	34	989	6	0.6	0.2-1.3	0.4	0.0-1.7
China, Shanxi	36	940	6	0.6	0.2-1.4	0.3	0.0-0.8
China, Shenzhen	30	1,516	6	0.4	0.1-0.9	0.3	0.0-0.6
Nepal, Bharatpur	33	1,061	2	0.2	0.0-0.7	0.2	0.0-0.8
Algeria, Zeralda	36	1,135	1	0.1	0.0-0.5	0.1	0.0-0.2
Iran, Tehran	38	892	0	0	0.0-0.4	0.0	0.0-0.4
Total	34	12,164	274	2.2	2.0-2.5	1.4	1.0-1.83

[a]Standardized to world population in CI5 [22]

Table 2 Prevalence ratios (PR) for HCV positivity and corresponding 95% confidence intervals (CI) according to selected women's characteristics

Risk factor	N tested	HCV positive N (%)	Adjusted PR[a]	95% CI
Age	12,164			
<35	6,249	79 (1.3)	1	-
35-44	2,894	78 (2.7)	1.86	1.39-2.50
≥45	3,021	117 (3.9)	2.84	2.18-3.71
χ_1^2 for trend			$p < 0.001$	
Education level	12,156			
None	1,713	24 (1.4)	1	-
Primary	1,552	21 (1.3)	0.96	0.52-1.77
Secondary and higher	8,891	229 (2.6)	0.86	0.46-1.60
Lifetime number of sexual partners[b]	10,926			
0	1,086	1 (0.1)	0.21	0.03-1.55
1	7,513	146 (1.9)	1	-
2	1,305	60 (4.6)	1.12	0.84-1.49
3+	1,022	65 (6.4)	1.08	0.81-1.44
χ_1^2 for trend			$p = 0.367$	
Number of births (parity)	11,199			
Nulliparous	2,207	21 (0.9)	1	-
1	3,228	55 (1.7)	1.68[d]	0.98-2.90
2	2,644	75 (2.8)	1.81[d]	1.01-3.26
3+	3,120	119 (3.8)	1.84[d]	1.01-3.38
χ_1^2 for trend			$p = 0.171$	
Induced abortion[c]	9,166			
0	5,433	95 (1.7)	1	-
1	1,750	46 (2.6)	0.97	0.69-1.37
2+	1,983	112 (5.6)	1.24	0.93-1.66
χ_1^2 for trend			$p = 0.121$	
Smoking status	12,153			
Never	10,860	235 (2.2)	1	-
Ever	1,293	38 (2.9)	1.21	0.88-1.66
HPV DNA-positive	9,984			
No	8,264	183 (2.2)	1	-
Yes	1,720	65 (3.8)	1.04	0.80-1.36

[a]Adjusted for age (5-year groups) and geographical area, as appropriate
[b]Algeria excluded because of missing data
[c]Algeria and Guinea excluded because of missing data
[d]Combined PR for ≥ 1 versus 0 = 1.73 (1.02-2.93)

countries, but the rise between women <35 to those 35-44 years of age was especially steep in Pakistan. Increases in HCV positivity in parous women were only observed in Mongolia and Pakistan and did not meet statistical significance (Table 3).

Age-specific HCV prevalence estimates are shown by study country in Fig. 1, in order of highest to lowest HCV prevalence among women aged ≥45 years, and are plotted against country-specific estimates of female HCV-related liver cancer incidence rates. Age-specific increases in HCV prevalence were observable in Mongolia, Pakistan, Guinea, Poland and China. HCV prevalence estimates in women aged ≥45 years correlated well with female HCV-related liver cancer incidence rates, ranging between the extremes of Mongolia (28.4% HCV prevalence versus 20.9 cases of HCV liver cancer per 100,000 women) and Iran (0.0% HCV prevalence versus 0.2 cases of HCV liver cancer per 100,000 women). The only slight exception to this

Table 3 HCV positivity by age and number of births, separately for Mongolia, Pakistan and China

Risk factor	Mongolia			Pakistan			China		
	N tested	HCV positive N (%)	Adjusted PR[a] and 95% CI	N tested	HCV positive N (%)	Adjusted PR[a] and 95% CI	N tested	HCV positive N (%)	Adjusted PR[a] and 95% CI
Age	1,075			963			3,445		
<35	511	55 (10.8)	1	479	7 (1.5)	1	1,915	5 (0.3)	1
35-44	289	54 (18.7)	1.74 (1.23-2.45)	254	12 (4.7)	3.23 (1.29-8.11)	755	4 (0.5)	2.03 (0.55-7.54)
≥45	275	78 (28.4)	2.63 (1.93-3.60)	230	12 (5.2)	3.57 (1.42-8.95)	775	9 (1.2)	4.45 (1.49-13.2)
χ_1^2 for trend			p < 0.001			p = 0.005			p = 0.007
Number of births	1,056			955			3,225		
0	228	16 (7.0)	1	136	1 (0.7)	1	942	2 (0.2)	1
≥1	828	169 (20.4)	1.62 (0.86-3.04)	819	30 (3.7)	3.06 (0.39-24.1)	2,283	16 (0.7)	0.48 (0.06-3.82)

[a]Adjusted for age (5 years groups), as appropriate

correlation was Pakistan, which showed a high HCV prevalence (5.2%) in comparison to a relatively low estimate of female HCV-related liver cancer (1.3 cases per 100,000 women).

Discussion

Benefiting from a standardized population-based sampling protocol and a validated serological assay, we describe important variation in HCV seroprevalence in women around the world and robustly confirm the absence of a sexual transmission route for HCV infection. Crude population-based HCV prevalence ranged from 17% in Mongolia down to 0% in Iran and correlated with country-specific estimates of female HCV-related liver cancer incidence, which are also highest in Mongolia (20.9 per 100,000 women) and lowest in Iran (0.2 per 100,000 women) in women aged ≥45 years. Furthermore, when available, our estimates were compatible with previous population-based estimates of HCV prevalence in the evaluated countries.

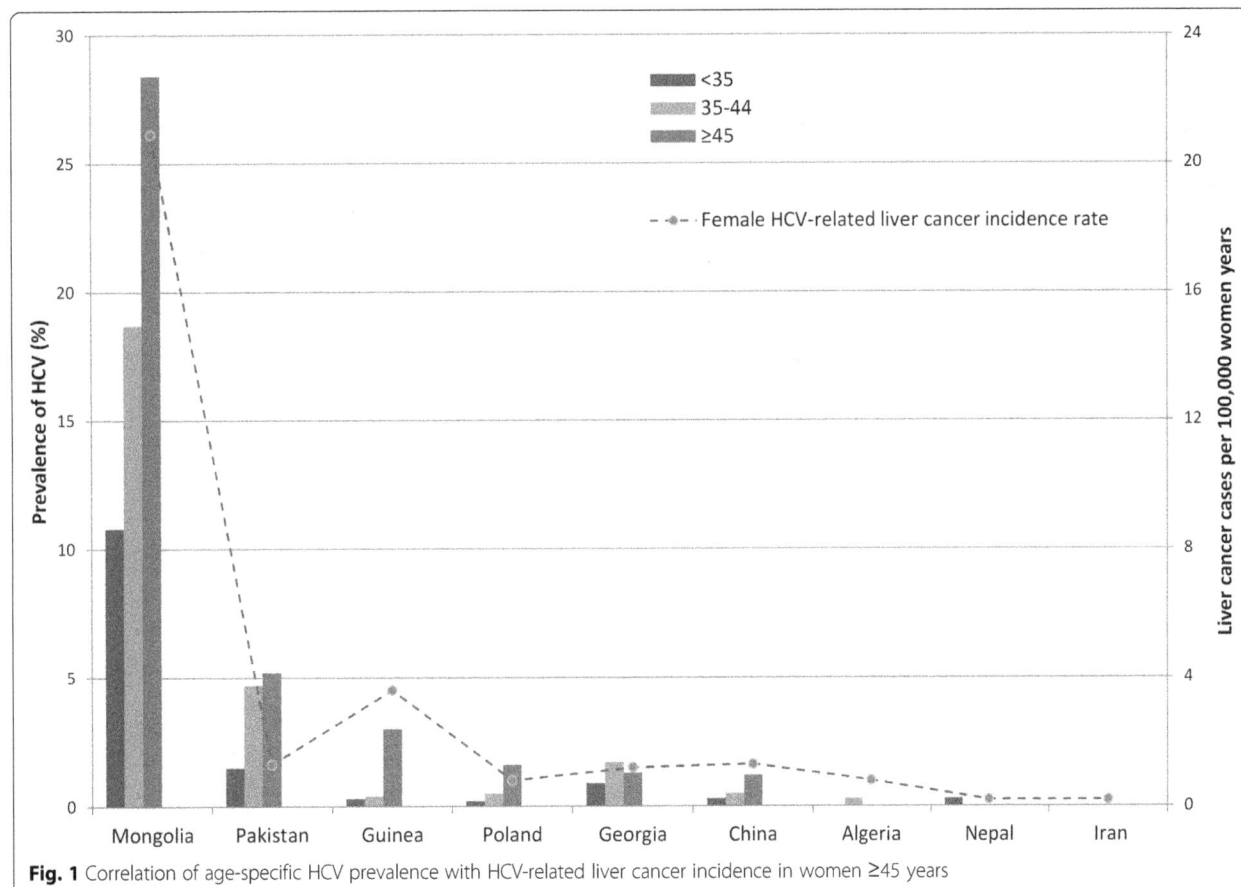

Fig. 1 Correlation of age-specific HCV prevalence with HCV-related liver cancer incidence in women ≥45 years

The extreme HCV prevalence in Mongolia was expected and has been previously described [7]. Indeed, Mongolia has the highest burden of HCV-related liver cancer in the world [23], driven by a long-lasting epidemic due to iatrogenic transmission of HCV through mass vaccination campaigns (e.g. smallpox, polio [25], blood transfusions [26, 27]) and extensive use of injected treatments [28]. At the lower extreme, we confirm an anti-HCV prevalence of less than 1% reported from a wide-range of other population-based studies in Iran [29], where a low fraction of liver cancers are estimated to be attributable to HCV [30].

The relatively high HCV prevalence found in Karachi, Pakistan (~5% in women aged 45+ years) is similar to that in previous large population-based surveys in Karachi [31, 32] and nationwide in Pakistan [33]. Indeed, HCV was reported to be the predominant cause of liver cancer in Pakistan [34, 35]. Given this high HCV prevalence, however, current estimates of HCV-related liver cancer incidence in Pakistani women are lower than expected. This may be due to limitations in liver cancer incidence data for Pakistan [24], or to a more recent iatrogenic spread of the virus compared to, for instance, Mongolia. Indeed the proportion of HCV-positive hepatocellular carcinoma is still increasing in Pakistan [34].

HCV prevalence estimates were highly consistent across the three Chinese sites (0.4-0.6%) and compatible with estimates of 0.4-1.0% in large population-based surveys of women performed since 2006 [36–39]. HCV prevalence is especially low below age 45. Thus, improvements in transfusion practices implemented in China in the mid-1990s, notably prohibition of paid donations of plasma and blood that were associated with mass transmission of HCV and HIV, appear to have largely controlled the HCV epidemic. Indeed, population-based HCV prevalence [36], and proportion of liver cancer attributed to HCV [34], appears to be relatively low and decreasing over time in China.

HCV prevalence in women in Tbilisi, Georgia (1.3%) is compatible with that from a previous population-based survey in which the vast majority of HCV infections in Tbilisi were observed to occur among male intravenous drug users [40]. Indeed, increasing intravenous drug use is feared to be an important source of recent HCV transmission in many former Soviet republics [41]. Estimates of 0.8% HCV prevalence in Warsaw, Poland are similar to that in a nationwide study of 42,274 women (0.8% [42]), and with that modelled from meta-analytical data [43].

No population-based data are available for Algeria, but our HCV prevalence estimates (0.1%) compare well to the 0.2% and 0.6% reported among 1,000 [44] and 3,044 [45] pregnant women, respectively. This would suggest Algeria to have an HCV prevalence similar to its neighbors Morocco and Tunisia [46], and much lower than in Egypt [2], for which much more population-based data is available.

No population-based data are available for Nepal, but our HCV prevalence estimate of 0.2% compares well to the 0.1% reported among 2,007 female blood donors [47], suggesting that Nepal has largely escaped an epidemic of HCV to date.

Lastly, this study provides the first report on HCV infection in Guinea, for which the 0.9% HCV prevalence is lower than previous regional estimates for West sub-Saharan Africa (2.8% [1] and 5.3% [2]), which are nonetheless very sensitive to the lack of relevant data from this region of the world. Lower HCV prevalence among women aged under 45 years in Guinea may represent a cohort effect of reduced HCV transmission in younger generations.

HCV infection increased with age in most countries, presumably due to accumulating risk of exposure. This confirms steady increases up to the age of 60 years reported in a meta-analysis of age-specific HCV infection from Mongolia and Poland [43], and in large studies in China [36–39].

Given the orientation of the surveys towards studying HPV, questionnaires did not include variables that would be useful to studying specific iatrogenic transmission routes. Nevertheless, to our knowledge, this is the first study to suggest the existence of a possible association between HCV infection and parity, which persisted even after adjustment for center and age, which may represent a risk of HCV transmission by medical interventions/hospitalizations linked to childbirth. On the other hand, we were able to robustly confirm the absence of sexual transmission of HCV in the general female population, through the null association with number of sexual partners, and presence of cervical HPV infection, as proxies of sexual intercourse.

Our data arises entirely from females in selected towns, and may not be representative of males or other areas in the same country. In most populations around the world, HCV prevalence in females has been estimated to be similar or lower than that in males [43]. However, at least Mongolia [43] and China [38] may represent exceptions to this rule. In any case, we propose that our population-based sampling procedures provide a more representative picture than studies limited to typically young pregnant women or blood donors.

HCV genotypes are known to vary between the different worldwide regions represented by this study. Nevertheless, the cross-reactivity of serological assays for NS3 and Core proteins of genotypes 1a, 1b and 2a does not suggest that their performance should be affected by the existence of HCV serotypes [7]. Furthermore, the assay was shown to be highly reproducible when a large subset of samples were re-tested on a second occasion, and has been well-validated against commercial HCV tests [7] and for use with dried blood spots [19]. Taken together, we believe that this protocol represents a useful model for obtaining HCV prevalence data from low- and middle-income settings where data is scarce, for both men and women alike. Indeed, DBS do not require blood centrifugation and allow storage and shipment at ambient temperature, thus facilitating field work for seroepidemiological studies in environments with limited technical infrastructure, and the research serological assay is both high-throughput and cost-effective.

Conclusions

HCV prevalence varied enormously across the female populations represented in our study. Medical interventions/hospitalizations linked to childbirth may have represented a route of HCV transmission, at least in some settings, but not sexual intercourse. Combining dried blood spot collection with high-throughput HCV assays can facilitate seroepidemiological studies in LMIC where data is otherwise scarce. Indeed, the availability of population-based HCV estimates is going to become increasingly relevant in the next years, as countries consider the cost and public health priority of going beyond the prevention of HCV transmission by ensuring safety of medical interventions, towards screen-and-treat approaches that can benefit from a new generation of highly performant oral HCV treatment regimens [5].

Abbreviations

CI: confidence interval; DBS: dried blood spot; DKFZ: German Cancer Research Center; HCV: hepatitis C virus; HPV: human papillomavirus virus; IARC: International Agency for Research on Cancer; LMIC: low and middle-income countries; MFI: median R-phycoerythrin fluorescence intensity; PR: prevalence ratio

Acknowledgements
We would like to thank Vanessa Tenet for data management and analysis.

Funding
Not applicable.

Authors' contributions
GMC conceived the study, supervised the data analysis and drafted the manuscript, in collaboration with SF. BD, TW and M Pawlita developed and performed the HCV assay. YLQ, DK, DH, NK, NK, SAR, ATS and WZ are the local principal investigators for each of the study centres responsible for acquiring the primary epidemiological data and samples. M Plummer was responsible for estimates of HCV-related liver cancer rates. All authors read, gave feedback and approved the final version of the manuscript.

Competing interests
The authors declare they have no competing interests.

Author details
[1]International Agency for Research on Cancer, 150 cours Albert Thomas, 69372 Lyon Cedex 08, France. [2]Infection, Inflammation and Cancer Program, German Cancer Research Center (DKFZ), Heidelberg, Germany. [3]Cancer Institute of the Chinese Academy of Medical Sciences, Beijing, China. [4]Iv. Javakhishvili Tbilisi State University, Tbilisi, Georgia. [5]Institut National de Sante Publique, Algiers, Algeria. [6]Department of Obstetrics and Gynaecology, Centre Hospitalier Universitaire de Donka, Conakry, Guinea. [7]Infertility and Reproductive Health Research Centre, Shahid Beheshti University of Medical Sciences, Tehran, Iran. [8]Department of Surgery, The Aga Khan University, Karachi, Pakistan. [9]Centre de Recherche du CHUM, Département de Médecine Sociale et Préventive Université de Montréal, Quebec, Canada. [10]Kist Medical College, Lalitpur, Nepal. [11]The Maria Sklodowska-Curie Memorial Cancer Center and Institute of Oncology, Warsaw, Poland.

References
1. Mohd Hanafiah K, Groeger J, Flaxman AD, Wiersma ST. Global epidemiology of hepatitis C virus infection: new estimates of age-specific antibody to HCV seroprevalence. Hepatology. 2013;57:1333–42. doi:10.1002/hep.26141.
2. Gower E, Estes C, Blach S, Razavi-Shearer K, Razavi H. Global epidemiology and genotype distribution of the hepatitis C virus infection. J Hepatol. 2014; 61:S45–57. doi:10.1016/j.jhep.2014.07.027.
3. Petruzziello A, Marigliano S, Loquercio G, Cozzolino A, Cacciapuoti C. Global epidemiology of hepatitis C virus infection: An up-date of the distribution and circulation of hepatitis C virus genotypes. World J Gastroenterol. 2016; 22:7824–40. doi:10.3748/wjg.v22.i34.7824.
4. Lozano R, Naghavi M, Foreman K, Lim S, Shibuya K, Aboyans V, et al. Global and regional mortality from 235 causes of death for 20 age groups in 1990 and 2010: a systematic analysis for the Global Burden of Disease Study 2010. Lancet. 2012;380:2095–128. doi:10.1016/s0140-6736(12)61728-0.
5. WHO. Global health sector strategy on viral hepatitis 2016–2021. Geneva: WHO Press; 2016.
6. IARC. 2012. Biological agents. IARC Monogr Eval Carcinog Risks Hum 100B:1-475. http://monographs.iarc.fr/ENG/Monographs/vol100B/index.php. Accessed 27 July 2016
7. Dondog B, Schnitzler P, Michael KM, Clifford G, Franceschi S, Pawlita M, et al. Hepatitis C Virus Seroprevalence in Mongolian Women Assessed by a Novel Multiplex Antibody Detection Assay. Cancer Epidemiol Biomarkers Prev. 2015;24:1360–5. doi:10.1158/1055-9965.epi-15-0351.
8. Dai M, Bao YP, Li N, Clifford GM, Vaccarella S, Snijders PJF, et al. Human papillomavirus infection in Shanxi Province, People's Republic of China: a population-based study. Br J Cancer. 2006;95:96–101.
9. Li LK, Dai M, Clifford GM, Yao WQ, Arslan A, Li N, et al. Human papillomavirus infection in Shenyang City, People's Republic of China: A population-based study. Br J Cancer. 2006;95:1593–7.
10. Wu RF, Dai M, Qiao YL, Clifford GM, Liu ZH, Arslan A, et al. Human papillomavirus infection in women in Shenzhen City, People's Republic of China, a population typical of recent Chinese urbanisation. Int J Cancer. 2007;121:1306–11.
11. Dondog B, Clifford GM, Vaccarella S, Waterboer T, Unurjargal D, Avirmed D, et al. Human papillomavirus infection in Ulaanbaatar, Mongolia: a population-based study. Cancer Epidemiol Biomarkers Prev. 2008;17:1731–8.
12. Bardin A, Vaccarella S, Clifford GM, Lissowska J, Rekosz M, Bobkiewicz P, et al. Human papillomavirus infection in women with and without cervical cancer in Warsaw, Poland. Eur J Cancer. 2008;44:557–64.
13. Keita N, Clifford GM, Koulibaly M, Douno K, Kabba I, Haba M, et al. HPV infection in women with and without cervical cancer in Conakry, Guinea. Br J Cancer. 2009;101:202–8.
14. Sherpa AT, Clifford GM, Vaccarella S, Shrestha S, Nygard M, Karki BS, et al. Human papillomavirus infection in women with and without cervical cancer in Nepal. Cancer Causes Control. 2010;21:323–30.
15. Raza SA, Franceschi S, Pallardy S, Malik FR, Avan BI, Zafar A, et al. Human papillomavirus infection in women with and without cervical cancer in Karachi, Pakistan. Br J Cancer. 2010;102:1657–60.
16. Hammouda D, Clifford GM, Pallardy S, Ayyach G, Chekiri A, Boudrich A, et al. Human papillomavirus infection in a population-based sample of women in Algiers, Algeria. Int J Cancer. 2011;128:2224–9.

17. Alibegashvili T, Clifford GM, Vaccarella S, Baidoshvili A, Gogiashvili L, Tsagareli Z, et al. Human papillomavirus infection in women with and without cervical cancer in Tbilisi, Georgia. Cancer Epidemiol. 2011;35:465–70.

18. Khodakarami N, Clifford GM, Yavari P, Farzaneh F, Salehpour S, Broutet N, et al. Human papillomavirus infection in women with and without cervical cancer in Tehran, Iran. Int J Cancer. 2012;131:E156–61.

19. Waterboer T, Dondog B, Michael KM, Michel A, Schmitt M, Vaccarella S, et al. Dried blood spot samples for seroepidemiology of infections with human papillomaviruses, Helicobacter pylori, Hepatitis C Virus, and JC Virus. Cancer Epidemiol Biomarkers Prev. 2012;21:287–93.

20. Jacobs MV, Walboomers JM, Snijders PJ, Voorhorst FJ, Verheijen RH, Fransen-Daalmeijer N, et al. Distribution of 37 mucosotropic HPV types in women with cytologically normal cervical smears: the age-related patterns for high-risk and low-risk types. Int J Cancer. 2000;87:221–7.

21. Waterboer T, Sehr P, Michael KM, Franceschi S, Nieland JD, Joos TO, et al. Multiplex human papillomavirus serology based on in situ-purified glutathione s-transferase fusion proteins. Clin Chem. 2005;51:1845–53.

22. Doll R, Payne P, Waterhouse J. Cancer Incidence in Five Continents: A Technical Report. Berlin: Springer-Verlag (for UICC); 1966.

23. Plummer M, de Martel C, Vignat J, Ferlay J, Bray F, Franceschi S. Global burden of cancers attributable to infections in 2012: a synthetic analysis. Lancet Glob Health. 2016;4:e609–e616. doi:10.1016/S2214-109X(16)30143-7.

24. Ferlay J, Soerjomataram I, Ervik M, Dikshit R, Eser S, Mathers C, et al. 2013. GLOBOCAN 2012 v1.0, Cancer Incidence and Mortality Worldwide: IARC CancerBase No. 11 [Internet]. on International Agency for Research on Cancer. http://gco.iarc.fr/today/home. Accessed 27 July 2016.

25. Kurbanov F, Tanaka Y, Elkady A, Oyunsuren T, Mizokami M. Tracing hepatitis C and Delta viruses to estimate their contribution in HCC rates in Mongolia. J Viral Hepat. 2007;14:667–74.

26. Tsatsralt-Od B, Takahashi M, Nishizawa T, Inoue J, Ulaankhuu D, Okamoto H. High prevalence of hepatitis B, C and delta virus infections among blood donors in Mongolia. Arch Virol. 2005;150:2513–28.

27. Tserenpuntsag B, Nelson K, Lamjav O, Triner W, Smith P, Kacica M, et al. Prevalence of and risk factors for hepatitis B and C infection among Mongolian blood donors. Transfusion. 2010;50:92–9.

28. Logez S, Soyolgerel G, Fields R, Luby S, Hutin Y. Rapid assessment of injection practices in Mongolia. Am J Infect Control. 2004;32:31–7.

29. Taherkhani R, Farshadpour F. Epidemiology of hepatitis C virus in Iran. World J Gastroenterol. 2015;21:10790–810. doi:10.3748/wjg.v21.i38.10790.

30. Hajiani E, Masjedizadeh R, Hashemi J, Azmi M, Rajabi T. Risk factors for hepatocellular carcinoma in Southern Iran. Saudi Med J. 2005;26:974–7.

31. Abdullah F, Pasha H, Memon A, Shah U. Increasing frequency of anti-hcv seropositivity in a cross-section of people in Karachi, Pakistan. Pak J Med Sci. 2011;27:767–70.

32. Afzal MS. 2016. Are efforts up to the mark? A cirrhotic state and knowledge about HCV prevalence in general population of Pakistan. Asian Pacific Journal of Tropical Medicine 9:616-618. doi:http://dx.doi.org/10.1016/j.apjtm.2016.04.013.

33. Qureshi H, Bile KM, Jooma R, Alam SE, Afridi HU. Prevalence of hepatitis B and C viral infections in Pakistan: findings of a national survey appealing for effective prevention and control measures. East Mediterr Health J. 2010;16(Suppl):S15–23.

34. de Martel C, Maucort-Boulch D, Plummer M, Franceschi S. 2015. Worldwide relative contribution of hepatitis B and C viruses in hepatocellular carcinoma. Hepatology 62:1190-1200. doi:10.1002/hep.27969 [doi].

35. Alavian SM, Haghbin H. Relative Importance of Hepatitis B and C Viruses in Hepatocellular Carcinoma in EMRO Countries and the Middle East: A Systematic Review. Hepat Mon. 2016;16, e35106. doi:10.5812/hepatmon.35106.

36. Chen Y, Li L, Cui F, Xing W, Wang L, Jia Z, et al. A sero-epidemiological study on hepatitis C in China. Chin J Epidemiol. 2011;32:888–91.

37. Lu J, Zhou Y, Lin X, Jiang Y, Tian R, Zhang Y, et al. General epidemiological parameters of viral hepatitis A, B, C, and E in six regions of China: a cross-sectional study in 2007. PLoS One. 2009;4, e8467. doi:10.1371/journal.pone.0008467.

38. Ke X, Liguo Z, Fenyang T, Changjun B, Yefei Z, Minquan C, et al. Rate of infection and related risk factors on hepatitis C virus in three counties of Jiangsu province. Chin J Epidemiol. 2014;35:1212–7.

39. Zhou M, Li H, Ji Y, Ma Y, Hou F, Yuan P. Hepatitis C virus infection in the general population: A large community-based study in Mianyang, West China. Biosci Trends. 2015;9:97–103. doi:10.5582/bst.2015.01033.

40. Stvilia K, Tsertsvadze T, Sharvadze L, Aladashvili M, del Rio C, Kuniholm MH, et al. Prevalence of hepatitis C, HIV, and risk behaviors for blood-borne infections: a population-based survey of the adult population of T'bilisi, Republic of Georgia. J Urban Health. 2006;83:289–98. doi:10.1007/s11524-006-9032-y.

41. Kelly JA, Amirkhanian YA. The newest epidemic: a review of HIV/AIDS in Central and Eastern Europe. Int J STD AIDS. 2003;14:361–71. doi:10.1258/095646203765371231.

42. Walewska-Zielecka B, Religioni U, Juszczyk G, Czerw A, Wawrzyniak Z, Soszyński P. Diagnosis of hepatitis C virus infection in pregnant women in the healthcare system in Poland: Is it worth the effort? Medicine (Baltimore). 2016;95, e4331. doi:10.1097/md.0000000000004331.

43. Saraswat V, Norris S, de Knegt RJ, Sanchez Avila JF, Sonderup M, Zuckerman E, et al. Historical epidemiology of hepatitis C virus (HCV) in select countries - volume 2. J Viral Hepat. 2015;22 Suppl 1:6–25. doi:10.1111/jvh.12350.

44. Ayed Z, Houinato D, Hocine M, Ranger-Rogez S, Denis F. Prevalence of serum markers of hepatitis B and C in blood donors and pregnant women in Algeria. Bull Soc Pathol Exot. 1995;88:225–8.

45. Aidaoui M, Bouzbid S, Laouar M. Seroprevalence of HIV infection in pregnant women in the Annaba region (Algeria). Rev Epidemiol Sante Publique. 2008;56:261–6. doi:10.1016/j.respe.2008.05.023.

46. Fadlalla FA, Mohamoud YA, Mumtaz GR, Abu-Raddad LJ. The epidemiology of hepatitis C virus in the Maghreb region: systematic review and meta-analyses. PLoS One. 2015;10, e0121873. doi:10.1371/journal.pone.0121873.

47. Tiwari BR, Ghimire P, Kandel SR, Rajkarnikar M. Seroprevalence of HBV and HCV in blood donors: A study from regional blood transfusion services of Nepal. Asian J Transfus Sci. 2010;4:91–3. doi:10.4103/0973-6247.67026.

7

Rare bacterial isolates causing bloodstream infections in Ethiopian patients with cancer

Balew Arega[1,2], Yimtubezinash Wolde-Amanuel[2], Kelemework Adane[3*], Ezra Belay[4], Abdulaziz Abubeker[5] and Daniel Asrat[2]

Abstract

Background: In recent years, saprophytic bacteria have been emerging as potential human pathogens causing life-threatening infections in patients with malignancies. However, evidence is lacking concerning such bacteria, particularly in sub-Saharan countries. This study was designed to determine the spectrum and drug resistance profile of the rare bacterial pathogens causing bloodstream infections (BSIs) in febrile cancer patients at a referral hospital in Ethiopia.

Methods: Between December 2011 and June 2012, blood samples were collected from 107 patients with cancer in Tikur Anbessa hospital. Culturing was performed using the blood culture bottles and solid media and the microorganisms were identified using the gram staining and APINE identification kits (Biomerieux, France). The disk diffusion method was used for the antimicrobial susceptibility testing.

Results: Overall, 13 (12.2%) rare human pathogens were isolated from 107 adult febrile cancer patients investigated. *Aeromonas hydrophilia* species (a fermentative gram-negative rod) was the predominant isolate, 30.8% (4/13), followed by *Chryseomonas luteola* 15.4% (2/13), *Sphignomonas poucimobilis* 15.4% (2/13), *and Pseudomonas fluorescens* 15.4% (2/13). Of the nine isolates tested for a nine set of antibiotics, 89% were resistant to amoxicillin-clavulanic acid, ampicillin, and trimethoprim-sulphamethoxazole.

Conclusions: This study revealed the emergence of saprophytic bacteria as potential drug-resistant nosocomial pathogens in Ethiopian patients with cancer. As these pathogens are ubiquitous in the environment, infection prevention actions should be strengthened in the hospital and early diagnosis and treatment with appropriate antibiotics are warranted for those already infected.

Keywords: Bloodstream infections, Cancer patients, Drug resistance, Ethiopia, Rare bacteria

Background

Patients with cancer are at a high risk of infection and often the focus of the infection is not apparent. Bloodstream infections (BSIs) have been the leading complications in such patients [1, 2]. In adult patients with malignancies, the crude mortality rates of BSIs range from 18%-42% [3, 4]. A variety of factors including frequent hospitalization, exposure to invasive procedures, use of broad-spectrum antibiotics and chemotherapy make cancer patients more susceptible to BSIs [1, 5]. Chemotherapy renders cancer patients to be neutropenic making them more susceptible to potentially life-threatening BSIs [6, 7].

Bacteria are the primary causative agents of BSIs [8, 9]. The gram-positive pathogens such as *Staphylococcus aureus* (prevalence of *S. aureus* ranging from 18% - 35%) [10, 11] and the gram-negative bacteria such as *E. coil* (13% - 23.1%), *K. pneumoniae* (4.6% - 12%) , and/or *P.aeruginosa* (6% - 12.5%) [10, 12, 13] had been reported as the common pathogens causing BSIs in cancer patients. However, in recent years, saprophytic bacteria have been emerging as potential human pathogens causing life-threatening infections in patients with malignancies. A case report from Delhi State Cancer Institute, for example, indicated that *Aeromonas hydrophila*, a saprophyte in the soil, caused a serious soft tissue infection in a woman with

* Correspondence: ingoldmlt@gmail.com
[3]Department of Microbiology and Immunology, College of Health Sciences, Mekelle University, P.O.Box 1872, Mekelle, Ethiopia
Full list of author information is available at the end of the article

breast malignancy [14]. A study from Texas Children's Hospital isolated the plant pathogen *Pantoea agglomerans* from a blood culture of children [15]. Another study from Egypt had also reported the rare bacterial pathogen *Chryseobacterium meningosepticum* from blood cultures of patients with cancer [16].

The spectrum and drug resistance profile of the pathogens causing BSIs in patients with cancer have been reported to show significant fluctuations in different geographical areas and time points [8, 17]. Data regarding the emerging saprophytic potential nosocomial pathogens is limited, particularly in sub-Saharan countries, despite the escalating burden of cancer. This study therefore aimed at determining the spectrum and drug resistance profile of the rare bacterial pathogens causing BSIs in febrile cancer patients at a referral hospital in Ethiopia.

Methods
Study setting, design, and populations
This cross-sectional study was conducted at Tikur Anbessa (Black Lion) referral teaching hospital in Addis Ababa, Ethiopia between December 2011 and June 2012. Tikur Anbessa Hospital is the largest hospital in Ethiopia and is a referral site for patients from all parts of the country. To date, this hospital is the only hospital providing cancer chemotherapy and radiotherapy service in Ethiopia. Cancer patients attending the hospital were our study populations. Providing written informed consent, being an age of $\geq$ 18 years and not being under antibiotic treatment during the study time were the inclusion criteria for this study. All inpatient and outpatient adult febrile cancer patients ($n = 107$) attending the Internal Medicine Department and Oncology-Radiotherapy Center of the hospital during the study period were included in the study conveniently.

Specimen collection
From each patient included in the study, venous blood was drawn aseptically. Two sets (one-bottle set) of 10 ml for each patient were collected within 24 hours. Then, we poured blood samples into the blood-culture bottles and we incubated them aerobically at 37 °C. We inspected these cultures daily for up to 7 days. Sociodemographic and other relevant data were also collected using structured questionnaire.

Blood culture and identification
We performed gram staining for broths that showed visible growth (as evidenced by the appearance of turbidity, growing colonies on top of the red cells ('cotton balls'), hemolysis, and /or gas bubbles). If growth was not detected within 24-hours, we undertook blind sub-

culturing to recover pathogenic microorganisms. For bottles that did not show growth until 7 days, we performed terminal sub-culturing. Preliminary identification of the pathogens from the tubes that showed growth was done by gram staining.

Then, we sub-cultured the organisms on Blood agar, Chocolate agar, and MacConkey agar. We incubated these cultures aerobically at 37^0C and growth was inspected for up to 24-48 hours. We used APINE identification kits (Biomerieux, France) to identify the non-fermentative gram-negative bacilli.

Antimicrobial susceptibility testing
We used the disk diffusion method for antimicrobial susceptibility testing following standard operating procedures. We prepared suspensions equivalent to a 0.5 McFarland standard by mixing 3-5 bacterial colonies from a pure culture with 5 ml of saline. We then distributed the bacterial suspension evenly over the entire surface of Mueller-Hinton agar using a sterile cotton swab. The inoculated Muller-Hinton plates were left at room temperature for 3-5 minutes to dry and a nine set of antibiotic discs (Oxoid) were dispensed on the surface of each plate. The antibiotics used included amoxicillin-clavulanate (AMC) (30µg), chloramphenicol (C) (30 µg), tetracycline (TTC) (30 µg), trimethoprim-sulphamethoxazole (SXT) (25µg), ceftriaxone (CRO) (30 µg), ampicillin (AMP) (10 µg), nalidixic acid (NA) (30 µg), gentamicin (CN) (10 µg), and ciprofloxacin (CIP) (5 µg). After incubation of the plates at 37^0C for 24-48 hours, we measured the diameters of the zone of inhibition to the nearest millimeter using a caliper. The isolates were then classified as sensitive, intermediate, and resistant according to the standardized table supplied by the Clinical Laboratory Standard Institute (CLSI). *E. coli* (ATCC-25922) and *P.aeruginosa* (ATCC-27853) were used as standard reference strains for quality control of the culture and antimicrobial susceptibility testing.

Data analysis
Data were entered using Epi Data entry version 3.1 software and analyzed using SPSS version 16. Descriptive statistics was used to depict the frequencies and proportions.

Results
Patient profiles
The study population has been previously described (in press). Briefly, of 107 adult febrile cancer patients enrolled, 52 (48.6%) were males and 55 (51.4%) females with a mean age of 35.5 $\pm$ 14.64 years. The majority of the study participants, 81 (75.7%), suffered from leukemia and 56 (52.3%) were neutropenic. More than half of the neutropenic patients were with leukemia. Seventy-six (71%) of them had taken cancer therapy in which all received chemotherapy; none had received

radiation therapy. About 57% (61/107) had received antibiotics previously of which 64% (39/61) received ceftriaxone, 18% (11/61) ceftriaxone, and vancomycin and the remaining 18% (11/61) received ceftriaxone, vancomycin, and ciprofloxacin. None of the 107 patients investigated had either central intravenous device or indwelling intravenous devices during our investigation, but 76% (81/107) had total parenteral nutrition (TPN) devices.

Bacterial isolates and their drug susceptibility pattern

Of 107 adult febrile cancer patients investigated for BSIs, 71 bacterial pathogens were isolated of which 13 (18.3%) were rare human pathogens. The characteristics and drug resistance profile of other pathogens have been previously described (in press). Out of the 13 rare bacterial pathogens, the majority 30.8% (4/13) were *Aeromonas hydrophilia* species (a fermentative gram-negative rod). *Chryseomonas luteola, Sphignomonas poucimobilis, and Pseudomonas fluorescens* each accounted two isolates while *Chryseobacterium meningosepticum, Pantoea agglomerans,* and *Serratia ficaria* accounted one isolate for each. The antimicrobial susceptibility results were available for nine of the 13 (69.2%) isolates. Eighty-nine percent of these isolates were resistant to amoxicillin-clavulanic acid, ampicillin, and trimethoprim-sulphamethoxazole (Table 1).

Discussion

This study is the first to describe the rare bacterial isolates as causes of BSIs in Ethiopian patients with cancer. The fermentative gram-negative rod, *Aeromonas*

hydrophilia species, was the most predominant isolate of the rare bacteria isolated. Previous studies from Egypt had also reported this pathogen as an agent of BSIs in patients with hematological malignancy [18, 19]. *Aeromonas* species are widely distributed in the aquatic environment and patients acquire infection by oral consumption or direct contact with contaminated water or seafood [20]. *Aeromonas* may cause serious fatal infections such as hepatobiliary infection, invasive skin and soft tissue infections, primary bacteremia, burn infections, pleuropulmonary infection, meningitis and endocarditis in the immunocompromised patient [21, 22]. Though *Aeromonas* isolates are susceptible to a broad range of antibiotics, some species may produce beta-lactamase which makes them resistant to ampicillin and first-generation cephalosporins [23]. In this study, all the four isolates were resistant to amoxicillin-clavulanic acid, ampicillin, and trimethoprim-sulphamethoxazole suggesting the emergence of this saprophytic pathogen as a drug resistant potential nosocomial pathogen in Ethiopia.

Chryseomonas luteola, a saprophyte found in the soil and water, has only rarely been reported as a human bacterial pathogen [24, 25]. In a case report from a Moroccan University Hospital, this bacterium was indicated causing serious infection in a newborn with a respiratory failure [24]. In the current study, we isolated two *Chryseomonas luteola* pathogens from neutropenic patients with non-Hodgkin lymphoma. In the previous reports, *Chryseomonas luteola* isolates showed variable sensitivity to ampicillin,

Table 1 Susceptibility patterns of the rare bacteria isolated from blood cultures of febrile cancer patients at Tikur Anbessa specialized hospital, Addis Ababa, Ethiopia; December 2011 and June 2012

Organisms		Antimicrobial drugs, n (%)								
		AMC	AMP	C	CRO	SXT	TTC	CIP	NA	CN
Aeromonas hydrophilia (n=4)	S	-	-	1 (25)	1 (25)	-	-	3 (75)	2 (50)	4 (100)
	I	-	-	1 (25)	-	-	1 (25)	-	-	-
	R	4 (100)	4 (100)	2 (50)	3 (75)	4 (100)	3 (75)	1 (25)	2 (50)	-
Chryseomonas luteola (n=2)	S	-	-	-	-	-	2 (100)	2 (100)	2 (100)	2 (100)
	I	-	-	-	-	-	-	-	-	
	R	2 (100)	2 (100)	2 (100)	2 (100)	2 (100)	-	-	-	-
Pseudomonas fluorescens (n=2)	S	-	-	1 (50)	2 (100)		1 (50)	1 (50)	1 (50)	2 (100)
	I	-	-	-	-	-	-	-	-	-
	R	2 (100)	2 (100)	1 (50)	-	2 (100)	1 (50)	1 (50)	1 (50)	-
Serracia ficaria (n=1)	S	1 (100)	1 (100)	1 (100)	-	1 (100)	1 (100)	1 (100)	-	-
	I	-	-	-	-	-	-	-	-	
	R	-	-	-	-	-	1 (100)	-	-	1 (100)
Total (n = 9)	S	1 (11.1)	1 (11.1)	3 (33.3)		1 (11.1)	3 (33.3)	7 (77.8)	5 (62.5)[a]	8 (88.9)
	I	-	-	1 (11.1)		-	1 (11.1	-	-	
	R	8 (88.9)	8 (88.9)	5 (55.6)		8 (88.9)	5 (55.5)	2 (22.2)	3 (37.5)[a]	1 (11.1)

[a] = the denominator is 8, *S* Sensitive, *I* Intermediate, *R* Resistant, *AMC* Amoxicillin-clavulanic acid, *AMP* Ampicillin, *C* Chloramphenicol, *CRO* Ceftriaxone, *SXT* Trimethoprim-sulphamethoxazole, *TTC* Teteracycline, *CIP* Ciprofloxacin *GN* Gentamycin, *NA* Nalidixic acid

tetracycline, and co-trimoxazole. In this study, both isolates were resistant to five of the nine antibiotics tested including amoxicillin-clavulanic acid, ampicillin, chloramphenicol, ceftriaxone, and trimethoprim-sulphamethoxazole. This also suggests the emergence of this bacterium as a potential nosocomial pathogen in Ethiopia.

Chryseobacterium meningosepticum was isolated from a blood culture of a leukemic patient. This bacterium was already defined as etiology of bloodstream infection among cancer patients by the Infectious Diseases Society of America [26]. A study from Egypt had also reported this bacterium from blood cultures of patients with cancer [16]. *Chryseobacterium meningosepticum* is found in soil and can survive in chlorine-treated municipal water supplies [27] and could colonize patients via contaminated medical devices involving fluids (respirators, intubation tubes, incubators for newborns, ice chests, syringes, intravascular catheters, etc) [28, 29] and cause severe infections in immunocompromised people and in children [16, 28].

Two isolates of *Sphignomonas poucimobilis* were also observed in this study; one from a 40-year-old female patient with acute leukemia and the other from a 24-year-old female patient with chronic lymphocytic leukemia. These non-fermenting gram-negative bacilli create a significant problem in clinical settings, being the most widespread cause of nosocomial infections. They are opportunistic pathogens that take advantage of underlying conditions and diseases [30]. According to a review of the case reports by Lin *et al*, about 42 isolates of *S.poucimobilis* were indicated as agents of BSIs in cancer patients (mostly in patients with hematological malignancy) [30]. The existence of this bacterium in our setting could pose a challenge in managing and treating patients appropriately as standard methods to undertake antibiotic susceptibility testing are not on hand for this pathogen [30].

Pantoea agglomerans, a very a rare fermentative gram-negative pathogen, was also isolated in our study as an agent of BSIs in patients with acute myeloid leukemia. Previously, this pathogen was isolated from patients with hematological malignancy in Belgium [31]. *Pantoea agglomerans* is a plant pathogen widely distributed in the soil [32]. A review of case reports indicated that *P.agglomerans* was mostly associated with penetrating trauma by vegetative material and catheter-related bacteremia in immunocompromised patients and in children in the hospital [15].

Serratia ficaria has been isolated from human clinical samples in rare instances [33]. Although its pathogenicity was always questionable, *S. ficaria* was later found to be able to cause severe infections (septicemia) or deep suppurations such as gallbladder empyema [34]. Thus, *S. ficaria* is an opportunistic pathogen responsible for colonization or serious infections in compromised patients. In this study, we isolated this organism from a 24-year-old female patient with acute lymphocytic leukemia. Another study in France also isolated *Serratia ficaria* from a blood of 83-year-old adenocarcinoma patient [34]. Other case reports [33, 35] also reported this bacterium from a blood culture of patients with underlying disease other than neoplasm. In previous reports, *S. ficaria* was usually susceptible to numerous antibiotics but always resistant to cephalothin (cefazolin was the prophylactic antibiotic in the present case) [34]. In our study, the *S. ficaria* isolate was susceptible to seven of the nine antibiotics tested while it was resistant to teteracycline and nalidixic acid. We didn't test it against cephalothin (cefazolin).

We also recovered two isolates of *Pseudomonas fluorescens* from blood cultures of male febrile neutropenic patients with hematological malignancy. Previously, *P. fluorescens was* reported from a bone marrow transplant patients with hematological malignancies, who became colonized with the organism from a contaminated water dispenser that supplied bottled natural spring water in a hospital [36]. The case holds also true in our setting where the patients didn't have adequate access to clean water supply. A previous study showed that *P. fluorescens* strains isolated from cancer patients were susceptible to gentamicin, neomycin, tetracyclines, polymyxin B, and colistin and resistant to chloramphenicol, ampicillin, and narrow-spectrum cephalosporin [37, 38]. In the current study, both of our isolates were resistant to amoxicillin-clavulanic acid, ampicillin, and trimethoprim-sulphamethoxazole and one of the strains were resistant to teteracycline, ciprofloxacillin and nalidixic acid. This is of some concern because these classes of antibiotics are commonly recommended for the management of neutropenic sepsis in hematological malignancies.

To mention some of the limitations: first we used only aerobic culture techniques; anaerobic microorganisms that might have been contributing for BSIs were not defined. The fact that we took only blood sample might also have limited the range of bacterial pathogens to be isolated.

Conclusions

This study revealed the emergence of saprophytic bacteria as potential drug-resistant nosocomial pathogens in Ethiopian patients with cancer. The majority of the isolates were resistant to the commonly used chemotherapic antibiotics imposing a challenge to the health care program. As these pathogens are ubiquitous in the environment, infection prevention actions should be strengthened in the hospital and early diagnosis and treatment with appropriate antibiotics are warranted for those already infected.

Acknowledgments
The authors are thankful to all staff members of the Internal Medicine and Oncology-radiotherapy center of Tikur Anbesa Hospital for their collaboration during the data collection. We would also like to thank the School of Graduate study of Addis Ababa University for financing this project.

Funding
This study was financially supported by the School of Graduate Studies of Addis Ababa University. The funder had no role in study design, data collection, and analysis, decision to publish, or preparation of the manuscript.

Authors' contributions
BA, DA, and YW were involved in the study conception and design, culturing and drug susceptibility testing, data analysis and drafting of the manuscript. KA was involved in the data analysis, drafting and writing up of the manuscript and correction of the comments. EB involved in writing up of the manuscript. All authors have read and approved the final version of the manuscript.

Competing interests
The authors declare that there is no any competing interest.

Author details
[1]College of Health Sciences, Debremarkos University, P.O.Box 269, Debremarkos, Ethiopia. [2]Department of Microbiology, Immunology & Parasitology, School of Medicine, College of Health Sciences, Addis Ababa University, Churchill Avenue, P.O. Box 9086, Addis Ababa, Ethiopia. [3]Department of Microbiology and Immunology, College of Health Sciences, Mekelle University, P.O.Box 1872, Mekelle, Ethiopia. [4]Department Medical Biochemistry, College of Health Sciences, Mekelle University, P.O.Box 1872, Mekelle, Ethiopia. [5]Department of Internal Medicine, School of Medicine, College of Health Sciences, Addis Ababa University, Churchill Avenue, P.O. Box 9086, Addis Ababa, Ethiopia.

References
1. Walshe LJ, Malak SF, Eagan J, Sepkowitz KA. Complication rates among cancer patients with peripherally inserted central catheters. *Journal of Clinical Oncology.* 2002;20(15):3276–81.
2. Wisplinghoff H, Bischoff T, Tallent SM, Seifert H, Wenzel RP, Edmond MB. Nosocomial bloodstream infections in US hospitals: analysis of 24,179 cases from a prospective nationwide surveillance study. *Clinical Infectious Diseases.* 2004;39(3):309–17.
3. Fayyaz M, Mirza IA, Ikram A, Hussain A, Ghafoor T, Shujat U. Pathogens Causing Blood Stream Infections and their Drug Susceptibility Profile in Immunocompromised Patients. *Journal of the College of Physicians and Surgeons Pakistan.* 2013;23(12):848–51.
4. Butt T, Afzal RK, Ahmad RN, Salman M, Mahmood A, Anwar M. Bloodstream infections in febrile neutropenic patients: bacterial spectrum and antimicrobial susceptibility pattern. *J Ayub Med Coll Abbottabad.* 2004;16(1):18–22.
5. Leibovici L, Shraga I, Drucker M, Konigsberger H, Samra Z, Pitlik S. The benefit of appropriate empirical antibiotic treatment in patients with bloodstream infection. *JOURNAL OF INTERNAL MEDICINE-OXFORD-.* 1998;244: 379–86.
6. Crawford J, Dale DC, Lyman GH. Chemotherapy-induced neutropenia. *Cancer.* 2004;100(2):228–37.
7. Cebon J, Layton JE, Maher D, Morstyn G. Endogenous hemopoietic growth factors in neutropenia and infection. *British journal of hematology.* 1994; 86(2):265–74.
8. Ramphal R. Changes in the etiology of bacteremia in febrile neutropenic patients and the susceptibilities of the currently isolated pathogens. *Clinical infectious diseases.* 2004;39(Supplement 1):S25–31.
9. Rolston KV, Bodey GP. Bacterial Infections in Cancer Patients. Cancer Supportive Care: Advances in Therapeutic Strategies. 2008;6:73.
10. Mutnick AH, Kirby JT, Jones RN. CANCER resistance surveillance program: initial results from hematology–oncology centers in North America. Annals of Pharmacotherapy. 2003;37(1):47–56.
11. Nejad ZE, Ghafouri E, Farahmandi-Nia Z, Kalantari B, Safari F. Isolation, identification, and profile of antibiotic resistance of bacteria in patients with cancer. Iranian Journal of Medical Sciences. 2015;35(2):109–15.
12. Chen C-Y, Tang J-L, Hsueh P-R, Yao M, Huang S-Y, Chen Y-C, et al. Trends and antimicrobial resistance of pathogens causing bloodstream infections among febrile neutropenic adults with hematological malignancy. *Journal of the Formosan Medical Association=. Taiwan yi zhi.* 2004;103(7):526–32.
13. Zahid KF, Hafeez H, Afzal A. Bacterial spectrum and susceptibility patterns of pathogens in adult febrile neutropenic patients: a comparison between two time periods. *J Ayub Med Coll Abbottabad.* 2009;21(4):146–9.
14. Baruah FK, Ahmed NH, Grover RK. Surgical site infection caused by Aeromonas hydrophilia in a patient with underlying malignancy. *Journal of clinical and diagnostic research: JCDR.* 2015;9(1):DD01.
15. Cruz AT, Cazacu AC, Allen CH. Pantoea agglomerans, a plant pathogen causing human disease. *Journal of Clinical Microbiology.* 2007;45(6):1989–92.
16. El-Mahallawy HA, El-Wakil M, Moneer MM, Shalaby L. Antibiotic resistance is associated with longer bacteremic episodes and worse outcome in febrile neutropenic children with cancer. *Pediatric blood & cancer.* 2011;57(2):283–8.
17. Montassier E, Batard E, Gastinne T, Potel G, de La Cochetière M. Recent changes in bacteremia in patients with cancer: a systematic review of epidemiology and antibiotic resistance. *European journal of clinical microbiology & infectious diseases.* 2013;32(7):841–50.
18. Baskaran ND, Gan GG, Adeeba K, Sam I-C. Bacteremia in patients with febrile neutropenia after chemotherapy at a university medical center in Malaysia. *International Journal of Infectious Diseases.* 2007;11(6):513–7.
19. Ashour HM, El-Sharif A. Microbial spectrum and antibiotic susceptibility profile of gram-positive aerobic bacteria isolated from cancer patients. *Journal of Clinical Oncology.* 2007;25(36):5763–9.
20. Igbinosa IH, Igumbor EU, Aghdasi F, Tom M, Okoh AI. Emerging Aeromonas species infections and their significance in public health. *The Scientific World Journal.* 2012;2012
21. Okumura K, Shoji F, Yoshida M, Mizuta A, Makino I, Higashi H. Severe sepsis caused by Aeromonas hydrophila in a patient using tocilizumab: a case report. *J Med Case Rep.* 2011;5:499.
22. Janda JM, Abbott SL. The genus Aeromonas: taxonomy, pathogenicity, and infection. *Clinical microbiology reviews.* 2010;23(1):35–73.
23. Medeiros AA. Evolution and dissemination of β-lactamases accelerated by generations of β-lactam antibiotics. *Clinical Infectious Diseases.* 1997; 24(Supplement 1):S19–45.
24. Chihab W, Alaoui AS, Amar M. Chryseomonas luteola identified as the source of serious infections in a Moroccan University Hospital. *Journal of clinical microbiology.* 2004;42(4):1837–9.
25. Kostman JR, Solomon F, Fekete T. Infections with Chryseomonas luteola (CDC group Ve-1) and Flavimonas oryzihabitans (CDC group Ve-2) in neurosurgical patients. *Review of Infectious Diseases.* 1991;13(2):233–6.
26. Hugues W, Armstrong D, Bodey G, Bow E, Brown A, Calandra T. Guidelines for the use of antimicrobial agents in neutropenic patients with cancer. *Clin Infect Dis.* 2002;34(6):730–51.
27. Bloch KC, Nadarajah R, Jacobs R. Chryseobacterium meningosepticum: An Emerging Pathogen Among Immunocompromised Adults Report of 6 Cases and Literature Review. *Medicine.* 1997;76(1):30–41.
28. Güngör S, Özen M, Akinci A, Durmaz R. A Chryseobacterium meningosepticum outbreak in a neonatal ward. *Infection Control & Hospital Epidemiology.* 2003;24(08):613–7.
29. Vandamme P, Bernardet J-F, Segers P, Kersters K, Holmes B. NOTES: New Perspectives in the Classification of the Flavobacteria: Description of Chryseobacterium gen. nov., Bergeyella gen. nov., and Empedobacter nom. rev. *International Journal of Systematic and Evolutionary Microbiology.* 1994;44(4):827–31.
30. Lin J-N, Lai C-H, Chen Y-H, Lin H-L, Huang C-K, Chen W-F, et al. Sphingomonas paucimobilis bacteremia in humans: 16 case reports and a literature review. *Journal of Microbiology, Immunology and Infection.* 2010; 43(1):35–42.

31. Mebis J, Jansens H, Minalu G, Molenberghs G, Schroyens W, Gadisseur A, et al. Long-term epidemiology of bacterial susceptibility profiles in adults suffering from febrile neutropenia with hematologic malignancy after antibiotic change. *Infection and drug resistance.* 2010;3:53.

32. Andersson A, Weiss N, Rainey F, Salkinoja-Salonen M. Dust-borne bacteria in animal sheds, schools and children's day care centres. *Journal of applied microbiology.* 1999;86(4):622–34.

33. Anahory T, Darbas H, Ongaro O, Jean-Pierre H, Mion P. Serratia ficaria: a misidentified or unidentified rare cause of human infections in fig tree culture zones. *Journal of clinical microbiology.* 1998;36(11):3266–72.

34. Darbas H, Jean-Pierre H, Paillisson J. Case report and review of septicemia due to Serratia ficaria. *Journal of clinical microbiology.* 1994;32(9):2285–8.

35. Gill V, Farmer J, Grimont P, Asbury M, McIntosh C. Serratia ficaria isolated from a human clinical specimen. *Journal of clinical microbiology.* 1981;14(2):234–6.

36. Wong V, Levi K, Baddal B, Turton J, Boswell TC. Spread of Pseudomonas fluorescens due to contaminated drinking water in a bone marrow transplant unit. *Journal of clinical microbiology.* 2011;49(6):2093–6.

37. Moody MR, Young VM, Kenton DM. In vitro antibiotic susceptibility of pseudomonads other than Pseudomonas aeruginosa recovered from cancer patients. *Antimicrobial agents and chemotherapy.* 1972;2(5):344–9.

38. Kenneth V, Rolston I. Infections in Cancer Patients with Solid Tumors: A Review. Infect Dis Ther. 2017;6(1):69–83.

8

LPS promotes resistance to TRAIL-induced apoptosis in pancreatic cancer

Katharina Beyer[1,2*†], Lars Ivo Partecke[1†], Felicitas Roetz[1†], Herbert Fluhr[4], Frank Ulrich Weiss[3], Claus-Dieter Heidecke[1] and Wolfram von Bernstorff[1]

Abstract

Background: Though TRAIL has been hailed as a promising drug for tumour treatment, it has been observed that many tumour cells have developed escape mechanisms against TRAIL-induced apoptosis. As a receptor of LPS, TLR 4, which is expressed on a variety of cancer cells, can be associated with TRAIL-resistance of tumour cells and tumour progression as well as with the generation of an anti-tumour immune response.

Methods: In this study, the sensitivity to TRAIL-induced apoptosis as well as the influence of LPS-co-stimulation on the cell viability of the pancreatic cancer cell lines PANC-1, BxPC-3 and COLO 357 was examined by FACS analyses and a cell viability assay. Subsequently, the expression of TRAIL-receptors was detected via FACS analyses. Levels of osteoprotegerin (OPG) were also determined using an enzyme-linked immunosorbent assay.

Results: PANC-1 cells were shown to be resistant to TRAIL-induced apoptosis. This was accompanied by significantly increased osteoprotegerin levels and a significantly decreased expression of DR4.
In contrast, TRAIL significantly induced apoptosis in COLO 357 cells and to a lesser degree in BxPC-3 cells. Co-stimulation of COLO 357 as well as BxPC-3 cells combining TRAIL and LPS resulted in a significant decrease in TRAIL-induced apoptosis. In COLO 357 cells TRAIL-stimulation decreased the levels of OPG thereby not altering the expression of the TRAIL-receptors 1–4 resulting in a high susceptibility to TRAIL-induced apoptosis. Co-stimulation with LPS and TRAIL completely reversed the effect of TRAIL on OPG levels reaching a 2-fold increase beyond the level of non-stimulated cells resulting in a lower susceptibility to apoptosis.
In BxPC-3, TRAIL stimulation decreased the expression of DR4 and significantly increased the decoy receptors TRAIL-R3 and TRAIL-R4 leading to a decrease in TRAIL-induced apoptosis. OPG levels remained unchanged. Co-stimulation with TRAIL and LPS further enhanced the changes in TRAIL-receptor-expression promoting apoptosis resistance.

Conclusions: Here it has been shown that TRAIL-resistance in pancreatic cancer cells can be mediated by the inflammatory molecule LPS as well as by different expression patterns of functional and non-functional TRAIL-receptors.

Keywords: TRAIL, LPS, Pancreas cancer, Apoptosis, Cell lines

* Correspondence: katharina.beyer2@charite.de
The present work was partly presented at the 44th European Pancreatic Club Meeting. This article contains parts of the thesis of F. Rötz.
†Equal contributors
[1]Department of General, Visceral, Thoracic and Vascular Surgery, Universitätsmedizin Greifswald, Greifswald, Germany
[2]Department of General, Visceral and Vascular Surgery, Charité Universitätsmedizin Berlin, Campus Benjamin Franklin, Hindenburgdamm 30, 12203 Berlin, Germany
Full list of author information is available at the end of the article

Background

Pancreatic cancer remains a devastating disease which displays resistance to even the most aggressive treatment regime [1]. There is increasing evidence that the development and progression of exocrine pancreatic cancer can be promoted by chronic inflammation [2–4]. This connection of inflammation with tumour progression can be mediated by components of the bacterial cell wall like lipopolysaccharide (LPS) from gram-negative bacteria [5]. LPS interacts with immune cells of the tumour microenvironment which, in turn, is especially important in tumour development and progression [2, 6]. Additionally, LPS can directly interact with pancreatic cancer cells increasing the invasive ability of these cells [5]. LPS is recognized by the Toll-like receptor (TLR) 4. TLRs are a family of pattern recognition receptors exerting an important role in host defence against infections [7]. Apart from the expression of TLR4 by cells of the immune system, TLRs have been linked to several cancers including pancreatic cancer [5, 8–14]. In these tumours, LPS can lead to activation of NFkB thus promoting cancer progression and chemoresistance [13].

TNF-related apoptosis inducing ligand (TRAIL) is involved in tumour surveillance. It induces apoptosis upon binding to its receptors death receptor (DR) 4 (TRAIL-receptor 1) and DR5 (TRAIL-receptor 2). Additionally, there are three more TRAIL receptors lacking a functionally active death domain: TRAIL-receptor (TRAIL-R) 3 (decoy receptor 1 or DcR1), TRAIL-R 4 (decoy receptor 2 or DcR2) and the soluble receptor osteoprotegerin (OPG). Thus, they are unable to transmit apoptosis-inducing signals [15]. Several factors determine whether a cell becomes apoptotic following TRAIL-binding: Firstly, many cells express these decoy-receptors inhibiting TRAIL at the membrane level: TRAIL-R3 (DcR1) competes for TRAIL binding, sequestering TRAIL in lipid rafts. TRAIL-R4 (DcR2) inhibits activation of caspase 8 through the formation of heteromeric complexes [16]. Secondly, the cell cycle progression can change the balance of pro- and anti-apoptotic proteins. These proteins collectively help to regulate the signal generated by binding of TRAIL to DR4 or DR5. Thus, a preponderance of anti-apoptotic proteins may result in TRAIL-resistance [17]. Especially members of the Bcl-2 family, cFLIP and IAPs (inhibitor of apoptosis proteins) contribute to TRAIL receptor-signal-transduction pathways leading to TRAIL resistance [17–19].

Despite TRAIL-R1/2 – expression, most pancreatic cancer cells show resistance to TRAIL-induced apoptosis [20–23] mediated by a high activation level of NF-kappaB [24] which enhances the expression of inhibitors of apoptosis like XIAP and FLIP [20–23].

In human colon cancer cell lines, it has been detected by Tang et al. [25] that LPS binding to TLR-4 did not affect the expression of TLR4 nor proliferation of respective cell lines. However, LPS activated NFkB thereby inducing resistance to TRAIL-induced apoptosis [25].

For human lung cancer cell lines, it has been shown that TLR 4 ligation by LPS led to production of anti-inflammatory cytokines as well as resistance of human lung cancer cells to TNFa- and TRAIL-mediated apoptosis. Furthermore, binding of LPS to its receptor TLR4 can activate NFkB thereby promoting resistance to TRAIL – induced apoptosis [26].

In the present study, the effects of LPS stimulation on TRAIL-induced apoptosis in several pancreatic cancer cell lines were examined.

Methods

Cell lines

The human pancreatic cancer cell lines PANC-1 and BxPC-3 were obtained from the ATCC (*American Type Culture Collection, Manassas, VA, USA*). The cell line COLO 357 was obtained from ECACC (European Collection of Authenticated Cell Cultures, London, UK). Cells were maintained in RPMI 1640 (Gibco cell culture, Karlsruhe, Germany) supplemented with 10% heat-inactivated fetal bovine serum (FCS) (PAA, Pasching, Austria) and 1% penicilline/streptomycine (Gibco cell culture) at 37 °C in a 5% CO_2 atmosphere at 85% humidity.

LPS and TRAIL stimulation

Human recombinant TRAIL (purity 95%, endotoxin level < 1.0 EU per 1 g protein) was purchased from Biomol (Hamburg, Germany) and dissolved in RPMI medium. Lipopolysaccharide (E. coli) was purchased from Sigma Aldrich (Munich, Germany). Cells were seeded in six well plates. After 12 h, respective amounts of TRAIL (100 ng/ml or 300 ng/ml) and/or LPS (1 µg/ml) were added and cells were stimulated for 24 h.

Detection of apoptotic cells

Apoptotic cell death was assessed using an Annexin V Apoptosis Detection Kit (BD Bioscience, Heidelberg, Germany) according to manufacturer's instructions. Annexin V-positive cells were detected by flow cytometry (FACS Canto, Becton Dickinson, Heidelberg, Germany).

To confirm the results, a propidium iodide cell cycle analysis was performed. For this assay, cells were harvested, stored on ice and washed three times with 2% FCS in PBS. A total of 10^5 cells were fixed in 70% ethanol and incubated with 0.025 M sodium citrate and 0.067 M disodium phosphate. The pellets were washed with PBS plus 5% FCS, resuspended in 30 µl RNase (1 mg/mL; Qiagen, Hilden, Germany) and stained with 25 µg/mL propidium iodide (Sigma Aldrich). Apoptosis was measured by flow cytometry (FACS Canto, Becton

Dickinson, Heidelberg, Germany) employing a standard protocol as described before [27]. In detail, cells were stored on ice and washed 3 times with 2% fetal calf serum (Biochrom) in PBS. A total of 10^5 cells were fixed in 70% ethanol and incubated with 0.025 M sodium citrate and 0.067 M disodium phosphate at pH 7.8 at room temperature. The pellets were washed with PBS plus 5% FCS, resuspended in 30 µL RNase (1 mg/mL; Qiagen, Hilden, Germany) and stained with 25 g/mL propidium iodide (Sigma Aldrich, Munich, Germany). Apoptosis was measured by FlowCytometry (FACS Canto, Becton Dickinson). Debris were gated out in the FSC versus SSC plot. Singlets were manually gated in the FL2A versus FL2W plot. The hypodiploid DNA peaks in singlevariable DNA histograms were identified. Data were analysed using BD CellQuest Pro.

Cell viability assay
A Cell Titer Blue Assay (Promega, Mannheim, Germany) was performed according to the manufacturer's instructions. In brief, Cell Titer Blue substrates were added and plates were incubated for 4 h at 37 °C. Subsequently, fluorescence (excitation at 544 nm and emission at 590 nm) was measured on a plate reader. Triplicates were run for each measurement and means were calculated. Controls without cells were run in parallel.

FACS analyses of TRAIL-receptors
After stimulation cells were harvested using accutase (Sigma Aldrich) and washed with PBS. After blocking with FcBlock (BD Bioscience, Heidelberg, Germany) cells were labelled with appropriate antibodies according to the manufacturer's instructions. Purified mouse monoclonal antibodies of anti-human DR4, anti-human DR5, anti-human DcR1 and anti-human DcR2 as well as appropriate secondary antibodies and isotype controls were purchased from Pierce (ThermoFisher Scientific, Schwerte, Germany). FACS analyses were performed using the above flow cytometer. FACS data were analysed using WinMDI.

Osteoprotegerin ELISA
Levels of osteoprotegerin within the cell culture supernatants were detected using an osteoprotegerin – ELISA (Bender MedSystems, Vienna, Austria) according to the manufacturer's recommondations.

Real time quantitative PCR
After stimulation of respective cell lines, cells were harvested and washed with PBS. RNA was extracted using an RNeasy kit (Qiagen, Hilden, Germany) and quantified by spectrophotometry. Subsequently, cDNA was prepared using an RT2 PCR Array first strand kit (Qiagen).

Respective primers (i.e. TLR4, GAPDH and becta-actin) (Qiagen) were used according to the manufacturer's recommandations. Realtime PCR amplification was conducted using an ABI Prism 7000 (ThermoFisher Scientific). Data were analysed using a SuperArray PCR Data analyses software using the comparative threshold method. Data were normalized to the house keeping genes GAPDH and beta-actin.

Statistics
Results were statistically analysed using the program Graph Pad Prism for Macintosh. The Mann Whitney U test was employed to compare means of values of experiments in order to test two independent samples. An ANOVA test was employed to compare more than two independent samples. A p-value below 0.05 was considered to be statistically significant. All data are expressed as mean standard error of the mean.

Results
TRAIL – stimulation decreased viability of COLO 357 and BxPC-3 whereas viability of PANC-1 cells remained almost unchanged
To determine the impact of TRAIL-stimulation on cell viability, cell cultures of PANC-1, BxPC-3 and COLO 357 were TRAIL-stimulated for 24 h and cell viability was determined by a CellTiter Blue Assay. In COLO 357 cells, the mean fluorescence intensity (MFI) ratio was 43256 ± 5347 without stimulation. TRAIL-stimulation decreased the MFI ratio in a dose-dependent manner (10 ng/ml: 33701 ± 3486 ($p = 0.17$, $n = 5$); 100 ng/ml 11213 ± 2784 ($p = 0.0007$ when compared to non-stimulated control; $p = 0.001$ when compared to 10 ng/ml TRAIL; $n = 5$); 300 ng/ml 7276 ± 589 ($p = 0.0002$ when compared to non-stimulated control, $p = 0.0001$ when compared to 10 ng/ml TRAIL, $p = 0.01$ when compared to 100 ng/ml TRAIL; $n = 5$; Fig. 1a).

In BxPC-3 cell cultures, stimulation with 10 ng/ml TRAIL did not significantly alter the cell viability (MFI ratio 29644 ± 1356 versus 31537 ± 479, $p = 0.22$; $n = 5$; Fig. 1a). However, higher concentrations of TRAIL led to decreased amounts of viable cells (100 ng/ml TRAIL: 18292 ± 1189 ($p = 0.0002$ when compared to non-stimulated control, $p = 0.0001$ when compared to 10 ng/ml TRAIL); 300 ng/ml TRAIL: 11853 ± 589 ($p = 0.0001$ when compared to non-stimulated control, $p = 0.0001$ when compared to 10 ng/ml TRAIL, $p = 0.0012$ when compared to 100 ng/ml TRAIL); $n = 5$; Fig. 1a). The pancreatic cancer cell line PANC-1 was the most resistant pancreatic cancer cell line of those tested. TRAIL-stimulation with at least 300 ng/ml did significantly reduce cell viability but only to a minor degree (without stimulation: 59872 ± 548; 10 ng/ml TRAIL: 58714 ± 1125; 100 ng/ml TRAIL: 58562 ± 1593; 300 ng/ml

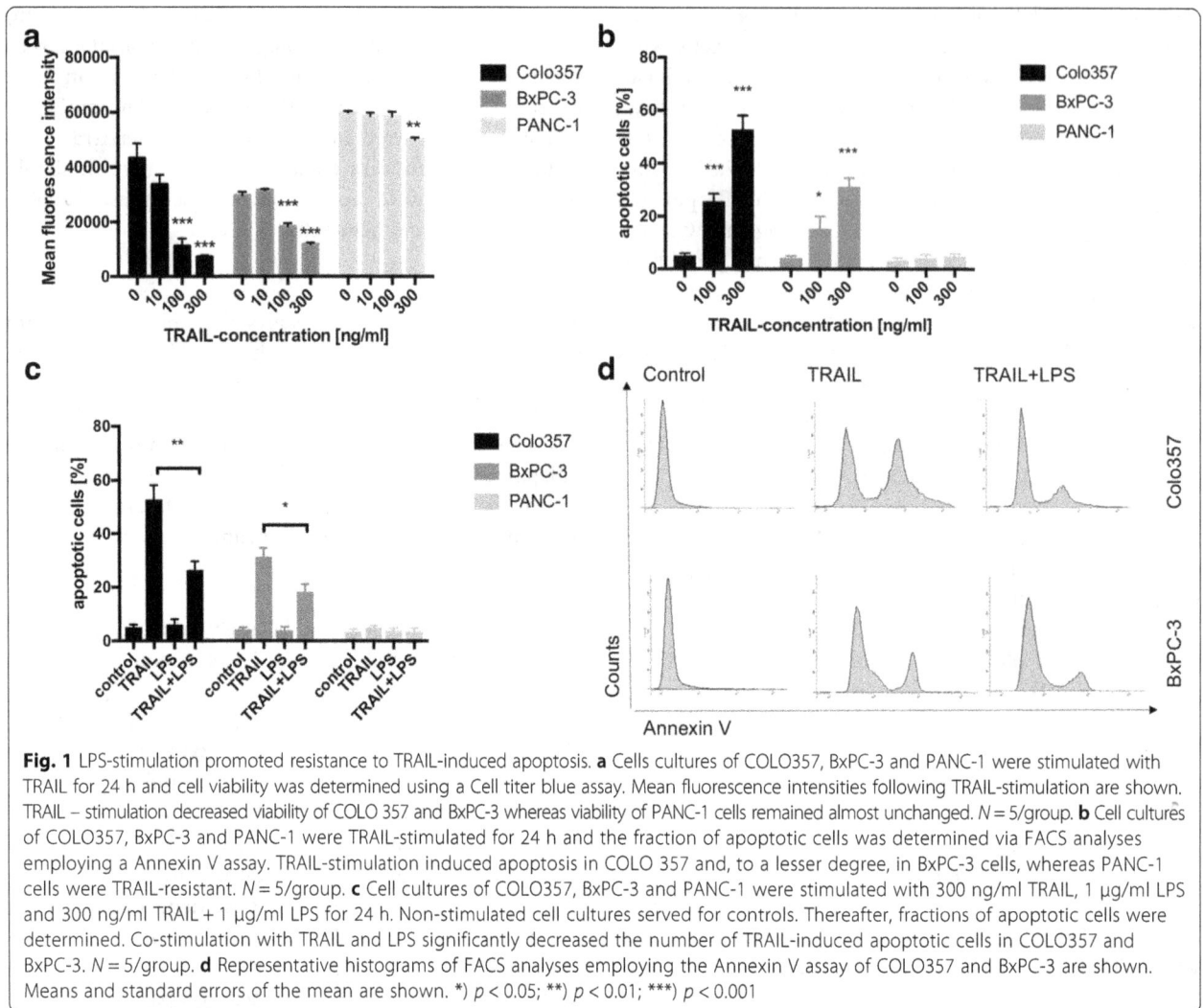

Fig. 1 LPS-stimulation promoted resistance to TRAIL-induced apoptosis. **a** Cells cultures of COLO357, BxPC-3 and PANC-1 were stimulated with TRAIL for 24 h and cell viability was determined using a Cell titer blue assay. Mean fluorescence intensities following TRAIL-stimulation are shown. TRAIL – stimulation decreased viability of COLO 357 and BxPC-3 whereas viability of PANC-1 cells remained almost unchanged. $N = 5$/group. **b** Cell cultures of COLO357, BxPC-3 and PANC-1 were TRAIL-stimulated for 24 h and the fraction of apoptotic cells was determined via FACS analyses employing a Annexin V assay. TRAIL-stimulation induced apoptosis in COLO 357 and, to a lesser degree, in BxPC-3 cells, whereas PANC-1 cells were TRAIL-resistant. $N = 5$/group. **c** Cell cultures of COLO357, BxPC-3 and PANC-1 were stimulated with 300 ng/ml TRAIL, 1 µg/ml LPS and 300 ng/ml TRAIL + 1 µg/ml LPS for 24 h. Non-stimulated cell cultures served for controls. Thereafter, fractions of apoptotic cells were determined. Co-stimulation with TRAIL and LPS significantly decreased the number of TRAIL-induced apoptotic cells in COLO357 and BxPC-3. $N = 5$/group. **d** Representative histograms of FACS analyses employing the Annexin V assay of COLO357 and BxPC-3 are shown. Means and standard errors of the mean are shown. *) $p < 0.05$; **) $p < 0.01$; ***) $p < 0.001$

TRAIL: 49993 ± 783 ($p = 0.001$ when compared to 300 ng/ml TRAIL; $n = 5$) (Fig. 1a).

TRAIL-stimulation induced apoptosis in COLO 357 and, to a lesser degree, in BxPC-3 cells, whereas PANC-1 cells were TRAIL-resistant

The amounts of apoptotic cells induced by TRAIL-stimulation were detected by an Annexin V assay.

Whereas the fraction of apoptotic cells was only $5.1 \pm 0.94\%$ in non-stimulated cell cultures of COLO 357, TRAIL-stimulation for 24 h led to a dose-dependent induction of apoptosis ($25.7 \pm 2.89\%$ in COLO357 cell cultures stimulated with 100 ng/ml TRAIL ($p = 0.0001$) and $52.8 \pm 5.39\%$ following stimulation with 300 ng/ml TRAIL ($p < 0.0001$ when compared to non-stimulated control, $p = 0.0022$ when compared to 100 ng/ml TRAIL; $n = 5$, Fig. 1b).

When examining cell cultures of BxPC-3, TRAIL-stimulation with 100 ng/ml significantly enhanced the fraction of apoptotic cells ($4.2 \pm 0.78\%$ versus $15.43 \pm$

4.58%, $p = 0.042$; $n = 5$; Fig. 1b). This effect was further increased when stimulating with 300 ng/ml TRAIL reaching $31.32 \pm 3.27\%$ apoptotic cells ($p < 0.0001$ when compared to non-stimulated cells, $p = 0.0224$ when compared to 100 ng/ml TRAIL, $n = 5$).

In marked contrast, in PANC-1 cell cultures the fraction of apoptotic cells remained below 5% following TRAIL stimulation indicating that PANC-1 is a cell line resistant to TRAIL-induced apoptosis.

These results indicate that COLO 357 displays a high susceptibility towards TRAIL-induced apoptosis whereas PANC-1 cell cultures are TRAIL-resistant. Cultures of BxPC-3 cells display intermediate sensibilities against TRAIL-induced apoptosis.

These data were confirmed using a propidium iodide cell cycle assay (data not shown).

LPS stimulation inhibited TRAIL-induced apoptosis

To assess an effect of LPS stimulation on apoptosis induction by TRAIL, respective cell cultures were stimulated with 300 ng/ml TRAIL, 1 µg/ml LPS and 300 ng/ml TRAIL + 1 µg/ml LPS. Thereafter, fractions of apoptotic cells were determined. In the TRAIL-resistant pancreatic cancer cell line PANC-1, co-stimulation with LPS and TRAIL did not lead to any significant alterations in the fraction of apoptotic cells. Thus, there were $3.28 \pm 1.0\%$ apoptotic cells without stimulation. LPS-stimulation revealed $3.8 \pm 0.9\%$ apoptotic cells. Stimulation with 300 ng/ml TRAIL and LPS resulted in $3.5 \pm 1.3\%$ apoptotic cells.

In non-stimulated COLO 357 cells, there were $5.1 \pm 0.94\%$ cells apoptotic. TRAIL-stimulation led to $52.8 \pm 5.39\%$ apoptotic cells ($p < 0.0001$, $n = 5$) whereas LPS-stimulation revealed $6.1\% \pm 1.90\%$ apoptotic cells ($n = 5$, $p = 0.66$ when compared to non-stimulated cells, Fig. 1c). Co-stimulation with TRAIL and LPS partially reversed the effect of TRAIL on apoptosis-induction revealing $26.4 \pm 3.21\%$ apoptotic cells ($n = 5$, $p = 0.003$ when compared to TRAIL-stimulated cell cultures; Fig. 1c).

In BxPC-3 cultures, there were $4.2 \pm 0.78\%$ apoptotic cells. TRAIL treatment led to $31.32 \pm 3.27\%$ apoptotic cells ($n = 5$, $p < 0.0001$). Co-stimulation with TRAIL and LPS significantly decreased the number of apoptotic cells

reaching $18.3 \pm 2.84\%$ ($n = 5$, $p = 0.0169$ when compared to TRAIL-stimulated cell cultures) whereas stimulation with LPS alone did not have an impact on apoptosis ($3.9 \pm 1.3\%$, Fig. 1c).

In PANC-1 cells TRAIL-stimulation decreased the expression of DR4, DR5 and DcR2 as well as increasing the expression of osteoprotegerin (OPG)

As shown by FACS analyses, PANC-1 cells expressed the TRAIL-receptors DR4, DR5, DcR1 and DcR2 (Fig. 2a,b). Additionally, significant amounts of OPG were detected in the supernatants of PANC-1 cell cultures (Fig. 2c). Following TRAIL-stimulation, the expression of the death receptors DR4 and DR5 by PANC-1 cells was decreased. For DR4 the mean fluorescence intensity (MFI) was 1397 ± 145.8 for non-stimulated cell cultures, whereas TRAIL-stimulated cell cultures showed a mean fluorescence intensity of 436.8 ± 76.0 ($p = 0.0001$, $n = 6$/group). For DR5 the mean fluorescence intensity was 1025 ± 77.8 in non-stimulated cells, whereas TRAIL-stimulation led to a mean fluorescence intensity of 663.6 ± 72.5 ($p = 0.005$, $n \geq 7$/group). The expression of DcR1 remained unchanged following

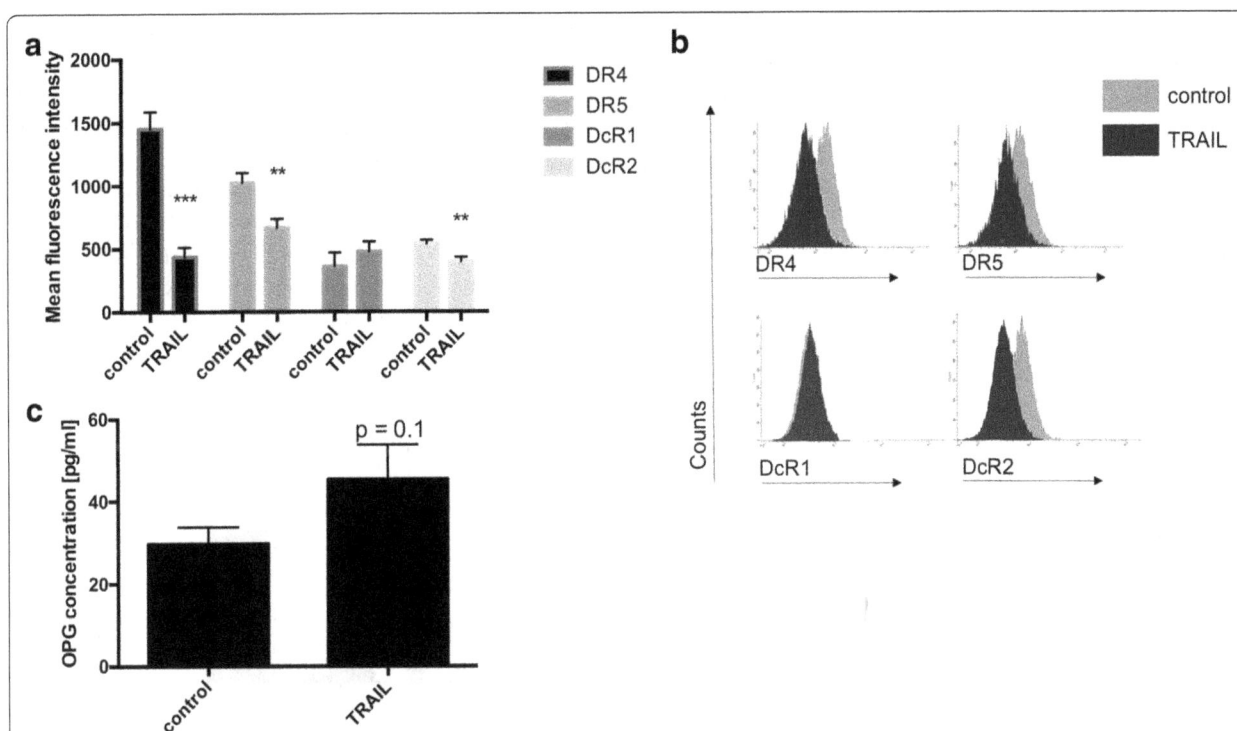

Fig. 2 TRAIL-stimulation decreased the expression of DR4, DR5 and DcR2 as well as increasing the expression of osteoprotegerin (OPG) in PANC-1 cells. Cultures of PANC-1 cells were stimulated with 300 ng/ml TRAIL for 24 h. The expression of the TRAIL-receptors 1–4 was detected by FACS analyses. The concentrations of OPG within the supernatants were determined by ELISA. **a** The expression of respective TRAIL-receptors is expressed as mean fluorescence intensity. TRAIL-stimulation of PANC-1 cells led to significantly decreased expressions of DR4 (TRAIL receptor 1), DR5 (TRAIL receptor 2) and DcR2 (TRAIL receptor 4) whereas the expression of DcR1 (TRAIL receptor 3) remained unaltered. N ≥ 6/group. **b** Representative histograms show the expression of TRAIL-receptors 1 – 4 in TRAIL-stimulated PANC-1 cells and unstimulated controls. **c** The concentration of OPG within the cell culture supernatant increased following TRAIL-stimulation. N = 7/group. Means and standard errors of the mean are shown. *) $p < 0.05$; **) $p < 0.01$; ***) $p < 0.001$

TRAIL-stimulation (MFI 361.4 ± 108.4, $n = 5$ versus 477.0 ± 77.5, $n = 7$, $p = 0.39$). In contrast, the expression of DcR2 significantly decreased following TRAIL-treatment. The MFI of DcR2 was 537.5 ± 28.9 in non-stimulated cell cultures but decreased to 396.8 ± 25.3 following TRAIL-stimulation ($p = 0.009$; Fig. 2a).

The levels of OPG within the cell culture supernatants of PANC-1 cell cultures were 29.71 ± 4.1 pg/ml in non-stimulated controls. TRAIL-stimulation increased the concentration of OPG within the supernatants revealing 45.29 ± 8.5 ($n = 7$, $p = 0.1$).

LPS stimulation significantly affected the impact of TRAIL on TRAIL-receptor-expression

As shown by FACS analyses, COLO 357 cells expressed the TRAIL-receptors 1–4. Neither TRAIL-stimulation alone nor LPS-stimulation alone significantly altered the expression of TRAIL-receptors by COLO 357 cells (Fig. 3a). In contrast, TRAIL-stimulation significantly decreased the levels of OPG: Whereas the concentration of OPG in the cell culture supernatants was 18.67 ± 3.8 pg/ml in non-simulated cell cultures, TRAIL stimulation decreased the OPG secretion reaching 10.60 ± 1.5 pg/ml ($p = 0.06$). This effect was significantly reversed by co-stimulation with LPS: Co-stimulation with TRAIL and LPS increased the OPG concentration reaching 37.83 ± 6.4 pg/ml ($p = 0.0044$ when compared to TRAIL-stimulated COLO 357 cultures, $n = 6$/group, Fig. 3b).

In contrast, in BxPC-3 cells neither stimulation with TRAIL alone nor co-stimulation with TRAIL and LPS significantly altered the levels of OPG: The concentration of OPG within supernatants of BxPC-3 cultures was 11.0 ± 1.1 pg/ml without stimulation and 8.9 ± 1.3 pg/ml following TRAIL-stimulation ($n = 8$/group, $p = 0.66$ when compared to non-stimulated cell cultures). After co-

stimulation with TRAIL and LPS, the concentration of OPG was determined as 7.5 ± 0.8 pg/ml ($n = 8$/group, $p = 0.25$ when compared to TRAIL-stimulated cell cultures, Fig. 4b).

However, TRAIL stimulation significantly decreased the expression of DR4 whereas the expression of DR5 was increased albeit not to a significant degree (DR4: 1908 ± 296.6 for non-stimulated cell cultures versus 722.4 ± 86.0 for TRAIL-stimulated cell cultures, $n = 6$, $p = 0.0009$; DR5: 866.2 ± 77.6 versus 1018 ± 22.0, $p = 0.08$). In contrast, the expression of the decoy receptors DcR1 and DcR2 was increased in TRAIL-stimulated BxPC-3 cell cultures. The mean fluorescence intensity for DcR1 was 783.9 ± 46.7 for non-stimulated cultures of BxPC-3 and TRAIL-treatment significantly increased the expression of DcR1 reaching a mean fluorescence intensity of 1083.0 ± 52.7 ($n = 7$, $p = 0.0009$). Regarding the expression of DcR2 in BxPC-3 cell cultures, the mean fluorescence intensity was 287.4 ± 24.5. This was significantly increased following TRAIL-stimulation to a mean fluorescence intensity of 522.3 ± 40.9 ($n = 8$, $p = 0.0002$, Fig. 4a).

Co-stimulation with TRAIL and LPS significantly further decreased the expression of DR4 and further increased the expression of DcR2 by BxPC-3 cell cultures: The expression of DR4 by BxPC-3 cell cultures decreased from 722.4 ± 86.0 in TRAIL-stimulated cell cultures to 440.0 ± 81.6 in cell cultures co-stimulated with LPS and TRAIL ($n = 6$, $p = 0.03$, Fig. 4a).

Regarding the expression of DcR2 by BxPC-3 cell cultures, the mean fluorescence raised from 522.3 ± 40.9 in TRAIL-stimulated cell cultures to 631.8 ± 69.0 following co-stimulation with TRAIL and LPS ($n = 8$, $p = 0.1$). However, this effect did not reach significance.

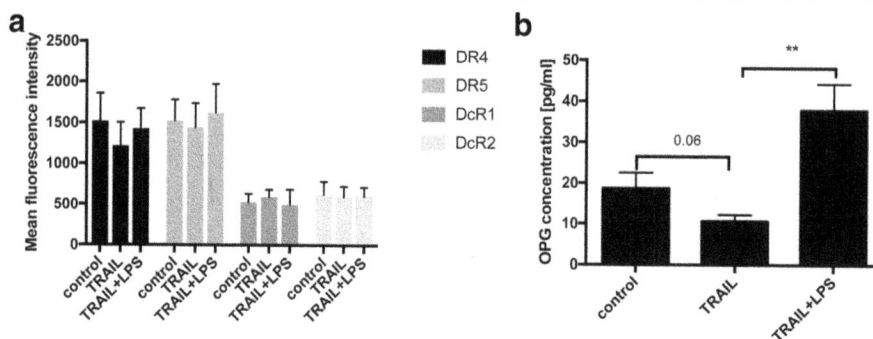

Fig. 3 Co-stimulation of COLO357 cultures with LPS and TRAIL increased OPG-levels. Cultures of COLO357 were stimulated with 300 ng/ml TRAIL, 1 μg/ml LPS and 300 ng/ml TRAIL + 1 μg/ml LPS for 24 h. Non-stimulated cell cultures served as controls. The concentration of OPG within the supernatants of respective cell cultures was measured by ELISA. The expression of the TRAIL-receptors 1–4 was determined via FACS analysis. **a** The expression of respective TRAIL-receptors was determined by FACS analysis. Data are expressed as mean fluorescence intensity. $N = 5$/group. **b** Concentrations of OPG within the supernatants of COLO357 cultures are depicted. Whereas TRAIL-stimulated cultures displayed a trend toward decreased OPG-levels, co-stimulation with LPS and TRAIL increased OPG-levels when compared to non-stimulated controls. $N = 6$/group. Means and standard errors of the means are shown. **) $p < 0.01$

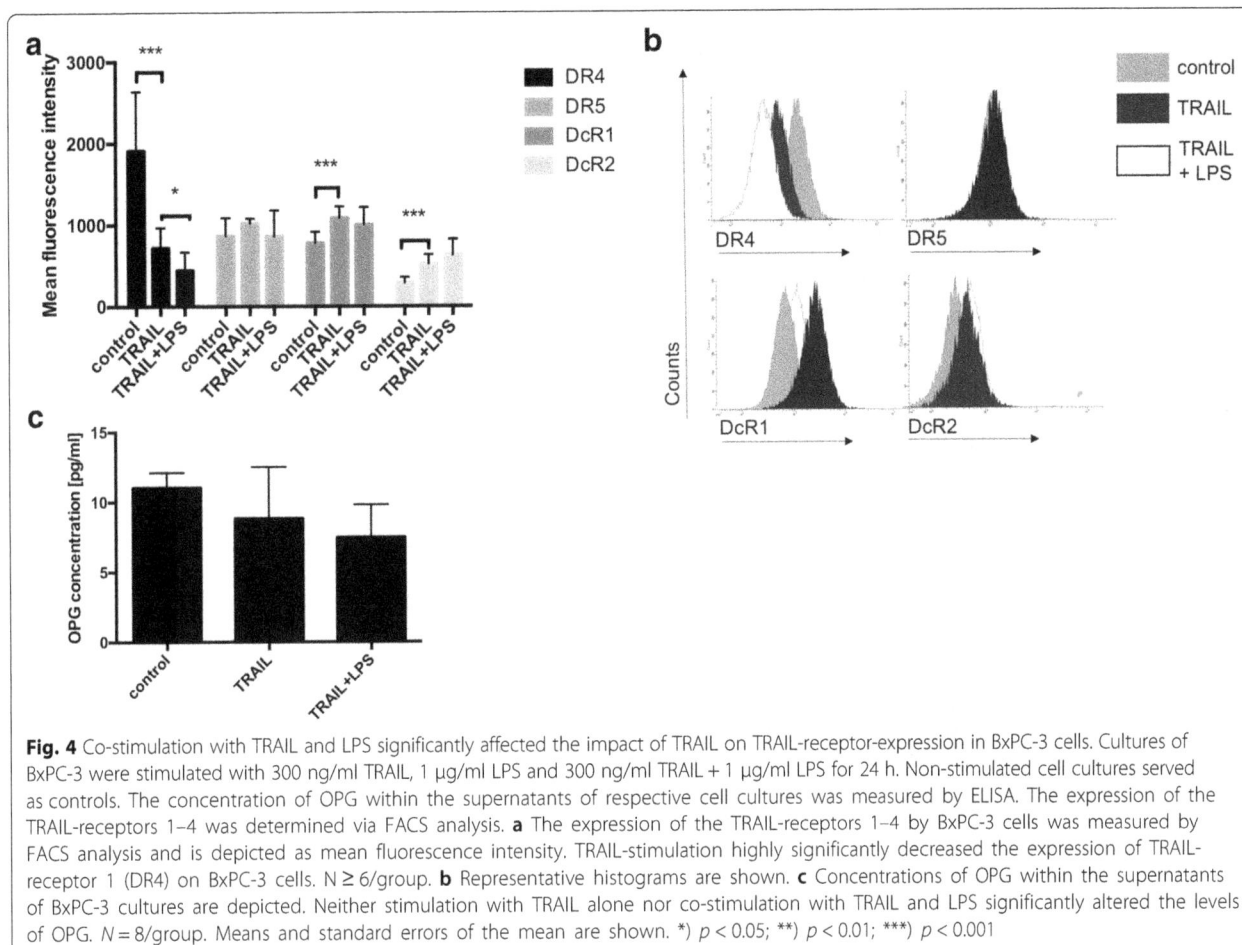

Fig. 4 Co-stimulation with TRAIL and LPS significantly affected the impact of TRAIL on TRAIL-receptor-expression in BxPC-3 cells. Cultures of BxPC-3 were stimulated with 300 ng/ml TRAIL, 1 µg/ml LPS and 300 ng/ml TRAIL + 1 µg/ml LPS for 24 h. Non-stimulated cell cultures served as controls. The concentration of OPG within the supernatants of respective cell cultures was measured by ELISA. The expression of the TRAIL-receptors 1–4 was determined via FACS analysis. **a** The expression of the TRAIL-receptors 1–4 by BxPC-3 cells was measured by FACS analysis and is depicted as mean fluorescence intensity. TRAIL-stimulation highly significantly decreased the expression of TRAIL-receptor 1 (DR4) on BxPC-3 cells. N ≥ 6/group. **b** Representative histograms are shown. **c** Concentrations of OPG within the supernatants of BxPC-3 cultures are depicted. Neither stimulation with TRAIL alone nor co-stimulation with TRAIL and LPS significantly altered the levels of OPG. $N = 8$/group. Means and standard errors of the mean are shown. *) $p < 0.05$; **) $p < 0.01$; ***) $p < 0.001$

Co-stimulation with LPS and TRAIL did not significantly influence the expression of neither DR5 nor DcR1 when compared to TRAIL-stimulated cell cultures. Regarding the expression of DR5 by BxPC-3 cells, the mean fluorescence intensity was 1017.5 + – 22.0 in TRAIL-stimulated cell cultures. In co-stimulated cell cultures the mean fluorescence intensity was 861.4 ± 112.3 ($p = 0.2$, $n = 8$). Regarding the expression of DcR1, the mean fluorescence intensity was 1083.43 ± 52.7 ($n = 7$) in TRAIL-stimulated cells and 1001.0 ± 75.7 in co-stimulated cell cultures of BxPC-3 ($n = 8$) ($p = 0.4$; Fig. 4a).

Pancreatic cancer cell lines expressed TLR4 and TRAIL-stimulation decreased the expression of TLR4

As TLR4 is the receptor for LPS, we investigated the expression of this receptor in pancreatic cancer cell lines. As shown by RT-PCR, all of the investigated pancreatic cancer cell lines expressed TLR4. Yet, TRAIL-stimulation decreased the expression of TLR4 in all investigated cell lines: TRAIL-stimulation of PANC-1 cell cultures led to a 3.2-fold decrease in the expression of TLR4 (Fig. 5a). In BxPC-3 cells, TRAIL-stimulation

decreased the TLR4 expression 4.4-fold (Fig. 5b). Co-stimulation with LPS and TRAIL further decreased the expression of TLR4 resulting in a 35.3-fold decrease when compared to non-stimulated cultures of BxPC-3 cells (Fig. 5b). In COLO 357 cells, TRAIL-stimulation induced a 31.1-fold decrease in the expression of TLR4. Co-stimulation with TRAIL and LPS further decreased TLR4 reaching a 933.3 fold decrease when compared to non-stimulated COLO 357 cell cultures ($n = 5$/group, Fig. 5c).

Discussion

In this study, it could be shown that LPS-stimulation inhibited TRAIL-induced apoptosis in pancreatic cancer cell lines by modulating the expression patterns of respective TRAIL-receptors.

TRAIL is a member of the TNF superfamily and was initially thought to selectively induce apoptosis in cancer cells [28]. However, more recently it has been discovered that TRAIL also exerts a negative impact on immune cells [27, 29, 30] demonstrating promotion of tumour growth in a murine model of pancreatic cancer [31].

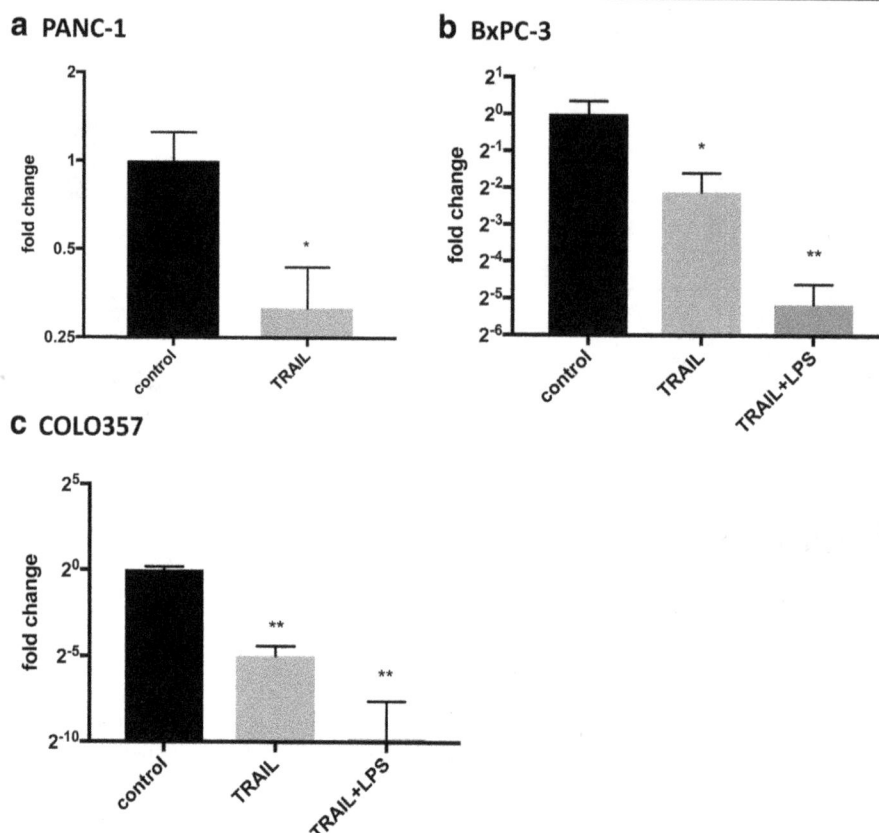

Fig. 5 TRAIL-stimulation decreased the mRNA-levels of TLR4. Cultures of PANC-1 (**a**), BxPC-3 (**b**) and COLO357 (**c**) were stimulated with 300 ng/ml TRAIL and 300 ng/ml TRAIL + 1 μg/ml LPS for 24 h. Non-stimulated cell cultures served as controls. TLR4 mRNA levels were measured by quantitative realtime-PCR. Data were normalized to mRNA expression of a housekeeping gene, *GAPDH*, and shown as fold change compared to untreated cells. Means and standard errors of the mean are shown. *) $p < 0.05$; **) $p < 0.01$

To avoid excessive apoptosis induction following TRAIL-stimulation, many tumour cells developed several mechanisms to counteract TRAIL-induced apoptosis. Several mechanisms can involve different steps of the TRAIL signalling pathway. Firstly, NF-kB mediated survival mechanisms have been discovered involving genes like X-linked inhibitor of apoptosis (XIAP). Secondly, the expression pattern of different TRAIL-receptors can contribute to TRAIL-resistance. Whereas the expression of TRAIL-R1 (DR4) and TRAIL-R2 (DR5) contributes to TRAIL-induced apoptosis [32, 33], these effects can be counteracted through the binding of TRAIL to the decoy receptors DcR1, DcR2 and osteoprotegerin [34]. Variations in the expression of these receptors will thus influence the impact on TRAIL-induced apoptosis.

Previously it has been shown that sensitivity to TRAIL-induced apoptosis may differ between cell lines of pancreatic cancer cells: PANC-1 has been detected to be TRAIL-resistant, whereas the cell line BxPC-3 appears to be TRAIL-sensitive. This effect was contributed to KRAS mutations in PANC-1 cell lines [22, 35]. This

present study confirmed the finding: COLO 357 displayed a high sensitivity to TRAIL-induced apoptosis, BxPC-3 displayed an intermediate sensitivity and PANC-1 cells were resistant to TRAIL-induced apoptosis.

Previous results could confirm the expression of the TRAIL-receptors DR4, DR5, DcR1, DcR2 and osteoprotegerin showing that these receptors were expressed by all investigated cell lines [22]. Additionally, it could be shown that all investigated cell lines secreted osteoprotegerin (OPG). However, there were significant differences between the investigated cell lines regarding the regulation of the expression of TRAIL-receptors following TRAIL-stimulation. In the TRAIL-resistant cell line PANC-1, TRAIL-stimulation significantly decreased the expression of the death receptors DR4 and DR5 whereas the secretion of osteoprotegerin was significantly increased. The levels of OPG in PANC-1 cell cultures were highest, confirming reports linking K-RAS mutations in pancreatic cancer cells with levels of osteoprotegerin [36]. Remarkably, in the present study TRAIL-stimulation increased OPG-levels thereby decreasing the expression of death receptors. Levels of OPG were lowest in the KRAS wild type cell line BxPC-3. TRAIL-stimulation had no influence on OPG secretion. However, the expression of DR4 was decreased following TRAIL-stimulation and the expression of the decoy receptors DcR1 and DcR2 was increased resulting in an intermediate resistant phenotype. In contrast, the cell line COLO 357 displayed a high sensitivity to TRAIL-mediated apoptosis. Following TRAIL-treatment the levels of OPG were decreased whereas the expression pattern of the receptors DR4, DR5, DcR1 and DcR2 did not alter.

Toll-like receptors are a major class of pattern recognition receptors which recognize highly conserved microbial structures called pathogen-associated molecular patterns (PAMPs) allowing the immune system to identify a variety of pathogens [7]. Therefore, TLRs are able to detect pathogens and subsequently initiate an immediate immune response.

TLR4 which binds LPS was the first Toll-like receptor to be identified. Therefore, it plays an important role in innate immunity. Thus, the activation of TLR4 by bacterial LPS mounts a pro-inflammatory reaction yielding in the elimination of the pathogen [37].

Apart from their expression on immune cells, Toll-like receptors have been identified in many other cell types including endothelial cells, myocytes and thyreocytes. Additionally, TLR expression has been found on pancreatic beta-cells, alpha-cells and even ductal cells [38].

In pancreatic ductal adenocarcinoma an increased expression of TLR4 has been detected compared to adjacent normal tissue [39]. In this study, we have confirmed and expanded these investigations showing that all investigated pancreatic cancer cell lines expressed Toll-like receptor 4.

TLR4 appears to act as a double-edged sword as it has been linked to both cancer inhibition and growth [40]. Whereas TLR4-/- mice showed decreased tumour growth in a murine model of pancreatic cancer, inhibition of MyD88 accelerated tumour development [41] as well as an increased TLR4 expression correlated with tumour size, lymph node involvement, venous invasion and pathological stage [39]. Most reports regarding pancreatic cancer and TLRs however focus on interactions of respective ligands with immune cells of the tumour's microenvironment. With lung cancer cells it has been shown that TLR4-signalling promoted resistance towards TRAIL-induced apoptosis and that this effect could be induced by LPS-stimulation [26]. For the pancreatic cancer cell lines PANC-1 and AsPC-1 it has been demonstrated that LPS-stimulation increased the invasive ability of respective cell lines through NFkB signalling [5].

This study showed an effect of LPS-signalling on the sensitivity to TRAIL-induced apoptosis in pancreatic cancer cell lines. This effect has been detected in all investigated TRAIL-sensitive cell lines and showed a strong reduction of TRAIL-induced apoptosis. In BxPC-3 cells, this effect was accompanied by an increase in the expression of DcR1 and a decrease of DR4-expression whereas the expression of DR5 and DcR2 remained unchanged when compared to TRAIL-stimulation. There were no changes detected in the secretion of OPG. In contrast, in COLO 357 cells the expression of the TRAIL-receptors was not changed comparing TRAIL-stimulated cell cultures with cell cultures stimulated with TRAIL and LPS. However, there was a significant increase in the level of osteoprotegerin contributing to TRAIL-resistance following co-stimulation [36].

Despite this fundamental role of LPS on TRAIL-function, the significance of TLR4 in this context has yet to be analysed. All cell lines expressed TLR4 but its level of expression was significantly reduced by TRAIL-stimulation. Therefore, only small numbers of functional TLR4s are required for LPS-mediated TRAIL-inhibition.

In summary, TLR4 was expressed on all analysed pancreatic cancer cell lines. LPS-stimulation decreased TRAIL-induced apoptosis. The decreased resistance to TRAIL-induced apoptosis was accompanied by alteration in the patterns expression of TRAIL-receptors. Future TRAIL-therapeutic strategies must be aimed at restoring TRAIL sensitivity by increasing functional TRAIL-receptors, blocking decoy receptors and other TRAIL-binding proteins as well as by counter-acting the inflammatory micro-milieu in pancreatic cancer. The role of LPS and TLR4 has to be further elucidated in future studies.

Conclusions

In this study, it has been shown that TRAIL-resistance in pancreatic cancer cells can be mediated by the inflammatory molecule LPS as well as by different expression patterns of functional and non-functional TRAIL-receptors.

Abbreviations
DR: Death receptor; ELISA: Enzyme-linked immunosorbent assay;
LPS: Lipopolysaccharide; MFI: Mean fluorescence intensity; OPG: Osteoprotegerin;
PCR: Polymerase chain reaction; TLR: Toll-like receptor; TRAIL: TNF-related
apoptosis inducing ligand; TRAIL-R: TRAIL-receptor

Acknowledgements
The authors wish to thank Antje Janetzko and Doreen Biedenweg for
excellent technical assistance.

Funding
Not applicable.

Authors' contributions
KB, LIP, CDH and WB designed and supervised the experiments. KB and FR
analyzed and interpreted the data. FR, HF and LIP performed FACS analyses.

FR, UW and LIP performed cell viability assays and ELISAs. KB performed PCR analyses. KB and WB wrote the manuscript. All authors read and approved the final manuscript.

Competing interests

The authors declare that they have no competing interests.

Author details

[1]Department of General, Visceral, Thoracic and Vascular Surgery, Universitätsmedizin Greifswald, Greifswald, Germany. [2]Department of General, Visceral and Vascular Surgery, Charité Universitätsmedizin Berlin, Campus Benjamin Franklin, Hindenburgdamm 30, 12203 Berlin, Germany. [3]Department of Obstetrics and Gynaecology, Universitätsklinikum Heidelberg, Heidelberg, Germany. [4]Department of Medicine A, Universitätsmedizin Greifswald, Greifswald, Germany.

References

1. Schneider G, Siveke JT, Eckel F, Schmid RM. Pancreatic cancer: basic and clinical aspects. Gastroenterology. 2005;128:1606–25.
2. Coussens LM, Werb Z. Inflammation and cancer. Nature. 2002;420:860–7.
3. Farrow B, Evers BM. Inflammation and the development of pancreatic cancer. Surg Oncol. 2002;10:153–69.
4. Greer JB, Whitcomb DC. Inflammation and pancreatic cancer: an evidence-based review. Curr Opin Pharmacol. 2009;9:411–8.
5. Ikebe M, Kitaura Y, Nakamura M, Tanaka H, Yamasaki A, Nagai S, Wada J, Yanai K, Koga K, Sato N, et al. Lipopolysaccharide (LPS) increases the invasive ability of pancreatic cancer cells through the TLR4/MyD88 signaling pathway. J Surg Oncol. 2009;100:725–31.
6. Kusmartsev S, Gabrilovich DI. Immature myeloid cells and cancer-associated immune suppression. Cancer Immunol Immunother. 2002;51:293–8.
7. Medzhitov R. Toll-like receptors and innate immunity. Nat Rev Immunol. 2001;1:135–45.
8. Ahmed A, Redmond HP, Wang JH. Links between Toll-like receptor 4 and breast cancer. Oncoimmunology. 2013;2, e22945.
9. Huang HY, Zhang ZJ, Cao CB, Wang N, Liu FF, Peng JQ, Ren XJ, Qian J. The TLR4/NF-kappaB signaling pathway mediates the growth of colon cancer. Eur Rev Med Pharmacol Sci. 2014;18:3834–43.
10. Li XM, Su JR, Yan SP, Cheng ZL, Yang TT, Zhu Q. A novel inflammatory regulator TIPE2 inhibits TLR4-mediated development of colon cancer via caspase-8. Cancer Biomark. 2014;14:233–40.
11. Rakhesh M, Cate M, Vijay R, Shrikant A, Shanjana A. A TLR4-interacting peptide inhibits lipopolysaccharide-stimulated inflammatory responses, migration and invasion of colon cancer SW480 cells. Oncoimmunology. 2012;1:1495–506.
12. Tang X, Zhu Y. TLR4 signaling promotes immune escape of human colon cancer cells by inducing immunosuppressive cytokines and apoptosis resistance. Oncol Res. 2012;20:15–24.
13. Zhou L, Qi L, Jiang L, Zhou P, Ma J, Xu X, Li P. Antitumor activity of gemcitabine can be potentiated in pancreatic cancer through modulation of TLR4/NF-kappaB signaling by 6-shogaol. AAPS J. 2014;16:246–57.
14. Wu Y, Lu J, Antony S, Juhasz A, Liu H, Jiang G, Meitzler JL, Hollingshead M, Haines DC, Butcher D, et al. Activation of TLR4 is required for the synergistic induction of dual oxidase 2 and dual oxidase A2 by IFN-gamma and lipopolysaccharide in human pancreatic cancer cell lines. J Immunol. 2013; 190:1859–72.
15. Mahalingam D, Szegezdi E, Keane M, de Jong S, Samali A. TRAIL receptor signalling and modulation: Are we on the right TRAIL? Cancer Treat Rev. 2009;35:280–8.
16. Shirley S, Morizot A, Micheau O. Regulating TRAIL receptor-induced cell death at the membrane : a deadly discussion. Recent Pat Anticancer Drug Discov. 2011;6:311–23.
17. Holoch PA, Griffith TS. TNF-related apoptosis-inducing ligand (TRAIL): a new path to anti-cancer therapies. Eur J Pharmacol. 2009;625:63–72.
18. Lecis D, Drago C, Manzoni L, Seneci P, Scolastico C, Mastrangelo E, Bolognesi M, Anichini A, Kashkar H, Walczak H, Delia D. Novel SMAC-mimetics synergistically stimulate melanoma cell death in combination with TRAIL and Bortezomib. Br J Cancer. 2010;102:1707–16.
19. Giaisi M, Kohler R, Fulda S, Krammer PH, Li-Weber M. Rocaglamide and a XIAP inhibitor cooperatively sensitize TRAIL-mediated apoptosis in Hodgkin's lymphomas. Int J Cancer. 2012;131:1003–8.
20. Buneker CK, Yu R, Deedigan L, Mohr A, Zwacka RM. IFN-gamma combined with targeting of XIAP leads to increased apoptosis-sensitisation of TRAIL resistant pancreatic carcinoma cells. Cancer Lett. 2012;316:168–77.
21. Mori T, Doi R, Kida A, Nagai K, Kami K, Ito D, Toyoda E, Kawaguchi Y, Uemoto S. Effect of the XIAP inhibitor Embelin on TRAIL-induced apoptosis of pancreatic cancer cells. J Surg Res. 2007;142:281–6.
22. Ibrahim SM, Ringel J, Schmidt C, Ringel B, Muller P, Koczan D, Thiesen HJ, Lohr M. Pancreatic adenocarcinoma cell lines show variable susceptibility to TRAIL-mediated cell death. Pancreas. 2001;23:72–9.
23. Li Y, Jian Z, Xia K, Li X, Lv X, Pei H, Chen Z, Li J. XIAP is related to the chemoresistance and inhibited its expression by RNA interference sensitize pancreatic carcinoma cells to chemotherapeutics. Pancreas. 2006;32:288–96.
24. Khanbolooki S, Nawrocki ST, Arumugam T, Andtbacka R, Pino MS, Kurzrock R, Logsdon CD, Abbruzzese JL, McConkey DJ. Nuclear factor-kappaB maintains TRAIL resistance in human pancreatic cancer cells. Mol Cancer Ther. 2006;5:2251–60.
25. Tang W, Wang W, Zhang Y, Liu S, Liu Y, Zheng D. Tumour necrosis factor-related apoptosis-inducing ligand (TRAIL)-induced chemokine release in both TRAIL-resistant and TRAIL-sensitive cells via nuclear factor kappa B. FEBS J. 2009;276:581–93.
26. He W, Liu Q, Wang L, Chen W, Li N, Cao X. TLR4 signaling promotes immune escape of human lung cancer cells by inducing immunosuppressive cytokines and apoptosis resistance. Mol Immunol. 2007; 44:2850–9.
27. Cziupka K, Busemann A, Partecke LI, Potschke C, Rath M, Traeger T, Koerner P, von Bernstorff W, Kessler W, Diedrich S, et al. Tumor necrosis factor-related apoptosis-inducing ligand (TRAIL) improves the innate immune response and enhances survival in murine polymicrobial sepsis. Crit Care Med. 2010;38:2169–74.
28. Lemke J, von Karstedt S, Zinngrebe J, Walczak H. Getting TRAIL back on track for cancer therapy. Cell Death Differ. 2014;21:1350–64.
29. Beyer K, Poetschke C, Partecke LI, von Bernstorff W, Maier S, Broeker BM, Heidecke CD. TRAIL induces neutrophil apoptosis and dampens sepsis-induced organ injury in murine colon ascendens stent peritonitis. PLoS One. 2014;9, e97451.
30. Beyer K, Stollhof L, Poetschke C, von Bernstorff W, Partecke LI, Diedrich S, Maier S, Broker BM, Heidecke CD. TNF-related apoptosis-inducing ligand deficiency enhances survival in murine colon ascendens stent peritonitis. J Inflamm Res. 2016;9:103–13.
31. Beyer K, Normann L, Sendler M, Kading A, Heidecke CD, Partecke LI, von Bernstorff W. TRAIL Promotes Tumor Growth in a Syngeneic Murine Orthotopic Pancreatic Cancer Model and Affects the Host Immune Response. Pancreas. 2016;45:401–8.
32. Yu R, Albarenque SM, Cool RH, Quax WJ, Mohr A, Zwacka RM. DR4 specific TRAIL variants are more efficacious than wild-type TRAIL in pancreatic cancer. Cancer Biol Ther. 2014;15:1658–66.
33. Stadel D, Mohr A, Ref C, MacFarlane M, Zhou S, Humphreys R, Bachem M, Cohen G, Moller P, Zwacka RM, et al. TRAIL-induced apoptosis is preferentially mediated via TRAIL receptor 1 in pancreatic carcinoma cells and profoundly enhanced by XIAP inhibitors. Clin Cancer Res. 2010;16:5734–49.
34. Walczak H. Death receptor-ligand systems in cancer, cell death, and inflammation. Cold Spring Harb Perspect Biol. 2013;5:a008698.
35. Sahu RP, Batra S, Kandala PK, Brown TL, Srivastava SK. The role of K-ras gene mutation in TRAIL-induced apoptosis in pancreatic and lung cancer cell lines. Cancer Chemother Pharmacol. 2011;67:481–7.
36. Kanzaki H, Ohtaki A, Merchant FK, Greene MI, Murali R. Mutations in K-Ras linked to levels of osteoprotegerin and sensitivity to TRAIL-induced cell death in pancreatic ductal adenocarcinoma cells. Exp Mol Pathol. 2013;94:372–9.
37. Vaure C, Liu Y. A comparative review of toll-like receptor 4 expression and functionality in different animal species. Front Immunol. 2014;5:316.

38. Garay-Malpartida HM, Mourao RF, Mantovani M, Santos IA, Sogayar MC, Goldberg AC. Toll-like receptor 4 (TLR4) expression in human and murine pancreatic beta-cells affects cell viability and insulin homeostasis. BMC Immunol. 2011;12:18.

39. Zhang JJ, Wu HS, Wang L, Tian Y, Zhang JH, Wu HL. Expression and significance of TLR4 and HIF-1alpha in pancreatic ductal adenocarcinoma. World J Gastroenterol. 2010;16:2881–8.

40. Mai CW, Kang YB, Pichika MR. Should a Toll-like receptor 4 (TLR-4) agonist or antagonist be designed to treat cancer? TLR-4: its expression and effects in the ten most common cancers. Onco Targets Ther. 2013;6:1573–87.

41. Vaz J, Andersson R. Intervention on toll-like receptors in pancreatic cancer. World J Gastroenterol. 2014;20:5808–17.

9

Prevalence and characteristics of Epstein–Barr virus-associated gastric carcinomas in Portugal

Célia Nogueira[1,2,3*] (iD), Marta Mota[1,3], Rui Gradiz[4,5], Maria Augusta Cipriano[6], Francisco Caramelo[7], Hugo Cruz[1], Ana Alarcão[8], Francisco Castro e Sousa[9], Fernando Oliveira[9], Fernando Martinho[9], João Moura Pereira[10], Paulo Figueiredo[11†] and Maximino Leitão[5†]

Abstract

Background: Gastric cancer (GC) is one of the most common malignant tumors of the digestive tract and is the third leading cause of cancer death worldwide. Epstein–Barr virus (EBV) has been associated with approximately 10% of the total cases of gastric carcinomas. No previous study has analyzed the prevalence of EBV infection in gastric cancer of the Portuguese population.

Methods: In the present study, we have analyzed 82 gastric carcinoma cases and 33 healthy individuals (control group) from Coimbra region for the presence of EBV by polymerase chain reaction (PCR) and by in situ hybridization (ISH) for EBV-encoded small RNAs (EBERs). The status of *H. pylori* infection was assessed by serology and by PCR.

Results: EBV was detected by PCR in 90.2% of stomach cancer cases, whereas EBERs were detected in 11%. In our series, EBV-associated gastric carcinoma (EBVaGC) were significantly associated with gender and the majority of them presented lymph node metastasis. These cases were generally graded in more advanced pTNM stages and, non-surprisingly, showed worse survival. *H. pylori* infection was detected in 62.2% of the gastric cancers and 64.7% of these patients were CagA+. On the other hand, the *H. pylori* prevalence was higher in the EBV-negative gastric carcinomas (64.4%) than in those carcinoma cases with EBV+ (44.4%).

Conclusions: The present study shows that prevalence of EBVaGC among Portuguese population is in accordance with the worldwide prevalence. EBV infection seems to be associated to poorer prognostic and no relation to *H. pylori* infection has been found. Conversely, the presence of *H. pylori* seems to have a favourable impact on patient's survival. Our results emphasize that geographic variation can contribute with new epidemiological data on the association of EBV with gastric cancer.

Keywords: Gastric cancer, Epstein-Barr virus, *Helicobacter pylori*, Clinicopathologic feature, Prognosis

Background

Gastric cancer (GC) is one of the most frequent malignant tumors of the digestive tract and is the fifth most commonly diagnosed cancer and the third leading cause of cancer death worldwide (723,073 deaths, 8.8% of the total) [1]. As so, associations to other comorbidities, such as the Epstein-Barr virus and the *Helicobacter pylori* infection, are extremely important as they may be used either clinically as prognosis factor or in basic research to get a deeper understanding of the underlying mechanisms.

The Epstein-Barr virus (EBV) belongs to the *Herpesviridae* family and approximately 95% of the world's population is infected with it, being the oral route the principal way of infection [2]. In 1997, the International Agency for Research on Cancer (IARC) has classified EBV as a Group I carcinogen for Burkitt's lymphoma, nasopharyngeal carcinoma and for Hodgkin's and non- Hodgkin's lymphoma [3].

* Correspondence: cnogueira@fmed.uc.pt
†Equal contributors
[1]Microbiology, Faculty of Medicine of the University of Coimbra, 3004-504 Coimbra, Portugal
[2]CIMAGO, Faculty of Medicine of the University of Coimbra, 3001-301 Coimbra, Portugal
Full list of author information is available at the end of the article

The presence of EBV in a patient with gastric cancer was first reported in a case of lymphoepithelioma type by Burke et al. in 1990 [4]. Subsequently, Shibata and Weiss have identified the presence of EBV in 16% of gastric adenocarcinomas in USA [5].Unlike other EBV-associated malignancies, the EBV-associated gastric carcinoma (EBVaGC) is not endemic in any region yet is quite distributed worldwide. In fact, it is emerging as the most common among EBV-associated malignant neoplasms with more than 90,000 patients being estimated to develop GC in association with EBV annually (10% of total GC) [6–8].

H. pylori is the major causative agent of gastritis, peptic ulcer disease, mucosa-associated lymphoid tissue (MALT) lymphoma, and GC [9].The clinical outcome of H. pylori infection depends on bacterial virulence factors, host susceptibility, environmental and life-style factors [10]. Several H. pylori virulence genes have also been identified and among those cagA (cytotoxin-associated gene) is one of the most important gene. Infection with CagA strains is associated to higher risk of developing atrophic gastritis and gastric cancer [11, 12].

Some studies have addressed the question if exists a cooperative effect between EBV and H. pylori in GC but, their results are inconsistent and conflicting. The present study aims at determining the frequency of EBV-related gastric carcinoma in the Portuguese population and drawing both epidemiological and clinicopathological features of EBV-associated GC in this geographic area relating to H. pylori infection.

Methods

Patients and samples
A total of 82 patients with gastric cancer who underwent surgical resection at Coimbra University Hospital (HUC) and Regional Oncology Center of Coimbra, IPOFG, SA and 33 patients with non-cancer diseases (control group) who underwent routine surveillance endoscopy at Gastroenterology department of HUC by nonspecific complaints were enrolled in our study. Serum, tumor tissue and their corresponding adjacent non-cancerous mucosa was collected from each gastric cancer patient. Gastric tissue samples and serum were obtained from each individual of the control group.

This study was approved by Ethics Committee of the respective institutions and informed consent was obtained from all individuals. None of the patients received chemotherapy or radiation therapy before surgery. Patient overall survival times were calculated from the date of diagnosis to either the date of death or the last follow up, resulting in a follow-up period ranging from 1 to 55 months (mean, 36 months). Those cases lost to follow-up and those ending in death from any other

cause than gastric cancer (2 cases) were considered censored data during the analysis of survival rates.

Clinicopathologic data comprise patient age and gender as well as the anatomical site, histological classification according to the Lauren classification system [13], and pathological tumor stage (TNM stage; T: depth of tumor invasion, N: lymph node metastasis, M: distant metastasis) according to the American Joint Committee on Cancer (AJCC) system [14].

DNA extraction
DNA from tumor tissue and from non-cancerous mucosa was extracted and purified in MagNA Pure Compact equipment (Roche, Germany) using MagNA Pure Compact Nucleic Acid Isolation Kit I (Roche, Germany), according to manufacturer's instructions. Prior to extraction on the MagNA Pure Compact, tissues were disrupted in Magna Lyser (Roche, Germany) and treated with ATL buffer (QIAGEN, Spain) and proteinase K (QIAGEN, Spain) for 10 min at 65 °C. DNA concentration (A260) and purity (A260/A280) were determined spectrophotometrically (NanoDrop, Thermo Fisher Scientific). DNA was stored at −80 °C for further use.

EBV real-time PCR
EBV detection was performed using specific primers described by Drouet et al. (1999) [15] that amplify a segment of the BamH1W region.

Real-time PCR reactions were carried out on the SmartCycler instrument (Cepheid, USA) in a final volume of 20 µl, containing 2 µl of extracted DNA, 2 µl of FastStart SYBR Green Master kit (Roche, Germany) and 0.4 mM of each primer. Thermocycling conditions were a preheating step of 10 min at 95 °C followed by 45 cycles of 95 °C for 10 s, 59 °C for 5 s and 72 °C for 8 s. Fluorescence was measured at the end of each extension step. Melting analysis was achieved with continuous monitoring of fluorescence from 65 °C to 95 °C at a temperature transition rate of 0.2 °C. A specimen was considered positive if a single melting peak was measured between 88 °C and 89 °C. To validate the amplification process and exclude carryover contamination, positive and negative controls were included in each PCR run.

EBER1 in situ hybridization
The presence of EBV in gastric cells was identified by the expression of EBV-encode small RNA-1 (EBER1), the most abundant viral product in latently infected cells. In situ hybridization reactions were carried out in an automated system, the BOND -MAX ™ (Leica Microsystems, Wetzlar, Germany) using the staining protocol "ISH protocol A" with an enzymatic pre-treatment with the Bond Enzyme Pre-treatment Kit, according

to manufacturer's instructions. From paraffin-embedded tissues were cut 3 histological sections with 3 μm thick that were mounted on glass slides coated with 3-(amino-propyl) triethoxysilane (Sigma Diagnostics, St. Louis, USA) and used for hybridization with 3 different probes: the EBER Probe, the RNA Positive Control Probe and the RNA Negative Control Probe (Leica Microsystems, Wetzlar, Germany). A sample was considered EBER-1-positive when appeared a dark brown staining in the nuclei of tumor cells, under light microscopy. In each hybridization a positive control, Hodgkin's lymphoma EBV positive and a negative control, Hodgkin's lymphoma EBV negative were included. The cases with EBER1 positive signals were classified as EBVaGC group.

PCR amplification of *H. pylori* and *cagA* gene
Detection of *H. pylori* in gastric samples was accomplished by amplification of *H. pylori* flagella gene. For the *H. pylori*-positive samples, the presence of the *cagA* gene was assessed. Single type PCRs were performed with specific primers described elsewhere [16].

H. pylori serology
IgG antibodies against *H. pylori* were determined with an enzyme-linked immunosorbent assay (ELISA), using a commercial assay (HELICOBACTER PYLORI ELISA IgG, Vircell, Spain), with a sensitivity of 97% and specificity of 100%; according to the manufacturer's instructions.

Statistical analysis
The χ2 test and Fisher's exact test were used to test associations between categorical variables. Cases within the follow-up period were censored either at the time of death or at the last update of the subject. Survival curves were estimated using the Kaplan-Meier product-limit method, and the differences between the survival curves was tested using the log-rank test. All statistical analyses were performed using the Statistical Package for the Social Sciences, version 19 (SPSS Inc., Chicago, IL, USA), and a *p* value <0.05 was considered as statistically significant.

Results
Prevalence of EBV positive cases
We evaluated 82 patients (45 males and 37 females; mean age, 66.6; range, 39 to 88 years) with gastric carcinoma and 33 patients (13 males and 20 females; mean age 57.8; range, 30 to 82 years) with non-cancer diseases. Using PCR analysis, EBV DNA was detected in 90.2% of the patients with gastric carcinoma and in 27.3% of the individuals from the control group. However, in situ hybridization showed EBER expression in malignant cells in only 9 patients with gastric cancer (corresponding to 11%) and in one case of the control group (3%).

In one of the nine cases EBVaGC, the EBER expression was also detected in non-malignant gastric mucosa. The EBER expression in malignant cells was either uniformly positive or uniformly negative, suggesting that EBV infection may have occurred before malignant transformation and was transmitted to all daughter cells in the neoplastic clone.

Association between EBV status and clinicopathological characteristics
The clinicopathological characteristics of EBVaGC and EBV-negative gastric carcinomas (EBVnGC) patients are summarized in Table 1. Gender ratio (male/female) was 8:1 in EBVaGC and 1.03:1 in EBVnGC, revealing a

Table 1 Comparison of clinicopathological features between EBV positive gastric carcinomas and EBV negative gastric carcinomas

	EBV positive gastric carcinomas (*n* = 9)	EBV negative gastric carcinomas (*n* = 73)	*P* value
Gender			
Male	8	37	0.037
Female	1	36	
Age (years)			
Mean (range)	70.1 (60–81)	66.2 (39–88)	
18–39	0	1	0.279[§]
40–59	0	17	
≥ 60	9	55	
Tumor location			
Fundus + Body	2	17	1.0
Antrum	5	54	
Cardia	2	2	
Histological type			
Diffuse	2	18	1.0[§]
Intestinal	5	41	
Mixed	2	14	
Lymph node			
Positive	6	47	0.080
Negative	2	26	
pTNM Stage			
I + II	4	42	0.721
III + IV	4	31	
Survival			
≤ 36 months	6	39	0.191
> 36 months	3	32	
H. pylori			
Positive	4	47	0.288
Negative	5	26	

§ – *p* obtained by Monte Carlo

significant (p = 0.037) association where male shows predominance in EBV positive GC. Although there were no statistically significant differences, EBVaGC were more frequently associated with older age group, notably up to 100% of cases were older than 60 years old versus 75% of EBVnGC.

Regarding tumor localization, a tendency for the antrum was denoted in both groups, 55.6% in EBVaGC and 74% in EBVnGC; nonetheless, the percentage of tumors at proximal locations was higher in EBVaGC (44.4% vs. 26%). Tumor histology was not related to EBV status since in both groups intestinal type was predominant. Furthermore, the positivity of EBV was not significantly associated with either stage or survival, whilst a slight tendency of EBVaGC having a worse prognosis was noticed. This perception is based on the fact of EBVaGC patients present higher probability of having lymph node metastasis, were typically stratified in more advanced stages and showed poorer survival rates (Fig. 1). Although this trend could be biased by age, gender and the TNM status a deeper analysis

reveals that EBV+ subjects tend to present worse survival rate even correcting for that factors. Nonetheless, the attempted statistical models did not present statistical significance for the EBV groups.

Detection and genotyping of H. pylori

The presence of *H. pylori* DNA was identified in 62.2% (n = 51) of GC patients and in 54.5% (n = 18) of the control group. Comparing the clinicopathological characteristics between the GC *H.pylori* + against the GC *H. pylori*– significant differences due to gender, age, tumor location, histological classification, TMN stage and survival rate were not observed (Table 2). The gene *cagA* was detected in 64.7% (33/51) of the GC cases with *H. pylori* infection and in 38.9% (7/18) at the control group with *H. pylori* infection, which highlights a significant association between the *H. pylori* strains present in tumors to express gene *cagA* (p = 0.043). In fact, *H. pylori* strains found in tumors have about 3 times more probability of being CagA+ (OR: IC95% [1.01, 6.66]) than the *H. pylori* strains detected in gastric tissue of healthy individuals.

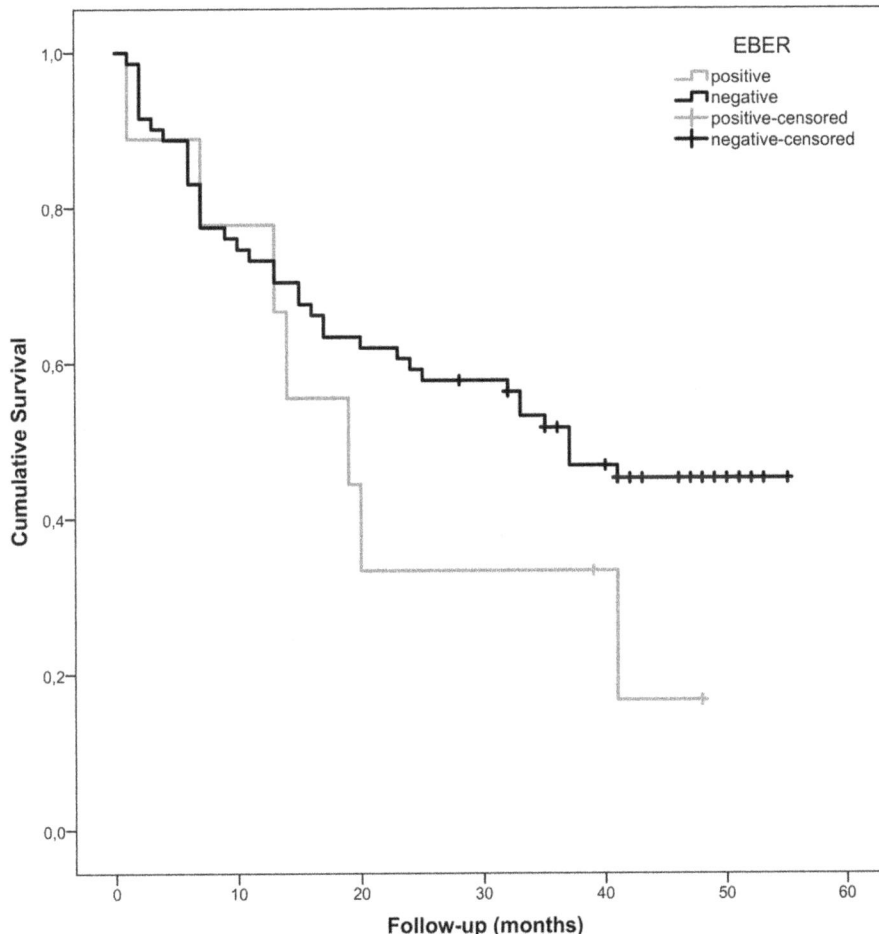

Fig. 1 Survival graph of EBV associated gastric cancer and non-EBV associated gastric cancer

Table 2 Comparison of clinicopathologic variables between *H. pylori*-positive and *H. pylori*-negative gastric cancer patients

	H. pylori positive	H. pylori negative	P value
Gender			
Male	28	17	0.996
Female	23	14	
Age (years)			
Mean (range)	66.0 (44–87)	67.7 (39–88)	
18–39	0	1	0.548§
40–59	11	6	
≥ 60	40	24	
Tumor location			
Fundus + Body	13	6	0.561
Antrum	36	23	
Cardia	2	2	
Histologicaltype			
Diffuse	13	7	0.851
Intestinal	29	17	
Mixed	9	7	
pTNM Stage			
I + II	29	17	0.780
III + IV	21	14	
Survival			
≤ 36 months	28	17	0.747
> 36 months	23	12	

§ – p obtained by Monte Carlo

Seroprevalence of *H. pylori* infection reveals higher rates in GC patients when compared to the control group (85.4% vs 57.6%, *p* = 0.001). The odds ratio of an individual *H. pylori* seropositive to have gastric cancer is about 4 times higher than an individual seronegative (95% CI: [1.71, 10.82]).

Concerning seroprevalence another relationship was observed, namely the association with clinical stage; the majority of *H. pylori* seropositive cases were graded in the less advanced tumors stages (I and II) (*p* = 0.002). The overall survival also follows this trend but with no statistical significance (Log Rank *p* = 0.201, Breslow *p* = 0.141), which is not altered if age, gender and stage status is taken into account.

No significant association was observed between the occurrence of *H. pylori* infection and EBVaGC, since of the nine EBVaGC cases four had *H. pylori* co-infection (*p* = 0.288); moreover the positivity of *H. pylori* in EBVnGC is higher (64.4%) than that found in EBVaGC (44.4%).

Discussion

Over the past 50 years there has been a decline in gastric cancer (GC) incidence and mortality, however, it still accounts for 6.8% of all malignant tumors [1].

In Portugal, the WHO data for 2012 indicate that the GC is the fifth most frequent malignancy, with 3018 new cases (1834 men and 1184 women), and the third most lethal cancer, as it was responsible for the death of 2285 Portuguese [1].

In the present study, we assessed the status of EBV by PCR and ISH and *H. pylori* infection by PCR and serology in 82 cases of primary gastric carcinomas and in 33 healthy individuals. To the best of our knowledge this is the first report presenting Portuguese casuistry regarding the association of EBV with stomach cancer and, simultaneously correlating the involvement of these two pathogens in gastric carcinogenesis. Using PCR we found that 90.2% of GC were EBV-positive; extremely high positivities of >80% were as well reported in three studies from India [17–19], where EBV detection was also accomplished by PCR; this may be due to the high sensitivity of PCR that amplified indiscriminately EBV DNA present in tumor cells and in tumor-infiltrating lymphocytes. To overcome this issue, it was used EBER in situ hybridization, which is the recommended technique for the detection of EBV in human tissue and tumors because of its high sensitivity and specificity to accurate localize the EBV-infected cells [20]. Hence, by ISH the EBV was detected in 11% of our cases, which is consistent with the prevalence of EBVaGC worldwide, since several studies in the literature report that approximately 10% of gastric carcinomas are associated with EBV [6, 8, 21, 22]. EBER expression was mainly restricted to the tumor tissue, as pointed out by others [23–25], however we found one EBVaGC case with EBER positivity in the non-neoplastic mucosa and one patient of the control group, with chronic pangastritis, was also EBV+ in epithelial cells. This is in line with the observations of others who detected EBV in precancerous lesions [5, 7, 22, 26]. Despite being quite rare, the EBV infection in non-neoplastic gastric mucosa indicates that EBV enters the gastric epithelium at an early stage of gastric carcinogenesis preceding the clonal growth of EBV-infected cells and subsequently the development to carcinoma.

In our study, we found that patients with EBV-positive tumors are predominantly male (8: 1), as corroborated by the majority of published reports [5, 6, 20, 23, 24, 27, 28]. This highest incidence in men can be attributed to both genetic status and lifestyle factors. Earlier studies indicate that eating salty or spicy foods, frequently drinking coffee and high-temperature drinks, exposure to wood dust and/or iron filings and smoking are risk factors for developing EBVaGC [6, 29].

Concerning histological classification and topographic distribution we found a prevalence of intestinal type and tumors located in the antrum, which is consistent with others studies [5, 26, 30] but in disagreement in what regards the characteristic of EBVaGC [20, 24].

Although it has been proposed that the presence of EBV in gastric cancers is associated with a better prognosis [31], former reports are inconsistent. Our results point in the direction that the presence of EBV is a marker of poor prognosis since the majority of our cases have lymph node involvement, are grouped in more advanced stages and, as so, have worse survival.

Taken together, these variations between data might be explained by the contribution of local risk factors, such as geographical and environmental aspects, along with the size and features of the cohort.

It is estimated that *H. pylori* infects half the world population [11, 32, 33] and is responsible for more than 60% of gastric cancer cases [34, 35]. In this series the prevalence of *H. pylori* for both groups, patients with carcinoma and controls, fall within the described in the literature. In the control group *H. pylori* detection rates (DNA - 54.6%, seroprevalence - 57.6%), are close to the average of *H. pylori* infection rate reported worldwide (50%). In GC patients the *H. pylori* DNA was found in 62.2% of the cases, which is also in agreement with its involvement in more than 60% of the total gastric tumors. On the other hand, the serologic positivity was 85.4% which is in line with the value found in another Portuguese study (85.5%) in patients with stomach cancer [36]. These differences in detection rates may be explained by the spontaneous disappearance of the *Helicobacter pylori* during malignant transformation of gastric epithelium, perhaps due to lack of nutrients needed by this bacterium; however, the tumor still occurs after the effective eradication of *H. pylori*; this occurrence has also been described in other studies [37].

In the current study, statistical comparison between the 2 groups revealed that seropositive *H. pylori* status is associated to increasing risk of developing gastric cancer [38, 39] and that *H. pylori cagA+* strains are more aggressive than *H. pylori cagA-* strains, being also linked to stomach adenocarcinoma progression [11, 12]. Regarding the prognostic value of *H. pylori* status we found a significant association between positive *H. pylori* status and better outcome, since the tumors *H. pylori* + are stratified in early pTNM stages, as observed by others [40–42]. A plausible explanation for this fact is that *H. pylori* may contribute to a more efficient immune response against the tumor by triggering a type-1 T-helper-cell response [43], or it was also suggested that *Helicobacter pylori* antigens mimic the surface molecules of gastric epithelial cells and that would activate a cross-reactivity of autoantibodies against the tumor cells [44]. The involvement of the microsatellite instability is also highlighted, because it has been related with a higher rate of *H. pylori* infection and a better postoperative survival [45].

It has been suggested that EBV and *H. pylori* can be influenced by each other or cooperated together, in a direct or indirect way, in gastric carcinogenesis. In the present study no statistical association was found between EBV infection and *H. pylori* infection once there is no evidence of an *H. pylori* co-participation in the 11% of the GCs that are EBV positive by EBER-ISH. In fact, several studies that address the effect and interaction between them do not detected any association [20, 23, 46–49]. However, there are others publications showing synergism between EBV and *H. pylori* in the pathogenesis of gastric diseases [30, 50–53]. In point of fact, it is suggested two possible mechanisms, first an additional inflammatory response in co-infection and increased tissue damaging by both *H. pylori* and EBV. The studies by Cárdenas-Mondragón et co-workers give evidence of this mechanism; in pediatrics patients they demonstrated that co-infection with EBV and *H. pylori* CagA+ is more associated with severe gastritis than cases with single *H. pylori* CagA+ infection [52], as well as the study with Latin American patients confirm that EBV co-participates with *H. pylori* to induce severe inflammation and increase the risk of progression to intestinal-type GC [53]. The second mechanism pointed out is based on gene products interaction. An in vitro study found that EBV reactivation occurs by the PLCγ signalling pathway and *H. pylori* toxin CagA strongly activates PLCγ [54]. On the other hand, Saju et al. suggested that host protein SHP1 dephosphorylates CagA, thus preventing its oncogenic activity; however EBV co-infection causes SHP1 methylation and prevents its dephosphorylation activity of CagA and thereby increasing the oncogenic potential of CagA [55].

Conclusion

We identified 9 cases of EBVaGC (11%) corresponding to the average prevalence of EBVaGC worldwide. EBVaGC was associated with male predominance and seems to emerge as a factor of poor prognosis, while *H. pylori* infection appears to have a protective role in the outcome of GC patients. This results highlight that geographic variation can contribute with new epidemiological data on the association of EBV with GC.

Abbreviations
AJCC: American Joint Committee on Cancer; *cagA*: cytotoxin-associated gene; EBERs: EBV-encoded small RNAs; EBV: Epstein–Barr virus; EBVaGC: EBV-associated gastric carcinoma; EBVnGC: EBV-negative gastric carcinomas; ELISA: enzyme-linked immunosorbent assay; GC: Gastric cancer; HUC: Coimbra University Hospital; IARC: International Agency for Research on Cancer; ISH: In situ hybridization; MALT: mucosa-associated lymphoid tissue; PCR: polymerase chain reaction; WHO: World Health Organization

Acknowledgements
The authors would like to thank the patients and the supporting staff in this study. We are indebted to Professor Lina Carvalho from Faculty of Medicine of the University of Coimbra for kindly allow us to use the Bond Max equipment.

Funding

This research did not receive any specific grant from funding agencies in the public, commercial, or not-for-profit sectors.

Authors' contributions

Study concept and design: CN, ML; experimental work: CN, MM, HC, AA, PF; provided patients samples: RG, MAC, FCS, FO, FM, JMP, PF, ML; data collection and interpretation of the results: CN, RG, MAC, PF; statistical analysis: FC; wrote the manuscript: CN; critical revision of the manuscript: RG, FC, PF, ML. The final version of the manuscript was approved by all authors.

Competing interests

The authors declare that they have no competing interests.

Author details

[1]Microbiology, Faculty of Medicine of the University of Coimbra, 3004-504 Coimbra, Portugal. [2]CIMAGO, Faculty of Medicine of the University of Coimbra, 3001-301 Coimbra, Portugal. [3]Medical Microbiology, Centre for Neuroscience and Cell Biology of the University of Coimbra, 3004-504 Coimbra, Portugal. [4]Physiopathology, Faculty of Medicine of the University of Coimbra, 3004-504 Coimbra, Portugal. [5]Gastroenterology, University Hospitals of Coimbra, 3000-075 Coimbra, Portugal. [6]Pathological Anatomy, University Hospitals of Coimbra, 3000-075 Coimbra, Portugal. [7]Laboratory of Biostatistics and Medical Informatics, IBILI, Faculty of Medicine of the University of Coimbra, 3000-548 Coimbra, Portugal. [8]Pathology Institute, Faculty of Medicine of the University of Coimbra, 3004-504 Coimbra, Portugal. [9]Department of Surgery, University Hospitals of Coimbra, 3000-075 Coimbra, Portugal. [10]Surgery, Regional Oncology Center of Coimbra, IPOFG, 3000-075 Coimbra, Portugal. [11]Histopathology, Regional Oncology Center of Coimbra, IPOFG, 3000-075 Coimbra, Portugal.

References

1. Ferlay J, Soerjomataram I, Ervik M, Dikshit R, Eser S, Mathers C, et al. GLOBOCAN 2012 v1.0, cancer incidence and mortality worldwide: IARC CancerBase no. 11 [internet]. Lyon, France: International Agency for Research on Cancer; 2013. Available from: http://globocan.iarc.fr. accessed on 20 July 2016

2. Rickinson AB, Kieff E. Epstein-Barr virus. In: Knipe DM, Howley PM, editors. Fields Virology. Vol. 2, 4th ed.; Lippincott–Williams & Wilkins; 2001. p.2579.

3. International Agency for Research on Cancer, World Health Organization. Epstein-Barr virus and Kaposi sarcoma herpes virus/human herpes virus 8. In: IARC monographs on the evaluation of carcinogenic risks to humans. Vol. 70. Lyon: IARC Press; 1997.

4. Burke AP, Yen TS, Shekitka KM, Sobin LH. Lymphoepithelial carcinoma of the stomach with Epstein-Barr virus demonstrated by polymerase chain reaction. Modern Pathol. 1990;3:377–80.

5. Shibata D, Weiss LM. Epstein Barr-virus-associated gastric adenocarcinoma. Am J Pathol. 1992;140:769–74.

6. Camargo MC, Koriyama C, Matsuo K, Kim WH, Herrera-Goepfert R, Liao LM, et al. Case–case comparison of smoking and alcohol risk associations with Epstein–Barr virus-positive gastric cancer. Int J Cancer. 2014;134:948–53.

7. Shinozaki-Ushiku A, Kunita A, Fukayama M. Update on Epstein-Barr virus and gastric cancer (review). Int J Oncol. 2015;46:1421–34.

8. Liu Y, Yang W, Pan Y, Ji J, Lu Z, Ke Y. Genome-wide analysis of Epstein-Barr virus (EBV) isolated from EBV-associated gastric carcinoma (EBVaGC). Oncotarget. 2016;7:4903–14.

9. Blaser MJ. Hypothesis: the changing relationships of Helicobacter pylori and humans: implications for health and disease. J Infect Dis. 1999;79:1523–30.

10. Palli D, Masala G, Del Giudice G, Plebani M, Basso D, Berti D, et al. CagA+ Helicobacter pylori infection and gastric cancer risk in the EPIC-EURGAST study. Int J Cancer. 2007;120:859–67.

11. Abadi ATB, Kusters JG. Management of Helicobacter pylori infections. BMC Gastroenterol. 2016;16:94.

12. Blaser MJ, Perez-Perez GI, Kleanthous H, Cover TL, Peek RM, Chyou PH, et al. Infection with Helicobacter pylori strains possessing cagA is associated with an increased risk of developing adenocarcinoma of the stomach. Cancer Res. 1995;55:2111–5.

13. Lauren P. The two histological main types of gastric carcinoma: diffuse and so-called intestinal-type carcinoma. An attempt at a histo-clinical classification. Acta Pathol Microbiol Scand. 1965;64:31–49.

14. AJCC Cancer Staging Manual. In: American Joint Committee on Cancer. Stomach. 6th ed. New York: NY: Springer; 2002. p. 99–106.

15. Drouet E, Brousset P, Fares F, Icart J, Verniol C, Meggetto F, et al. High Epstein-Barr virus serum load and elevated titers of anti-ZEBRA antibodies in patients with EBV-harboring tumor cells of Hodgkin's disease. J Med Virol. 1999;57:383–9.

16. Podzorski RP, Podzorski DS, Wuerth A, Tolia V. Analysis of the vacA, cagA, cagE, iceA, and babA2 genes in Helicobacter pylori from sixty-one pediatric patients from the Midwestern United States. Diagn Micr Infec Dis. 2003;46:83–8.

17. Saxena A, Nath Prasad K, Chand Ghoshal U, Krishnani N, Roshan Bhagat M, Husain N. Association of Helicobacter pylori and Epstein-Barr virus with gastric cancer and peptic ulcer disease. Scand J Gastroentero. 2008;43:669–74.

18. Shukla SK, Prasad KN, Tripathi A, Singh A, Saxena A, Ghoshal UC, et al. Epstein-Barr virus DNA load and its association with Helicobacter pylori infection in gastroduodenal diseases. Braz J Infect Dis. 2011;15:583–90.

19. Shukla SK, Prasad KN, Tripathi A, Ghoshal UC, Krishnani N, Husain N. Expression profile of latent and lytic transcripts of epstein–barr virus in patients with gastroduodenal diseases: a study from northern India. J Med Virol. 2012;84:1289–97.

20. Lee JH, Kim SH, Han SH, An JS, Lee ES, Kim YS. Clinicopathological and molecular characteristics of Epstein-Barr virus-associated gastric carcinoma: a meta-analysis. J Gastroen Hepatol. 2009;24:354–65.

21. zur Hausen A, Brink AA, Craanen ME, Middeldorp JM, Meijer CJ, van den Brule AJ. Unique transcription pattern of Epstein-Barr virus (EBV) in EBV-carrying gastric adenocarcinomas: expression of the transforming BARF1 gene. Cancer Res. 2000;60:2745–8.

22. Herrera-Goepfert R, Akiba S, Koriyama C, Ding S, Reyes E, Itoh T, et al. Epstein-Barr virus-associated gastric carcinoma: evidence of age-dependence among a Mexican population. World J Gastroentero. 2005;11:6096–103.

23. Murphy G, Pfeiffer R, Camargo MC, Rabkin CS. Meta-analysis shows that prevalence of Epstein-Barr virus-positive gastric cancer differs based on sex and anatomic location. Gastroenterology. 2009;137:824–33.

24. Corvalan A, Koriyama C, Akiba S, Eizuru Y, Backhouse C, Palma M, et al. Epstein-Barr virus in gastric carcinoma is associated with location in the cardia and with a diffuse histology: a study in one area of Chile. Int J Cancer. 2001;94:527–30.

25. Chen XZ, Chen H, Castro FA, Hu JK, Brenner H. Epstein–Barr virus infection and gastric cancer: a systematic review. Medicine. 2015;94:e792.

26. Zhao J, Jin H, Cheung KF, Tong JH, Zhang S, Go MY, et al. Zinc finger E-box binding factor 1 plays a central role in regulating Epstein-Barr virus (EBV) latent-lytic switch and acts as a therapeutic target in EBV-associated gastric cancer. Cancer. 2012;118:924–36.

27. van Beek J, zur Hausen A, Klein Kranenbarg E, van de Velde CJ, Middeldorp JM, van den Brule AJ, et al. EBV-positive gastric adenocarcinomas: a distinct clinico-pathologic entity with a low frequency of lymph node involvement. J Clin Oncol. 2004;22:664–70.

28. Genitsch V, Novotny A, Seiler CA, Kröll D, Walch A, Langer R. Epstein–Barr virus in gastro-esophageal adenocarcinomas–single center experiences in the context of current literature. Front Oncol. 2015;5:73.

29. Koriyama C, Akiba S, Minakami Y, Eizuru Y. Environmental fators related to Epstein-Barr virus-associated gastric cancer in Japan. J Exp Clin Canc Res. 2005;24:547–53.

30. Lima VP, de Lima MA, André AR, Ferreira MV, Barros MA, Rabenhorst SH. H pylori (CagA) and Epstein-Barr virus infection in gastric carcinomas: correlation with p53 mutation and c-Myc, Bcl-2 and Bax expression. World J Gastroentero. 2008;14:884–91.

31. Liu X, Liu J, Qiu H, Kong P, Chen S, Li W, et al. Prognostic significance of Epstein-Barr virus infection in gastric cancer: a meta-analysis. BMC Cancer. 2015;15:782.

32. Atherton JC, Blaser MJ. Coadaptation of Helicobacter pylori and humans: ancient history, modern implications. J Clin Invest. 2009;119:2475–87.

33. Backert S, Blaser MJ. The role of CagA in the gastric biology of Helicobacter pylori. Cancer Res. 2016;76:4028–31.

34. Bornschein J, Selgrad M, Warnecke M, Kuester D, Wex T, Malfertheiner P. H. Pylori infection is a key risk factor for proximal gastric cancer. Digest Dis Sci. 2010;55:3124–31.

35. Leja M, Axon A, Brenner H. (2016). Epidemiology of Helicobacter pylori infection. Helicobacter. 2016;21:3–7.

36. Peleteiro B, Lopes C, Figueiredo C, Lunet N. Salt intake and gastric cancer

risk according to Helicobacter pylori infection, smoking, tumour site and histological type. Br J Cancer. 2011;104:198–207.

37. Kokkola A, Kosunen TU, Puolakkainen P, Sipponen P, Harkonen M, Laxen F, et al. Spontaneous disappearance of Helicobacter pylori antibodies in patients with advanced atrophic corpus gastritis. APMIS. 2003;111:619–24.

38. Nomura A, Stemmermann GN, Chyou PH, Kato I, Perez-Perez GI, Blaser MJ. Helicobacter pylori infection and gastric carcinoma among Japanese Americans in Hawaii. New Engl J Med. 1991;325:1132–6.

39. Crew KD, Neugut AI. Epidemiology of gastric cancer. World J Gastroentero. 2006;12:354–62.

40. Kang SY, Han JH, Ahn MS, Lee HW, Jeong SH, Park JS, et al. Helicobacter pylori infection as an independent prognostic factor for locally advanced gastric cancer patients treated with adjuvant chemotherapy after curative resection. Int J Cancer. 2012;130:948–58.

41. Marrelli D, Pedrazzani C, Berardi A, Corso G, Neri A, Garosi L, et al. Negative Helicobacter pylori status is associated with poor prognosis in patients with gastric cancer. Cancer. 2009;115:2071–80.

42. Wang F, Sun G, Zou Y, Zhong F, Ma T, Li X. Protective role of Helicobacter pylori infection in prognosis of gastric cancer: evidence from 2454 patients with gastric cancer. PLoS One. 2013;8:e62440.

43. Bamford KB, Fan X, Crowe SE, Leary JF, Gourley WK, Luthra GK, et al. Lymphocytes in the human gastric mucosa during Helicobacter pylori have a T helper cell 1 phenotype. Gastroenterology. 1998;114:482–92.

44. Xue LJ, Su QS, Yang JH, Lin Y. Autoimmune responses induced by Helicobacter pylori improve the prognosis of gastric carcinoma. Med Hypotheses. 2008;70: 273–6.

45. Wu MS, Lee CW, Sheu JC, Shun CT, Wang HP, Hong RL, et al. Alterations of BAT-26 identify a subset of gastric cancer with distinct clinicopathologic features and better postoperative prognosis. Hepato-gastroenterol. 2002;49: 285–9.

46. Kim Y, Shin A, Gwack J, Ko KP, Kim CS, Park SK, et al. Epstein-Barr virus antibody level and gastric cancer risk in Korea: a nested case-control study. Br J Cancer. 2009;101:526–9.

47. Luo B, Wang Y, Wang XF, Gao Y, Huang BH, Zhao P. Correlation of Epstein-Barr virus and its encoded proteins with Helicobacter pylori and expression of c-met and c-myc in gastric carcinoma. World J Gastroenterol. 2006;12: 1842–8.

48. de Souza CR, de Oliveira KS, Ferraz JJ, Leal MF, Calcagno DQ, Seabra AD, et al. Occurrence of Helicobacter pylori and Epstein-Barr virus infection in endoscopic and gastric cancer patients from northern Brazil. BMC Gastroenterol. 2014;14:179.

49. Camargo MC, Kim KM, Matsuo K, Torres J, Liao LM, Morgan DR, et al. Anti-Helicobacter pylori antibody profiles in Epstein-Barr virus (EBV)-positive and EBV-negative gastric cancer. Helicobacter. 2016;21:153–7.

50. Minoura-Etoh J, Gotoh K, Sato R, Ogata M, Kaku N, Fujioka T, et al. Helicobacter pylori associated oxidant monochloramine induces reactivation of Epstein-Barr virus (EBV) in gastric epithelial cells latently infected with EBV. J Med Microbiol. 2006;55:905–11.

51. Ferrasi AC, Pinheiro NA, Rabenhorst SH, Caballero OL, Rodrigues MA, de Carvalho F, et al. Helicobacter pylori and EBV in gastric carcinomas: methylation status and microsatellite instability. World J Gastroentero. 2010;16:312–9.

52. Cárdenas-Mondragón MG, Carreon-Talavera R, Camorlinga-Ponce M, Gomez-Delgado A, Torres J, Fuentes-Panana EM. Epstein Barr virus and Helicobacter pylori co-infection are positively associated with severe gastritis in pediatric patients. PLoS One. 2013;8:e62850.

53. Cárdenas-Mondragón MG, Torres J, Flores-Luna L, Camorlinga-Ponce M, Carreón-Talavera R, Gomez-Delgado A, et al. Case-control study of Epstein–Barr virus and Helicobacter pylori serology in Latin American patients with gastric disease. Br J Cancer. 2015;112:1866–73.

54. Churin Y, Al-Ghoul L, Kepp O, Meyer TF, Birchmeier W, Naumann M. Helicobacter pylori CagA protein targets the c-met receptor and enhances the motogenic response. J Cell Biol. 2003;161:249–55.

55. Saju P, Murata-Kamiya N, Hayashi T, Senda Y, Nagase L, Noda S. Host SHP1 phosphatase antagonizes Helicobacter pylori CagA and can be downregulated by Epstein-Barr virus. Nat Microbiol. 2016;1:16026.

10

Major and ancillary magnetic resonance features of LI-RADS to assess HCC

Vincenza Granata[1], Roberta Fusco[1*], Antonio Avallone[2], Orlando Catalano[1], Francesco Filice[1], Maddalena Leongito[3], Raffaele Palaia[3], Francesco Izzo[3] and Antonella Petrillo[1]

Abstract

Liver Imaging Reporting and Data System (LI-RADS) is a system for interpreting and reporting of imaging features on multidetector computed tomography (MDCT) and magnetic resonance (MR) studies in patients at risk for hepatocellular carcinoma (HCC). American College of Radiology (ACR) sustained the spread of LI-RADS to homogenizing the interpreting and reporting data of HCC patients. Diagnosis of HCC is due to the presence of major imaging features. Major features are imaging data used to categorize LI-RADS-3, LI-RADS-4, and LI-RADS-5 and include arterial-phase hyperenhancement, tumor diameter, washout appearance, capsule appearance and threshold growth. Ancillary are features that can be used to modify the LI-RADS classification. Ancillary features supporting malignancy (diffusion restriction, moderate T2 hyperintensity, T1 hypointensity on hapatospecifc phase) can be used to upgrade category by one or more categories, but not beyond LI-RADS-4. Our purpose is reporting an overview and update of major and ancillary MR imaging features in assessment of HCC.

Keywords: HCC, LI-RADS, Magnetic resonance imaging

Background

Hepatocellular carcinoma (HCC) is one of the most common human solid malignancies worldwide [1, 2]. The most important risk factor for the development of HCC is liver cirrhosis, regardless of its etiology [1]. Among patients with cirrhosis, those with chronic viral infection (hepatitis B and C) and high alcohol intake have the highest risks of HCC development. Imaging surveillance is a widely accepted tool that increases the likelihood of early detection of HCC and an accurate detection and characterization of focal liver nodule on patient at risk for HCC is mandatory since the management of HCC patients differs to other malignant or benign nodules [2]. According to National Comprehensive Cancer Network (NCCN) [3] and the guidelines of European Association for the Study of the Liver (EASL) and American Association for the Study Liver Diseases (AASLD), diagnostic criteria, to characterize HCC, can

* Correspondence: r.fusco@istitutotumori.na.it
[1]Radiology Division, "Istituto Nazionale Tumori - IRCCS - Fondazione G. Pascale", Via Mariano Semmola, Naples, Italy
Full list of author information is available at the end of the article

only be applied to cirrhotic patients and should be based on the detection of the typical hallmark of HCC (hypervascular in the arterial phase with washout in the portal venous or delayed phases) [4]. However, the current imaging-based criteria have several limitations, including the lack of established consensus regarding the exact definitions of imaging features, binary categorization (either definite or not definite HCC), and failure to address non-HCC malignancies and vascular invasion [5]. Therefore American College of Radiology (ACR) sustained the spread of Liver Imaging Reporting and Data System (LI-RADS) to homogenizing the interpreting, reporting and data collection of HCC imaging [6]. LI-RADS is a scheme for interpreting and reporting of imaging features on multidetector computed tomography (CT) and magnetic resonance (MR) studies in patients at risk for hepatocellular carcinoma (HCC) [5-7]. In the current (v. 2014) LI-RADS [6], the diagnosis of HCC is based on the presence of major imaging features. These are features used to categorize LI-RADS- category 3 (LR-3), LI-RADS- category 4 (LR-4), and LI-RADS- category 5 (LR-5) and include arterial-phase hyperenhancement, tumor diameter, washout appearance, capsule appearance, and threshold growth [6]. Ancillary features are imaging features that can be used to change the LI-RADS category [5]. Ancillary features favoring malignancy (diffusion restriction, moderate T2 hyperintensity, T1 hypointensity on hepatospecific phase) can upgrade category, but not beyond LR-4. In contrast, ancillary features favoring benignity can decrease category [5, 6].

As required in most clinical trials, MDCT presents the key imaging modality in the patient assessment. This is due to its wide availability, standardization, and ability to scan the whole abdomen and chest in one setting. MRI plays a role in HCC assessment of patients with contraindication to iodine contrast medium [8]. However, considering the evidences on the accuracy of the various imaging modalities on HCC assessment [9], so as the guidelines of the European Society of Gastrointestinal and Abdominal Radiology (ESGAR) Working Group [10], MRI is the technique to choose in pre-treatment setting. It is a valuable diagnostic tool providing lesion morphological and functional data, thanks to hepatospecific contrast medium and DW sequences [11–14].

To standardize imaging technique among institutions, LI-RADS outlines technical requirements for MRI. Precontrast, arterial phase, portal venous phase, and delayed phase are all required for MRI with extracellular agents. Each phase contributes to characterization of LI-RADS major features. For MRI with hepatobiliary agents, a delay of 15–20 min for gadoxetic acid and a delay of 1 h for gadobenate dimeglumine consistently provide high-quality hepatobiliary phase imaging. In the setting of cirrhosis increasing the delay for hepatobiliary phase imaging to 30 min or more for gadoxetic acid and 2–3 h for gadobenate dimeglumine may improve parenchymal enhancement somewhat [6]. Although the delayed phase cannot be used to evaluate washout appearance, it can be used to evaluate capsule appearance, a major feature of HCC. Also, the delayed phase and hepatobiliary phase can be used to evaluate hypointensity on both sequences; these are ancillary features favoring malignancy and so can be used to upgrade the category. Late arterial phase is strongly preferred over early arterial phase, as HCC enhancement usually is greater in the late than in the early phase, and some HCCs show hyperenhancement only in the late arterial phase [6]. Unenhanced T1-weighted (T1-W) out of phase (OP)/in phase (IP) is required. T1-W OP/IP allows identification of fat and iron and is necessary for assessment of some ancillary features. T2-W sequences are required, improving distinction between solid and nonsolid lesions and are necessary for assessment of some ancillary LI-RADS features. DWI is suggested but not required [6].

Our purpose is reporting an overview and update of major and ancillary MR imaging features in assessment of HCC.

Methods
This overview and update is the result of autonomous studies without protocol and registration number.

Search criterion
Several electronic dataset were searched: PubMed (US National Library of Medicine, http://www.ncbi.nlm.nih.gov/pubmed), Scopus (Elsevier, http://www.scopus.com/), Web of Science (Thomson Reuters, http://apps.webof knowledge.com/) and Google Scholar (https://scholar.google.it/). The following search criteria have been used: "hepatocellular carcinoma" AND "diffusion magnetic resonance imaging" AND "characterization, "hepatocellular carcinoma" AND "dynamic contrast enhanced magnetic resonance imaging" AND "characterization, "hepatocellular carcinoma" AND "EOB-GD-DTPA contrast medium" AND "characterization, "hepatocellular carcinoma" AND "multimodal imaging" AND "characterization". The search covered the years from January 2000 to January 2017. Moreover, the reference lists of the found papers were analysed for papers not indexed in the electronic databases.

All titles and abstracts were analysed and exclusively the studies reporting MRI, EOB-GD-DTPA MRI, DWI results in the characterization of HCC were retained.

The inclusion criteria were: clinical study evaluating MR assessment of HCC, clinical study evaluating functional MR imaging criteria in the assessment of patients with HCC, and clinical study evaluating DWI and EOB-GD-DTPA to assessing HCC patient. Articles published in the English language from January 2000 to January 2017 were included. Exclusion criteria were unavailability of full text, general overview articles and congress abstracts; studies with lesion higher than 20 mm. There was not define a minimum number of patients as an inclusion criteria.

Results
By using the search terms described earlier, we identified 5181 studies from January 2000 to January 2017. To identify additional relevant studies, the reference lists of the retrieved studies were checked manually. 1955 studies used other diagnostic techniques than MRI, EOB-GD-DTPA-MRI and DWI, 726 have different topic respect to characterization; 309 did not have sufficient data (case report, review, letter to editors); 2128 corresponded to more than one criteria so 63 articles were included at the end (Fig. 1).

Discussion
Early diagnosis is a critical step in the management of HCC patients. The identification of the specific vascular

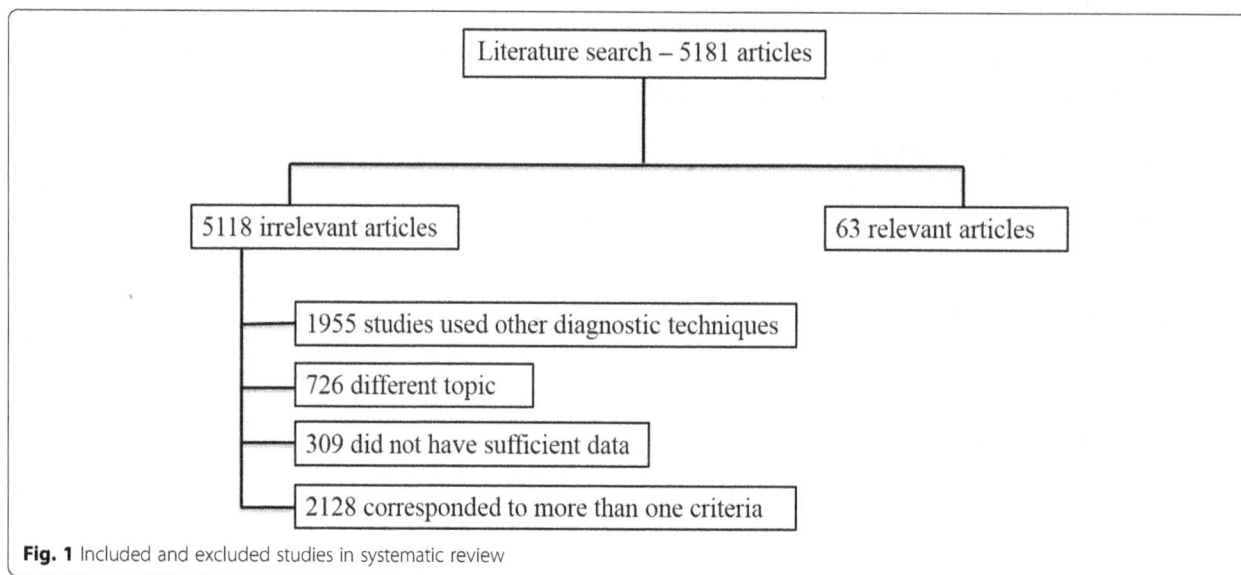

Fig. 1 Included and excluded studies in systematic review

profile characterized by contrast arterial uptake followed by washout in the venous phases has allowed defining the non-invasive diagnostic criteria for HCC according to AASLD and EASL-EORTC guidelines [4, 5]. The typical hallmark has 100% specificity when demonstrated on dynamic contrast study, both on CT than on MRI, in patients at high risk of HCC [1]. However, arterial hyperehnancement and wash out appearance have a sensitivity rate of 50–60% in lesion smaller than 2 cm and thus a biopsy is still needed [15]. The typical vascular profile is correlated to hemodynamic changes in nodule during hepatocarcinogenesis, and to understand the hemodynamics of HCC is important for the accurate diagnostic analysis, because there is an intense correlation between their hemodynamics and pathophysiology [16]. Angiogenesis such as sinusoidal capillarization and unpaired arteries shows gradual increase during carcinogenesis from high-grade dysplastic nodule to classic hypervascular HCC. In accordance with this angiogenesis, the intranodular portal supply is decreased, whereas the intranodular arterial supply is first decreased during the early stage and then increased in parallel with increasing grade of malignancy of the lesion. On the other hand, the main drainage vessels of hepatocellular nodules change from hepatic veins to hepatic sinusoids and then to portal veins, mainly due to disappearance of the hepatic veins from the nodules [16]. The nodule appearance on arterial phase relative, considering the intra-lesion arterial supply, can be categorized into four types. Type I when the nodule is isodense to the surrounding cirrhotic liver parenchyma, and it is due to the same intranodular arterial blood supply relative to the surrounding liver. Type II, when the nodule is hypodense to the surrounding cirrhotic liver parenchyma, indicating decreased arterial

blood supply. Type III a part of the nodule demonstrating hyperdensity due a partially increased arterial supply and type IV entirely hyperdense indicating entirely increased arterial supply [16, 17]. These findings reveal the significant correlation or strong tendency between type I and low grade dysplastic nodule and early HCC, type II and high grade dysplastic nodule and early HCC, type III and well differentiated HCC and type IV and moderately or poorly differentiated HCC [16, 17]. Also in early HCC, there is not perinodular enhancement on portal or equilibrium phase of contrast study, but it is definite in hypervascular classical HCC.

During hepatocarcinogenesis multi-step changes of drainage vessels and peritumoral enhancement occurred. In dysplastic nodules or early HCCs, the main drainage route from the tumor is intranodular or perinodular hepatic vein. However, because hepatic veins disappear from the tumor during very early stage of hepatocarcinogenesis, drainage vessels change to hepatic sinusoids. This drainage was well visualized in the late phase of contrast studies. Histological examination revealed continuity between a tumor sinusoid and a portal venule in the pseudocapsule (encapsulated HCC) or surrounding hepatic sinusoids (HCC without pseudocapsule). In moderately differentiated HCC with pseudocapsule formation, the communication between tumor sinusoids and the surrounding hepatic sinusoids are also blocked, and then, the portal venules in the pseudo-capsule finally become the main drainage vessel from the tumor. In accordance with the changes of the drainage vessels, thin to thick corona enhancement appears surrounding the tumor. Corona enhancement is thicker in encapsulated HCC and thin in HCC without pseudocapsule [16].

Arterial phase hyperenhancement

Arterial phase hyperenhancement is an essential prerequisite for definitely HCC (LR-5), but it is non-specific. In fact considering the hepatocarcinogenesis this feature may be not present, so as it may be observed in benign entities such as dysplastic nodules and arterio-portal shunts [1, 2]. Holland et al. showed, in proven HCC patients, that the majority (93%) of hypervascular lesions on arterial phase that were not detected on T2-W and portal and/or equilibrium phase of contrast study were non-neoplastic [18]. Conversely, Kim et coworkers [19] demonstrated that the most significant findings associated with HCC, in nodules smaller than 20 mm, were arterial phase hypernhancement. Ehman et al. demonstrated that arterial hypenhancement was the most commonly observed major criterion on 159 (86%) of 184 proven HCC, and was seen slightly more frequently at CT vs. MRI (87 vs. 86%, $p = 1.00$). Between the two readers, there was agreement on arterial phase characteristics in 156 (95%) cases ($\kappa = 0.75$) [20]. Conversely Burrel et al. [21] showed that sensitivity of MR was superior to CT to detect HCC (58/76 [76%] versus 43/70 [61%], respectively). Sensitivity of MR for detection of additional nodules decreased with size (>20 mm: 6/6 [100%]; 10–20 mm: 16/19 [84%]; <10 mm: 7/22 [32%]) and was superior to CT for nodules 10 to 20 mm (84 vs. 47%). Non specific hypervascular nodules >5 mm at MR were HCC in two thirds of the cases [21]. Special attention must be given to perfusion alterations, common condition in cirrhotic livers that may be false positive. These are areas of arterial hyperenhancement most frequently caused by arterioportal shunts [22, 23]. These alterations are usually peripheral, wedge shaped, and isointense relative to the surrounding parenchyma on T1- and T2-W MR images, and can be confidently characterized as LR-1. Perfusion alterations can also be nodular and it is difficult to distinguish from a true lesion [18, 23]. Areas of nodular arterial hyperenhancement seen exclusively during the arterial phase are more appropriately categorized as LR-2 [13, 18], but if corresponding others observations (eg, hyperintensity T2 signal or restricted diffusion) should be categorized as either LR-3 or LR-4 depending on its size and nonvascular features. Some areas of perfusion alteration can occur secondary to focal liver lesions, including HCC [24].

Arterial hyperenhancement is the most considerable feature in patients with HCC (Fig. 2) and is considered to be the most important feature for imaging diagnosis [25–27]. This feature reflects the neoangiogenesis, which is associated with the stepwise process of carcinogenesis and becomes the dominant blood supply in overt HCC lesions [16, 17].

Washout appearance

Washout appearance is a reduction in contrast-enhancement relative to liver from an earlier to a later phase resulting in hypoenhancement in portal or delayed phase [28]. This may reflect multiple concomitant phenomena: rapid venous drainage, reduced portal venous supply and later enhancement of the background liver especially with hepatobiliary agents [28]. Jang et al. reported a variation in the timing of washout

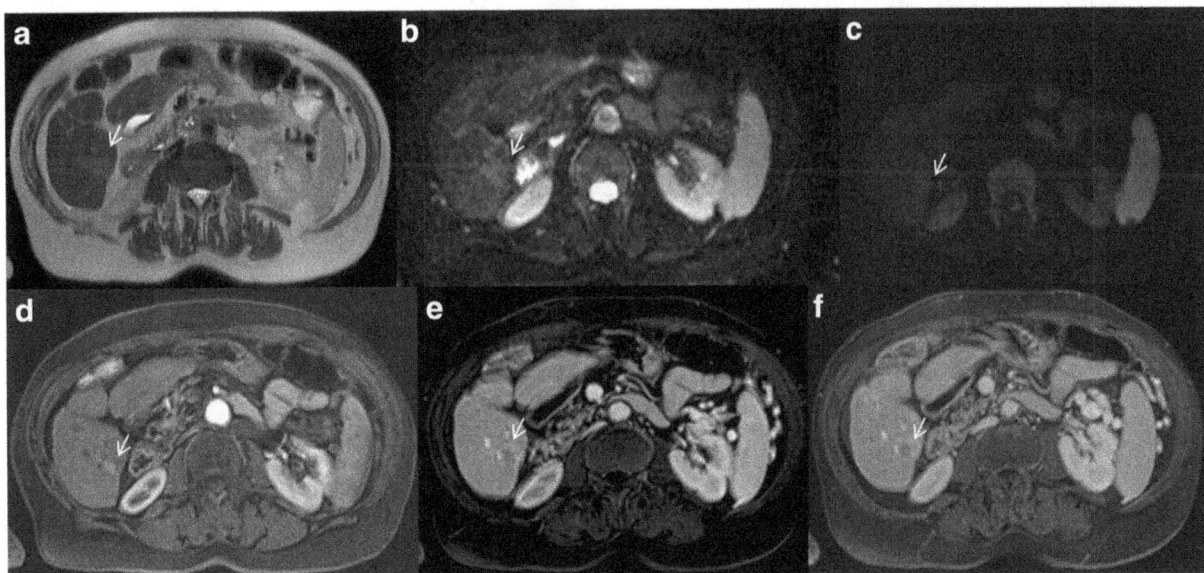

Fig. 2 Man 73 years old with typical HCC on VI hepatic segment. The HCC is hyperintense (*arrow*) on T2-W sequences (**a**), shows (*arrows*) restrict diffusion (**b**: b50 s/mm^2, **c**: b800 s/mm^2). After contrast medium injection, the nodule is hypervascular (*arrow*) on arterial phase (**d**), with wash-out appearance (*arrow*) on portal phase (**e**) and capsule appearance (*arrow*) on equilibrium phase (**f**) of contrast study with Gd-BT-DO3A

in the portal venous and delayed phases [29]. He reported, in a pilot study on enhancement of 112 histologically proven HCCs, that arterial phase hyperenhancement was present on 74 (77, 96%) and portal washout within 90 s on 72 (74, 97%) in the majority of moderately differentiated HCC. However, the authors found that well differentiated and poorly differentiated HCCs had an atypical enhancement patterns where 25 out of 97 (26%) showed washout between 91 and 180 s and 21 out of 97 (22%) showed late washout between 180 and 300 s [29]. Choi et al. [30] demonstrated as HCCs smaller than 1.5 cm showed typical features less frequently than HCCs 1.5 cm or larger in diameter. In subgroup analyses, HCCs with diameters between 1 and 1.5 cm showed similar MRI findings to HCCs with diameters 1 cm or less but significantly different findings compared with HCCs with diameters from 1.5 to 2 cm and 2–3 cm [31]. Portal or later hypoenhancement is considered a strong predictor of HCC, particularly when combined with arterial phase hyperenhancement [30]. Conversely Granito et al. [32] demonstrated that the most interesting result of their study was the finding of 8 HCC nodules, seven of which lacked the typical vascular pattern, which appeared as hypointense nodules on hepatobiliary phase with wash- out on portal phase, not preceded by arterial hyperenhancement (Fig. 3) [32]. This radiological pattern (wash-out and hypointense signal on hepatobiliary phase) could correspond to an early stage of

carcinogenesis characterized by a reduction in both portal venous and arterial supplies [32]. The presence of wash out is a crucial step on LI-RADS decision tree for LR- 3–5 observations [1–3]. Becker et al. showed as the diameter and washout criteria using a step wise LI-RADS decision tree for LR- 3–5 observations allowed faster categorization with better inter-observer reliability while maintaining the excellent diagnostic accuracy of the most recent LI-RADS v2014 [33]. Fibrotic tissue in cirrhotic hepatic parenchyma typically shows hypointensity signal on portal or delayed phase of contrast study that may cause a false appearance of hypoenhancement of a regenerative nodule when these are surrounded by fibrosis. In some cases, fibrotic tissue may even mimic a delayed enhancing capsule or pseudo-capsule [34].

Capsule appearance

Capsule appearance is defined as a peripheral rim of smooth hyperenhancement in the portal or delayed phase (Fig. 3). The rim of enhancement is not always a true tumor capsule, but may represent a pseudocapsule corresponding to fibrous tissue and dilated sinusoids around a nodule [16, 17, 28]. Anis and coworkers showed as the capsule appearance has a high positive predictive value for HCC in at-risk patients [35]. Dioguardi Burgio et al. [36] showed as hyperintense capsule was present either on portal phase in 11/46 and in 24/25 HCCs imaged with gadoxetic acid and gadobenate dimeglumine-enhanced

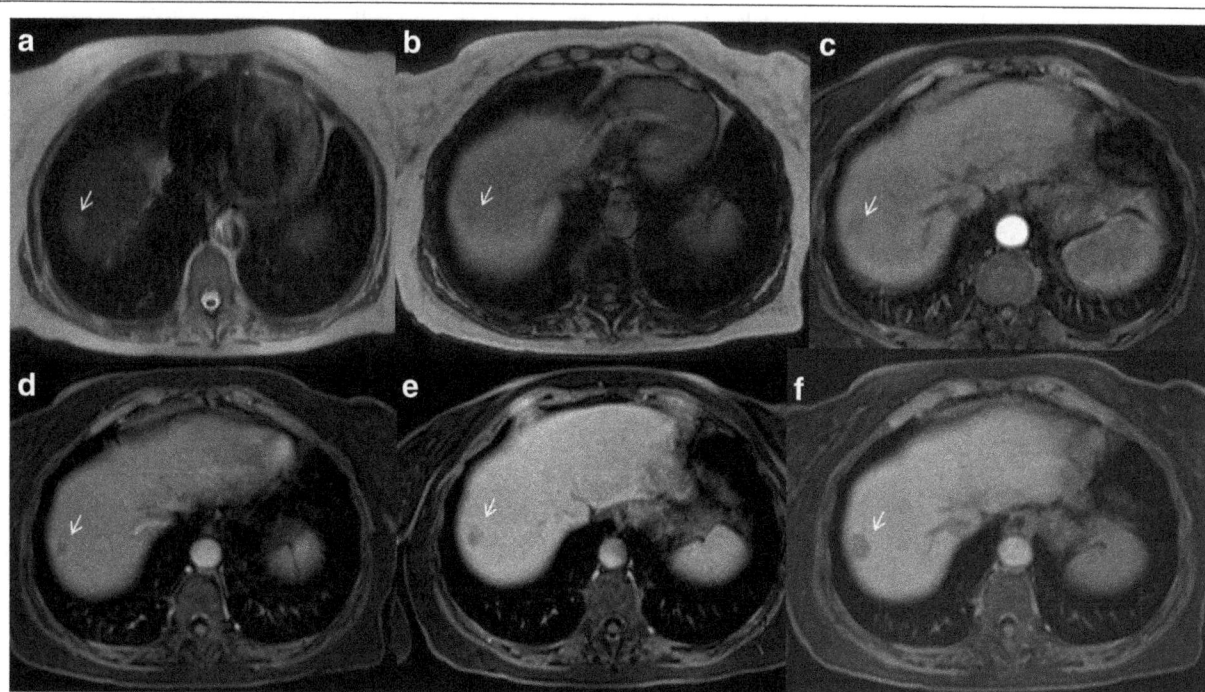

Fig. 3 Woman 73 years old with atypical HCC on VII-VIII hepatic segment. The HCC is hyperintense (*arrow*) on T2-W sequences (**a**) and hypointense (*arrow*) on T1-W sequences (**b**: out-of-phase). During arterial phase (**c**), it is not hypervascular (*arrow*), while there is wash-out appearance (*arrow*) and capsule appearance (*arrow*) on portal phase (**d**), on equilibrium phase (**e**) and hepatospecific phase (**f**) of contrast study

MR imaging, respectively (24 vs. 96%). A hypointense capsule appearance was present on hepatobiliary phase in 8/ 46 and 0/22 HCCs evaluated with gadoxetic acid and gadobenate dimeglumine-enhanced MR imaging, respectively (17 vs. 0%) [36]. Conversely to Dioguardi Burgio et al. that analyzed two different contrast media, Zhang et al. [37] compared diagnostic accuracy of CT and MRI to predicting of malignancy and showed that CT against MR produced false-negative findings of pseudo-capsule by 42.9% with an underestimated LI-RADS score by 16.9% for LR- 3, 37.3% for LR- 4, and 8.5% for LR- 5. CT produced significantly lower accuracy (54.3 versus 67.8%) and sensitivity (31.6 versus 71.1%) than MRI in the prediction of malignancy [37]. Also Corwin et al. [38] compared the diagnostic accuracy of CT respected to MR to grading LI-RADS. The most important finding of this study was that nearly half (42%) of observations were significantly upgraded on MRI compared with CT, and approximately one third of upgrades were to category 4, 5, or 5 V. The most common reason for the upgrade by MRI was the visualization of arterial hyperenhancement or a delayed enhancing capsule not seen on CT [38]. It is clear that these features should be correctly identified since they are major features on LI-RADS.

Hypointense signal on hepatobiliary phase

Hepatobiliary contrast agents are widely used in the evaluation of patients at high risk for HCC. GD-EOB-DTPA is a liver-specific agent, taken up by hepatocytes. It can be injected as an intravenous bolus, providing data about lesion vascularity in the different phases of contrast circulation. Additionally functional data can be obtained in the delayed, hepatobiliary phase [39]. Recently, the LI-RADS system incorporated the hepatobiliary phase appearance of observations as an ancillary feature that may be used to favor malignancy or benignity [40, 41]. Two ancillary features favoring malignancy on hepatobiliary phase include observation hypointensity, which is defined as the intensity of an observation lesser than the surrounding liver parenchyma, and hypointense rim, which is thought to correlate to a capsule (Fig. 4) [40, 41]. Conversely, iso-intensity of an observation to background liver favors benignity [41]; however, the study must have an adequate hepatobiliary phase, defined by LI-RADS as liver parenchyma being unequivocally hyperintense to the intrahepatic vessels. It has been demonstrated that the use of Gd-EOB-DTPA improves detection of HCC with higher sensitivity and specificity when compared to the studies with extracellular agents [40, 41]. Despites the advantages, there are also several limits. Hepatobiliary agents cost more than traditional extracellular contrast agents. Hepatobiliary agents have been associated with acute transient dyspnoea, independent of other patient risk factors [42, 43]. This dyspnoea occurs during the arterial phase imaging, therefore, degrading the study and limiting the evaluation for hepatic arterial hyperenhancement that is typical of HCC [42, 43]. Also the uptake of contrast medium by hepatocytes depends on function and the presence of membrane transporters, which are downregulated in the setting of cirrhosis [44–46]. Therefore, the utility of these agents may be clarified in patients with hepatic dysfunction. There have been several studies

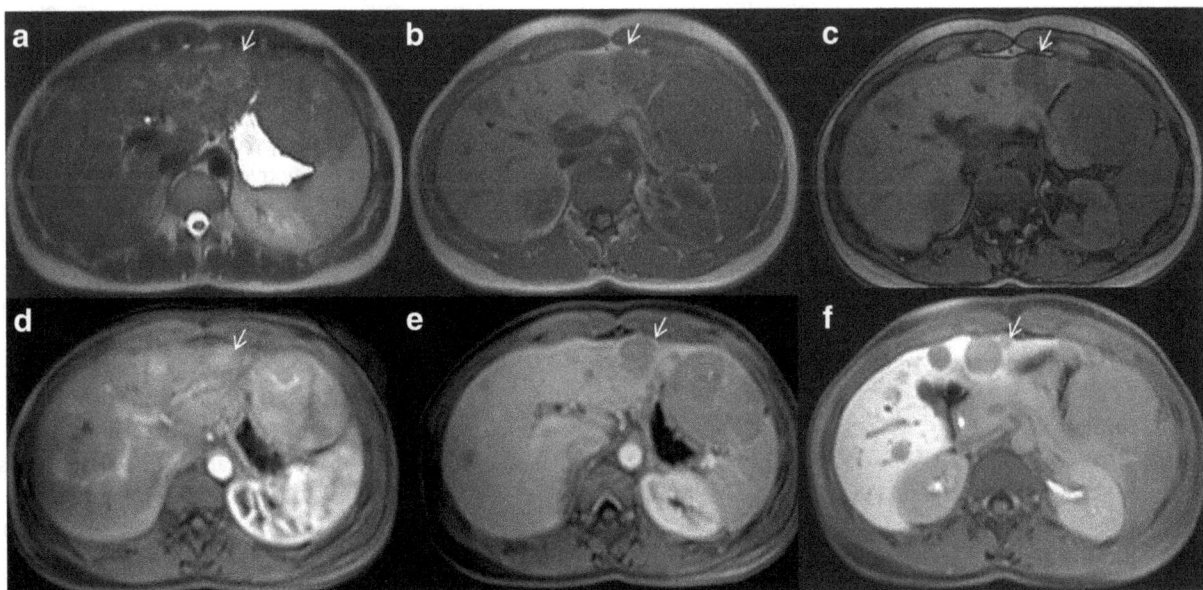

Fig. 4 Woman 44 years old with multiple nodules of HCC. The nodules are hyperintense (*arrow*) on T2-W sequences (**a**), hypointense (*arrow*) on T1-W sequences (**b**: in-of-phase; **c**: out-of-phase), hypervascular (*arrow*) on arterial phase (**d**), with wash-out and capsule appearance (*arrow*) on portal phase (**e**) and hypointense signal (*arrow*) on hepatospecific phase (**f**) of contrast study with EOB-GD-DTPA

examining correlation of liver enhancement during the hepatobiliary phase with Child Pugh class, Model for End-stage Liver Disease (MELD) score, and various laboratory factors [47, 48]; however, no definitive cut-off values have been established for clinical parameters. As a suboptimal hepatobiliary phase would negate the advantage of these agents respect to extracellular agents [49]. Despite these limits several researches have demonstrated that EOB-GD-DTPA can favor the detection and the characterization of HCC nodule [50–56]. According to Golfieri et al. [53], during the hepatospecific phase, typical HCC and early HCC appear hypointense, whereas low-grade dysplastic or regenerative nodules appear as iso- or hyperintense lesions. The diagnostic accuracy of EOB-MRI for the diagnosis of early HCC is approximately 95–100% [53]. One third of hypovascular hypointense nodules in hepatospecific phase become hypervascular 'progressed' HCC, with a 1 and 3-year. Therefore, the authors suggested that these hypovascular nodules should be strictly followed up or definitely treated as typical HCC [53]. In the study by Ahn et al. [54], 9 out of 84 HCCs (10.7%) were exclusively identified by hepatospecific phase and three were early HCCs, while in Golfieri et al. [55] 19 out of 20 early HCC remained unclassified at dynamic MRI alone because of atypical behavior and were diagnosed only in the hepatospecific phase. Golfieri et al. [56], in a pilot study, suggested that in atypical cirrhotic nodule, hypointensity in the hepatospecific phase is the most relevant diagnostic sign for differentiating low-risk from high-risk nodules, since the reduction of Gd-EOB-DTPA uptake seems to occur at an early stage of hepatocarcinogenesis which precedes the reduction of portal blood flow and nodule arterialization [56]. In fact an experimental study showed a gradual loss of the ability of hepatocytes to take up Gd-EOB-DTPA during hepatocarcinogenesis, according to the progression from dysplastic nodules to poorly differentiated HCC [57]. However, several authors documented that 5–10% of human HCCs can show a paradoxical uptake of Gd-EOB-DTPA in the hepatobiliary phase, appearing as iso- or hyperintense, whereas some dysplastic nodules can exhibit hypointensity [58–61]. However, according to Golfieri et al. [56], for atypical HCC hepatospecific phase hypointensity should be used as the second marker of malignancy.

T2-W Hyperintensity

According to LI-RADS, T2-W hyperintensity is an ancillary imaging features (Fig. 5). Park et al. [17] showed that dysplastic nodules and HCCs cannot be distinguished on the basis of signal intensity characteristics on unenhanced MRI, since their signal intensities are similar on T1- and T2-W sequences. However, dysplastic nodules are almost never hyperintense on T2-W, early HCCs are mostly isointense on T2-W,

while higher grade (moderately or poorly) of HCC is associated with high signal intensity on T2-W images, although the signal intensity may also be related with tumor vascularity and peliotic changes [17]. Previous study demonstrated that T2-W hyperintensity was a highly specific marker of nodule malignancy, although poorly sensitive [27–62]. Golfieri et al. [56] showed that, compared to hypointensy on hepatospecific phase, T2-W hyperintensity was a poor predictor of malignancy in the early stages of HCC. Conversely to Golfieri [56], Ouedraogo et al. [63] demonstrated that the addition of T2-W hyperintensity to the AASLD criteria increased the detection rate of HCC, especially nodules smaller than 20 mm. In fact the sensitivity of MRI increased from 67.6 to 79%. Sofue et al. [64] evaluated the imaging features in MRI that are associated with upgrade of LI-RADS category observations to category 5, and demonstrated that the risk factors in the 56 LR-4 observations that upgraded to LR-5 were mild-moderate T2 hyperintensity ($P < 0.001$; hazard ratio = 1.84) and growth ($P < 0.001$; hazard ratio = 3.71). Although mild-moderate T2 hyperintensity was the most useful risk factor for predicting upgrade, actual risk level was only mildly elevated. Hwang et al. [65] compared the diagnostic performance of DWI and T2-W images, in differentiating between hypovascular HCC and dysplastic nodules seen as hypointense nodules at hepatobiliary phase. They showed that hyperintensity on T2-W and DWI were significant features for differentiating hypovascular HCCs from dysplastic nodules ($P < 0.05$), while there was no significant difference in mean ADC between hypovascular HCCs (1.06 ± 0.13) and dysplastic nodules (1.09 ± 0.13). The sensitivity of DWI was higher than T2-W (72.0% [18 of 25] versus 40.0% [10 of 25]). Hyperintensity on T2-W and DWI could be a useful imaging tool to differentiate hypovascular HCCs from dysplastic nodules seen as hypointense nodules in the hepatobiliary phase. Kim et al. [66] evaluated the most predictive finding among hyperintensity on T2-W, DWI, washout, capsular enhancement, and hypointensity on gadoxetic acid-enhanced hepatobiliary phase images in the detailed characterization of arterial phase enhancing nodules 1 cm in diameter and smaller. They showed that for hypervascular lesions 1 cm in diameter or smaller, T2-weighted images have the highest sensitivity among tests with an odds ratio statistically separable from 1 for differentiating HCC from benign hypervascular lesions 1 cm or smaller. Conversely Hussain et al. [67] concluded that T2-W images do not provide added diagnostic value in the detection and characterization of focal lesions because the heterogeneity and hyperintense fibrotic septa in the cirrhotic liver parenchyma can obscure moderately hyperintense HCC on T2-W images and that 42–53% of HCCs may be iso-intense to hypointense on T2-weighted images. Other

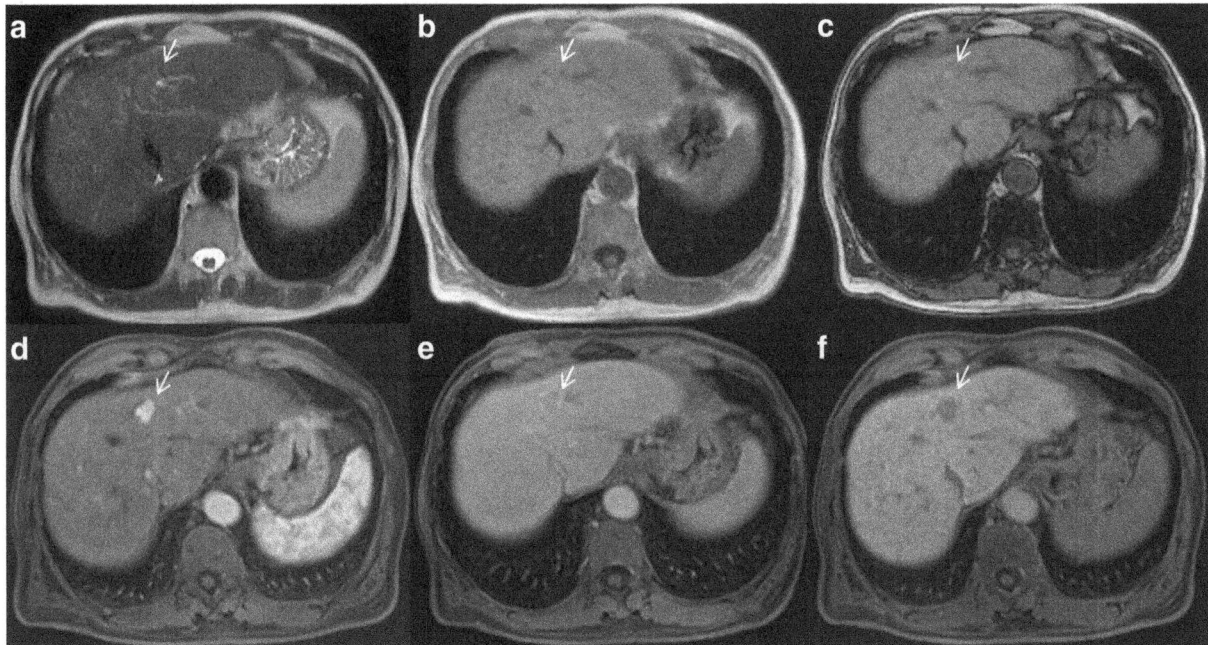

Fig. 5 Man 74 years old with HCC on II hepatic segment. The HCC is hyperintense (*arrow*) on T2-W sequence (**a**), isointense (*arrow*) on T1-W (**b**: in-of-phase) with peripheral fat suppression (*arrow*) on T1-out of phase (**c**). During arterial phase of contrast study (**d**) with EOB-GD-DTPA, the HCC shows hyperenhancement (*arrow*), with wash-out and capsule appearance (*arrow*) on portal phase (**e**). During hepatospecific phase (**f**) of contrast study the HCC is hypointense (*arrow*)

researches also have reported that the combined use of hyperintensity on T2-W images improves differentiation of small non solid benign lesions from solid malignant tumors in the liver [68, 69].

Restricted diffusion

The role of DWI in HCC patient has been evaluated by different studies [70–76]. Lee et al. [72] demonstrated that the addition of DWI to the gadoxetic acid-enhanced MRI could be a guideline in differentiating between HCCs and dysplastic nodules. In their study, 86 HCCs (84.3%) showed hyperintensity on DWI, whereas only three dysplastic nodules (13.0%) showed this feature. So they concluded that hyperintensity on DWI was highly indicative of HCC in patients with chronic hepatitis or cirrhosis. Also Piana et al. [73] showed that enhancement in the arterial phase and hyperintensity on DWI were found to be significantly more sensitive criteria for HCC than conventional criteria (77–76 vs. 60% for all HCCs and 66–60 vs. 37% for HCCs smaller than 20 mm). Sensitivity was even higher when enhancement in the arterial-dominant phase and washout (in the portal venous and/or equilibrium phases) or hyperintensity on DWI was used (84–85% for all HCCs and 71–74% for HCCs smaller than 20 mm). Granata et al. [74] demonstrated that that DWI could be used to predict the histological grade of HCC; in fact they found that there was a good correlation between ADC and grading,

between perfusion fraction (fp) and grading, and between tissue pure diffusivity (Dt) and grading. Nakanishi et al. [75] showed not only the usefulness of DWI for histological grading, but also the possibility to use ADC as a preoperative prediction of early HCC recurrence within 6 months of operation. Conversely, Nasu et al., in a series of 125 resected HCCs (sizes range: 0.8–15 cm), found no correlation between histological grade and ADC (using b factors of 0 and 500 s/mm^2), although the DWI and Signal Intensity of the HCCs increased in higher grade [76]. Sutherland et al. [77] compared ultrasound screening with DWI for detecting HCC. The sensitivity, specificity, positive predictive value and negative predictive values for US were 100, 90, 23 and 100%, respectively, while for MRI were 83, 98, 63 and 99%. The major advantage of DWI over US screening in this study has been the low false-positive rate of DWI. In fact US had false-positive studies 20 times (10%) while DWI had three false-positive examinations (2%). The reasons for the low false-positive rate of DWI include: not depicting macro regenerative and low grade dysplastic nodules and not depicting focal fatty heterogeneity, also the ability to correctly classify benign nodules as cavernous haemangiomas which usually have elevated apparent diffusion coefficient (ADC) values. They concluded that more studies are needed to validate the DWI as a screening tool and therefore it should replace US as a cost-effective screening tool

[77]. DWI could be used as a helpful diagnostic tool for HCC in patients with chronic liver disease, since DWI can accurately detect HCC in patients with chronic liver disease regardless of the lesion size (Fig. 6). A potential reason for the better accuracy of DWI is that this does not rely on morphologic features only. Malignant tissues tend to be hypercellular with an accumulation of macromolecular proteins leaving a small extracellular space resulting in a decrease of the ADC value [78]. The major limits of DWI are the different parameters used in DWI sequences which may affect the results of ADC calculation. The different b values, selection method, bias of patient selection, pathological characteristic of lesions and measurement of ADC values may be reduced the reproducibility of the data, however all analyzed studies showed that the mean ADC value of malignant lesions was lower than that of benign lesions [70–80].

Other ancillary features (intalesional fat, corona enhancement, mosaic architecture and iron sparing in iron overloaded)

MR imaging diagnosis of HCC is based mainly on assessment of vascularity, capsule appearance, and signal intensity in the hepatobiliary phase. MR imaging also permit assessment of ancillary imaging features, that can be divided into those that favor the diagnosis of HCC specifically (intralesional fat, corona enhancement, nodule-in-nodule architecture, and mosaic architecture) and those that favor the diagnosis of malignancy but are not specific for HCC (mild-moderate T2 hyperintensity, restricted diffusion, and lesional iron sparing) [5–7, 81].

Intralesional fat is the presence of lipid within a nodule in higher concentration than in the hepatic parenchyma [6]. This feature can be detected at MR by observing signal loss on out-of-phase compared with in-phase T1-weighted GRE images. In a patient at risk for HCC, the detection of intralesional fat in a solid nodule raises

concern for malignancy or premalignancy. In fact, this feature does not establish the diagnosis of HCC, however, as the differential diagnosis includes high-grade dysplastic nodule and occasionally low-grade dysplastic nodule [82].

Corona enhancement is a feature of hypervascular, progressed HCC and refers to enhancement of the venous drainage area in the peritumoral parenchyma [16]. It is as a rim ("corona") of enhancement around a progressed, hypervascular HCC in the late arterial phase or early portal venous phase, with fading to isoenhancement at subsequent phases. This feature begins a few seconds after tumor enhancement, so that corona and tumor enhancement may appear to overlap. This overlap may cause the tumor to appear larger than it really is. Its presence helps to differentiate small hypervascular HCCs from pseudolesions, however it is not a feature of early HCC [16, 82].

Mosaic architecture refers to the presence within a mass of randomly distributed internal nodules differing in enhancement, intensity, often separated by fibrous septa. This feature is characteristic of large HCCs and reflects the mosaic configuration observed at pathologic evaluation. It is unusual in tumors other than HCC [82].

Lesional iron sparing refers to relative paucity of iron in a solid mass compared with that of background iron-overloaded liver. This feature raises concern for premalignancy or malignancy because high-grade dysplastic nodules and HCCs characteristically are iron "resistant". However it is not specific for high-grade dysplastic nodule or HCC, but other non-HCC malignancies may have this appearance [82].

Conclusion

Early diagnosis is a critical step in the management of HCC patients. The identification of the specific vascular profile characterized by contrast arterial uptake followed by washout in the venous phases has 100% specificity when demonstrated on dynamic contrast study, in

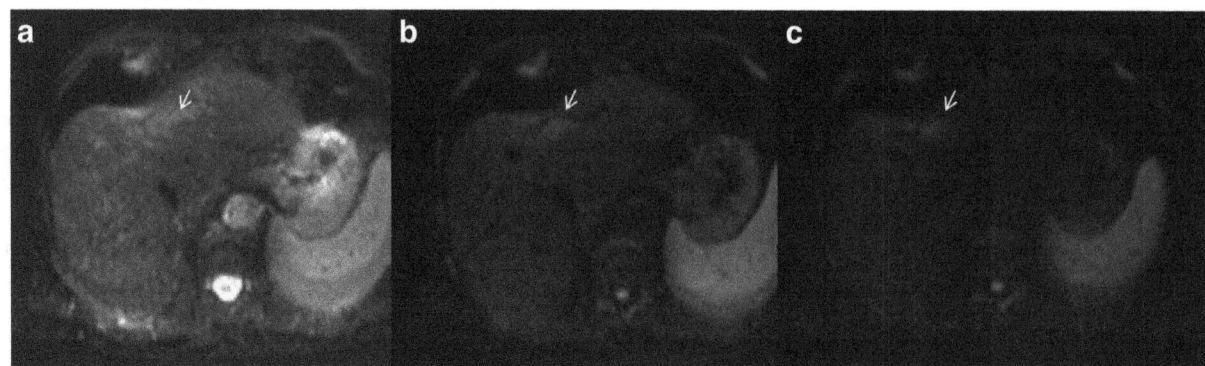

Fig. 6 The same patient of Fig. 5. Restricted diffusion. The nodule (arrow) shows hyperintense signal on b0 s/mm^2 (**a**), on b 500 s/mm^2 (**b**) and on b 800 s/mm^2(**c**)

patients at high risk of HCC. Although the arterial phase hyperenhancement is an essential prerequisite for definitely HCC, it is not sufficient for LR-5 categorization. Hypointensity on hepatospecific phase and wash-out appearance are the most relevant diagnostic sign for differentiating low-risk from high-risk nodules in patients at risk for HCC. Therefore the use of EOB-GD-DTPA should be considered in this category of patients. The capsule appearance, T2-W hyperintensity and restricted diffusion have a high positive predictive value for HCC and may be associated to other imaging features for LIRADS characterization.

Acknowledgements

The authors are grateful to Alessandra Trocino, librarian at the National Cancer Institute of Naples, Italy. Moreover, for the collaboration, authors are grateful to Maria Bruno, Laura Galeani, Rita Guarino, Leandro Eto and Assunta Zazzaro.

Funding

Not applicable.

Authors' contributions

VG conceived of the study, and participated in its design, coordination and drafting of the manuscript. RF participated in the studies collection and drafted the manuscript. AA, OC, FF, ML, RP, FI, AP participated in the studies collection. All authors read and approved the final manuscript.

Competing interests

The authors have no conflict of interest to be disclosed. The authors confirm that the article is not under consideration for publication elsewhere. Each author has participated sufficiently to take public responsibility for the manuscript content.

Author details

[1]Radiology Division, "Istituto Nazionale Tumori - IRCCS - Fondazione G. Pascale", Via Mariano Semmola, Naples, Italy. [2]Abdominal Oncology Division, "Istituto Nazionale Tumori - IRCCS - Fondazione G. Pascale", Via Mariano Semmola, Naples, Italy. [3]Hepatobiliary Surgery Division, "Istituto Nazionale Tumori - IRCCS - Fondazione G. Pascale", Via Mariano Semmola, Naples, Italy.

References

1. Bruix J, Sherman M. Management of hepatocellular carcinoma: An update. Hepatology. 2011;53:1020–2.
2. Izzo F, Albino V, Palaia R, et al. Hepatocellular carcinoma: preclinical data on a dual-lumen catheter kit for fibrin sealant infusion following loco-regional treatments. Infect Agent Cancer. 2014;9(1):39.
3. NCCN Clinical Practice Guidelines in Oncology on hepatobiliary cancer. Version 2016. http://www.nccn.org.
4. European Association for Study of Liver. European Organisation for Research and Treatment of Cancer. EASL-EORTC clinical practice guidelines: management of hepatocellular carcinoma. Eur J Cancer. 2012;48(5):599–641. doi:10.1016/j.ejca.2011.12.021. Erratum in: Eur J Cancer. 2012 May; 48(8): 1255–6.
5. An C, Rakhmonova G, Choi JY, et al. Liver imaging reporting and data system (LI-RADS) version 2014: understanding and application of the diagnostic algorithm. Clin Mol Hepatol. 2016;22(2):296–307.
6. American College of Radiology. Liver Imaging Reporting and Data System Version 2014. ACR Web site < http://www.acr.org/Quality-Safety/Resources/LIRADS >. Accessed 15 Apr 2016.
7. Santillan CS, Tang A, Cruite I, et al. Understanding LI-RADS: a primer for practical use. Magn Reson Imaging Clin N Am. 2014;22:337–52.
8. Schima W, Ba-Ssalamah A, Kurtaran A, et al. Post-treatment imaging of liver tumours. Cancer Imaging. 2007;7(Spec No A):S28–36.
9. Granata V, Petrillo M, Fusco R, et al. Surveillance of HCC Patients after Liver RFA: Role of MRI with Hepatospecific Contrast versus Three-Phase CT Scan-Experience of High Volume Oncologic Institute. Gastroenterol Res Pract. 2013;2013:469097.
10. Neri E, Bali MA, Ba-Ssalamah A, et al. ESGAR consensus statement on liver MR imaging and clinical use of liver-specific contrast agents. Eur Radiol. 2016;26:921–31.
11. Granata V, de Lutio di Castelguidone E, Fusco R, et al. Irreversible electroporation of hepatocellular carcinoma: preliminary report on the diagnostic accuracy of magnetic resonance, computer tomography, and contrast-enhanced ultrasound in evaluation of the ablated area. Radiol Med. 2016;121(2):122–31.
12. Prince MR, Zhang H, Zou Z, et al. Incidence of immediate gadolinium contrast media reactions. AJR Am J Roentgenol. 2011;196(2):W138–43.
13. Izzo F, Palaia R, Albino V, et al. S. Hepatocellular carcinoma and liver metastases: clinical data on a new dual-lumen catheter kit for surgical sealant infusion to prevent perihepatic bleeding and dissemination of cancer cells following biopsy and loco-regional treatments. Infect Agent Cancer. 2015;10:11.
14. Granata V, Fusco R, Catalano O, et al. Percutaneous ablation therapy of hepatocellular carcinoma with irreversible electroporation: MRI findings. AJR Am J Roentgenol. 2015;204(5):1000–7.
15. Forner A, Vilana R, Ayuso C, et al. Diagnosis of hepatic nodules 20 mm or smaller in cirrhosis: Prospective validation of the noninvasive diagnostic criteria for hepatocellular carcinoma. Hepatology. 2008;47:97–104.
16. Matsui O, Kobayashi S, Sanada J, et al. Hepatocelluar nodules in liver cirrhosis: hemodynamic evaluation (angiography-assisted CT) with special reference to multi-step hepatocarcinogenesis. Abdom Imaging. 2011;36(3):264–72.
17. Park YN, Kim MJ. Hepatocarcinogenesis: imaging-pathologic correlation. Abdom Imaging. 2011;36:232–43.
18. Holland AE, Hecht EM, Hahn WY, et al. Importance of small (< or = 20-mm) enhancing lesions seen only during the hepatic arterial phase at MR imaging of the cirrhotic liver: evaluation and comparison with whole explanted liver. Radiology. 2005;237(3):938–44.
19. Kim TK, Lee KH, Jang HJ, et al. K. Analysis of gadobenate dimeglumine-enhanced MR findings for characterizing small (1-2-cm) hepatic nodules in patients at high risk for hepatocellular carcinoma. Radiology. 2011;259(3):730–8.
20. Ehman EC, Behr SC, Umetsu SE, et al. Rate of observation and inter-observer agreement for LI-RADS major features at CT and MRI in 184 pathology proven hepatocellular carcinomas. Abdom Radiol (NY). 2016;41(5):963–9.
21. Burrel M, Llovet JM, Ayuso C, et al. Barcelona Clínic Liver Cancer Group. MRI angiography is superior to helical CT for detection of HCC prior to live transplantation: an explant correlation. Hepatology. 2003;38(4):1034–42.
22. Brancatelli G, Baron RL, Peterson MS, et al. Helical CT screening for hepatocellular carcinoma in patients with cirrhosis: frequency and causes of false-positive interpretation. AJR Am J Roentgenol. 2003;180(4):1007–14.
23. Yu JS, Kim KW, Jeong MG, et al. Non- tumorous hepatic arterial-portal venous shunts: MR imaging findings. Radiology. 2000;217(3):750–6.
24. Colagrande S, Centi N, Galdiero R, et al. Transient hepatic intensity differences. 1. Those associated with focal lesions. AJR Am J Roentgenol. 2007;188(1):154–9.
25. Sharma P, Kalb B, Kitajima HD, et al. Optimization of single injection liver arterial phase gadolinium enhanced MRI using bolus track real-time imaging. J Magn Reson Imaging. 2011;33(1):110–8.
26. Hecht EM, Holland AE, Israel GM, et al. Hepatocellular carcinoma in the cirrhotic liver: gadolinium-enhanced 3D T1-weighted MR imaging as a stand-alone sequence for diagnosis. Radiology. 2006;239(2):438–47.
27. Willatt JM, Hussain HK, Adusumilli S, Marrero JA. MR imaging of hepatocellular carcinoma in the cirrhotic liver: challenges and controversies. Radiology. 2008;247(2):311–30.
28. Efremidis SC, Hytiroglou P. The multistep process of hepatocarcinogenesis in cirrhosis with imaging correlation. Eur Radiol. 2002;12:753–64.
29. Jang HJ, Kim TK, Burns PN, Wilson SR. Enhancement patterns of

hepatocellular carcinoma at contrast-enhanced US: comparison with histologic differentiation. Radiology. 2007;244(3):898–906.

30. Marrero JA, Hussain HK, Nghiem HV, et al. Improving the prediction of hepatocellular carcinoma in cirrhotic patients with an arterially-enhancing liver mass. Liver Transpl. 2005;11(3):281–9.

31. Choi MH, Choi JI, Lee YJ, et al. MRI of Small Hepatocellular Carcinoma: Typical Features Are Less Frequent Below a Size Cutoff of 1.5 cm. AJR Am J Roentgenol. 2016;27:1–8.

32. Granito A, Galassi M, Piscaglia F, et al. Impact of gadoxetic acid (Gd-EOB-DTPA)-enhanced magnetic resonance on the non-invasive diagnosis of small hepatocellular carcinoma: a prospective study. Aliment Pharmacol Ther. 2013;37(3):355–63.

33. Becker AS, Barth BK, Marquez PH, et al. Increased interreader agreement in diagnosis of hepatocellular carcinoma using an adapted LI-RADS algorithm. Eur J Radiol. 2017;86:33–40.

34. Fowler KJ, Brown JJ, Narra VR. Magnetic resonance imaging of focal liver lesions: approach to imaging diagnosis. Hepatology. 2011;54(6):2227–37.

35. Anis M. Imaging of hepatocellular carcinoma: new approaches to diagnosis. Clin Liver Dis. 2015;19(2):325–40.

36. Dioguardi Burgio M, Picone D, Cabibbo G, et al. MR-imaging features of hepatocellular carcinoma capsule appearance in cirrhotic liver: comparison of gadoxetic acid and gadobenate dimeglumine. Abdom Radiol (NY). 2016; 41(8):1546–54.

37. Zhang YD, Zhu FP, Xu X, et al. Liver Imaging Reporting and Data System: Substantial Discordance Between CT and MR for Imaging Classification of Hepatic Nodules. Acad Radiol. 2016;23(3):344–52.

38. Corwin MT, Fananapazir G, Jin M, et al. Differences in Liver Imaging and Reporting Data System Categorization Between MRI and CT. AJR Am J Roentgenol. 2016;206(2):307–12.

39. Granata V, Cascella M, Fusco R, et al. Immediate adverse reactions to gadolinium-based MR contrast media: a retrospective analysis on 10,608 examinations. Biomed Res Int. 2016;2016:3918292.

40. Hope TA, Fowler KJ, Sirlin CB, et al. Hepatobiliary agents and their role in LI-RADS. Abdom Imaging. 2015;40(3):613e25.

41. Ahn SS, Kim MJ, Lim JS, et al. Added value of gadoxetic acid-enhanced hepatobiliary phase MR imaging in the diagnosis of hepatocellular carcinoma. Radiology. 2010;255(2):459e66.

42. Davenport MS, Viglianti BL, Al-Hawary MM, et al. Comparison of acute transient dyspnea after intravenous administration of gadoxetate disodium and gadobenate dimeglumine: effect on arterial phase image quality. Radiology. 2013;266(2):452e61.

43. Kim SY, Park SH, Wu EH, et al. Transient respiratory motion artifact during arterial phase MRI with gadoxetate disodium: risk factor analyses. AJR Am J Roentgenol. 2015;204(6):1220e7.

44. Tsuda N, Harada K, Matsui O. Effect of change in transporter expression on gadolinium-ethoxybenzyl-diethylenetriamine pentaacetic acid-enhanced magnetic resonance imaging during hepatocarcinogenesis in rats. J Gastroenterol Hepatol. 2011;26(3):568e76.

45. Kim T, Murakami T, Hasuike Y, et al. Experimental hepatic dysfunction: evaluation by MRI with Gd-EOB-DTPA. J Magn Reson Imaging. 1997;7(4):683e8.

46. Nassif A, Jia J, Keiser M, et al. Visualization of hepatic uptake transporter function in healthy subjects by using gadoxetic acid-enhanced MR imaging. Radiology. 2012;264(3):741e50.

47. Kim H, Kim MJ, Park MS, et al. Potential conditions causing impairment of selective hepatobiliary enhancement of gadobenate dimeglumine-enhanced delayed magnetic resonance imaging. J Comput Assist Tomogr. 2010;34(1):113e20.

48. Chernyak V, Kim J, Rozenblit AM, et al. Hepatic enhancement during the hepatobiliary phase after gadoxetate disodium administration in patients with chronic liver disease: the role of laboratory factors. J Magn Reson Imaging. 2011;34(2):301e9.

49. Esterson YB, Flusberg M, Oh S, et al. Improved parenchymal liver enhancement with extended delay on Gd-EOB-DTPA-enhanced MRI in patients with parenchymal liver disease: associated clinical and imaging factors. Clin Radiol. 2015;70(7):723e9.

50. Tong HF, Liang HB, Mo ZK, et al. Quantitative analysis of gadoxetic acid-enhanced magnetic resonance imaging predicts histological grade of hepatocellular carcinoma. Clin Imaging. 2017;43:9–14.

51. Jeon I, Cho ES, Kim JH, et al. Feasibility of 10-Minute Delayed Hepatocyte Phase Imaging Using a 30° Flip Angle in Gd-EOB-DTPA-Enhanced Liver MRI for the Detection of Hepatocellular Carcinoma in Patients with Chronic Hepatitis or Cirrhosis. PLoS One. 2016;11(12):e0167701.

52. Toyoda H, Kumada T, Tada T, et al. Non-hypervascular hypointense nodules on Gd-EOB-DTPA-enhanced MRI as a predictor of outcomes for early-stage HCC. Hepatol Int. 2015;9(1):84–92.

53. Golfieri R, Garzillo G, Ascanio S, Renzulli M. Focal lesions in the cirrhotic liver: their pivotal role in gadoxetic acid-enhanced MRI and recognition by the Western guidelines. Dig Dis. 2014;32(6):696–704.

54. Ahn SS, Kim MJ, Lim JS, et al. Added value of gadoxetic acid-enhanced hepatobiliary phase MR imaging in the diagnosis of hepatocellular carcinoma. Radiology. 2010;255:459–66.

55. Golfieri R, Renzulli M, Lucidi V, et al. Contribution of the hepatobiliary phase of Gd-EOB-DTPA-enhanced MRI to Dynamic MRI in the detection of hypovascular small (≤2 cm) HCC in cirrhosis. Eur Radiol. 2011;21(6):1233–42.

56. Golfieri R, Grazioli L, Orlando E, et al. Which is the best MRI marker of malignancy for atypical cirrhotic nodules: hypointensity in hepatobiliary phase alone or combined with other features? Classification after Gd-EOB-DTPA administration. J Magn Reson Imaging. 2012;36(3):648–57.

57. Tsuda N, Kato N, Murayama C, et al. Potential for differential diagnosis with gadolinium- ethoxybenzyl-diethylenetriamine pentaacetic acid-enhanced magnetic resonance imaging in experimental hepatic tumors. Invest Radiol. 2004;39:80–8.

58. Huppertz A, Haraida S, Kraus A, et al. Enhancement of focal liver lesions at gadoxetic acid-enhanced MR imaging: correlation with histopathologic findings and spiral CT-initial observations. Radiology. 2005;234:468–78.

59. Saito K, Kotake F, Ito N, et al. Gd- EOB-DTPA enhanced MRI for hepatocellular carcinoma: quantitative evaluation of tumor enhancement in hepatobiliary phase. Magn Reson Med Sci. 2005;4:1–9.

60. Lee SA, Lee CH, Jung WY, et al. Paradoxical high signal intensity of hepatocellular carcinoma in the hepatobiliary phase of Gd-EOB- DTPA enhanced MRI: initial experience. Magn Reson Imaging. 2011;29:83–90.

61. Kudo M. Will Gd-EOB-MRI change the diagnostic algorithm in hepatocellular carcinoma? Oncology. 2010;78 Suppl 1:87–93.

62. Kim JI, Lee JM, Choi JY, et al. The value of gadobenate dimeglumine-enhanced delayed phase MR imaging for characterization of hepatocellular nodules in the cirrhotic liver. Invest Radiol. 2008;43:202–10.

63. Ouedraogo W, Tran-Van Nhieu J, et al. Evaluation of noninvasive diagnostic criteria for hepatocellular carcinoma on pretransplant MRI (2010): correlation between MR imaging features and histological features on liver specimen]. J Radiol. 2011;92(7–8):688–700.

64. Sofue K, Burke LM, Nilmini V, et al. Liver imaging reporting and data system category 4 observations in MRI: Risk factors predicting upgrade to category 5. J Magn Reson Imaging. 2017. doi:10.1002/jmri.25627.

65. Hwang J, Kim YK, Jeong WK, et al. Nonhypervascular Hypointense Nodules at Gadoxetic Acid-enhanced MR Imaging in Chronic Liver Disease: Diffusion-weighted Imaging for Characterization. Radiology. 2015;276(1):137–46.

66. Kim JE, Kim SH, Lee SJ, Rhim H. Hypervascular hepatocellular carcinoma 1 cm or smaller in patients with chronic liver disease: characterization with gadoxetic acid-enhanced MRI that includes diffusion-weighted imaging. AJR Am J Roentgenol. 2011;196(6):W758–65.

67. Hussain HK, Syed I, Nghiem HV, et al. T2- weighted MR imaging in the assessment of cirrhotic liver. Radiology. 2004;230:637–44.

68. Kim YK, Lee YH, Kim CS, Han YM. Added diagnostic value of T2-weighted MR imaging to gadolinium-enhanced three-dimensional dynamic MR imaging for the detection of small hepatocel- lular carcinomas. Eur J Radiol. 2008;67:304–10.

69. Brancatelli G, Federle MP, Blachar A, Grazioli L. Hemangioma in the cirrhotic liver: diagnosis and natural history. Radiology. 2001;219:69–74.

70. Shankar S, Kalra N, Bhatia A, et al. Role of Diffusion Weighted Imaging (DWI) for Hepatocellular Carcinoma (HCC) Detection and its Grading on 3 T MRI: A Prospective Study. J Clin Exp Hepatol. 2016;6(4):303–10.

71. Xu PJ, Yan FH, Wang JH, et al. Contribution of diffusion-weighted magnetic resonance imaging in the characterization of hepatocellular carcinomas and dysplastic nodules in cirrhotic liver. J Comput Assist Tomogr. 2010;34(4):506–12.

72. Lee MH, Kim SH, Park MJ, et al. Gadoxetic acid-enhanced hepatobiliary phase MRI and high-b-value diffusion-weighted imaging to distinguish well-

differentiated hepatocellular carcinomas from benign nodules in patients with chronic liver disease. AJR Am J Roentgenol. 2011;197(5):W868–75.

73. Piana G, Trinquart L, Meskine N, et al. New MR imaging criteria with a diffusion-weighted sequence for the diagnosis of hepatocellular carcinoma in chronic liver diseases. J Hepatol. 2011;55:126–32.

74. Granata V, Fusco R, Catalano O, et al. Intravoxel incoherent motion (IVIM) in diffusion-weighted imaging (DWI) for Hepatocellular carcinoma: correlation with histologic grade. Oncotarget. 2016;7(48):79357–64.

75. Nakanishi M, Chuma M, Hige S, et al. Relationship between diffusion-weighted magnetic resonance imaging and histological tumor grading of hepatocellular carcinoma. Ann Surg Oncol. 2012;19(4):1302–9.

76. Nasu K, Kuroki Y, Tsukamoto T, et al. Diffusion-weighted imaging of surgically resected hepatocellular carcinoma: imaging characteristics and relationship among signal intensity, apparent diffusion coefficient, and histopathologic grade. AJR Am J Roentgenol. 2009;193:438–44.

77. Sutherland T, Watts J, Ryan M, et al. Diffusion-weighted MRI for hepatocellular carcinoma screening in chronic liver disease: Direct comparison with ultrasound screening. J Med Imaging Radiat Oncol. 2017;61(1):34–9.

78. Koh D, Collins DJ. Diffusion-weighted MRI in the body: applications and challenges in oncology. AJR Am J Roentgenol. 2007;188:1622–35.

79. Scialpi M, Palumbo B, Pierotti L, et al. Detection and characterization of focal liver lesions by split-bolus multidetector-row CT: diagnostic accuracy and radiation dose in oncologic patients. Anticancer Res. 2014;34(8):4335–44.

80. Sforza V, Martinelli E, Ciardiello F, et al. Mechanisms of resistance to anti-epidermal growth factor receptor inhibitors in metastatic colorectal cancer. World J Gastroenterol. 2016;22(28):6345–61.

81. Granata V, Fusco R, Avallone A, Filice F, Tatangelo F, Piccirillo M, Grassi R, Izzo F, Petrillo A. Critical analysis of the major and ancillary imaging features of LI-RADS on 127 proven HCCs evaluated with functional and morphological MRI: Lights and shadows. Oncotarget. 2017. doi:10.18632/oncotarget.17227.

82. Choi JY, Lee JM, Sirlin CB. CT and MR imaging diagnosis and staging of hepatocellular carcinoma: part II. Extracellular agents, hepatobiliary agents, and ancillary imaging features. Radiology. 2014;273(1):30–50.

11

Worldwide malaria incidence and cancer mortality are inversely associated

Li Qin[1†], Changzhong Chen[3†], Lili Chen[1], Ran Xue[4], Ming Ou-Yang[2], Chengzhi Zhou[2], Siting Zhao[1], Zhengxiang He[1], Yu Xia[5], Jianxing He[2], Pinghua Liu[4], Nanshan Zhong[2*] and Xiaoping Chen[1*]

Abstract

Background: Investigations on the effects of malaria infection on cancer mortality are limited except for the incidence of Burkitt's lymphoma (BL) in African children. Our previous murine lung cancer model study demonstrated that malaria infection significantly inhibited tumor growth and prolonged the life span of tumor-bearing mice. This study aims to assess the possible associations between malaria incidence and human cancer mortality.

Methods: We compiled data on worldwide malaria incidence and age-standardized mortality related to 30 types of cancer in 56 countries for the period 1955–2008, and analyzed their longitudinal correlations by a generalized additive mixed model (GAMM), adjusted for a nonlinear year effect and potential confounders such as country's income levels, life expectancies and geographical locations.

Results: Malaria incidence was negatively correlated with all-cause cancer mortality, yielding regression coefficients (log scale) of −0.020 (95%CI: −0.027,-0.014) for men ($P < 0.001$) and-0.020 (95%CI: −0.025,-0.014) for women ($P < 0.001$). Among the 29 individual types of cancer studied, malaria incidence was negatively correlated with colorectum and anus (men and women), colon (men and women), lung (men), stomach (men), and breast (women) cancer.

Conclusions: Our analysis revealed a possible inverse association between malaria incidence and the mortalities of all-cause and some types of solid cancers, which is opposite to the known effect of malaria on the pathogenesis of Burkitt's lymphoma. Activation of the whole immune system, inhibition of tumor angiogenesis by *Plasmodium* infection may partially explain why endemic malaria might reduce cancer mortality at the population level.

Keywords: Malaria incidence, Cancer mortality, Generalized additive mixed model (GAMM), Epidemiological data, Regression analysis

Background

Some parasites have been implicated as risk factors for certain cancers, including *Schistosoma haematobium* for bladder cancer and *Clonorchis sinensis* for liver cancer and bile duct cancer [1]. However, other parasites, such as *Trypanosoma cruzi*, *Toxoplasma gondii*, *Toxocara Canis*, and *Acanthamoeba castellani*, have been suggested to improve the survival of cancer-bearing mice

* Correspondence: nanshan@vip.163.com; chen_xiaoping@gibh.ac.cn
[†]Equal contributors
[2]State Key Laboratory of Respiratory Disease, Guangzhou Institute of Respiratory Disease, First Affiliated Hospital, Guangzhou Medical University, 151 Yanjiang Road, 510120 Guangzhou, China
[1]State Key Laboratory of Respiratory Disease, Guangzhou Institutes of Biomedicine and Health, Chinese Academy of Sciences, 190 Kaiyuan Avenue, Guangzhou Science Park, 510530 Guangzhou, China
Full list of author information is available at the end of the article

[2]. Regarding malaria parasites specifically, there are two opposing viewpoints. In 1981, Greentree proposed that malaria infection might enhance the host's immune system and could serve as an adjuvant to conventional cancer therapy [3]. In contrast, in 1990, Eze suggested that malaria infection might trigger the production of reactive oxygen species or could activate oncogenes and eventually lead to cancer [4]. One previous study suggested that malaria incidence and all-cancer mortality might be positively correlated [5]. The author compared malaria incidence data from 1994 with all-cancer mortality for the period 1950–1994 in United States. However the results were limited because the time spans for cancer mortality and malaria incidence did not match, and there were many potential confounders, particularly due

to variations in economic development and immigration across the states. In 1994, the entire United States had fewer than 1000 imported cases of malaria, and it is known that immigrants usually target more economically advanced cities. It has been known that a positive correlation exists between malaria infection and the incidence of Burkitt's lymphoma (BL) in African children [6, 7]. However, no study has systematically examined the correlation between endemic malaria and the incidences or mortality rates of other cancers.

Some reports using animal models have suggested a link between malaria infection and the incidences or mortality rates of certain cancers. Trager et al. reported that the plasma of malaria-infected chickens could inhibit a chicken Rous I tumor [8]. Contradictory results have been reported for liver cancer and malaria in rat models [9, 10]. We recently demonstrated that malaria infection inhibited tumor growth and metastasis and prolonged the survival of tumor-bearing mice in a murine Lewis lung cancer (LLC) model [11]. *Plasmodium yoelii* 17XNL (a benign form of a murine malaria parasite) infection inhibited tumor angiogenesis in mice and induced innate and adaptive antitumor responses in LLC-bearing mice, leading to the induction of antitumor and anti-metastatic activities.

To examine whether such an association also exists in humans, we systematically analyzed malaria and all-cause cancer and 29 individual cancer statistical data in 56 countries from WHO publications and databases for the period 1955–2008.

Methods

Malaria data

Data regarding malaria cases for the following time periods were collected from the following sources: 1955–1964, WHO Epidemiological and Vital Statistics Report (1966); 1962–1981, WHO World Health Statistics Annual (1983); 1982–1997, WHO Weekly Epidemiological Record (1999); and 1990–2008, WHO 2009 annual report. In the event of a short overlap between two reports, data from the later report were used. We compiled worldwide malaria data from 218 countries for the period 1955–2008. Worldwide population data for 228 countries during the period 1955–2008 were obtained from the International Database of the U.S. Census Bureau (http://www.census.gov). The malaria incidence was calculated by dividing the number of reported malaria cases by the country's overall population; malaria incidence data were produced for 170 countries in this way.

Cancer data

Age-standardized mortality data on all-cause cancer and 29 individual types of cancer (1955–2008) from 194 countries were obtained from the WHO cancer mortality database (http://www-dep.iarc.fr/WHOdb/WHOdb.htm); the database provides statistics separately for each gender. As shown in Additional file 1: Table S1, merging the cancer mortality data (1955–2008) with the malaria incidence data provided combined data for 56 countries. Income information for these 56 countries was obtained from the World Bank database (http://data.worldbank.org/country). Data on life expectancies at birth (both sexes combined) and location data from the 56 countries were obtained from a publication of the Population Division of the United Nations Department of Economic and Social Affairs (World Population Prospects: The 2012 Revision; http://esa.un.org/wpp/).

Epidemiological data analysis

Using longitudinal malaria incidence and cancer mortality data from 56 countries, we examined trends in malaria incidence and all-cause cancer mortality for each country via linear regression. We then applied a generalized additive mixed model (GAMM) to examine the association between malaria incidence and cancer mortality. GAMM has the ability to set a random intercept to fit a wide range of cancer mortality rates among countries, to examine the nonlinear relationship between malaria incidence and cancer mortality, and to adjust for a nonlinear year effect and potential confounders such as country's income levels, life expectancies and geographical locations.

We first examined the distributions of the malaria incidence and cancer mortality rates and then log-transformed the malaria incidence and cancer mortality rates before inputting the rates into the models. All the analyses were performed using Empower software (www.empowerstats.com, X&Y solutions, Inc., Boston, MA) and R software (http://www.R-project.org).

Results

Of the 56 countries examined, the data integrity was different from country to country. The 56 countries provide average 23-year data, while Venezuela has 50-year data, but both Barbados and Kuwait have only 6-year data. Twenty nine countries provide the data of 1955–1981, 9 countries provide the data of 1982–2008, 18 countries have the data of 1955–2008. Thirty four countries locate in Asia/Africa/Latin America, among them 3 (Egypt, Mauritius and South Africa) in Africa, and 22 in Eruope/North America/Oceania. Twenty five countries were classified as high-income (high), and 31 were classified as low- and middle-income (low).

We first drew a smooth curve fitting the malaria incidence and the all-cause cancer mortality. The year 1981 was defined as a turning point; in this year, the malaria incidence increased, and the all-cause cancer mortality decreased significantly. We thus divided the study period into two periods: 1955–1981 and 1982–2008 in the following analysis. In addition, 24 countries showed a significant (P <0.05) increasing trend (up) in malaria incidence, 8 countries showed a significant decreasing trend (down) in malaria incidence, and 24 countries showed a non-significant change over the years (no change). We summarized the malaria incidence and all-cause cancer mortality data for the 56 countries from 1955–2008 in Table 1.

Spline smoothing by the GAMM showed a linear inverse relationship between malaria incidence and all-cause cancer mortality. A further analysis using the linear term of malaria incidence showed that a 10-fold increase in malaria incidence was associated with a lower log-transformed all-cause cancer mortality (−0.31 [95% CI:-0.37,-0.25], P <0.001, for men and −0.32 [95% CI:-0.37,-0.26], P <0.001, for women; Table 2). After adjusting for year, life expectancy at birth, income level, and geographical locations, this negative relationship persisted (regression coefficients: −0.20 [95% CI:-0.27,-0.14], P <0.001, for men and −0.20 [95% CI:-0.25,-0.14], P <0.001, for women). A stratified analysis showed an inverse relationship between malaria incidence and all-cause cancer mortality regardless of time periods, national income levels, geographical locations, or the malaria incidence trend (Table 2).

We then analyzed 29 individual types of cancer, and found that the inverse relationship between malaria incidence and cancer mortality was significant for colorectum and anus (both men and women), colon (both men and women), lung (men), stomach (men) and breast (women) cancer (Table 3). For other individual cancers, the correlation was not as significant as for these cancers. Detailed analyses of other cancer types are given in Additional file 2: Table S2.

The epidemiological analysis suggested that an inverse relationship exists between malaria incidence and mortality due to colorectum and anus, colon, lung, breast and stomach cancer; however, no significant correlations were found between malaria incidence and other cancers.

Discussion

In the present study, we utilized WHO cancer and malaria data to conduct longitudinal (1955–2008) analyses to assess the relationship between these diseases. Our analyses indicate that endemic or epidemic malaria may decrease mortality for some solid cancers, including colon cancer both in men and women, lung and stomach cancer in men, and breast cancer in women. Country-specific cancer incidence and mortality are associated with many factors, such as ethnicity, habits, customs, the level of economic development, the level of health care, and the level of cancer diagnosis and

treatment. The geographical distribution of the countries is also a potential confounding factor. Malaria is widely transmitted in Africa, Asia, and Latin America but has a low incidence in industrialized countries. Another potential confounding factor is the effect of time. To reduce the effects of these confounding factors, a GAMM was used to analyze the longitudinal data. A random intercept effect for each country in the GAMM regression analysis was used to accommodate the variations in cancer mortality across different countries. After adjusting for year, life expectancy at birth, national income level, and geographical locations, the inverse relationship between malaria incidence and all-cause cancer mortality persisted. Recent studies have demonstrated that some antimalarial drugs, such as artemisinin and chloroquine, have antitumor activities [12, 13]; thus, malaria treatment in endemic areas may affect cancer mortality, as well. However, although artemisinin was only used in clinics after the 1990s [14, 15], our analysis indicated that the negative relationship between malaria incidence and all-cause cancer mortality existed before the 1990s, during the period 1955–1981. Thus, the clinical use of artemisinin should not be a major confounder. Chloroquine may have been widely used throughout the entire period 1955–2008, but it was used only for short-term (3-day) treatment of malaria; thus, it is unlikely to have significantly affected cancer mortality. Furthermore, our murine Lewis lung cancer (LLC) model studies have demonstrated that 3-day treatment with a clinically relevant dose of chloroquine does not improve the survival of tumor-bearing mice (data not shown). Therefore, it is less likely that the observed inverse relationship between malaria incidence and cancer mortality was caused by the confounding factors discussed above.

Increased levels of economic development and increased life span typically decrease malaria incidence and increase cancer mortality. Thus, in countries with low levels of malaria and controlled endemic malaria, an inverse relationship between malaria incidence and cancer mortality would be observed merely through a simple analysis. To address this issue, we included a year variable spline smoothing term in the model to control for this time effect. We also conducted simulation analyses to estimate class I errors and the statistical power using data from 8 countries with decreasing malaria incidence. The estimated probability of this finding being due to chance was <0.035, and the power to detect our observed effect (−0.03) was 0.752. We also stratified the countries by trends in malaria incidence (up, down or no change). Negative correlations between malaria incidence and cancer mortality were observed in each stratum. Another potential time effect was the changing population structure over time because aging that relates

Table 1 Characteristics of malaria incidence and all-cause cancer mortality in 56 countries

| Country | Period | N | Malaria incidence | | All cancers | | | |
| | | | | | Male | | Female | |
			Median (Min-Max)	Yr. ratio[a]	Median (Min-Max)	Yr. ratio	Median (Min-Max)	Yr. ratio
Argentina	1966-2008	43	1.80 (0.26-7.08)	0.97	152.62 (132.01-199.59)	0.99	95.59 (86.39-124.56)	0.99
Armenia	1982-2008	22	4.84 (0–37.91)	1.24*	135.54 (115.84-150.75)	1.01	80.115 (69.29-90.5)	1.01
Australia	1955-1981	27	1.29 (0.39-4.30)	1.07*	151.21 (128.66-164.78)	1.01	98.43 (95.23-101.73)	1.00
Austria	1955-1981	26	0.08 (0.01-1.24)	1.15*	189.84 (181.83-199.04)	1.00	128.935 (113.45-138.06)	0.99
Azerbaijan	1982-2007	22	4.7 (0.28-161.40)	1.1	116.3 (77.16-149.99)	0.98	64.825 (47.8-79.77)	0.99
Barbados	1976-1981	6	0.60 (0.40-2.82)	0.75	125.56 (118.13-141.62)	1.01	102.3 (90.87-107)	0.98
Belgium	1955-1981	21	0.05 (0.01-0.60)	1.14*	195.63 (153.64-216.35)	1.01	117.84 (111.95-126.6)	1.00
Belize	1971-1999	21	1505.52 (26.4-4696.7)	1.15*	58.13 (26.39-147.75)	1.02	55.69 (36.51-131.28)	1.01
Brazil	1979-2008	28	281.77 (124.94-404.38)	1.01	93.62 (85.36-103.3)	1.01	67.41 (63.96-72.99001)	1.00
Bulgaria	1964-1981	17	0.15 (0.05-4.74)	1.28*	128.08 (117.99-142.31)	0.99	81.82 (77.03-89.66)	0.99
Canada	1955-1981	24	0.03 (0–2.57)	1.22*	150.21 (134.13-162.86)	1.01	109.23 (104.19-115.47)	1.00
Colombia	1955-2008	39	301.58 (81.42-588.20)	1.01	96.9 (61.78-103.77)	1.01	85.15 (71.38-97.2)	1.00
Costa Rica	1961-2008	47	34.45 (4.54-279.67)	1	103.62 (87.74-124.21)	1.00	88.79 (65.97-100.72)	1.00
Cuba	1970-1981	12	1.29 (0.01-5.90)	1.61*	133.21 (123.91-139.03)	0.99	92.24 (85.03-95.82)	0.99
Denmark	1955-1981	26	0.33 (0.11-2.15)	1.09*	165.54 (151.26-181.88)	1.00	135.72 (125.75-145.28)	1.00
Dominican Republic	1970-2005	31	14.05 (3.15-83.90)	1	42.58 (34.04-61.54)	1.01	39.33 (34.97-51.95)	1.00
Ecuador	1977-2008	29	362.59 (34.07-890.54)	0.98	71.42 (55.09-78.69)	1.00	71.52 (59.06-78.98)	1.00
Egypt	1955-2008	17	0.10 (0.01-474.70)	0.85*	41.35 (22.02-50.13)	1.01	26.23 (13.32-33.14)	1.02
El Salvador	1958-2008	34	147.79 (0.55-1924.15)	0.88*	39.99 (21.8-60.4)	1.02	54.05 (34.52-68.83)	1.01
Finland	1965-1981	15	0.09 (0.02-0.47)	1.16*	184.27 (177.38-195.1)	0.99	98.47 (94.04-106.99)	0.99
France	1955-1981	24	0.04 (0–1.03)	1.14*	185.97 (149.46-207.7)	1.01	100.655 (94.08-106.6)	0.99
Georgia	1990-2007	16	0.43 (0.02-9.25)	1.43*	79.99 (62.51-102.93)	1.00	52.14 (41.88-66.36)	1.00
Greece	1961-1981	21	0.55 (0.30-1.77)	0.96*	125.41 (116.45-145.84)	1.01	75.95 (71.89-82.94)	1.01
Guatemala	1963-2008	25	445.36 (69.81-1004.5)	1.01	67.03 (38.95-78.97)	1.02	75.595 (50.07-84.01)	1.01
Hungary	1955-1981	27	0.06 (0.01-0.46)	0.98	170.12 (130.85-214.48)	1.02	121.71 (114.18-129.34)	1.00
Ireland	1955-1981	17	0.07 (0.03-0.98)	1.13*	158.37 (128.77-169.4)	1.01	121.11 (107.84-130.69)	1.01
Israel	1975-1981	7	0.48 (0.27-1.16)	1.24*	131.36 (118.82-137.7)	0.99	113.88 (107.84-116.67)	0.99
Italy	1955-1981	27	0.07 (0.01-0.43)	1.11*	160.04 (123.09-187.98)	1.02	100.25 (96.73-103.36)	1.00
Japan	1955-1981	27	0.03 (0.01-0.07)	1.03	143.55 (125.39-149.85)	1.00	94.36 (84.6-99.17)	0.99
Kuwait	1975-1981	6	11.93 (7.15-16.04)	0.88*	94.08 (89.14-142.41)	0.95	73.56 (56.31-85.91)	1.02
Kyrgyzstan	1990-2008	19	0.27 (0–54.73)	1.34	103.2 (95.9-139.63)	0.98	66.97 (62.79-79.04)	1.00
Mauritius	1961-1989	29	5.57 (1.26-67.34)	1.08	96.93 (72.36-134.73)	1.01	68.86 (55.38-84.72)	0.99
Mexico	1969-2008	32	22.03 (2.14-174.16)	0.9*	73.52 (51.76-76.71)	1.01	68.87 (64.13-73.67)	1.00
New Zealand	1955-1981	26	0.48 (0.09-2.23)	1.04	157.77 (134.46-175.78)	1.01	114.795 (108.98-124.02)	1.00
Nicaragua	1973-2008	25	524.44 (13.95-1679.01)	0.94	49.55 (15.79-59.14)	1.04	52.13 (21.9-61.56)	1.03
Norway	1955-1981	21	0.08 (0.03-1.39)	1.15*	134.65 (124.81-145.52)	1.01	101.08 (97.48-110.9)	1.00
Panama	1955-2008	47	53.18 (5.81-670.11)	0.96*	73.97 (57.86-91.1)	1.01	66 (55.64-81.41)	1.00
Paraguay	1988-2008	15	21.94 (6.34-187.26)	0.94	72.11 (66.2-74.86)	1.00	63.07 (58.71-65.54)	1.00
Peru	1966-2007	30	179.07 (16.11-984.90)	1.08*	63.9 (40.08-74.8)	1.00	65.13 (38.9-77.01)	1.00
Philippines	1988-2008	15	54.54 (24.62-249.58)	0.91*	92.9 (78.82-100.9)	1.01	65.715 (57.07-71.5)	1.01
Poland	1959-1981	22	0.04 (0.01-0.10)	1.04*	153.43 (103.15-181.65)	1.02	102.625 (81.88-106.09)	1.01
Portugal	1955-1981	27	1.38 (0.04-10.35)	1.05	121.39 (89.41-133.25)	1.01	84.4 (75.34-90.29)	1.00

Table 1 Characteristics of malaria incidence and all-cause cancer mortality in 56 countries *(Continued)*

Romania	1963-1981	13	0.08 (0.02-0.10)	1.03	127.47 (124.17-131.21)	1.00	86.39 (83.02-98.06)	0.99
Singapore	1963-1981	19	11.53 (7.05-22.80)	0.98	171.88 (157.07-207.55)	1.01	100.32 (91.53-116.34)	1.01
South Africa	1988-2008	17	30.16 (13.08-143.40)	0.97	136.65 (121.25-145.78)	0.99	84.31 (70.13-87.88)	1.01
Spain	1955-1981	27	0.09 (0.02-8.57)	0.94*	134.17 (105.68-151.66)	1.01	86.23 (79.24001-91.09)	1.00
Suriname	1971-2008	26	2058.43 (152.56-14273.09)	1.12*	69.16 (34.15-95.24)	1.00	65.26 (26.55-95.75)	0.99
Sweden	1955-1981	27	0.30 (0.05-1.48)	1.14*	131.41 (117.91-148.03)	1.01	109.24 (101.89-113.42)	1.00
Switzerland	1955-1981	22	0.12 (0.02-2.15)	1.19*	174.17 (169.64-183.12)	1.00	111.08 (102.52-123.75)	0.99
Tajikistan	1982-2005	22	75.25 (3.32-4508.57)	1.46*	71.17 (52.63-110.44)	0.97	52.985 (36.33-69.2)	0.98
Thailand	1959-2006	27	175.6 (41.84-843.59)	0.99	58.68 (13.05-89.11)	1.04	36.42 (10.44-56.02)	1.04
Trinidad and Tobago	1955-1981	8	20.54 (0.27-213.59)	0.8	93.44 (83.49-116.19)	1.00	106.055 (88.44-123.58)	0.99
Turkmenistan	1990-1998	9	0.29 (0.03-3.21)	1.39	102.3 (87.32-132.92)	0.95	66.835 (55.55-81.32)	0.96
United Kingdom	1962-1981	20	0.54 (0-3.65)	1.41*	186.43 (180.55-189.06)	1.00	120.165 (114.59-123.92)	1.00
Uruguay	1963-1978	8	0.04 (0.03-0.15)	0.95	200.58 (192.12-205.04)	1.00	126.605 (119.13-133.04)	0.99
Venezuela	1955-2007	50	66.1 (7.5-249.34)	1.04*	98.74 (89.01-113.05)	1.00	94.185 (77.43-141.76)	0.99

Notes: [a]Yr. ratio: annual change ratio calculated as 10^β, where β is the regression coefficient of the annual log-transformed malaria incidence or cancer mortalities. *$P < 0.05$

to cancer mortality may also relate to malaria incidence. To address this issue, we stratified the years into two segments, 1955–1981 and 1982–2008, to narrow the aging effect. Negative correlations between malaria incidence and cancer mortality were still observed during each time period.

There are three limitations to the present study. First, cancer mortality and malaria incidence data were obtained from WHO publications and databases. Different countries may use different reporting criteria for the malaria incidence data. In addition, we were unable to obtain age-standardized malaria incidence data from existing databases. For cancer mortality, although the data were age-standardized for the countries studied, medical care and cancer reporting systems varied across countries and may have changed over time; these factors may affect the comparability of cancer mortality data between countries and years. Although our analysis using the GAMM approach maximally accommodated the limitations of existing data by primarily examining

Table 2 Regression analysis of the relationship between all-cancer mortality and malaria incidence, 1955–2008

Model	Male	Female
Basic model	−0.31 (−0.37, −0.25) ***	−0.32 (−0.37, −0.26) ***
Adjusted model	−0.20 (−0.27, −0.14) ***	−0.20 (−0.26, −0.14) ***
Period		
1955-1981	−0.11 (−0.16, −0.05) ***	−0.05 (−0.10, 0.00) **
1982-2008	−0.24 (−0.34, −0.15) ***	−0.11 (−0.19, −0.03) **
Income		
Low	−0.28 (−0.37, −0.18) ***	−0.25 (−0.34, −0.16) ***
High	−0.11 (−0.15, −0.06) ***	−0.07 (−0.11, −0.03) ***
Geographical location		
Asia/Africa/Latin America	−0.27 (−0.36, −0.18) ***	−0.24 (−0.33, −0.16) ***
Europe/North America/Oceania	−0.16 (−0.20, −0.12) ***	−0.10 (−0.13, −0.06) ***
Malaria incidence trend		
Down	−0.20 (−0.31, −0.08) ***	−0.25 (−0.36, −0.13) ***
No change	−0.13 (−0.26, 0.00) *	−0.06 (−0.18, 0.06)
Up	−0.21 (−0.32, −0.10) ***	−0.03 (−0.12, 0.07)

Notes

1. Both malaria incidence and cancer mortality data were log transformed. The results shown are 10 times the regression coefficients and 95% confidence intervals

2. The basic model was adjusted for year; the adjusted model was adjusted for year, life expectancy at birth, national income level and geographical location

3. ***$P < 0.001$; **$P < 0.01$; *$P < 0.05$

Table 3 Regression analysis of the relationship between mortality rates associated with 5 individual types of cancer and malaria incidence, 1955–2008

Cancer	Basic model	Adjusted model	Period	
			1955-1981	1982-2008
Colon				
Male	−0.72 (−0.87, −0.56) ***	−0.52 (−0.68, −0.36) ***	−0.31 (−0.48, −0.14) ***	−0.59 (−0.81, −0.38) ***
Female	−0.87 (−1.02, −0.72) ***	−0.63 (−0.78, −0.48) ***	−0.39 (−0.54, −0.24) ***	−0.64 (−0.86, −0.43) ***
Colon, rectum and anus				
Male	−0.51 (−0.62, −0.41) ***	−0.37 (−0.47, −0.26) ***	−0.25 (−0.37, −0.13) ***	−0.41 (−0.58, −0.25) ***
Female	−0.58 (−0.68, −0.48) ***	−0.42 (−0.52, −0.32) ***	−0.34 (−0.46, −0.22) ***	−0.45 (−0.60, −0.29) ***
Lung				
Male	−0.36 (−0.46, −0.25) ***	−0.20 (−0.32, −0.09) ***	−0.24 (−0.35, −0.12) ***	−0.54 (−0.71, −0.37) ***
Breast				
Female	−0.46 (−0.56, −0.37) ***	−0.30 (−0.40, −0.20) ***	−0.20 (−0.29, −0.10) ***	−0.32 (−0.45, −0.19) ***
Stomach				
Male	−0.66 (−0.76, −0.55) ***	−0.39 (−0.50, −0.28) ***	−0.31 (−0.40, −0.21) ***	−0.23 (−0.37, −0.08) ***

Notes
1. Both malaria incidence and cancer mortality data were log transformed. The results are 10 times the regression coefficients and the 95% confidence intervals
2. The basic model was adjusted for year; the adjusted model was adjusted for year, life expectancy at birth, national income level and geographical location
3. ***P <0.001

trends over time within each country instead of across countries, such limitations could not be completely eliminated by our data analysis. Second, we do not have other countries' data, especially the data from malaria high endemic countries in Africa. Therefore the impact of endemic malaria on cancer mortality in our analysis may mainly reflect *vivax* malaria that prevails outside Africa, not *falcipuram* malaria that prevails in Africa, even though all four species of human malaria parasite (*Plasmodium vivax, falcipuram, ovale and malariae*) contain pathogen-associated molecular patterns (PAMPs [16]) that can trigger the antitumor immune response (see below). Third, the positive relationship between the incidence of Burkitt's lymphoma in African children and *falciparum* malaria has been well established, because this malaria causes a prolonged expansion of B cell in the germinal centers and therefore provides more time for DNA damage and MYC oncogene translocation that ultimately leads to Burkitts lymphoma [17], but we were unable to obtain mortality or incidence data for this tumor from WHO publications or databases. Thus, our analysis model lacks information that could be used to establish a positive relationship between malaria incidence and cancer mortality; such information would be important for validating our model further.

Malaria infection may serve to enhance immune surveillance mechanisms against some types of solid cancers. During the course of malaria, *Plasmodium* PAMPs [16] as danger signals are detected by the host immune cells' sensors called pattern recognition receptors (PRRs) which include the toll-like receptors (TLRs) [18] at the membrane of endosomes or on the cell surface, RIG-I-like receptors (RLRs) [19] and NOD-like receptors (NLRs) [20] localized in cytoplasm. The *Plasmodium* PAMPs include the known glycosylphosphatidylinositol anchors (GPI anchors) [21], haemozoin [22] and immunostimulatory nucleic acid motifs [23] and other unknown molecules [24]. The PRRs activated by *Plasmodium* PAMPs trigger distinct transcriptional programs and stimulate multiple downstream pathways to induce systemic immune responses [25], including release of pro-inflammatory and Th1-type cytokines such as TNF-α, IL-1β, IL-2, IL-6, IL-12, type I and type II IFNs [25, 26], activation of NK cells, NKT cells, γ/δ T cells, macrophages and dendritic cells (DCs), afterwards activation of CD4+ and CD8+ T cells [26, 27] that counteract the tumor immune-suppressive microenvironment that contains TGF-β, IL-10, regulatory T cells (Tregs) and myeloid-derived suppressive cells (MDSCs) [28, 29], then turn the immune-suppressive milieu to immune-supportive milieu, finally may transform the tumor into an effective tumor vaccine [30, 31]. On the other hand, malaria damage-associate molecular patterns (DAMPs), such as the known intrinsic uric acid, microvesicles and haem [31–33] also induce similar immune activity. Indeed, our previous study demonstrated that blood-stage malaria exhibits anti-tumor effects by inducing a potent anti-tumor innate immune response, including the secretion of IFN-γ and TNF-α and the activation of NK cells. Our murine lung cancer model studies also demonstrated that malaria infection induced adaptive anti-tumor immunity by increasing tumor-specific T-cell proliferation and the cytolytic activity of CD8+ T cells and increased the infiltration of these cells into tumor tissues. In these studies, we found that in approximately 10% of lung cancer (LLC)-bearing mice infected with malaria parasite, the tumor regressed and did not regrow when the mice were re-inoculated with the same cancer cells, most likely because of the long-term memory of specific antitumor cellular immunity [11]. Study by Deng XF and colleagues demonstrated that attenuated liver-stage *Plasmodium* inoculation induced antitumor innate immune response, including secretion of TNF-α, IL-6/12 and IFN-γ and antitumor adaptive immunity with increasing cytolytic activity of CD8+ T cells [34]. Our unpublished data suggest that blood-stage *Plasmodium* infection significantly decreases the numbers of MDSCs in breast cancer (4 T1)-bearing mice or Tregs in lung cancer (LLC)-bearing mice. In addition, our previous study indicated that malaria infection significantly inhibited tumor angiogenesis in mice [11]. A review by Hobohm [35] suggested that the fever induced by malaria infection may cause an increase in tumor cell death. Based on our previous study and our unpublished data, parasitemia is required to effectively inhibit tumor growth. However, in mice, *Plasmodium* infection causes only a short-term infection without fever. Repeated *Plasmodium* infection is difficult to observe in murine models [36]. In humans lacking effective antimalarial treatment, *Plasmodium* infection can cause long-term parasitemia that is accompanied by a high fever in the acute phase, and this syndrome can recur many times throughout the life span [37]. Therefore, a naturally acquired *Plasmodium* infection by mosquito bite would produce liver-stage and blood-stage malaria that sequentially stimulate the immune systems to turn the tumor into the effective tumor vaccine, in combination with fever during the acute phase and the inhibition of tumor angiogenesis. In medical literature, febrile infection was linked to spontaneous regression of tumor [38], and malaria is a typical febrile infection. Other pathogen infections may have similar impact on cancer mortality or morbidity [39, 40], due to a similar mechanism of PAMPs-triggered antitumor immunity [41], but malaria parasite may be more significant than other pathogens, because malaria contains two stages (liver and blood) of infection, manifests typical high fever paroxysms during acute phase and may last longer period if not treated with effective antimalarial drugs. In addition, malaria is a well-documentary infectious disease in WHO databases and publications partially due to easily to be diagnosed by fever paroxysm and a simple blood smear test. Other pathogen infections lack well-documentary data in WHO databases or publications for analysis. In summary, some or all of these above mentioned factors and mechanisms may explain why endemic malaria might reduce cancer mortality at the population level.

Conclusion

We report an inverse association between malaria incidence and the mortality rates of all-cause and several types of solid cancers. However, because this study is a descriptive retrospective analysis, we are unable to draw a causal relationship between malaria and the mortality rates of some cancers. More well-defined prospective epidemiological studies are required to confirm this relationship. We recommend that public health officials in the WHO and in individual countries coordinate malaria control programs and cancer epidemiological studies in the future. In addition, more comprehensive mechanistic studies should be conducted.

Abbreviations

BL: Burkitt's lymphoma; CI: Coefficience interval; CSA: Chondroitine Sulfate A.; DCs: Dendritic cells; GAMM: Generalized additive mixed model; GPI: Glycosylphosphatidylinositol anchors; LLC: Lewis lung cancer; MDSCs: Myeloid-derived suppressive cells; NLRs: NOD-like receptors; PAMPs: Pathogen-associated molecular patterns; Pf: Plasmodium falciparum; PRRs: Pattern recognition receptors; RLRs: RIG-I-like receptors; TLRs: Toll-like receptors; Tregs: regulatory T cells; WHO: World Health Organization

Acknowledgments

We are grateful to Dr. Hongbing Tang, Professor Nan Hong and Miss Wanwan Xu for their help with preparing the data and performing statistical analyses. Special thanks are given to the Malaria Research and Reference Reagent Resource Center (MR4) for providing the non-lethal *P. yoelii* 17XNL strain. P Liu thanks Boston University for sabbatical leave and support to conduct collaborative malaria research in X Chen's laboratory.

Funding

This study was supported by Natural Science Foundation of China (NSFC) (No. 81673003, 31570925,81372451, 31501046), the Guangzhou Municipal Funds of Science and Technology (No.2014Y2-00076, 201504010016), and the National High Technology Research and Development Program (No.2014AA020544).

Authors' contributions

L Qin, X Chen, N Zhong, and C Chen conceived and designed the research. L Qin, C Chen, L Chen, and R Xue analyzed the data. C Chen, Y Xia, Z He, M Ou-yang, J He, S Zhao and C Zhou contributed materials/analysis tools. L Qin, C Chen, P Liu, and X Chen wrote the paper. All authors read and approved the final manuscript.

Authors' information

L Qin, X Chen, and S Zhao are faculty from State Key Laboratory of Respiratory Disease, Guangzhou Institutes of Biomedicine and Health, Chinese Academy of Sciences, Guangzhou, China. L Chen and Z He are PhD student of Guangzhou Institutes of Biomedicine and Health, Chinese Academy of Sciences, Guangzhou, China. C Chen is faculty of Channing Laboratory, Brigham and Women's Hospital, Boston, USA. N Zhong, M Ou-yang, C Zhou and J He are the faculty from State Key Laboratory of Respiratory Disease, First Affiliated Hospital, Guangzhou Medical University, Guangzhou, China. P Liu is faculty of Chemistry Department, Boston University, Boston, USA. R Xue is master student of Boston University, Boston, USA. Y Xia is faculty of Department of Bioengineering, McGill University, Montreal, Canada.

Competing interests

The authors declare that they have no competing interests.

Author details

[1]State Key Laboratory of Respiratory Disease, Guangzhou Institutes of Biomedicine and Health, Chinese Academy of Sciences, 190 Kaiyuan Avenue, Guangzhou Science Park, 510530 Guangzhou, China. [2]State Key Laboratory of Respiratory Disease, Guangzhou Institute of Respiratory Disease, First Affiliated Hospital, Guangzhou Medical University, 151 Yanjiang Road, 510120 Guangzhou, China. [3]Channing Laboratory, Brigham and Women's Hospital, 181 Longwood Ave, Boston, MA 02115, USA. [4]Boston University, Boston, MA 02215, USA. [5]Department of Bioengineering, McGill University, Montreal, QC H3A 0C3, Canada.

References

1. de Martel C, Ferlay J, Franceschi S, Vignat J, Bray F, Forman D, Plummer M. Global burden of cancers attributable to infections in 2008. A review and synthetic analysis. Lancet Oncol. 2012;13(6):607–15.
2. Darani HY, Yousefi M. Parasites and cancers: parasite antigens as possible targets for cancer immunotherapy. Future Oncol. 2012;8(12):1529–35.
3. Greentree LB. Malariotherapy and cancer. Med Hypotheses. 1981;7(1):43–9.
4. Eze MO, Hunting DJ, Ogan AU. Reactive oxygen production against malaria–a potential cancer risk factor. Med Hypotheses. 1990;32(2):121–3.
5. Lehrer S. Association between malaria incidence and all cancer mortality in fifty U.S. States and the district of Columbia. Anticancer Res. 2010;30(4):1371–3.
6. Whittle HC, Brown J, Marsh K, Greenwood BM, Seidelin P, Tighe H, et al. T-cell control of Epstein-Barr virus-infected B cells is lost during P. Falciparum malaria. Nature. 1984;312(5993):449–50.
7. Rochford R, Cannon MJ, Moormann AM. Endemic Burkitt's lymphoma: a polymicrobial disease? Nat Rev Microbiol. 2005;3(2):182–7.
8. Trager W, McGhee RB. Inhibition of chicken tumor I by plasma from chickens infected with an avian malaria parasite. Proc Soc Exp Biol Med. 1953;83(2):349–52.
9. Angsubhakorn S, Bhamarapravati N, Sahaphong S, Sathiropas P. Reducing effects of rodent malaria on hepatic carcinogenesis induced by dietary aflatoxin B1. Int J Cancer. 1988;41(1):69–73.
10. Angsubhakorn S, Sathiropas P, Bhamarapravati N. Enhancing effects of rodent malaria on aflatoxin B1-induced hepatic neoplasia. J Cancer Res Clin Oncol. 1986;112(2):177–9.
11. Chen L, He Z, Qin L, Li Q, Shi X, Zhao S, et al. Antitumor effect of malaria parasite infection in a murine lewis lung cancer model through induction of innate and adaptive immunity. PLoS One. 2011;6(9).
12. Kimura T, Takabatake Y, Takahashi A, Isaka Y. Chloroquine in cancer therapy: a double-edged sword of autophagy. Cancer Res. 2013;73(1):3–7.
13. Tilaoui M, Mouse HA, Jaafari A, Zyad A. Differential effect of artemisinin against cancer cell lines. Nat prod bioprospecting. 2014;4(3):189–96.
14. White NJ. The treatment of malaria. N Engl J Med. 1996;335(11):800–6.
15. Karbwang J, Na-Bangchang K, Thanavibul A, Bunnag D, Chongsuphajaisiddhi T, Harinasuta T. Comparison of oral artesunate and quinine plus tetracycline in acute uncomplicated falciparum malaria. Bull World Health Organ. 1994;72(2):233–8.
16. Takeuchi O, Akira S. Pattern recognition receptors and inflammation. Cell. 2010;140(6):805–20.
17. Robbiani DF, Deroubaix S, Feldhahn N, Oliveira TY, Callen E, Wang Q, et al. *Plasmodium* infection promotes genomic instability and AID-dependent B cell lymphoma. Cell. 2015;162(4):727–37.
18. Schroder K, Tschopp J. The inflammasomes. Cell. 2010;140(6):821–32.
19. O'Neill LA, Golenbock D, Bowie AG. The history of toll-like receptors - redefining innate immunity. Nat Rev Immunol. 2013;13(6):453–60.
20. Barbalat R, Ewald SE, Mouchess ML, Barton GM. Nucleic acid recognition by the innate immune system. Annu Rev Immunol. 2011;29:185–214.
21. Durai P, Govindaraj RG, Choi S. Structure and dynamic behavior of toll-like receptor 2 subfamily triggered by malarial glycosylphosphatidylinositols of plasmodium falciparum. FEBS J. 2013;280(23):6196–212.
22. Kalantari P, DeOliveira RB, Chan J, Corbett Y, Rathinam V, Stutz A, et al. Dual engagement of the NLRP3 and AIM2 inflammasomes by plasmodium-derived hemozoin and DNA during malaria. Cell Rep. 2014;6(1):196–210.
23. Sharma S, DeOliveira RB, Kalantari P, Parroche P, Goutagny N, Jiang Z, et al. Innate immune recognition of an AT-rich stem-loop DNA motif in the plasmodium falciparum genome. Immunity. 2011;35(2):194–207.
24. Liehl P, Zuzarte-Luis V, Chan J, Zillinger T, Baptista F, Carapau D, et al. Host-cell sensors for plasmodium activate innate immunity against liver-stage infection. Nat Med. 2014;20(1):47–53.
25. Gazzinelli RT, Kalantari P, Fitzgerald KA, Golenbock DT. Innate sensing of malaria parasites. Nat Rev Immunol. 2014;14(11):744–57.
26. Punsawad C. Effect of malaria components on blood mononuclear cells involved in immune response. Asia Pac j Trop Biomed. 2013;3(9):751–6.
27. Inoue S, Niikura M, Mineo S, Kobayashi F. Roles of IFN-gamma and gammadelta T cells in protective immunity against blood-stage malaria. Front Immunol. 2013;4:258.
28. Smyth MJ, Ngiow SF, Ribas A, Teng MW. Combination cancer immunotherapies tailored to the tumour microenvironment. Nat Rev Clin Oncol. 2016;13(3):143–58.
29. van der Burg SH, Arens R, Ossendorp F, van Hall T, Melief CJ. Vaccines for established cancer: overcoming the challenges posed by immune evasion. Nat Rev Cancer. 2016;16(4):219–33.
30. van den Boorn JG, Hartmann G. Turning tumors into vaccines: co-opting the innate immune system. Immunity. 2013;39(1):27–37.
31. Figueiredo RT, Fernandez PL, Mourao-Sa DS, Porto BN, Dutra FF, Alves LS, et al. Characterization of heme as activator of toll-like receptor 4. J Biol Chem. 2007;282(28):20221–9.
32. Mantel PY, Marti M. The role of extracellular vesicles in plasmodium and other protozoan parasites. Cell Microbiol. 2014;16(3):344–54.
33. Gallego-Delgado J, Ty M, Orengo JM, van de Hoef D, Rodriguez A. A surprising role for uric acid: the inflammatory malaria response. Curr Rheumatol Rep. 2014;16(2):401.
34. Deng X, Dong Z, Quanxing L, Yan D, Xu W, Qian C, et al. Antitumor effect of intravenous immunization with malaria genetically attenuated sporozoites through induction of innate and adaptive immunity. Int J Clin Exp Pathol. 2016;9(2):978–86.
35. Hobohm U. Fever and cancer in perspective. Cancer Immunol Immunother: CII. 2001;50(8):391–6.
36. Dascombe MJ, SJIMA, editors. The absence of fever in rat malaria is associated with increased turnover of 5-hydroxytryptamine in the brain. Temperature regulation: advances in pharmacological sciences. Boston: Basel; 1994. p. 47–52.
37. Fernando SD, Gunawardena DM, Bandara MR, De Silva D, Carter R, Mendis KN, et al. The impact of repeated malaria attacks on the school performance of children. AmJTrop Med Hyg. 2003;69(6):582–8.
38. Hoption Cann SA, van Netten JP, van Netten C. Dr william Coley and tumour regression. A place in history or in the future. Postgrad Med J. 2003; 79(938):672–80.
39. Mastrangelo G, Fadda E, Milan G. Cancer increased after a reduction of infections in the first half of this century in Italy: etiologic and preventive implications. Eur J Epidemiol. 1998;14(8):749–54.
40. Keef R, Jonas WB, Knogler W, Stenzinger W. Fever, cancer incidence and spontaneous remissions. Neuroimmunomodulation. 2011;9(2):55-64.
41. Kucerova P, Cervinkova M. Spontaneous regression of tumour and the role of microbial infection–possibilities for cancer treatment. Anticancer Drugs. 2016;27(4):269–77.

12

Introduction of p16^{INK4a} as a surrogate biomarker for HPV in women with invasive cervical cancer in Sudan

Hina Sarwath[1], Devendra Bansal[2], Nazik Elmalaika Husain[3], Mahmoud Mohamed[1], Ali A. Sultan[2] and Shahinaz Bedri[1*]

Abstract

Background: Cervical cancer is the fourth most common cancer in women worldwide with highest incidence reported in Eastern Africa in 2012. The primary goal of this study was to study the expression of p16^{INK4a} in squamous cell carcinoma (SCC) of the cervix by immunohistochemistry (IHC) and determine relation with clinico-pathological parameters. This study further explored the correlation of p16^{INK4a} immunostaining with another proliferation marker, Ki-67 and to study if human papillomavirus (HPV) IHC can be used as a marker for detection of virus in high-grade dysplasia.

Methods: A total of 90 samples, diagnosed for cervical cancer, were included in the study. Fixed Paraffin Embedded (FFPE) tissue sections were stained with anti-p16^{INK4a}, anti-Ki-67 and anti-HPV antibodies using automated immunohistochemistry platform (ASLink 48-DAKO).

Results: Immunohistochemical protein expression of p16^{INK4a} positivity was found to be highest in SCC (92.2%, $n = 71$) than other HPV tumors (76.9%, $n = 10$). The majority of cases (97.4%) were p16^{INK4a} positive in the age group 41–60 years. In addition, a statistically significant difference between p16^{INK4a} and HPV was observed among total cervical tumor cases and SCC cases.

Conclusions: As expected staining of invasive cervical cancer with anti-HPV showed rare positivity because HPV heralds active infection in dysplastic lesions and not of frank cervical carcinoma. In contrast, anti-p16^{INK4a} IHC results showed positive correlation in SCC and other cervical tumors.

Keywords: Cervical cancer, Human Papillomavirus, p16^{INK4a}, Ki-67, Immunohistochemistry, Sudan

Background

Cervical cancer continues to be a major public health problem in less developed regions of the world and ranked at fourth position among various cancers in women with estimated age standardized rates over 30 per 100, 000 women [1]. Global prevalence of cervical cancer is estimated 11.7%, out of which Sub-Saharan Africa was reported most affected region with highest prevalence rates (24%) [2]. It has been well documented that developed nations have significantly reduced the incidence and mortality rates of cervical cancer by successful implementation and sustenance of population wide primary screening programs using the cytological Pap smear and HPV DNA testing [3]. In contrast, data published by the WHO / ICO HPV Information Center reports that frequency of cervical cancer rises steadily in Sudan where 2.7% of women from the total population harbor 82–94% of high-risk HPV subtypes 16, 18, 45, 52 and 58 in the age group ranging between 15 and 44 years of age [4–7]. In Sudan, the current and commonest diagnostic method used to detect high-grade cervical dysplasia is the visual inspection with acetic acid (VIA) test [8, 9]. Though, VIA method showed higher sensitivity to detect high-grade lesions than Pap test but it has a lower specificity and misdiagnosis of cervical cancer ranges ~20–50% of true disease [10, 11]. Currently, molecular assay such as

* Correspondence: shahinazbedri@gmail.com; shb2026@qatar-med.cornell.edu

[1]Department of Pathology and Laboratory Medicine, Weill Cornell Medicine – Qatar, Cornell University, Qatar Foundation - Education City, Doha, Qatar

HPV DNA testing has been standardized and being commonly used with cytology.

HPV mediated cervical carcinogenesis is a process divided into two stages: productive and transforming infections. Productive infections are short-term lesions, which regress spontaneously, however transforming infections with certain high risk-HPV (HR-HPV) progress to invasive cancer gradually (20–30 years) if not followed up. Histomorphological types of cervical cancers include squamous cell carcinoma (SCC), adenocarcinomas and neuroendocrine carcinomas. SCC represents the majority of cases diagnosed (80%) while the remainder cases are adenocarcinomas and other types [12, 13].

A previously published study from Sudan has reported that women are diagnosed in late stages with aggressive disease emphasizing lack of efficient screening tests [8]. To facilitate early detection and proper treatment, there is a need to evaluate and introduce robust molecular markers of functional biological relevance, which can track disease progression and help in patient stratification [12, 14].

Among the various biomarkers established to facilitate early screening is the cell cycle regulatory protein known as p16^{INK4a}, which has demonstrated to be highly sensitive and specific marker of high-grade squamous and glandular neoplasia of the cervix due to its overexpression in cancerous and precancerous cervical lesions [3, 15]. Moreover, p16^{INK4a} inhibits the phosphorylation of pRb mediated through cyclin dependent kinases and regulating mitotic transition of cell cycle from G1 to S phase [16, 17]. Alterations in this host cell proliferation pathway is due to interference of viral oncoproteins E6 and E7 causing erratic cell division which leads to enhanced expression and cellular accumulation of p16^{INK4a} in the basal and parabasal epithelial cells of HPV transformed lesions [18]. A recent meta-analysis study has shown that p16^{INK4a} over-expression using immunohistochemistry (IHC) is linked with increased and disease free survival hence proving to be a marker for prognosis [19]. Studies have also shown that HR-HPV DNA presence is elevated in low-grade cervical lesions indicating active viral multiplication in host cell. Immuno-staining of anti-HPV protein expression is detectable in initial transient cervical lesions but not in advanced lesions such as invasive SCC where p16^{INK4a} is over-expressed [20].

In addition, cellular proliferation marker that could be used in conjunction with p16^{INK4a} is Ki-67. HPV infected cells/lesions that overexpressed p16^{INK4a}, as a response to viral oncogenes will concomitantly express Ki-67 [18]. Several studies have shown the relation of Ki-67 antibody expression in malignant lesions such as vulva, penis, breast and uterine cervix [21, 22]. Localized in the nucleus, this non-histone cell proliferation antigen is expressed in all cell cycle phases except G0 [23]. Increased Ki-67 expression in

the basal layers of the dysplastic epithelium strongly correlates with lesion aggressiveness, and therefore can be used as predicator of proliferation and disease progression [24]. In addition, multiplexing p16^{INK4a} and Ki-67 in both SCC and adenocarcinoma (AC) can be a synergistic approach to quantitate each marker at a cellular level in tumor regions instead of the benign proliferative zones, thereby increasing diagnostic accuracy in both immunohisto-chemistry studies [25].

The present study aimed to determine the expression of p16^{INK4a} protein in SCC of the cervix by IHC and relate the findings with clinico-pathological characteristics, correlate p16^{INK4a} overexpression with proliferation marker Ki-67 and validate that anti-HPV immunostaining is not suitable for detecting presence of virus in high grade invasive carcinoma.

Methods

Study population and samples

The Joint Institutional Review Board (JIRB) of Weill Cornell Medicine - Qatar (WCM-Q) and Hamad Medical Corporation (HMC) Research Office, Qatar has approved the present study (Protocol no.-10,165/10). This is a retrospective cohort study with a total of 90 formalin-fixed paraffin-embedded (FFPE) cervical carcinoma tumors obtained from patients diagnosed at the pathology laboratory at the National Health Laboratory (NHL), Sudan between years 2004–2008. Clinicopathologic information such as age, tumor differentiation and diagnosis was obtained when available.

Histopathological analysis

All cervical biopsies were fixed in 10% neutral buffered formalin, dehydrated and paraffin embedded. FFPE specimens were sectioned on microtome (4 μm thickness) for both Hematoxylin & Eosin (H&E) staining and immuno-staining. H&E stained slides were examined for histopathologic diagnosis by experienced pathologist to record morphological alterations such as presence of koilocytotic cells, extent of keratinization and significant differentiation in the squamous epithelial cells (dysplasia).

Immunohistochemical staining and scoring

Immunostaining of FFPE tissue sections was performed using the Envision Flex™ protocol on ASLink48 (Dako, Glostrup, Denmark), as described previously [26]. The antibody titers and staining parameters were optimized on recommended control tissue according to the manufacturer's instructions (Dako, Glostrup, Denmark). The antibodies used in this study were: anti-p16^{INK4a} (dilution 1:3, clone E6H4, Roche, Tucson, AZ, USA), anti-HPV (dilution 1:50, clone K1H8, Dako, Glostrup, Denmark) and anti-human Ki-67 (dilution 1:200, clone MIB-1, Dako, Glostrup, Denmark). Briefly, after antigen retrieval the fixed tissue sections were blocked and incubated with primary antibodies for 20 min, washed, and secondary antibody coupled to HRP was added. The reaction was developed using DAB Chromogen (Dako, Glostrup, Denmark) and counterstained with Hematoxylin stain following dehydration in ethanol. Positive and negative tissue controls such as tonsil for p16^{INK4a}, Ki-67 and human condyloma tissue for HPV immunostaining were included in each run to validate the stain localization whereas the negative control was the same tissue section omitting primary antibody.

Scoring of immunostained tumor sections was performed by an experienced pathologist. Strong diffuse nuclear as well as cytoplasmic staining in the basal layers of the squamous epithelium is considered p16^{INK4a} positive. Depending on the distribution of the stain in the epithelium, positivity is scored as strong diffuse or high intensity (3^+), strong focal or moderate intensity (2^+) and weak sporadic or mild (1^+). For anti-HPV, positive staining in the nuclei of infected squamous cells and occasional staining of cytoplasm in koilocytotic & dysplastic epithelial cells was observed. All the cases were scored as positive or negative based if protein expression of HPV capsid protein (VP1) was observed. In case of anti-Ki-67 antigen, depending on the intensity and proportion of mitotic cells in the basal and parabasal cells of the squamous epithelium, scores were assigned as follows: <10- Negative, 10–30 cells- 1^+, 40–60 cells- 2^+, 70–100- 3^+.

Statistical analysis

Immunohistochemical intensity for each of the three markers irrespective of the score was designated as positive for presence and negative if absent. Results were presented using frequencies and percentages. Comparison between different groups was performed using ANOVA test, followed by Student's t-test. Sensitivity and specificity between p16^{INK4a} and HPV immunostaining were compared using McNemar's test and positive predictive value (PPV) and negative predictive value (NPV) were recorded. Two tailed test were used for analysis and p-value <0.05 was considered significant. The SPSS statistical package (IBM SPSS version 22.0.) was used for the statistical analysis.

Results

Demographic and clinical characteristics of the study population

This study includes 90 cases of cervical tumor biopsies from Sudan. Based on histology analysis, data in Table 1, 85.6% ($n = 77$) of women were diagnosed with squamous cell carcinoma (SCC) and 14.4% ($n = 13$) of other HPV associated tumors. In addition, tumor grade, which is the histopathologic differentiation of cancerous tissue,

Table 1 Demographic, clinico-pathological characteristics and frequency of different immunostaining profiles according to diagnosis among women from Sudan

	SCC n = 77[a] (%)	Other tumors n = 13 (%)	p value
Age (years)			
21–40	13 (18.6%)	3 (23.1%)	0.134
41–60	36 (51.4%)	3 (23.1%)	
61–80	21 (30.0%)	7 (53.8%)	
Pathological diagnosis			
Keratinizing	20 (26.0)		NA
Non-keratinizing	53 (68.8)		
No data	4 (5.2)	13 (100)	
p16^{INK4a} immunostaining			
Positive	71 (92.2)	10 (76.9)	0.119
Negative	6 (7.8)	3 (23.1)	
HPV immunostaining			
Positive	7 (9.1)	2 (15.4)	0.384
Negative	70 (90.9)	11 (84.6)	
Ki-67 immunostaining			
Positive	47 (61.0)	8 (61.5)	0.314
Negative	5 (6.5)	2 (15.4)	
No data	25 (32.5)	3 (23.1)	

[a]Age of 7 patients were not available

were classified into well differentiated, moderately and poorly differentiated. The age range among the studied population was 27–80 years with a mean age of 54.2 (±13.5) years. Furthermore, the individuals were categorized into 3 age groups (<40, 41–60, >60 years), in which majority (52.1%) of women were aged 41–60 years. However, age was not reported for seven patients in the study (Table 1). The degree of differentiation, an important classification in SCC cases revealed that the majority of samples were of non-keratinizing 68.8% ($n = 53$) subtypes, 26% ($n = 20$) were keratinizing carcinomas. Data were not available for four SCC cases (Table 1 and Fig. 1a, b).

Immunostaining

Immunohistochemistry (IHC) of FFPE tissue samples was performed using anti-p16^{INK4a}, Ki-67 and anti-HPV antibodies (Fig. 1c-k). Overexpression of p16^{INK4a} was found to be higher in SCC, 92.2% (n = 71) compared to other HPV tumors, 76.9% (n = 10) (Table 1). Furthermore, based on immunostaining intensity, we extended our analysis to evaluate and compare the test sensitivity between different immunostaining and diagnosis, we found a significant difference in p16^{INK4a} among SCC cases (sensitivity = 79.2%, specificity = 46.1%, PPV = 83.9%, NPV = 27.2%, $p = 0.049$) (Fig. 2a).

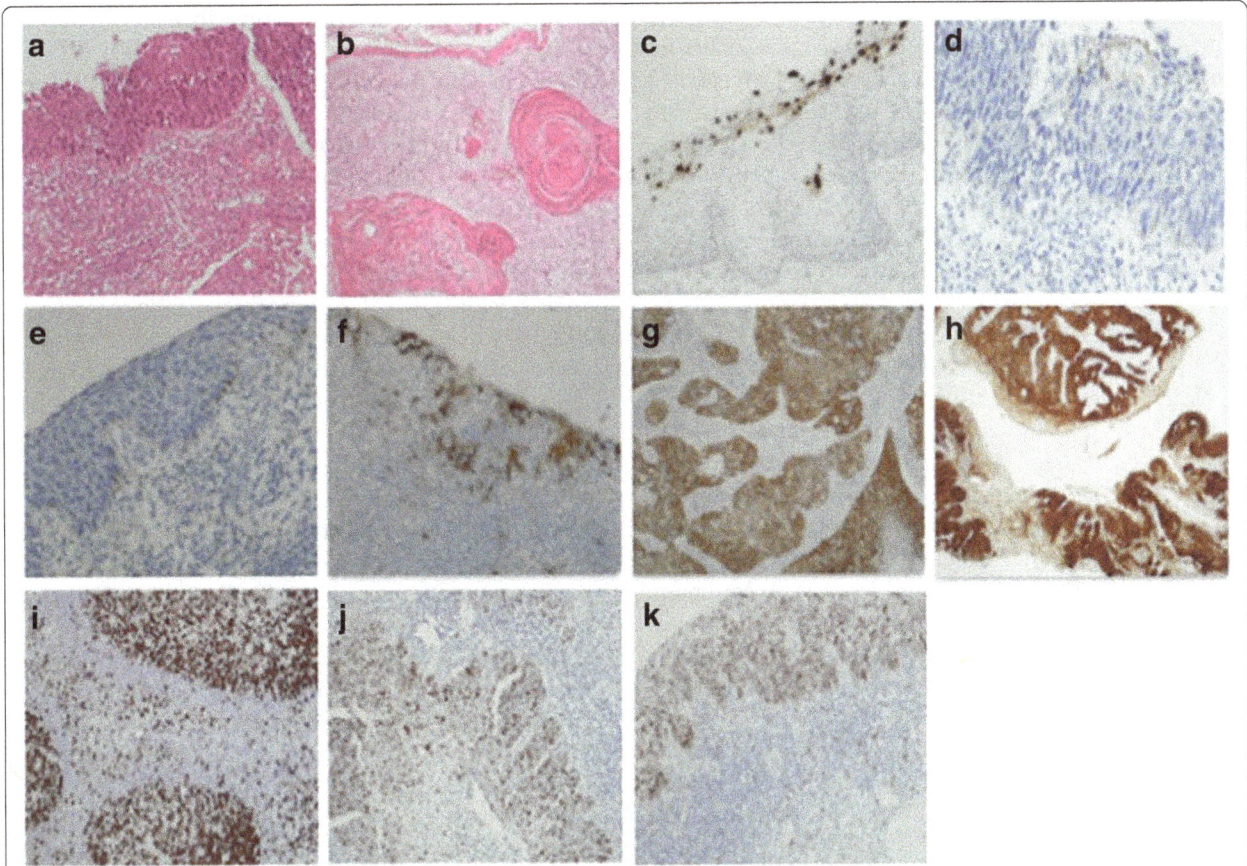

Fig. 1 Representative pictures of Hematoxylin & Eosin (H&E) and Immunohistochemical staining for p16^{INK4a}, HPV and Ki-67 in squamous cell carcinoma (SCC). **a** Non-keratinizing SCC (H&E) (**b**) Keratinizing SCC (H&E) (**c**) anti-HPV positive control (human condyloma) (**d**) anti-HPV positivity in other tumors (**e**) anti-HPV positivity in SCC (**f**) p16^{INK4a} positive control (tonsil) (**g**) p16^{INK4a} moderate intensity (focal) immunostaining in SCC (**h**) p16^{INK4a} high intensity (diffuse) immunostaining in SCC (**i**) Ki-67 positive control (tonsil) (**j**) Ki-67 proliferating epithelial cells in SCC (**k**) Ki-67 positivity in SCC (**a-k**: ×20)

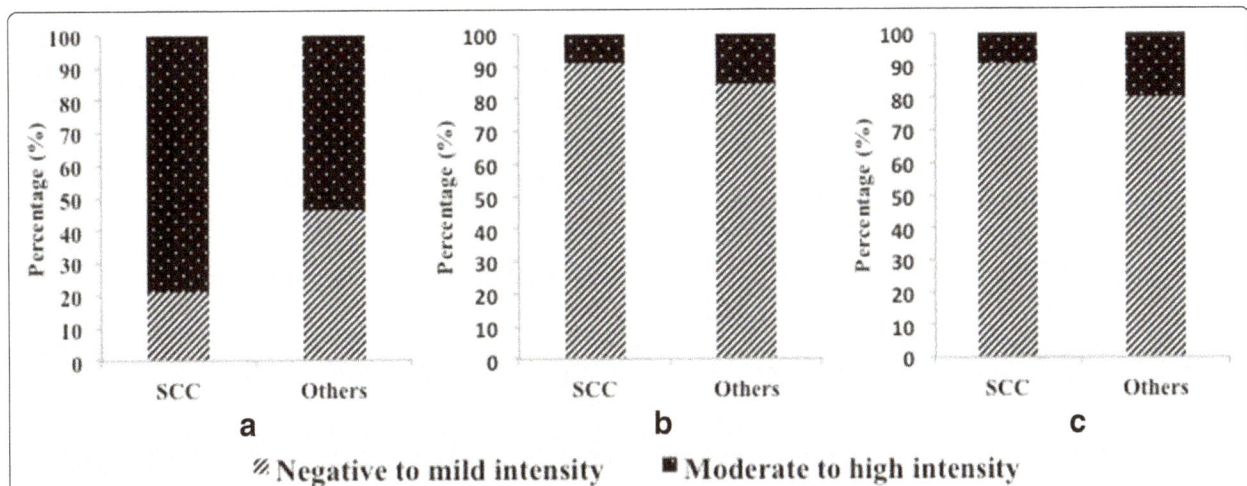

Fig. 2 Differential staining of (**a**) p16^{INK4a}, (**b**) HPV and (**c**) Ki-67 between SCC and other tumors

However, no significant difference was observed in HPV and Ki-67 immunostaining ($p = 0.484$ and $p = 0.329$), respectively (Fig. 2b, c). Additionally, an exact McNemar's test determined that there was a statistically significant difference between p16^{INK4a} and HPV among cervical tumor cases ($p = 0.011$) and SCC cases alone (p = 0.049) however; no significant difference was noted in other tumor cases ($p = 0.219$) (Table 2). Furthermore, no significant correlation was found between tumor grade and p16^{INK4a} immunostaining.

Of the total 90 samples collected in this study, Ki-67 immunoreaction was performed only in 68.9% ($n = 62$) cases (Table 1). Of these, 88.7% ($n = 55$) were found to be positive for Ki-67 immunostaining (Table 1). Furthermore, to correlate expression of p16^{INK4a} with a proliferation marker, Ki-67 according to the diagnosis, a significant difference was observed in other HPV associated tumors ($p = 0.019$) however, no significant association was found with SCC cases (Additional file 1: Table S1). According to age groups, the percentage frequency of p16^{INK4a} was significantly higher in the age group 41–60 years ($p = 0.001$), however, no association with age group was seen in Ki-67 and HPV immunostaining (Fig. 3).

Discussion

Meta-analysis studies have reported that cervical cancer incidence and mortality rates are rising in sub-Saharan Africa with an estimated prevalence of oncogenic HPV genotypes across all ages at 33.6% specifically in Eastern Africa [2]. The HPV distribution data in Africa reveals two peaks, one at <25 and another ≥45 years of age [2]. In the present study, we observed that 52.1% of women in age group between 41 and 60 years were diagnosed with SCC, a dominant histomorphological form in invasive cervical cancer [12]. According to the WHO guidelines, all women between ages of 35–45 years must be screened annually, which can significantly reduce mortality rates [27]. The degree of differentiation (keratinization) is

an important pathological feature in cervical tumors, indicates the site of infection in the cervical mucosal epithelium (squamo-columnar junction) and susceptible to HPV infection. In this study, majority of SCC cases were classified as non-keratinizing SCC, 68.8% and 26% were keratinizing SCC, this corroborates previous findings from Ethiopia [28].

Correlating p16^{INK4a} expression with clinico-pathological parameters, we found that p16^{INK4a} expression was directly proportional to the diagnosis of cervical tumors where 90.1% of SCC cases and 76.9% as Adenocarcinoma (AC) showed positive p16^{INK4a} expression, which is in agreement with previous studies [15, 29, 30]. However, Lin J et al. [19], reports that prognostic significance of p16^{INK4a} overexpression was not significantly associated with tumor grade nor tumor size, however p16^{INK4a} overexpression was highly associated with better prognosis and increased disease-free survival which, corroborates with previous studies [31, 32]. Additionally, in the present study, 9.9% ($n = 7$) of SCC cases and 23.1% ($n = 3$) of AC cases were p16^{INK4a} negative which has also been reported in previous studies [33, 34, 35]. Furthermore, absence of p16^{INK4a} expression in the cervical tumors does not indicate lack of HR- HPV or improper IHC technique but rather implicated due to silencing of the gene through mutations in the promoter regions resulting in transcription failure, epigenetic mechanisms and hyper methylation.

Molecular assays are the most sensitive for HPV detection in FFPE samples than IHC [32]. In the present study, the frequency of both p16^{INK4a} and HPV positive expression was seen in age group between 41 and 60 years (n = 3, 3.6%). The positive correlation of HPV expression with p16^{INK4a} intensity and dispersion on cervical carcinoma cases was reported in a study in Saudi Arabia [30]. However, majority (91.5%) of SCC cases were positive for p16^{INK4a}, but negative for HPV-1 derived capsid protein (VP1). The majority of cervical cancers does not have active dysplasia and therefore are limited in protein expression of HR-HPV.

To increase the reproducibility of diagnosis, p16^{INK4a} expression was compared with a cellular proliferation marker, Ki-67. To date, several studies have shown co-expression of p16^{INK4a} and Ki-67 when combined concurrently improve diagnostic accuracy and that Ki-67 expression increases linearly with tumor grade in SCC [25, 34, 36]. In this study, ~61% of SCC and AC cases were positive for Ki-67. Furthermore, the frequency of p16^{INK4a} and Ki-67 positive immunostaining when assessed individually was higher in the age group >40 and 6.6% ($n = 4$) were both positive for p16^{INK4a} and Ki-67. Several studies have shown that both p16^{INK4a} and Ki-67 proteins are co-expressed in most high-grade squamous lesions, which is also observed in this study. Ki-67 is employed as an objective marker indicating

Table 2 Distribution of p16^{INK4a} versus HPV immunoexpression in 90 cervical tumors cases according to diagnosis in women from Sudan

Diagnosis	HPV	p16^{INK4a}		p value$^{£}$
		Negative n (%)	Positive n (%)	
SCC	Positive	3 (18.8)	4 (6.6)	0.049$^{£}$
	Negative	13 (81.2)	57 (93.4)	
Others	Positive	1 (16.7)	1 (14.3)	0.219
	Negative	5 (83.3)	6 (85.7)	
Total	Positive	4 (18.2)	5 (7.4)	0.011$^{£}$
	Negative	18 (81.8)	63 (92.6)	

$^{£}$significant

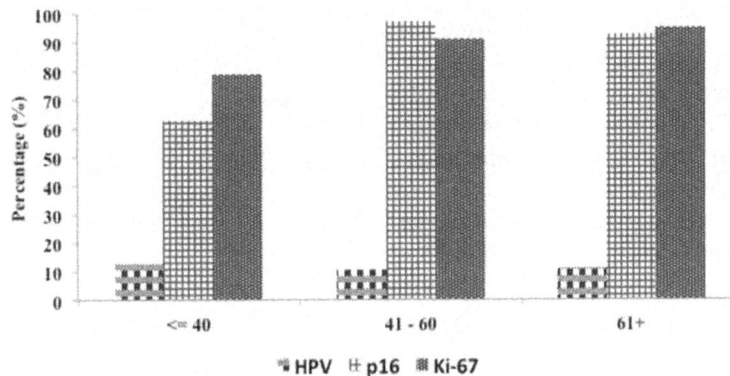

Fig. 3 Percentage of HPV, p16 ^{INK4a} and Ki-67 immunostaining according to age group. ($*p$ = 0.001)

aberrant cellular proliferation that facilitates measurement of advanced disease end point, which is progress of CIN to carcinoma. Hence, direct proportionality in Ki-67 expression in relation to tumor grade along with p16^{INK4a} is involved functionally in the process of HPV induced transformation and overexpressed in the epithelium [29, 36]. Furthermore, Ki-67 expression was found to be significantly different in cervical tumor lesions CIN2 and CIN3 [33] and also expressed in benign proliferative lesions and in basal cells of normal squamous mucosa [25].

In the present study, no correlation was found between p16^{INK4a} and Ki-67 with respect to HPV immunohistochemical protein expression, which is in agreement with previous report [29]. HPV detection rate using in situ hybridization (ISH) varied significantly between cervicitis and low grade SIL; in addition, significant correlation of HR-HPV status with histopathological grade was observed [37]. In contrast, p16INK4a and Ki67 was found useful to detect both LR and HR-HPV in precancerous lesions and distinguish between low grade SIL and high grade SIL [38].

Based on the tumor grade, it has been shown that in low-grade lesions, p16^{INK4a} is diffusely expressed in ~60% of CIN1 and mostly associated with HR-HPV genotypes, but HR-HPV presence was detected in p16^{INK4a} negative tumors [36, 39]. In addition, high incidence of HR-HPV has been observed among young women and most of these infections were transient and regress spontaneously [39]. We therefore concluded that p16^{INK4a} overexpression is already indicative of advanced viral interference progressing towards invasive cancer where aside from active viral replication there is significant morphological change occurring at histology, cellular and molecular level which can be visually scored. However, in invasive cervical cancer, the HPV protein expression was not detectable by IHC and HPV genotyping in FFPE tumor samples.

Currently, in Sudan precancerous cervical lesions are visually detected by VIA [8–10] unlike the Pap test, a primary screening method in industrialized nations, VIA has limitations to distinguish early morphological changes associated with neoplastic transformation. However, Pap test has not been implemented as a screening modality in low resource settings with no national HPV vaccination program [4]. Despite the increasing cancer related incidence and mortality rates, Sudan is burdened with other public health issues such as malaria, leprosy, tuberculosis, HIV/AIDS thereby causing lack of emphasis and knowledge about this disease [40]. Thus, introduction of such molecular biomarkers will prove beneficial in early detection and embarking on screening initiatives and reducing mortality [27]. Recently, WHO has recommended that HPV vaccination should be performed as part of national immunization programs for women between ages 13–26 years to effectively prevent disease [27]. In addition, it was suggested that boys should be included in HPV vaccination programs to overcome cost effectiveness in low resource settings [41]. Current treatment for invasive cervical cancer in sub-Saharan Africa is radiotherapy, which is a major challenge due to lack of both resources and primary screening facilities hence, resulting in progress to advanced disease stage when diagnosed [8, 40]. Thus, there is a need to establish frequent screening intervals of optimal target population as progression from low grade to invasive cervical cancer takes up to 20 years [27] and adopt algorithm models for cervical cancer prevention in developed countries to help in proper management of disease [41].

The strength of the present study lies in the use of IHC technique to study immunochemical staining along with H&E stain of SCC tumors for histopathology assessment. The monoclonal antibody clone used for p16^{INK4a}-E6H4 has been recommended specific antibody for exfoliated dysplastic cells both in histology tissue sections and cytology smears and that normal cervical epithelium, inflammatory or metaplastic lesions were not stained [14].

Limitations of this study are primarily the tissue quality, preservation and fixation of FFPE samples were not suitable to carry out analysis for HPV genotyping study. In addition, cut-off threshold for immune-positivity of p16^{INK4a} varies between pathologists, presenting a challenge as no standard parameters. Limited sample number for Ki-67 hence proper correlation with p16^{INK4a} in SCC cases could not be made. Larger cohort with proper diagnostic, survival data can help to correlate other clinical parameters.

Conclusions

In this preliminary study, we evaluate the clinical utility of p16INK4a as a surrogate marker using IHC technique in invasive cervical carcinoma among women in Sudan. Overall, p16^{INK4a} overexpression in squamous cell carcinoma was significant and differs from expression in other cervical tumors (AC). The immunostaining of p16^{INK4a} and HPV vary in the total sample positive and negative reaction, indicating that p16^{INK4a} is an effective way to detect invasive carcinoma than HPV. Proliferation marker, Ki-67 showed significant correlation with p16^{INK4a} in other HPV associated tumors. Lastly, significant correlation of p16^{INK4a} percentage frequency in age group 41–60 years where active advance transforming CIN occurs concludes that it is an appropriate surrogate marker to help in early screening of cervical neoplasia.

Abbreviations

AC: Adenocarcinoma; CIN: Cervical Intraepithelial Neoplasia; FFPE: Formalin-fixed paraffin embedded; H&E: Hematoxylin & Eosin; HMC: Hamad Medical Corporation; HPV: Human Papillomavirus; HR: High risk; IHC: Immunohistochemistry; LR: Low risk; NPV: Negative predictive value; PPV: Positive predictive value; SCC: Squamous cell carcinoma; SIL: Squamous Intraepithelial lesion; SPSS: Statistical package for the Social science; VIA: Visual inspection with acetic acid; WCM-Q: Weill Cornell Medicine-Qatar

Acknowledgements

We would like to acknowledge the support of the Human Histology Core and its personnel at WCM-Q. We are also grateful to Dr. Imad Bin Mujeeb and his team at the HMC-Anatomic Pathology Department for providing HPV Positive control tissue and facilitating with slides.

Funding

This publication was made possible by NPRP grant [NPRP-5-098-3-021] from the Qatar National Research Fund (a member of Qatar Foundation) and Weill Cornell Medicine-Qatar (WCM-Q) Histology Core grant [BMRP-5726005905]. The findings achieved herein are solely the responsibility of the author [s].

Authors' contributions

SB and AAS contributed to the conceptualization and design of the study. MM, HS, NH and SB assisted in the sample and preliminary clinicopathologic data collection. SB and NH confirmed the pathologic diagnosis. MM, HS and SB generated the data. HS, DB, MM and SB analyzed the data. SB, HS, DB and AAS wrote the manuscript. SB, AAS, MM, DB, NH, HS reviewed the manuscript. All the authors read and approved the final manuscript.

Competing interests

The authors declare that they have no competing interests.

Author details

[1]Department of Pathology and Laboratory Medicine, Weill Cornell Medicine – Qatar, Cornell University, Qatar Foundation - Education City, Doha, Qatar. [2]Department of Microbiology and Immunology, Weill Cornell Medicine – Qatar, Cornell University, Qatar Foundation - Education City, Doha, Qatar. [3]Faculty of Medicine, Omdurman Islamic University, P.O. Box 382, Omdurman, Sudan.

References

1. Torre LA, Bray F, Siegel RL, Ferlay J, Lortet-Tieulent J, Jemal A. Global cancer statistics, 2012. CA Cancer J Clin. 2015;65:87–108.

2. Bruni L, Diaz M, Castellsague X, Ferrer E, Bosch FX, de Sanjose S. Cervical human papillomavirus prevalence in 5 continents: meta-analysis of 1 million women with normal cytological findings. J Infect Dis. 2010;202:1789–99.

3. Sahasrabuddhe VV, Luhn P, Wentzensen N. Human papillomavirus and cervical cancer: biomarkers for improved prevention efforts. Future Microbiol. 2011;6:1083–98.

4. ICO Information Centre on HPV and Cancer. Sudan. Human Papillomavirus and related cancers, fact sheet. 2017. Available at http://www.hpvcentre.net/statistics/reports/SDN_FS.pdf. Accessed 28 May 2017.

5. Abate E, Aseffa A, El-Tayeb M, El-Hassan I, Yamuah L, Mihret W, et al. Genotyping of human papillomavirus in paraffin embedded cervical tissue samples from women in Ethiopia and the Sudan. J Med Virol. 2013;85:282–7.

6. Seoud M. Burden of human papillomavirus-related cervical disease in the extended middle east and north Africa-a comprehensive literature review. J Low Genit Tract Dis. 2012;16:106–20.

7. Mohammed EA, Alagib A, Babiker AI. Incidents of cancer in Sudan: past trends and future forecasts. Afr J Math Comput Sci Res. 2013;8:136–42.

8. Husain N, Helali T, Domi M, Bedri S. Cervical cancer in women diagnosed at the National Health Laboratory, Sudan: a call for screening. Afr J Online (AJOL). 2011;6:183–90.

9. Ibrahim A, Aro AR, Rasch V, Pukkala E. Cervical cancer screening in primary health care setting in Sudan: a comparative study of visual inspection with acetic acid and pap smear. Int J Womens Health. 2012;4:67–73.

10. Hassan FM, Khirelseed M. Cervical cancer screening among Sudanese women. Gulf J Oncolog. 2009;6:28–34.

11. Tambouret R. Screening for cervical cancer in low-resource settings in 2011. Arch Pathol Lab Med. 2013;137:782–90.

12. Steenbergen RD, Snijders PJ, Heideman DA, Meijer CJ. Clinical implications of (epi)genetic changes in HPV-induced cervical precancerous lesions. Nat Rev Cancer. 2014;14:395–405.

13. de Freitas AC, Gurgel AP, Chagas BS, Coimbra EC, do Amaral CM. Susceptibility to cervical cancer: an overview. Gynecol Oncol. 2012;126:304–11.

14. Burd EM. Human Papillomavirus laboratory testing: the changing paradigm. Clin Microbiol Rev. 2016;29:291–319.

15. Klaes R, Friedrich T, Spitkovsky D, Ridder R, Rudy W, Petry U, et al. Overexpression of p16INK4a as a specific marker for dysplastic and neoplastic epithelial cells of the cervix uteri. Int J Cancer. 2001;92:276–84.

16. McLaughlin-Drubin ME, Crum CP, Munger K. Human papillomavirus E7 oncoprotein induces KDM6A and KDM6B histone demethylase expression and causes epigenetic reprogramming. Proc Natl Acad Sci U S A. 2011;108:2130–5.

17. Bringold F, Serrano M. Tumor suppressors and oncogenes in cellular senescence. Exp Gerontol. 2000;35:317–29.

18. von Knebel DM, Reuschenbach M, Schmidt D, Bergeron C. Biomarkers for cervical cancer screening: the role of p16(INK4a) to highlight transforming HPV infections. Expert Rev Proteomics. 2012;9:149–63.

19. Lin J, Albers AE, Qin J, Kaufmann AM. Prognostic significance of overexpressed p16INK4a in patients with cervical cancer: a meta-analysis. PLoS One. 2014;9:e106384.

20. Calil LN, Edelweiss MI, Meurer L, Igansi CN, Bozzetti MC. p16INK4a And Ki67

expression in normal, dysplastic and neoplastic uterine cervical epithelium and human papillomavirus (HPV) infection. Pathol Res Pract. 2014;210:482–7.

21. Hemalatha A, Suresh TN, Kumar ML. Expression of vimentin inbreast carcinoma, its correlation with Ki67 and other histopathological param-eters. Indian J Cancer. 2013;50:189–94.

22. Herrero R, Castle PE, Schiffman M, Bratti MC, Hildesheim A, Morales J, et al. Epidemiologic profile of type-specific human papillomavirus infection and cervical neoplasia in Guanacaste. Costa Rica J Infect Dis. 2005;191:1796–807.

23. Ungureanu C, Teleman C, Socolov D, Anton G, Mihailovici MS. Evaluation of p16INK4a and Ki67 proteins expression in cervical intraepithelial neoplasia andtheir correlation with HPV-HR infection. Rev Med Chir Soc Med Nat Iasi. 2014;114:823–8.

24. Longatto Filho A, Utagawa ML, Shirata NK, Pereira SM, Namiyama GM, Kanamura CT, et al. Immunocytochemical expression of p16INK4A and Ki-67 incytologically negative and equivocal pap smears positive for oncogenic humanpapillomavirus. Int J Gynecol Pathol. 2005;24:118–24.

25. Samarawardana P, Singh M, Shroyer KR. Dual stain immunohistochemical localization of p16INK4A and ki-67: a synergistic approach to identify clinically significant cervical mucosal lesions. Appl Immunohistochem Mol Morphol. 2011;19:514–8.

26. Mohamed M, Sarwath H, Salih N, Bansal D, Chandra P, Husain NE, et al. CD8 ⁺ tumor infiltrating lymphocytes strongly correlate with molecular subtype and clinico-pathological characteristics in breast cancer patients from Sudan. Transl Med Commun. 2016;1:4.

27. Adewole IF, Abauleth YR, Adoubi I, Amorissani F, Anorlu RI, Awolude OA, et al. Consensus recommendations for the prevention of cervical cancer in sub-Saharan Africa. South Afr J Gynaecol Oncol. 2013;5:47–57.

28. Rashed MM, Bekele A. The prevalence and pattern of HPV-16 immunostaining in uterine cervical carcinomas in Ethiopian women: a pilot study. Pan Afr Med J. 2011;8:21.

29. Zhong P, Li J, Gu Y, Liu Y, Wang A, Sun Y, et al. P16 And Ki-67 expression improves the diagnostic accuracy of cervical lesions but not predict persistent high risk human papillomavirus infection with CIN1. Int J Clin Exp Pathol. 2015;8:2979–86.

30. Omran OM, AlSheeha M. Human Papilloma virus early proteins E6 (HPV16/18-E6) and the cell cycle marker P16 (INK4a) are useful PrognosticMarkers in uterine cervical Carcinomasin Qassim region-Saudi Arabia. Pathol Oncol Res. 2015;21:157–66.

31. Wang SS, Trunk M, Schiffman M, Herrero R, Sherman ME, Burk RD, et al. Validation of p16INK4a as a marker of Oncogenic HumanPapillomavirus infection in cervical biopsies from a population-based cohort in Costa Rica. Cancer Epidemiol Biomark Prev. 2004;13:1355–60.

32. Kalof AN, Cooper K. p16INK4a Immunoexpression: surrogate marker of high-risk HPV and high-grade cervical intraepithelial neoplasia. Adv Anat Pathol. 2006;13:190–4.

33. Cheah PL, Looi LM, Teoh KH, Mun KS, Nazarina AR. p16ᴵᴺᴷ⁴ᵃ Is a useful marker of human Papillomavirus integration allowing risk stratification for cervical malignancies. Asian Pacific J Cancer Prev. 2012;13:469–72.

34. Agoff SN, Lin P, Morihara J, Mao C, Kiviat NB, Koutsky LA. p16INK4a Expression correlates with degree of cervical Neoplasia: a comparison with Ki-67 expression and detection of high-risk HPV types. Mod Pathol. 2003; 16(7):665–73.

35. Volgareva G, Zavalishina L, Andreeva Y, Frank G, Krutikova E, Golovina D, et al. Protein p16 as a marker of dysplastic and neoplastic alterations in cervical epithelial cells. BMC Cancer. 2004;4:58.

36. Nam EJ, Kim JW, Hong JW, Jang HS, Lee SY, Jang SY, et al. Expression of the p16 and Ki-67 in relation to the grade of cervical intraepithelial neoplasia and high-risk human papillomavirus infection. J Gynecol Oncol. 2008;19: 162–8.

37. Zouheir Y, Fechtali T, Elgnaoui N. Human Papillomavirus genotyping and p16INK4a expression in cervical lesions: a combined test to avoid cervical cancer progression. J Cancer Prev. 2016;21:121–5.

38. Lim S, Lee MJ, Cho I, Hong R, Lim SC. Efficacy of p16 and Ki-67 immunostaining in the detection of squamous intraepithelial lesions in a high-risk HPV group. Oncol Lett. 2016;11:1447–52.

39. Negri G, Vittadello F, Romano F, Kasal A, Rivasi F, Girlando S, et al. P16INK4a Expression and progression risk of low-grade intraepithelial neoplasia of the cervix uteri. Virchows Arch. 2004;445:616–20.

40. Ntekim A. Cervical Cancer in Sub Sahara Africa, Topics on Cervical Cancer With an Advocacy for Prevention. Dr. R. Rajamanickam (Ed.), ISBN: 978–953–51-0183-3, InTech, 2012. Available at: https://cdn.intechopen. com/pdfs-wm/30747.pdf. Accessed 28 May 2017.

41. Kim JJ, Brisson M, Edmunds WJ, Goldie SJ. Modeling cervical cancer prevention in developed countries. Vaccine. 2008;26:76–86.

13

The potential role of infectious agents and pelvic inflammatory disease in ovarian carcinogenesis

Kasper Ingerslev[1][*], Estrid Hogdall[2], Tine Henrichsen Schnack[3], Wojciech Skovrider-Ruminski[4], Claus Hogdall[3] and Jan Blaakaer[1]

Abstract

Background: The etiological cause of ovarian cancer is poorly understood. It has been theorized that bacterial or viral infection as well as pelvic inflammatory disease could play a role in ovarian carcinogenesis.

Aim: To review the literature on studies examining the association between ovarian cancer and bacterial or viral infection or pelvic inflammatory disease.

Methods: Database search through MEDLINE, applying the medical subject headings: "Ovarian neoplasms", AND "Chlamydia infections", "Neisseria gonorrhoeae", "Mycoplasma genitalium", "Papillomaviridae", or "pelvic inflammatory disease". Corresponding searches were performed in EMBASE, and Web of Science. The literature search identified 935 articles of which 40 were eligible for inclusion in this review.

Results: Seven studies examined the association between bacterial infection and ovarian cancer. A single study found a significant association between chlamydial infection and ovarian cancer, while another study identified Mycoplasma genitalium in a large proportion of ovarian cancer cases. The remaining studies found no association. Human papillomavirus detection rates varied from 0 to 67% and were generally higher in the Asian studies than in studies from Western countries. Cytomegalovirus was the only other virus to be detected and was found in 50% of cases in a case-control study. The association between ovarian cancer and pelvic inflammatory disease was examined in seven epidemiological studies, two of which, reported a statistically significant association.

Conclusions: Data indicate a potential association between pelvic inflammatory disease and ovarian cancer. An association between ovarian cancer and high-risk human papillomavirus genotypes may exist in Asia, whereas an association in Western countries seems unlikely due to the low reported prevalence. Potential carcinogenic bacteria were found, but results were inconsistent, and further research is warranted.

Keywords: Ovarian cancer, Bacterial infection, Viral infection, Pelvic inflammatory disease, Carcinogenesis

Background

Ovarian cancer (OC) is a major threat to female health, with a global prevalence of 239,000 cases in 2012 [1]. Due to the lack of symptoms in early stage OC, advanced disease is often present at the time of diagnosis [2].

Almost 90% of OC originates from epithelial cells, which have been thought to arise from the surface mesothelial lining of the ovaries. However, recent research has indicated that a proportion of serous epithelial OC could originate in precancerous lesions called "serous tubal intraepithelial carcinomas" (STICs) located in the fimbriated end of the fallopian tubes [3]. This is an important finding because previous theories of ovarian carcinogenesis have been unable to explain the fact that precancerous lesions have never been identified in the ovaries [3].

The female internal genitalia and the peritoneal cavity are accessible to outside pathogens through the genital tract. The mesothelial lining of the peritoneal cavity is

---

* Correspondence: kasper.hjorth.ingerslev@rsyd.dk
[1]Department of Gynaecology and Obstetrics, Odense University Hospital, Denmark, Soendre Blvd. 29, 5000 Odense C, Denmark
Full list of author information is available at the end of the article

identical in both sexes. However, primary serous peritoneal cancer, which may represent a continuum with serous OC [3], occurs almost exclusively in female patients [4]. This suggests that extrinsic factors could play a crucial role in ovarian carcinogenesis. Furthermore, epidemiological studies have demonstrated that patients with tubal factor infertility have a higher risk of OC [5]. Since the fallopian tubes are often affected by pelvic inflammatory disease (PID), it is therefore highly relevant to consider the potential role of infectious agents in OC. Previous reviews have focused on human papillomavirus (HPV) and OC, but this review is the first to include studies on all bacterial and viral infections as well as studies on pelvic inflammatory disease (PID).

Material and methods

To review the existing literature on OC and infectious agents, we performed a systematic literature search by means of a database search for English language articles published in the period from 1980 to 2016. Using the Pubmed research tool, the keyword: "ovarian neoplasms" was by means of the Boolean logical "AND", combined with the following keywords: "Chlamydia infections"

(MeSH), "Neisseria gonorrhoeae" (MeSH), "Mycoplasma genitalium" (MeSH), "Papillomaviridae" (MeSH), "pelvic inflammatory disease" (MeSH). Correspondent searches were performed in EMBASE and Web of Science. The initial search identified 935 articles. After removal of 130 duplicates, 805 studies remained for further analysis. Contents were outside the scope of the present review in 740 articles that were excluded. The remaining 65 articles were subjected to full-text screening. Original studies, examining the association between infectious agents and ovarian cancer by use of tissue-based or serologic methods were included. Epidemiological studies examining the association between pelvic inflammatory disease and ovarian cancer were also included. Case-reports and reviews were excluded, leaving a total of 40 articles to be included in the review. More detailed information on the search strategy is given in the "Additional file 1" to this article.

Viral agents investigated in relation to ovarian carcinogenesis

Table 1 summarises the viruses investigated in relation to OC, and their potential oncogenic mechanisms.

Table 1 Carcinogenic mechanisms of investigated viruses in relation to ovarian cancer

Virus	Viral family	Key viral transforming factors	Mechanisms	Associated cancers
Human papillomavirus	*Papillomaviridae*	E6 E7	Inhibition of apoptosis Immune evasion Cell cycle arrest Immune evasion [8, 10, 11]	Anal/rectal cancer Cervical cancer Oro-pharyngeal cancer (Ovarian cancer)[a] Penile cancer Vaginal Vulvar cancer
Epstein bar virus	*Herpesviridae*	EBNA 1 EBNA 2 EBNA-3A Latent membrane protein 1	Inhibition of apoptosis B-cell growth transformation Cell cycle disruption Cell cycle disruption Inhibition of apoptosis Promotion of cell immortalisation [48, 49]	Burkitt lymphoma Gastric adenocarcinoma Hodgkin lymphoma Nasopharyngeal carcinoma Non-Hodgkin lymphoma (Ovarian cancer) Post-transplant lymphoproliferative disease
Cytomegalovirus	*Herpesviridae*	IE1/IE2 US28 gene	Inhibition of antiviral immune response Inhibition of apoptosis Enhanced proliferative signaling [44, 45]	Mucoepidermoid carcinoma of salivary glands (Ovarian cancer)
John Cunningham virus/ BK virus	*Polyomaviridae*	T-antigen/t-antigen	Cell cycle disruption Inhibition of apoptosis [56]	(Ovarian cancer)
Hepatitis C virus	*Flaviviridae*	(Indirect) (Direct) NS5B NOS2A NS3/4A protease	Chronic inflammation and oxidative stress Inhibition of antioxidant systems Cell cycle disruption Inhibition of apoptosis Inhibition of DDR response [51–53]	Hepatocellular carcinoma (Ovarian cancer)

DDR Double-stranded DNA Repair, *EBNA* Epstein Barr virus nuclear antigen, *IE* Immediate early genes, *NOS2A* Nitric oxide synthase 2A, *NS3/4A/5B* Nonstructural protein 3/4A/5B
[a]Causality is controversial and is still under investigation

Human papillomavirus infection

HPV infection is a prerequisite for cervical cancer development and is implicated in a range of other cancer forms such as vulvar, penile, anal, and oropharyngeal cancers. To date, The International Agency for Research on Cancer has classified 12 HPV subtypes as human carcinogens: HPV16/18/31/33/35/39/45/51/52/56/58/59 [6]. In HPV-induced tumorigenesis, the viral oncogenes E6 and E7 are integrated into the host cell DNA, allowing viral oncoproteins to be expressed by the cell [7]. The carcinogenic mechanisms of these oncoproteins involve the ability of E6 to form a trimeric complex with P53 and the cellular E3 ubiquitin ligase, E6AP. This complex induces proteasomal degradation of P53, which leads to inhibition of cell-regulatory mechanisms and apoptosis and, therefore, permits continuous cell proliferation despite irreparable DNA damage [8]. E7 can cause degradation of retinoblastoma protein, which is an important regulator of the cell cycle [9]. Furthermore, E7 can interact with several cell cycle regulators including cyclins, cyclin-dependent kinases, CDKs-inhibitors, cullin 2, histone deacetylase, AP-1, E2F1, and E2F6 [10]. These actions enable the virus to resume the replication-competent state within the infected cells, which is essential for viral DNA synthesis. E6 and E7 can also exhibit immunomodulatory effects by downregulating expression of various inflammatory cytokines and by reducing the production of antiviral interferons [11].

HPV is the most studied infectious agent in relation to OC, and the available studies are summarised below.

Six case-control studies, with 11–50 cases of OC, were identified that examined the relation between HPV and OC [12–17]. The applied methods of analysis were either tissue-based methods or serologic assays and included in-situ hybridisation, immunohistochemistry, enzyme-linked immunosorbent serologic assay (ELISA), southern blot hybridisation technique, and polymerase chain reaction (PCR)-based technologies. Only one study found a statistically significant association between HPV and OC [12]. This study was the largest and included 50 cases with OC and a control group with 30 patients with non- malignant ovarian lesions. In-situ hybridisation and immunohistochemistry were used to detect the HPV 16 E6 gene in the tumour specimens. The highest detection rates were obtained by in-situ hybridisation, with a prevalence of 52% among cases as compared to 6.7% among controls (OR: 16.7 95% CI: 3.2–71.4). The remaining smaller studies, found no or non-significant associations [13–17].

Twenty-two *case-series* and *cross-sectional* studies reporting on the prevalence of HPV in OC tissue were identified (Table 2). HPV 16 was most frequently found and was reported in eight studies, giving a combined

total of 60 cases. Ten studies did not find HPV in any of the samples [18–27]. The remaining studies reported a HPV prevalence ranging between 0.5 and 66.7% [28–39]. Interestingly, the reported HPV prevalence varied according to the geographical region. Among the 572 cases of OC in Europe and USA combined, 18 cases (3.1%) were positive for HPV DNA. Studies from the Middle East and Asia, with 347 combined cases of OC, reported 123 cases to be HPV DNA positive (35.4%).

Recently, sequencing data from The Cancer Genome Atlas (TCGA) database have been utilised to detect HPV oncogene expression in ovarian tumours. Using such data, Roos et al. concluded that six samples in 405 (1.5%) were positive for HPV18 oncogene expression [40]. However, Khoury et al. performed a similar analysis on 419 serous cystadenocarcinomas from the TCGA database and did not find signs of HPV infection [41]. Moreover, other studies present data that support potential HPV 18 contamination of the TCGA sequencing database and, consequently, question the validity of positive findings [42, 43].

Cytomegalovirus infection

Cytomegalovirus (CMV) is under increasing focus as a carcinogenic virus. It is speculated that rather than initiating malignant transformation, CMV can enhance the growth and migration of tumour cells through a process called "oncomodulation" [44]. For instance, the formation of metastasis may be aided by the capacity of CMV to adhere to and disrupt the endothelial cell integrity by activating β1α5 integrin on the surface of tumour cells [45]. However, data also indicate that CMV has inherent antiapoptotic and cell cycle modulatory effects [45]. A single study has examined the relation between OC and CMV. The study detected CMV infection in 12 (50%) out of 24 cases with OC and in three (50%) out of six cases of borderline ovarian tumours. No signs of CMV infection were found in the control group consisting of normal ovarian tissue [13]. These findings have not been confirmed by others.

Epstein-Barr virus and hepatitis C virus infection

Epstein-Barr virus (EBV) is present in more than 90% of the global adult population and causes latent infection in the host. [46] It exhibits tropism for epithelial cells, lymphocytes, and mesenchymal cells and is associated with a range of human cancers, including nasopharyngeal carcinoma (NPC) and lymphomas [47]. Its carcinogenic mechanisms include the actions of latent antigens that display effects similar to those of high-risk HPV oncogenes E6 and E7. An example is EBV nuclear antigen (EBNA)-1 that can induce proteasomal degradation of P53 and corresponding inhibition of apoptosis [48]. Likewise, EBNA-3A and -3C play an important role in

Table 2 Studies reporting on HPV prevalence in ovarian cancer tissue

Author & publication year	Detection method	HPV genotypes found	Number of cases of EOC	Number of HPV positive cases	HPV prevalence (%)
Ingerslev et al. (2016) [28]	PCR	18	191	1	0.5
Al-Shabanah et al. (2013) [29]	PCR	16,18,45	100	42	42.0
Malisic et al. (2012) [30]	PCR	16	54	4	7.4
Bilyk et al. (2011) [31]	PCR	16,18	53	9	16.9
Idahl et al. (2010) [18]	PCR		52	0	0
Giordano et al. (2008) [32]	PCR	Not specified	50	1	2.0
Wentzensen et al. (2008) [19]	PCR		74	0	0
Atalay et al. (2007) [33]	PCR	16,33	94	8	8.5
Quirk et al. (2006) [20]	PCR		16	0	0
Yang et al. (2003) [34]	PCR	16,18	56	19	33.9
Ip et al. (2002) [35]	PCR	16,18	60	6	10
Li et al. (2002) [36]	PCR	Not specified	39	26	66.6
Antilla et al. (1999) [21]	PCR		98	0	0
Chen et al. (1999) [22]	PCR		20	0	0
Strickler et al. (1998) [37]	ELISA	16	16	1	6.2
Zimna et al. (1997) [38]	PCR	18	18	7	38.8
Anwar et al. (1996) [23]	PCR		3	0	0
Runnebaum et al. (1995) [24]	PCR		26	0	0
Trottier et al. (1995) [25]	PCR		22	0	0
Lai et al. (1994) [39]	PCR	16,18	18	11	61.1
Beckmann et al. (1991) [26]	PCR		18	0	0
de Villiers (1986) [27]	Southern blot hybridisation		7	0	0

cell cycle regulation and EBNA-2 antigen is suspected to cause primary B-cell growth transformation and maintain human B-cell immortalisation [49]. Hepatitis C virus (HCV) is another investigated microorganism in relation to OC. Chronic HCV infection greatly increases the risk of subsequent hepatocellular carcinoma [50]. The mechanisms are not fully understood but may entail different pathways. The chronic inflammation enhances a pro-carcinogenic microenvironment through the release of nitric oxide (NO) and reactive oxygen species (ROS). This process is further mediated by the ability of HCV to increase the cellular generation of NO and ROS [51] and by its capacity to weaken the antioxidant defence of the host. [52] A more direct pathway involves the ability of HCV to impair phosphorylation of the ataxia telangiectasia mutated (ATM) kinase substrate, histone 2A.X, which plays a role in initiating cellular response to double-stranded DNA breaks [53]. Despite the obvious carcinogenic potential of EBV and HCV, only a single study has investigated their potential role in relation to OC. However, this study did not detect EBV or HCV in 419 serous cystadenocarcinomas from the TCGA database [41].

Polymyoma virus infection
Finally, a single study has analysed tissue samples for the presence of the BK virus and John Cunningham virus [18]. The oncogenic potential of polymyoma viruses has largely been attributed to viral proteins T-antigen and t-antigen through their interactions with various cellular proteins, including tumour suppressor proteins p53 and pRb [54, 55]. Furthermore, the capability of John Cunningham virus T- antigen to transform rodent cells has previously been demonstrated [56]. In the included study, however, polymyoma viruses were not detected in any of the ovarian cancer tissue samples, nor in the benign controls.

Bacterial agents investigated in relation to ovarian carcinogenesis
In relation to OC, previous research has focused on the potential association between *Chlamydia trachomatis (C. trachomatis), Mycoplasma genitalium (M. genitalium), and Neisseria gonorrhoeae (N. gonorrhoeae)* [13, 18, 57–61]. An overview of the potential carcinogenic mechanisms of these bacteria is provided in Table 3.

Table 3 Carcinogenic mechanisms of investigated bacteria in relation to ovarian cancer

Microorganism	Suspected mechanisms	Potentially associated cancers
Chlamydia trachomatis	Inhibition of apoptosis Production of reactive oxygen species Inhibition of DDR [62, 64]	Cervical squamous cell carcinoma Ovarian cancer
Neisseria Gonorrhoeae	DNA strand breaks. Inhibition of P53. Cell cycle disruption [68]	Bladder cancer Prostate cancer Ovarian cancer
Mycoplasma Genitalium	Acquisition of anchorage-independent growth Inhibition of apoptosis. Karyotypic entropy [69]	Ovarian cancer Prostate cancer

DDR Double-stranded DNA Repair

Chlamydia trachomatis infection

C. trachomatis is a small, obligate intracellular bacterium that has developed several mechanisms to improve its own survival and replication within the host. It can upregulate the production of reactive oxygen species (ROS) through the Mitochondrial Nod-like Family Member NLRX1 [62]. ROS production is normally a cellular defence mechanism against invading microorganisms. However, C. trachomatis can subvert cellular defences and use ROS to improve its own growth through activation of caspase-1 [62]. The resulting increased levels of ROS can lead to double-stranded DNA breaks in the infected cell. Furthermore, C. trachomatis can impair the DNA damage response (DDR) through inhibition of DDR proteins pATM and 53BP1 [63]. Despite the DNA damage, the chlamydia-infected cells continue to proliferate due to increased MAPK signalling and cyclin E expression [63]. Finally, C. trachomatis can initiate proteasomal degradation of P53 through interaction with the phosphorylated ubiquitin ligase Murine Double Minute 2, leading to inhibition of apoptosis [64]. Combined, these mechanisms promote bacterial survival, but they can also potentially lead to genomic instability, disruption of the cell cycle, and inhibition of apoptosis, all of which are among the hallmarks of cancer [65]. Therefore, C. trachomatis is a suitable candidate for ovarian carcinogenesis. However, the literature on the subject is scarce, and an association between C. trachomatis and OC has been found in only two studies.

One case-control study was based on fresh ovarian tissues from 39 women undergoing laparotomy [13]. The tissue samples, which included 24 cases of OC, six borderline tumours, and nine normal ovaries, were tested for the presence of C. trachomatis DNA by PCR techniques. C. trachomatis DNA was detected in 87.5% of the malignant tumours and 50% of the borderline ovarian tumours as compared to none of the benign ovarian tissue samples (OR = 32 (95% CI: 3.33, 307.65).

A study by Ness et al. included 117 women with OC and 171 healthy controls [60]. Serologic testing for IgG antibodies of the extracellular elementary bodies (EB) of C. trachomatis was performed. Patients with EOC were more likely to have high levels of C. trachomatis EB than the controls in adjusted analysis. In a subgroup analysis, the probability of having OC was insignificantly increased in patients with the highest levels of IgG EB antibodies compared to the group with the lowest levels (OR = 1.9 95% CI 0.9–3.9). However, these findings are controversial, since four other serologic studies with a total of 626 cases of OC found no association [57–59, 61]. Likewise, a single tissue-based study that included 51 OC cases did not find an association [18].

Neisseria gonorrhoeae & Mycoplasma genitalium infection

N. gonorrhoeae is a small, gram-negative diplococcus that infects epithelial cells and causes cervicitis/urethritis and PID. It has been associated with prostate and bladder cancer [66, 67]. One study has reported that N. gonorrhoeae can cause DNA strand breaks, affect the cell cycle progression, and can decrease the levels of P53 within infected cells [68].

M. genitalium is under increasing focus for its role in PID. Like N. gonorrhoeae, its propensity for malignant transformation of host cells is unclear. However, one study revealed that persistent infection of benign human prostate cells with M. genitalium resulted in increased migration/invasion [69]. Furthermore, it induced the acquisition of anchorage-independent growth, which allows cells to detach from the surrounding extracellular matrix and metastasise. Finally, it induced karyotypic entropy and malignant transformation proven by the formation of xenograft tumours in immune-compromised mice [69].

Very few studies have investigated the association between M. genitalium or N. gonorrhoeae and OC. Only one study reported an association, M. genitalium DNA being detected in 16 (59.3%) out of 27 samples by a combined PCR and ELISA technique. [70] However, in two separate studies, Idahl et al. found no association between *M. genitalium* or *N. gonorrhoeae* and OC [18, 57].

Pelvic inflammatory disease

Microorganisms that cannot directly induce cellular transformation may still play a role in OC oncogenesis due to the paradoxical effect of the host inflammatory response. It has long been recognised that the cells involved in innate and adaptive immune responses are recruited to the site of tumorigenesis. Here, they can release a multitude of tumour promoting inflammatory cytokines, chemokines, and ROS that can potentially facilitate tumour cell migration, metastasis, and angiogenesis [65]. Cancer has aptly been described as "a wound that does not heal [71]". Several conditions associated with pelvic inflammation such as perineal talc use and endometriosis have been demonstrated to increase the risk of OC [72]. Likewise, ovulation is speculated to induce focal damage and inflammation on the ovarian surface epithelium, and factors that reduce the number of lifetime ovulatory cycles have been shown to reduce the risk of OC [73]. Consequently, it has been speculated that PID could play a role in ovarian carcinogenesis, and the potential association between PID and OC have been investigated in seven case-control studies (Table 4). The majority of studies relied on patient-reported outcomes and identified cases of PID through interviews or questionnaires. Risch et al. reported a statistically significant association between PID and OC (odds ratio (OR) 1.53; 95% CI 1.10–2.13) [74]. Moreover, they found a dose-response effect in relation to repeated episodes of PID, implying a higher risk of OC with increasing episodes of PID (OR 1.88; 95% CI 1.13–3.12). A prospective, population-based study from Taiwan verified the diagnosis of PID by the International Statistical Classification of Diseases and Related Health Problems codes registered in a national database [75]. After 3 years of follow-up, a higher risk of OC was observed in the case group (hazard ratio (HR) 1.92; 95% CI 1.27–2.92)). In this study, the association was also stronger when analysis was restricted to cases exposed to more episodes of PID (HR 2.46; 95% CI 1.48–4.09) [75]. However, a statistically significant association between PID and OC could not be confirmed in any of the remaining studies [72, 74, 76–79].

Discussion

The reviewed studies were very heterogeneous in terms of study population, study design, and the analysis methods used.

However, based on the reviewed studies, it is fair to conclude that high-risk HPV is unlikely to be associated with OC in Western countries. Interestingly, a higher prevalence was consistently reported in Asia and the Middle East. This finding is supported by previous reviews focusing on HPV and ovarian cancer [80, 81] and a potential association may exist in these regions. The geographic variation could be caused by varying potency of HPV strains. Thus, it has been demonstrated that latent infection of the cervix uteri with the non- European variant of HPV 16 is associated with a 2- to 9-fold higher risk of cancer or high- grade cancer precursors, compared to infection with the European variant [82]. Differing genetic predispositions between ethnical groups may also be a factor because polymorphisms of the TP 53 gene or the promoter of the tumour necrosis factor alpha gene have been associated with increased vulnerability to HPV oncogenes [83, 84]. Lastly, environmental or life-style factors could play a role. For instance, the global incidence of EBV infection among adults is estimated to be over 90%, and there is strong evidence linking EBV infection to the development of NPC [47]. Despite the ubiquity of infection, the incidence of NPC is very low in most regions. However, dramatically elevated rates are observed in certain parts of Asia, and dietary factors, such as the intake of salt-preserved fish, are thought to play a role [85]. This

Table 4 Case-control studies on the association between PID and ovarian cancer

Author & publication year	Region	Data collection	Number of cases	Number of controls	Odds/Hazard- ratios (HR)
Rasmussen et al. (2013) [78]	Denmark	Interview	554	1.564	0.83 95% CI: 0.65–1.05
Lin et al. (2011) [75]	Taiwan	Database	67.936	135.872	1.92 95% CI: 1.27–2.92 (HR) 2.46 95% CI: 1.48–4.09[c] (HR)
Merritt et al. (2007) [76]	Australia	Questionnaire	1.576	1.509	1.15 95% CI: 0.85–1.57
Ness et al. (2000) [72]	USA	Interview	616	1.367	1.3 95% CI: 0.6–2.5
Parazzini et al. (1996) [79]	Italy	Questionnaire/interview	971	2.758	0.7 95% CI: 0.4–1.3
Risch et al. (1995) [74]	Canada	Interview	450	564	1.53 95% CI: 1.10–2.13[a] 1.88 95% CI: 1.13–3.12[b]
Shu et al. (1989) [77]	Hong Kong	Interview	172	172	3.0 95% CI: 0.3–30.2

[a]One episode of PID
[b]Two or more episodes of PID
[c]Five or more episodes of PID

underlines that, even though infection with oncogenic viruses is common, cancer is a rare event that can arise from a combination of genetic, environmental, and lifestyle factors.

Most of the epidemiological studies found an association between OC and PID, but only two studies reported a statistically significant association [74, 75]. It is noteworthy, however, that these studies also identified a dose- response effect. This is one of the key points in Hill's criteria for causation that state that a biological gradient must be present, with more exposure to the suspected agent leading to a larger effect [86]. These findings are supported by studies that found evaluated markers of inflammation such as CRP and interleukins to be significantly associated with an increased risk of OC [87]. A possible limitation to the reviewed studies is that they relied primarily on patient-reported outcomes, which may be subject to recall bias. Furthermore, due to the potential subclinical course of PID, patients can be unaware of previous episodes. This is supported by studies that have demonstrated a relatively high seroprevalence of chlamydia antibody titres in women that reported no history of PID, and this issue would tend to produce bias towards the null [88, 89].

Interestingly, CMV was reported in 50% of cases in a single study, but this finding requires confirmation in future and larger studies. No other viral agent was detected.

The only detected bacteria were *C. trachomatis and M. genitalium*. The results of this review do not support an association between *C. trachomatis* and OC, the majority of studies reporting negative results. The association between *M. genitalium* and OC was investigated and found in only a single study and more research is needed.

Several factors may account for the conflicting results. First of all, there may be no connection between the investigated infectious agents and OC. Secondly, the heterogeneity of analysis methods, study populations, and study designs may play a part. However, other explanations must be discussed. Importantly, it is unclear to what extent signs of microbiological agents are present in a tumour that arises decades after infection. For some oncogenic viruses, like high-risk HPV, expression of viral oncogenes is obligate for the maintenance of the malignant phenotype [90]. In these cases, viral genes will remain integrated and detectable in tumour cell DNA. But another potential mechanism is debated in the "hit and run" hypothesis. Here, integration of viral transforming genes and potential epigenetic reprogramming of host cells initiate tumorigenesis, but the viral gene expression is subsequently lost during neoplastic development [91]. Accordingly, it has been demonstrated that CMV oncogenes IE1 and IE2 can cooperate with adenovirus E1A gene to transform rat kidney cells. However, expression of the transforming oncogenes was absent in the clonal cell lines from the transformed foci [92].

Finally, other oncogenic agents act more indirectly by inducing chronic inflammation that may function as an initiator or promoter of carcinogenesis [93]. Consequently, the involved pathogen may no longer be present when cancer is diagnosed. For instance, despite the established role of HCV in hepatocellular carcinoma, only a minority of transformed hepatocytes contain viral RNA [94].

These examples highlight the fact that the abscense of microbiological agents in tumour tissue does not rule out their potential role in the transformation of host cells. These issues seem to strengthen the need for serologic studies. However, serologic methods are limited by the fact that antibody levels are likely to decline over time. In a study from Finland, 43% of women had declining *C. trachomatis* antibody titres 6 years after the diagnosis of PID [95]. Moreover, not all patients with prior chlamydial infection will have detectable antibodies [96].

These obstacles call for a revised strategy in the attempt to uncover the potential role of infectious agents in OC. It is fair to assume that signs of microbiological presence will be easier to detect when the interval between primary infection and investigation is short. Therefore, it seems more relevant to investigate precursor lesions for the presence of potential microbiological agents [91]. Until recently, this has been impossible due to the lack of a clearly defined premalignant lesion to OC. However, this has changed because increasing evidence indicates that STIC lesions in the distal fallopian tubes are precursor lesions to serous epithelial OC, which constitutes the majority of OC cases [3]. Yet, no explanation has been formulated as to why STIC lesions arise. Since the fallopian tubes are often affected and damaged by chronic PID, it is biological plausible that pathogens with transforming capacities, or the chronic inflammation they induce, could lead to subsequent neoplastic transformation. We therefore recommend that future studies focus on the detection of bacterial or viral agents in fallopian tube tissue samples with STIC lesions verified through the "Sectioning and Extensively Examining of the Fimbriated end" protocol.

Conclusion

The reviewed articles indicate a potential association between PID and OC. An association between OC and high-risk HPV genotypes may exist in Asia, whereas an association in Western countries seems unlikely due to the low reported prevalence. Two studies reported an association between bacterial agents and OC, but the majority of bacterial studies reported negative findings. However, the available literature was scarce and more studies are warranted.

Abbreviations

ATM: Ataxia telangiectasia mutated; *C. trachomatis*: *Chlamydia trachomatis*; CI: Confidence interval; CMV: Cytomegalovirus; DDR: Double-stranded DNA Repair.; EBNA: Epstein bar virus nuclear antigen; EBV: Epstein bar virus; ELISA: Enzyme-linked immunosorbent serologic assay; HCV: Hepatitis C virus; HPV: Human papillomavirus; HR: Hazard ratio; IE: Immediate early genes; *M. genitalium*: *Mycoplasma genitalium*; *N. Gonorrhoeae*: *Neisseria gonorrhoeae*; NO: Nitric oxide; NOS2A: Nitric oxide synthase 2A; NPC: Nasopharyngeal carcinoma; NS3/4A: Nonstructural protein 3/4A; OC: Ovarian cancer; PCR: Polymerase chain reaction; PID: Pelvic inflammatory disease; ROS: Reactive oxygen species; STIC: Serous tubal intraepithelial carcinoma; TCGA: Cancer Genome Atlas database

Acknowledgements

Not applicable.

Funding

The study was funded by several grant givers to the *"Danish Mermaid III Project"*. Please see list of individual grant givers at: http://www.mermaidprojektet.dk/en/about-the-mermaid-project/how-are-we-funded/. The grant givers had no influence on the study design, interpretation of data or in the writing or revision of the manuscript.

Authors' contributions

KI: devised the search strategy and performed the literature search and contributed to the development of the proposal, writing of the draft manuscript, and review of the manuscript. EH: contributed to the development of the proposal and participated in review of the manuscript. WS: contributed to the development of the proposal and review of the manuscript. THS: contributed to the development of the proposal and review of the manuscript. CH: contributed to the development of the proposal and review of the manuscript. JB: Contributed to the conception of the study and to the review and selection of studies as well as to the review of the manuscript. All authors have read and approved the final manuscript.

Competing interests

The authors declare that they have no competing interests.

Author details

[1]Department of Gynaecology and Obstetrics, Odense University Hospital, Denmark, Soendre Blvd. 29, 5000 Odense C, Denmark. [2]Department of Pathology, Herlev and Gentofte Hospital, Denmark, Herlev Ringvej 75, 2730 Herlev, Denmark. [3]Gynaecologic Clinic, Copenhagen University Hospital, Denmark, Blegdamsvej 9, 2100 Copenhagen, Denmark. [4]Department of Pathology, Herlev Hospital, Denmark, Herlev Ringvej 75, 2730 Herlev, Denmark.

References

1. Ferlay J, Soerjomataram I, Dikshit R, et al. Cancer incidence and mortality worldwide: sources, methods and major patterns in GLOBOCAN 2012. Int J Cancer. 2015;136:E359–86.
2. Maringe C, Walters S, Butler J, et al. Stage at diagnosis and ovarian cancer survival: evidence from the International Cancer Benchmarking Partnership. Gynecol Oncol. 2012;127:75–82.
3. Kurman RJ, Shih I. The origin and pathogenesis of epithelial ovarian cancer: a proposed unifying theory. Am J Surg Pathol. 2010;34:433–43.
4. Jermann M, Vogt P, Pestalozzi BC. "Peritoneal carcinoma in a male patient." Oncology 64.4. 2003;468–72.
5. Brinton LA, Lamb EJ, Moghissi KS, et al. Ovarian cancer risk associated with varying causes of infertility. Fertil Steril. 2004;82:405–14.
6. IARC Working Group on the Evaluation of Carcinogenic Risks to Humans. IARC monographs on the evaluation of carcinogenic risks to humans. Ingested nitrate and nitrite, and cyanobacterial peptide toxins. IARC Monogr Eval Carcinog Risks Hum. 2010;94:1–412. v,vii.
7. Chen Y, Williams V, Filippova M, et al. Viral carcinogenesis: factors inducing DNA damage and virus integration. Cancers. 2014;6:2155–86.
8. Bernard X, Robinson P, Nomine Y, et al. Proteasomal degradation of p53 by human papillomavirus E6 oncoprotein relies on the structural integrity of p53 core domain. PLoS One. 2011;6:e25981.
9. McLaughlin-Drubin ME, Münger K. The human papillomavirus E7 oncoprotein. Virology. 2009;384:335–44.
10. Boccardo E, Lepique AP, Villa LL. The role of inflammation in HPV carcinogenesis. Carcinogenesis. 2010;31:1905–12.
11. Richards KH, Doble R, Wasson CW, et al. Human papillomavirus E7 oncoprotein increases production of the anti-inflammatory interleukin-18 binding protein in keratinocytes. J Virol. 2014;88:4173–9.
12. Wu QJ, Guo M, Lu ZM, et al. Detection of human papillomavirus-16 in ovarian malignancy. Br J Cancer. 2003;89:672–5.
13. Shanmughapriya S, Senthilkumar G, Vinodhini K, et al. Viral and bacterial aetiologies of epithelial ovarian cancer. Eur J Clin Microbiol Infect Dis. 2012;31:2311–7.
14. Kuscu E, Ozdemir BH, Erkanli S, et al. HPV and p53 expression in epithelial ovarian carcinoma. Eur J Gynaecol Oncol. 2005;26:642–5.
15. Lai CH, Hsueh S, Lin CY, et al. Human papillomavirus in benign and malignant ovarian and endometrial tissues. Int J Gynecol Pathol. 1992;11:210–5.
16. Leake JF, Woodruff JD, Searle C, et al. Human papillomavirus and epithelial ovarian neoplasia. Gynecol Oncol. 1989;34:268–73.
17. Hisada M, van den Berg BJ, Strickler HD, et al. Prospective study of antibody to human papilloma virus type 16 and risk of cervical, endometrial, and ovarian cancers (United States). Cancer Causes Control. 2001;12:335–41.
18. Idahl A, Lundin E, Elgh F, et al. Chlamydia trachomatis, Mycoplasma genitalium, Neisseria gonorrhoeae, human papillomavirus, and polyomavirus are not detectable in human tissue with epithelial ovarian cancer, borderline tumor, or benign conditions. Am J Obstet Gynecol. 2010;202:71.e1,71.e6.
19. Wentzensen N, du Bois A, Kommoss S, et al. No metastatic cervical adenocarcinomas in a series of p16INK4a-positive mucinous or endometrioid advanced ovarian carcinomas: an analysis of the AGO Ovarian Cancer Study Group. Int J Gynecol Pathol. 2008;27:18–23.
20. Quirk JT, Kupinski JM, DiCioccio RA. Analysis of ovarian tumors for the presence of human papillomavirus DNA. J Obstet Gynaecol Res. 2006;32:202–5.
21. Anttila M, Syrjanen S, Ji H, et al. Failure to demonstrate human papillomavirus DNA in epithelial ovarian cancer by general primer PCR. Gynecol Oncol. 1999;72:337–41.
22. Chen TR, Chan PJ, Seraj IM, et al. Absence of human papillomavirus E6-E7 transforming genes from HPV 16 and 18 in malignant ovarian carcinoma. Gynecol Oncol. 1999;72:180–2.
23. Anwar K, Nakakuki K, Imai H, et al. Infection of human papillomavirus (HPV) and p53 over-expression in human female genital tract carcinoma. J Pak Med Assoc. 1996;46:220–4.
24. Runnebaum IB, Maier S, Tong XW, et al. Human papillomavirus integration is not associated with advanced epithelial ovarian cancer in German patients. Cancer Epidemiol Biomarkers Prev. 1995;4:573–5.
25. Trottier AM, Provencher D, Mes-Masson AM, et al. Absence of human papillomavirus sequences in ovarian pathologies. J Clin Microbiol. 1995;33:1011–3.
26. Beckmann AM, Sherman KJ, Saran L, et al. Genital-type human papillomavirus infection is not associated with surface epithelial ovarian carcinoma. Gynecol Oncol. 1991;43:247–51.
27. de Villiers E, Schneider A, Gross G, et al. Analysis of benign and malignant urogenital tumors for human papillomavirus infection by labelling cellular DNA. Med Microbiol Immunol (Berl). 1986;174:281–6.
28. Ingerslev K, Hogdall E, Skovrider-Ruminski W, et al. High-risk HPV is not associated with epithelial ovarian cancer in a Caucasian population. Infect Agent Cancer. 2016;11:1.
29. Al-Shabanah OA, Hafez MM, Hassan ZK, et al. Human papillomavirus genotyping and integration in ovarian cancer Saudi patients. Virol J. 2013;10:343. 422X-10-343.
30. Malisic E, Jankovic R, Jakovljevic K. Detection and genotyping of human papillomaviruses and their role in the development of ovarian carcinomas. Arch Gynecol Obstet. 2012;286:723–8.

31. Bilyk OO, Pande NT, Buchynska LG. Analysis of p53, p16(INK4a), pRb and Cyclin D1 expression and human papillomavirus in primary ovarian serous carcinomas. Exp Oncol. 2011;33:150–6.

32. Giordano G, D'Adda T, Gnetti L, et al. Role of human papillomavirus in the development of epithelial ovarian neoplasms in Italian women. J Obstet Gynaecol Res. 2008;34:210–7.

33. Atalay F, Taskiran C, Taner MZ, et al. Detection of human papillomavirus DNA and genotyping in patients with epithelial ovarian carcinoma. J Obstet Gynaecol Res. 2007;33:823–8.

34. Yang HJ, Liu VW, Tsang PC, et al. Comparison of human papillomavirus DNA levels in gynecological cancers: implication for cancer development. Tumour Biol. 2003;24:310–6.

35. Ip SM, Wong LC, Xu CM, et al. Detection of human papillomavirus DNA in malignant lesions from Chinese women with carcinomas of the upper genital tract. Gynecol Oncol. 2002;87:104–11.

36. Li T, Lu Z-M, Guo M, et al. p53 Codon 72 polymorphism (C/G) and the risk of human papillomavirus-associated carcinomas in China. Cancer. 2002;95:2571–6.

37. Strickler HD, Schiffman MH, Shah KV, et al. A survey of human papillomavirus 16 antibodies in patients with epithelial cancers. Eur J Cancer Prev. 1998;7:305–13.

38. Zimna K, Poreba E, Kedzia W, et al. Human papillomavirus (HPV) in upper genital tract carcinomas of women. Eur J Gynaecol Oncol. 1997;18:415–7.

39. Lai CH, Wang CY, Lin CY, et al. Detection of human papillomavirus RNA in ovarian and endometrial carcinomas by reverse transcription/polymerase chain reaction. Gynecol Obstet Invest. 1994;38:276–80.

40. Roos P, Orlando PA, Fagerstrom RM, et al. In North America, some ovarian cancers express the oncogenes of preventable human papillomavirus HPV-18. Sci Rep. 2015;5:8645.

41. Khoury JD, Tannir NM, Williams MD, et al. Landscape of DNA virus associations across human malignant cancers: Analysis of 3,775 cases using RNA-seq. J Virol. 2013;87:8916–26.

42. Kazemian M, Ren M, Lin JX, et al. Possible human papillomavirus 38 contamination of endometrial cancer rna sequencing samples in the cancer genome atlas database. J Virol. 2015;89:8967–73.

43. Cantalupo PG, Katz JP, Pipas JM. HeLa nucleic acid contamination in the cancer genome atlas leads to the misidentification of human papillomavirus 18. J Virol. 2015;89:4051–7.

44. Cinatl J, Scholz M, Kotchetkov R, et al. Molecular mechanisms of the modulatory effects of HCMV infection in tumor cell biology. Trends Mol Med. 2004;10:19–23.

45. Michaelis M, Doerr HW, Cinatl J. The story of human cytomegalovirus and cancer: increasing evidence and open questions. Neoplasia. 2009;11:1–9.

46. de-The G, Day NE, Geser A, et al. Sero-epidemiology of the Epstein-Barr virus: preliminary analysis of an international study - a review. IARC Sci Publ. 1975;11 Pt 2:3–16.

47. Coghill AE, Hildesheim A. Epstein-Barr virus antibodies and the risk of associated malignancies: review of the literature. Am J Epidemiol. 2014;180:687–95.

48. Grywalska E, Rolinski J. Epstein-barr virus–associated lymphomas. Semin Oncol. 2015;42:291–303.

49. Jha HC, Banerjee S, Robertson ES. The role of gammaherpesviruses in cancer pathogenesis. Pathogens. 2016;5:18.

50. Donato F, Tagger A, Gelatti U, et al. Alcohol and hepatocellular carcinoma: the effect of lifetime intake and hepatitis virus infections in men and women. Am J Epidemiol. 2002;155:323–31.

51. Mitchell JK, Lemon SM, McGivern DR. How do persistent infections with hepatitis C virus cause liver cancer? Curr Opin Virol. 2015;14:101–8.

52. Choi J, Corder NL, Koduru B, et al. Oxidative stress and hepatic Nox proteins in chronic hepatitis C and hepatocellular carcinoma. Free Radic Biol Med. 2014;72:267–84.

53. Duong FH, Christen V, Lin S, et al. Hepatitis C virus–induced up-regulation of protein phosphatase 2A inhibits histone modification and DNA damage repair. Hepatology. 2010;51:741–51.

54. Khalili K, Del Valle L, Otte J, et al. Human neurotropic polyomavirus, JCV, and its role in carcinogenesis. Oncogene. 2003;22:5181–91.

55. Caracciolo V, Reiss K, Khalili K, et al. Role of the interaction between large T antigen and Rb family members in the oncogenicity of JC virus. Oncogene. 2006;25:5294–301.

56. Barbanti-Brodano G, Sabbioni S, Martini F, et al. BK virus, JC virus and Simian Virus 40 infection in humans, and association with human tumors. Polyomaviruses and human diseases. New York: Springer; 2006:319–41.

57. Idahl A, Lundin E, Jurstrand M, et al. Chlamydia trachomatis and Mycoplasma genitalium plasma antibodies in relation to epithelial ovarian tumors. Infect Dis Obstet Gynecol. 2011;2011:824627.

58. Ness RB, Shen C, Bass D, et al. Chlamydia trachomatis serology in women with and without ovarian cancer. Infect Dis Obstet Gynecol. 2008;2008:219672.

59. Wong A, Maclean AB, Furrows SJ, et al. Could epithelial ovarian cancer be associated with chlamydial infection? Eur J Gynaecol Oncol. 2007;28:117–20.

60. Ness RB, Goodman MT, Shen C, et al. Serologic evidence of past infection with Chlamydia trachomatis, in relation to ovarian cancer. J Infect Dis. 2003;187:1147–52.

61. Martin DC, Khare VK, Miller BE, et al. Association of positive Chlamydia trachomatis and Chlamydia pneumoniae immunoglobulin-gamma titers with increasing age. J Am Assoc Gynecol Laparosc. 1997;4:583–6.

62. Abdul-Sater AA, Said-Sadier N, Lam VM, et al. Enhancement of reactive oxygen species production and chlamydial infection by the mitochondrial Nod-like family member NLRX1. J Biol Chem. 2010;285:41637–45.

63. Chumduri C, Gurumurthy RK, Zadora PK, et al. Chlamydia infection promotes host DNA damage and proliferation but impairs the DNA damage response. Cell Host Microbe. 2013;13:746–58.

64. Gonzalez E, Rother M, Kerr MC, et al. Chlamydia infection depends on a functional MDM2-p53 axis. Nat Commun. 2014;5:5201.

65. Hanahan D, Weinberg RA. Hallmarks of cancer: the next generation. Cell. 2011;144:646–74.

66. Michaud D, Platz E, Giovannucci E. Gonorrhoea and male bladder cancer in a prospective study. Br J Cancer. 2007;96:169–71.

67. Lian WQ, Luo F, Song XL, et al. Gonorrhea and prostate cancer incidence: an updated meta-analysis of 21 epidemiologic studies. Med Sci Monit. 2015;21:1902–10.

68. Vielfort K, Soderholm N, Weyler L, et al. Neisseria gonorrhoeae infection causes DNA damage and affects the expression of p21, p27 and p53 in non-tumor epithelial cells. J Cell Sci. 2013;126:339–47.

69. Namiki K, Goodison S, Porvasnik S, et al. Persistent exposure to Mycoplasma induces malignant transformation of human prostate cells. PLoS One. 2009;4:e6872.

70. Chan P, Seraj I, Kalugdan T, et al. Prevalence of Mycoplasma conserved DNA in malignant ovarian cancer detected using sensitive PCR-ELISA. Gynecol Oncol. 1996;63:258–60.

71. Dvorak HF. Tumors: wounds that do not heal. N Engl J Med. 1986;315:1650–9.

72. Ness RB, Grisso JA, Cottreau C, et al. Factors related to inflammation of the ovarian epithelium and risk of ovarian cancer. Epidemiology. 2000;11:111–7.

73. Li J, Fadare O, Xiang L, et al. Ovarian serous carcinoma: recent concepts on its origin and carcinogenesis. J Hematol Oncol. 2012;5:1.

74. Risch HA, Howe GR. Pelvic inflammatory disease and the risk of epithelial ovarian cancer. Cancer Epidemiol Biomarkers Prev. 1995;4:447–51.

75. Lin HW, Tu YY, Lin SY, et al. Risk of ovarian cancer in women with pelvic inflammatory disease: a population-based study. Lancet Oncol. 2011;12:900–4.

76. Merritt MA, Green AC, Nagle CM, et al. Talcum powder, chronic pelvic inflammation and NSAIDs in relation to risk of epithelial ovarian cancer. Int J Cancer. 2008;122:170–6.

77. Shu XO, Brinton LA, Gao YT, et al. Population-based case-control study of ovarian cancer in Shanghai. Cancer Res. 1989;49:3670–4.

78. Rasmussen CB, Faber MT, Jensen A, et al. Pelvic inflammatory disease and risk of invasive ovarian cancer and ovarian borderline tumors. Cancer Causes Control. 2013;24:1459–64.

79. Parazzini F, La Vecchia C, Negri E, et al. Pelvic inflammatory disease and risk of ovarian cancer. Cancer Epidemiol Biomarkers Prev. 1996;5:667–9.

80. Svahn MF, Faber MT, Christensen J, et al. Prevalence of human papillomavirus in epithelial ovarian cancer tissue. A meta-analysis of observational studies. Acta Obstet Gynecol Scand. 2014;93:6–19.

81. Rosa MI, Silva GD, de Azedo Simoes PW, et al. The prevalence of human papillomavirus in ovarian cancer: a systematic review. Int J Gynecol Cancer. 2013;23:437–41.

82. Hildesheim A, Wang SS. Host and viral genetics and risk of cervical cancer: a review. Virus Res. 2002;89:229–40.

83. Zhou X, Gu Y, Zhang S. Association between p53 codon 72 polymorphism and cervical cancer risk among Asians: a HuGE review and meta-analysis. Asian Pac J Cancer Prev. 2012;13:4909–14.

84. Liu L, Yang X, Chen X, et al. Association between TNF-α polymorphisms and cervical cancer risk: a meta-analysis. Mol Biol Rep. 2012;39:2683–8.

85. Chang ET, Adami HO. The enigmatic epidemiology of nasopharyngeal carcinoma. Cancer Epidemiol Biomarkers Prev. 2006;15:1765–77.

86. HILL AB. The environment and disease: association or causation? Proc R Soc Med. 1965;58:295–300.

87. Charbonneau B, Goode EL, Kalli KR, et al. The immune system in the pathogenesis of ovarian cancer. Crit Rev Immunol. 2013;33:137–64.

88. Bjercke S, Purvis K. Characteristics of women under fertility investigation with IgA/IgG seropositivity for Chlamydia trachomatis. Eur J Obstet Gynecol Reprod Biol. 1993;51:157–61.

89. Stamm WE, Holmes KK. Chlamydia trachomatis infections of the adult. Sex Transm Dis. 1999;3:407–22.

90. DeFilippis RA, Goodwin EC, Wu L, et al. Endogenous human papillomavirus E6 and E7 proteins differentially regulate proliferation, senescence, and apoptosis in HeLa cervical carcinoma cells. J Virol. 2003;77:1551–63.

91. Niller HH, Wolf H, Minarovits J. Viral hit and run-oncogenesis: genetic and epigenetic scenarios. Cancer Lett. 2011;305:200–17.

92. Shen Y, Zhu H, Shenk T. Human cytomagalovirus IE1 and IE2 proteins are mutagenic and mediate "hit-and-run" oncogenic transformation in cooperation with the adenovirus E1A proteins. Proc Natl Acad Sci U S A. 1997;94:3341–5.

93. Grivennikov SI, Greten FR, Karin M. Immunity, inflammation, and cancer. Cell. 2010;140:883–99.

94. Kandathil AJ, Graw F, Quinn J, et al. Use of laser capture microdissection to map hepatitis C virus–positive hepatocytes in human liver. Gastroenterology. 2013;145:1404,1413. e10.

95. Puolakkainen M, Vesterinen E, Purola E, et al. Persistence of chlamydial antibodies after pelvic inflammatory disease. J Clin Microbiol. 1986;23:924–8.

96. Bas S, Muzzin P, Ninet B, et al. Chlamydial serology: comparative diagnostic value of immunoblotting, microimmunofluorescence test, and immunoassays using different recombinant proteins as antigens. J Clin Microbiol. 2001;39:1368–77.

14

Aflatoxin B$_1$ inhibits the type 1 interferon response pathway via STAT1 suggesting another mechanism of hepatocellular carcinoma

Patrick W. Narkwa[1], David J. Blackbourn[2] and Mohamed Mutocheluh[1]*

Abstract

Background: Aflatoxin B$_1$ (AFB$_1$) contamination of food is very high in most sub-Saharan African countries. AFB$_1$ is known to cause hepatocellular carcinoma (HCC) by inducing mutation in the tumour suppressor gene TP53. The number of new HCC cases is high in West Africa with an accompanying high mortality. The type I interferon (IFN) pathway of the innate immune system limits viral infections and exerts its anti-cancer property by up-regulating tumour suppressor activities and pro-apoptotic pathways. Indeed, IFN-α is reported to show significant protective effects against hepatic fibrogenesis and carcinogenesis. However, the mechanism behind AFB$_1$ deregulation of the type I interferon (IFN) signalling pathway, with consequent HCC is largely unknown. This current study seeks to test the hypothesis that AFB$_1$ inhibits the type I IFN response by directly interfering with key signalling proteins and thus increase the risk of HCC in humans.

Methods: We evaluated the effects of AFB$_1$ on the type I IFN signalling pathway using IFN stimulated response element (ISRE)-based luciferase reporter gene assay. In addition, the effects of AFB$_1$ on the transcript levels of *JAK1*, *STAT1* and *OAS3* were assessed by real-time quantitative polymerase chain reaction (RT-qPCR) and confirmed by immunoblot assay.

Results: Our results indicated that AFB$_1$ inhibited the type I IFN signalling pathway in human hepatoma cell line HepG2 cells by suppressing the transcript levels of *JAK1*, *STAT1* and *OAS3*. AFB$_1$ also decreased the accumulation of STAT1 protein.

Conclusion: The inhibition of the type I IFN anti-cancer response pathway by AFB$_1$ suggest a novel mechanism by which AFB$_1$ may induce hepatocellular carcinoma in humans.

Keywords: Aflatoxin B$_1$, Hepatocellular carcinoma, STAT1, Type I interferon pathway, HepG2 cells, JAK1, ISRE

Background

The innate immune response is activated within few hours upon exposure of the human system to infectious agents and other toxic chemical compounds such as mycotoxins and works to protect the individual against the harmful effects of the chemical agents and the disease causing microorganisms. One component of the innate immune system that plays a key role in the first line of

* Correspondence: mmutocheluh.chs@knust.edu.gh; mutocheluh@gmail.com
[1]Department of Clinical Microbiology, School of Medical Sciences, Kwame Nkrumah University of Science and Technology, Kumasi, Ghana
Full list of author information is available at the end of the article

defence in eliminating pathogens and tumour cells is the IFN system. The type I IFNs for example in addition to their antiviral properties have been employed in the treatment of certain cancers such as Hairy cell Leukemia, AIDS-related Kaposi's sarcoma and other malignancies [1]. It has been reported that treatment of cells with IFN leads to the activation of the tumour suppressor gene p53 which plays a central role in the apoptosis of some tumour cells [1]. Indeed, Aziz and co-workers showed in their study that IFN-α has a significant protective effects against hepatic fibrogenesis and carcinogenesis [2]. Therefore any substance being component of pathogen or chemical produced by micro-organisms which tend to inhibit or suppress the type I IFN will weaken the innate immune system and predispose individuals to infections and cancers.

AFB$_1$, a lethal mycotoxin produced by *Aspergillus flavus* and *Aspergillus parasiticus* is a potent hepatocarcinogen in humans [3, 4] and in view of that it has been classified as group 1 human carcinogen by the International Agency for Research on Cancer (IARC) [5]. AFB$_1$ contamination of diet coupled with subsequent prolonged heavy exposure is a major risk factor for the development of HCC. Food meant for human and animal consumption have been reported to contain high levels of aflatoxins in some West African countries such as Ghana, Togo, Nigeria and Benin [6–8] largely due to sub-optimal farming practices, high humidity and poor storage conditions. For example in Ghana 83.3% of weanimix, food prepared locally from maize and groundnut for children have been reported to have aflatoxin levels higher than the national acceptable levels of 15 ppb [9]. Cereal based foods are staple in Ghana in particular and sub-Saharan Africa in general, it means many more people are exposed to high levels of aflatoxins and thus increasing their risk of HCC.

The incidence of HCC in the West African sub region is high with an annual death rate of about 200,000 [10]. In fact West Africa is ranked second, aside Eastern Asia as region affected most with HCC [10]. In West Africa, the death rate of HCC is almost equal to its incidence with most HCC sufferers dying within weeks of their diagnosis indicating the aggressive and dangerous nature of HCC [10, 11]. In addition to AFB$_1$, other risk factors that contribute to HCC include chronic HBV/HCV infection and heavy alcohol consumption. Information available indicates that the risk of HCC developing is amplified through the synergistic effects of aflatoxin ingestion and HBV infection. The risk of HCC in people with chronic HBV infection and also exposed to aflatoxin is up to 30 times greater than in individual exposed to either of the two factors only [12–14]. These two risk factors (aflatoxin and HBV) are common in underdeveloped countries of the world including Ghana [6, 15] suggesting that the risk of HCC is likely to be high in Ghana.

The role of AFB$_1$ in the pathogenesis of HCC, via mutation in the tumour suppressor gene p53 has been well established. However, information on how AFB$_1$ could deregulate other anti-cancer pathways such as the type I IFN signalling pathway as a way of causing HCC is very limited. This study was carried out to test the hypothesis that AFB$_1$ inhibits the type I IFN response pathway thus contributing to the pathogenesis of HCC. Results from this study could influence future therapeutic intervention for AFB$_1$-induced HCC and also broaden our knowledge of the role of AFB$_1$ in HCC immunobiology.

Methods
Reagents and chemicals
The AFB$_1$ used in the study was purchased from Sigma-Aldrich, USA (cat no A6636) and dissolved in dimethyl sulfoxide (DMSO) to a stock concentration of 3200 µM. The AFB$_1$ stock solution was divided into aliquots, wrapped in aluminium foil and stored frozen at −20 °C until used. The AFB$_1$ stock solution was diluted to the desired concentration in normal growth medium when necessary. The foetal bovine serum (FBS) was purchased from Sigma-Aldrich, USA. Dulbecco's Modified Eagles Medium (DMEM) (high glucose, L-glutamine, sodium pyruvate and 25 mM HEPES) was purchased from Science Cell. Minimum essential medium (MEM) non-essential amino acids was purchased from Sigma Aldrich, USA while penicillin-streptomycin was purchased from Gibco by Invitrogen, UK. Lipofectamine 2000 was purchased from Gibco by Life Technologies, UK (cat no 11668-019). The human recombinant interferon-alpha 2 (rIFN-α2) was purchased from PBL interferon source (cat no 11115-1). The stock solution of the human recombinant interferon-alpha 2 was diluted to working concentration using phosphate buffered saline containing 0.1% bovine serum albumen as a diluent. The STAT1 (cat no PA5-34504) and GAPDH (cat no QE 212271) primary antibodies were purchased from Thermo Scientific, USA. The secondary antibody conjugated to horse-radish peroxidase (cat no 31430) was purchased from Thermo Scientific, USA.

Cell culture
The cells used in this study were kindly donated by Professor David J. Blackbourn of the University of Surrey, UK. The cell lines used were human hepatoma cell line HepG2 (ECACC 85011430) and mouse fibroblast cell line L929 (NCTC) (ECACC 85103115). The HepG2 and the L929 cells were grown in DMEM high glucose containing L-glutamine, sodium pyruvate and HEPES supplemented with 10% v/v heat inactivated FBS, 1% v/v MEM non-essential amino acids, 100 IU/ml of penicillin and 100 µg/ml of streptomycin. The cultures were maintained at 37 °C in 5% carbon dioxide (CO_2) under humidified condition.

Cytotoxicity assay
HepG2 cells were grown to about 60% confluence and then treated with increasing concentrations of AFB$_1$ (0–3200 µM). Twenty four hours later, the AFB$_1$ containing medium was removed and fresh medium without AFB$_1$ was added. The cytotoxic effects was evaluated by an MTS based assay using Cell Titre 96 AQueous One Solution reagent (Promega, USA, cat no G358C) following the manufacturer's instruction.

Transient transfections and luciferase assays in HepG2 cells

Dual luciferase assays were performed according to our previous study [16]. Briefly, the cells were grown in duplicate wells of the 96-well plate until they reached about 80% confluence. The plasmids used in this study were kind gifts from Professor David J. Blackbourn (University of Surrey, UK). The DNA, pISRE-luc used in the study was extracted from *E.coli* strain HD5α using EndoFree Maxi Prep Kit (Qiagen, USA) following the manufacturer's instruction. The pISRE-luc expresses the firefly luciferase protein while pRLSV40 plasmid expresses the *Renilla* luciferase. The *Renilla* was included as internal control to which the pISRE-luc activity was normalized. A transfection mixture was prepared by diluting the plasmids DNA (pISRE-luc 500 ng: pRLSV40 1 ng) in serum and antibiotic free media and incubated at room temperature for 5 min. In addition, the Lipofectamine 2000 was also diluted in serum and antibiotic free media. After 5 min of incubation, the diluted DNA and Lipofectamine 2000 were mixed and incubated at room temperature for 20 min and then added to the designated wells and incubated at 37 °C in 5% CO_2 under humidified condition for 24 h.

For the experiment that involved the determination of the minimum concentration of rIFN-α that would induce the maximum activity of IFN-α-inducible pISRE-luc activity, the transfected cells were stimulated with increasing concentrations of rIFN-α (100–400 IU/ml). Twenty four hours later, luciferase assays were performed using the dual luciferase reporter assay system (Promega, USA, cat no E1960) following the manufacturer's protocol. After preparing the cell lysates, 20 μl of the aliquot was employed for luminescence measurement using Berthold Orion luminometer (Berthold Detection Systems, Germany).

For the experiment that involved the determination of the effects of AFB_1 on the type 1 IFN signalling pathway, the transfected cells were stimulated with rIFN-α (400 IU/ml) and simultaneously treated with increasing concentrations of AFB_1 (0.8–32 μM). Twenty four hours later, dual luciferase reporter gene assay was performed as described above.

Reverse transcriptase-quantitative polymerase chain reaction (RT-qPCR)

The cultured HepG2 cells were treated with AFB_1 and simultaneously stimulated with the rIFN-α for 24 h as described above. Total RNA was then extracted using Gene JET RNA purification kit (Thermo Scientific, Germany) following the instructions of the manufacturer. The quantity and the purity of the total RNA was verified by spectroscopy (Nano Drop 1000, Thermo Scientific). The purity was later confirmed by 1% agarose gel electrophoresis using ethidium bromide as stain.

Prior to the cDNA synthesis, any traces of genomic DNA present in the total RNA was removed by treating the total RNAs with double stranded (ds) DNase (Thermo Scientific, Germany) at 37 °C for 2 min followed by maintenance of the mixture on ice. The total RNAs were converted to cDNA using Moloney Murine Leukemia virus (M-Mul V) reverse transcriptase, oligo (dT) and random hexamer primers in a final reaction volume of 20 μl. The mixture was first incubated for 10 min at room temperature followed by further 15 min of incubation at 50 °C. The entire cDNA synthesis reaction was stopped by heating the mixture at 85 °C for 5 min. The cDNA was stored frozen at –80 °C until used in the qPCR.

JAK1, STAT1 and OAS3 target genes were amplified using the Maxima Probe/Rox qPCR master mix (Thermo Scientific, Germany). The primers and probes used were designed and synthesized by Biomers, Germany (Table 1).

The primers and probes of the target genes and the endogenous control (GAPDH) were labelled with different fluorescent reporter dyes at the 5′ end and quencher dyes at the 3′ end and this allowed the target genes to be amplified in the same tube in a duplex qPCR reaction.

After optimizing the primer and probe PCR conditions, a duplex qPCR was performed in a 25 μl reaction volume that contained 0.3 μM forward and reverse primers of the target genes, 0.2 μM of the target probes, 0.1 μM forward and reverse primers of the *GAPDH*, 0.2 μM of the *GAPDH* probe and 2.5 μl of 1:10 dilution

Table 1 Sequences of probes and primers

Name of gene	Sequence of primers and probes	Fluorophores
JAK1	Probe: 5′AGCAGTCAGTGTGGCG TCATTCTCC-3′ Forward primer 5′- CAATTGGCAT GGAACCAACGAC-3′ Reverse primer 5′-CAAATCATACT GTCCCTGAGCAAAC-3′	5′ FAM- 3′ BHQ-1
STAT1	Probe: 5′-CGCTCTGCTGTCTCCGC TTCCACTCC-3′ Forward primer: 5′GTTGCTGAATGT CACTGAACTTACC-3′ Reverse primer: 5′- AGCTGATCCAA GCAAGCATTGG-3′	5′ FAM- 3′ BHQ-1
OAS3	Probe 5′- AGCCTGGTGCCTGCCTTC AATGTCC-3′ Forward primer: 5′-TCCGCCTGACA TCCGTAGATC-3′ Reverse primer: 5′-TCCTCCGCAGCT CTGTGAAG-3′	5′ FAM- 3′ BHQ-1
GAPDH	Probe: 5′- CCGTTGACTCCGACCTTC ACCTTCC-3′ Forward primer: 5′- AGCCACATCGCT CAGACACC-3′ Reverse primer: 5′- TGACCAGGCGCC CAATACG-3′	5′HEX- 3′TAMRA

of the cDNA samples. The qPCR cycling conditions were as follows: 95 °C for 10 min for the first cycle (initial denaturation), 95 °C for 15 s for 40 cycles (denaturation) and 60 °C for 60 s for 40 cycles (annealing/extension). The qPCR reaction products were analyzed using Bio-Rad CFX 96 manager software (Bio-Rad, USA). The relative quantification of the target genes was calculated using the comparative CT method. The relative quantities of *JAK1*, *STAT1* and *OAS3* after normalization to the endogenous control (*GAPDH*) was given by $2^{-\Delta\Delta CT}$ as previously described [17].

Western blotting

To examine the effects of AFB_1 on the protein accumulation of STAT1, the cultured HepG2 cells were treated with AFB_1 and simultaneously stimulated with the rIFN-α for 24 h as described above. The cells were later harvested and lysed to extract total proteins using cold Radioimmunoprecipitation assay (RIPA) buffer (Thermo Scientific, Germany) containing freshly added protease and phosphatase inhibitor cocktails and ethylenediaminetetraacetic acid (EDTA) (Thermo Scientific, Germany) following a standard protocol. Aliquots of the protein samples were mixed with 2X sample buffer containing 2-beta mercaptoethanol and the mixture was heated for 5 min at 95 °C to denature the proteins. The proteins were separated by 10% sodium dodecyl sulfate polyacrylamide gel electrophoresis (SDS-PAGE) and then blotted onto 0.45 μM pore size polyvinylidene difluoride (PVDF) membranes (Bio-Rad Laboratories). The PVDF membranes were blocked in 5% non-fat dried milk in 1X Tris buffered saline with Tween-20 (TBST) before being incubated separately with STAT1 and GAPDH primary antibodies. Primary antibodies were used at the following dilutions: STAT1 (1:1000 dilution) and GAPDH (1:2500 dilution). The membranes were then incubated with the primary antibodies at 4 °C overnight. The secondary antibodies conjugated to horseradish peroxidase (Thermo Scientific, USA) were used at a dilution of 1:5000. The membranes were probed with the secondary antibody at room temperature with gentle shaking for 1 h after which bands were visualized by performing enhanced chemiluminescence using Pierce enhanced chemiluminescence (ECL) western blotting substrate (Thermo Scientific, USA). The images were captured with C-DIGIT blot scanner (Li-COR Bioscience, USA) and analyzed using image J software.

Results
Cytotoxic effects of AFB₁ and IFN concentration course
The AFB_1 is an extremely toxic compound which could not have been used directly on the cells. Therefore, the concentration of AFB_1 that was not toxic to the HepG2 cells was determined using MTS based assay as

described above. As shown in Fig. 1a, AFB_1 killed the HepG2 cells in a dose-dependent fashion after exposure to concentrations up to 3200 μM for 24 h followed by maintenance of cells in AFB_1 free media for 24, 48 and 72 h. The experiment established up to 10 μM of AFB_1 was not toxic to the cells and was therefore used in subsequent experiments. Next the concentration of rIFN-α required to induce maximal activity of the type I IFN response pathway was determined. It was observed that the pISRE-luc activity (a measure of the type I interferon activity) increased with increasing concentration of rIFN-α and peaked at concentrations of 200-400 IU/ml (Fig. 1b).

AFB₁ suppresses IFN-α induced ISRE signalling
To measure the effect of AFB_1 on the anti-cancer activity of the type I IFN response pathway, a luciferase reporter gene expressing pISRE-luc was employed. The pathway activation was induced with rIFN-α (400 IU/ml) through the transactivation of interferon stimulated response elements (ISRE). It is already established that the pathway is activated following the binding of IFN-α to the IFN-α receptors R1 and R2 on cells to trigger cascades of events leading to the transactivation of the ISRE as reviewed in Randall and Goodbourn [18].

The cultured HepG2 cells were stimulated with rIFN-α and simultaneously treated with AFB_1 as described above. As shown in Fig. 2, the activated pathway peaked at about five-fold above background or basal levels (see fourth bar; Fig. 2). It was noted that AFB_1 did not influence the pathway activity in anyway because cells treated with AFB_1 alone showed same background level of pathway activity as those cells in which the pathway was not activated; the so called 'none treated cells' (see first bar; Fig. 2).

The addition of AFB_1 to the cells in which the type I IFN response pathway was activated saw AFB_1 dose dependent inhibition of the pathway activity up to 54.8% in cells treated with 10 μM of AFB_1 and 68.2% in cells treated with 32 μM respectively (Fig. 2). The pathway activity was measured by the firefly luciferase pISRE-luc activities (Fig. 2).

The concentration of AFB_1 and rIFN-α used in the experiment were chosen based on the following: (i) at 10 μM of $AFB_1 \geq 90\%$ of the cells survived (Fig. 1a), (ii) between 200 and 400 IU/ml of rIFN-α induced the maximum activity of IFN-α inducible ISRE promoter i.e. a measure of the type I IFN response pathway (Fig. 1b). In the subsequent experiments, 10 μM of AFB_1 was used and that concentration was selected based on the fact it had the capacity to significantly inhibit the type I IFN induced signalling in HepG2 cells as measured by the firefly luciferase pISRE-luc activities (p-value ≤ 0.047) (Fig. 2).

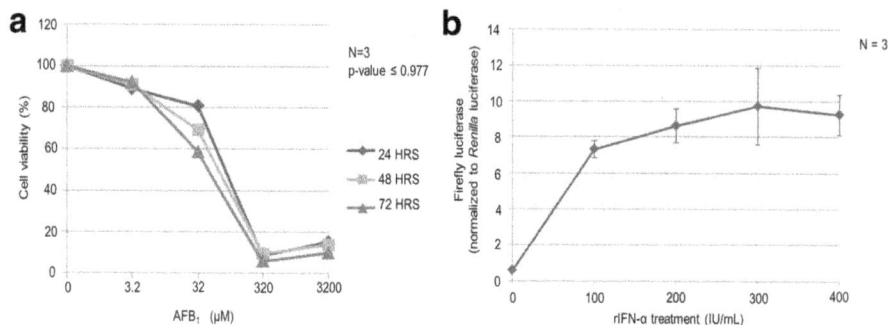

Fig. 1 Establishing the maximum non-toxic concentration of AFB_1 and maximum inducible concentration of rIFN-α (**a**) HepG2 cells were cultured at density of 5×10^4 cells per well of the 96-well plate until they reached 60% confluence. The cells were then treated with or without increasing amount of AFB_1 (0–3200 μM) for 24 h after which the AFB_1 containing media were replaced with fresh media. Cytotoxicity was evaluated by MTS-based assay at 24, 48 and 72 h. The viability of cells was calculated as ratio between AFB_1 treated cells and non-treated cells. Data are presented as mean and standard deviation of three independent experiments each performed in duplicate wells, p-value ≤ 0.977 as determined by one-way ANOVA. **b** Establishing the maximal IFN-α induction of ISRE driven luciferase reporter gene activity. HepG2 cells were cultured at density of 5×10^4 cells per well of the 96-well plate until they reached 80% confluence. The cells were transiently co-transfected with pISRE-luc (500 ng) and pRLSV40 (1 ng). At 24 h post-transfection, the cells were treated with increasing concentration of rIFN-α. Luciferase activity was measured 24 h later. The data are presented as mean and the standard deviation of three independent experiments each conducted in duplicate wells. There was no significant difference in pISRE-luc activity of cells treated with 300 and 400 IU/ml of rIFN-α (p-value ≤ 0.7527)

AFB$_1$ inhibits transcripts expression of JAK1, STAT1 and OAS3 genes

Having demonstrated at the luciferase reporter gene assay level that AFB_1 inhibits the type I IFN response signalling pathway, the next task was to test our hypothesis that AFB_1 would inhibit the transcripts of key signalling elements of the pathway. The JAK-STAT-ISRE arm of the type I IFN response pathway was chosen for the study because when activated it leads to the activation of interferon responsive genes such as OAS3 whose inhibition by AFB_1 was hypothesized in the current study.

RT-qPCR analysis of the transcripts levels of JAK1, STAT1 and OAS3 genes in the cultured HepG2 cells stimulated with or without rIFN-α (400 IU/ml) and simultaneously treated with or without AFB_1 (10 μM) was performed.

The cells in which the pathway was activated showed about 3-fold increase in the transcripts levels of JAK1 compared to background or basal levels. However, when AFB_1 was added to the cells in which the pathway was activated the transcripts levels of JAK1 reduced to almost half (49.1%, p-value ≤ 0.0001).

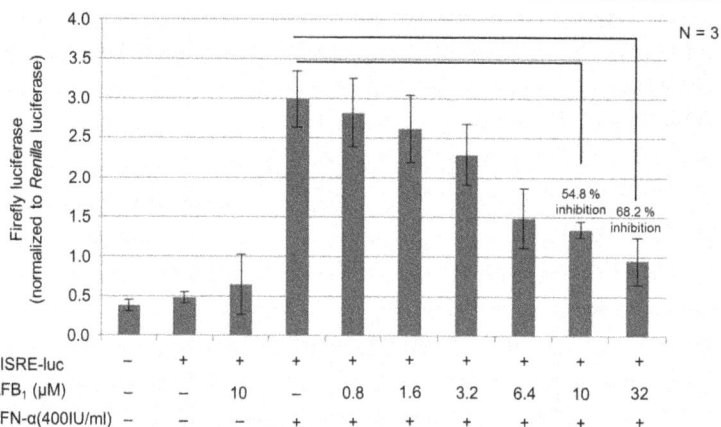

Fig. 2 AFB_1 inhibits IFN-α induced ISRE signalling in a dose dependent fashion. HepG2 cells were cultured at density of 5×10^4 cells per well of the 96-well plate until they reached 80% confluence. The cells were transiently co-transfected with pISRE-luc (500 ng) and pRLSV40 (1 ng). The pRL40-luc which constitutively expresses the *Renilla* luciferase was included as internal control to which pISRE-luc activity was normalized. At 24 h post-transfection, the cells were stimulated with or without rIFN-α and simultaneously treated with or without AFB_1. Transfected cells which were stimulated with rIFN-α but not treated with AFB_1 were calculated to have 100% pISRE-luc activity. The data are presented as mean normalized pISRE-luc activity and the standard deviation of three independent experiments each conducted in duplicate wells. There was a significant difference in pISRE-luc activity of cells stimulated with rIFN-α alone compared to cells stimulated with rIFN-α and simultaneously treated with 10 μM of AFB_1 (p-value ≤ 0.047)

Although the pathway activities in those experiments to assess the effect of *STAT1* and *OAS3* transcripts levels showed over 10-fold above background levels, similar pattern of results were seen for *STAT1* and *OAS3* because the transcripts levels were reduced by AFB$_1$ to 47% (*p*-value ≤ 0.03) and 39% (*p*-value ≤ 0.05) respectively (Fig. 3b & c).

Taken together, it was observed that AFB$_1$ significantly inhibited the mRNA expression levels of JAK1, STAT1 and OAS3 genes (Fig. 3). To be sure that HepG2 cells were responding to rIFN-α treatment and that the ISRE was functioning, a parallel experiment in which HepG2 cells were transiently transfected with pISRE-luc and pRLSV40-luc as described in Fig. 2 was conducted. At the time of harvest of the cells for RT-qPCR, aliquots of cell lysates from the parallel experiments were assayed for dual luciferase activity and the inhibition of ISRE activity was confirmed as described in Fig. 2 (data not shown).

AFB$_1$ inhibits STAT1 protein synthesis

Different post-transcriptional events could be involved in translating mRNAs into proteins [19] suggesting that lower mRNA levels might not necessarily corresponds to lower protein expression and vice versa. Therefore, western blot assay was employed to ascertain whether the inhibition of the mRNA expression level of STAT1 by AFB$_1$ would ultimately affect its translation into proteins as well (see Fig. 3).

Again the cultured HepG2 cells were stimulated and treated as described in Fig. 3. Protein extracts of HepG2 cells stimulated with or without rIFN-α and treated with AFB$_1$ (10 μM) were analysed by western blotting for

STAT1 using Glyceraldehyde 3-phosphate dehydrogenase (GAPDH) as a loading control. Briefly, cell lysates were prepared and thereafter, protein samples were separated on SDS-PAGE and immunoblotted with anti STAT1 and anti-GAPDH antibodies respectively. In order to ensure that the cells were functionally responding to stimulation and treatment at the time when the lysates were prepared, a parallel experiment in which the cells were transiently transfected with pISRE-luc and pRLSV40 as described in Fig. 3 were assayed for dual luciferase activity and the inhibition of the type I IFN response pathway activity by AFB$_1$ was confirmed (data not shown).

Consistent with the results shown in Fig. 3, STAT1 accumulation peaked in cells in which the type I IFN pathway was activated in the absence of AFB$_1$ (see Fig. 4; band 2 from right). However, on the contrary the STAT1 accumulation was substantially reduced in cells in which the pathway was activated in the presence of AFB$_1$ (see Fig. 4; band 1 from right). Again, cells in which the type I IFN pathway was not activated showed low background levels of STAT1 presence (see Fig. 4; bands 1 and 2 from left). Also consistent with Fig. 3 the protein levels of GAPDH were not affected by AFB$_1$ as their levels were shown to be equal in all cells regardless of the AFB$_1$ treatment or stimulation with rIFN-α.

Discussion

AFB$_1$ is a potent hepatocarcinogen [3, 4] which when ingested is metabolized by CYP450 class of enzymes in the liver to AFB$_1$, 8-9 exo epoxide [3, 4]. The AFB$_1$ 8-9 exo epoxide binds DNA and induces AGG to AGT transversion mutation at codon 249 in the tumour

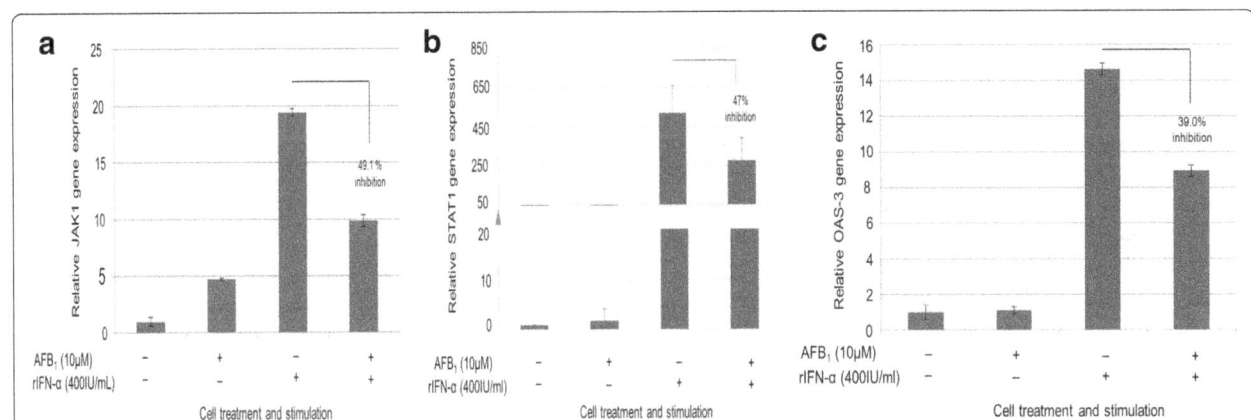

Fig. 3 AFB$_1$ inhibits the mRNA expression levels of the JAK1 (**a**), STAT1 (**b**) and OAS3. **c.** HepG2 cells were cultured at density of 5×10^4 cells per well of the 6-well plate until they reached 80% confluence. The cells were stimulated with or without rIFN-α (400 IU/ml) and simultaneously treated with or without AFB$_1$ (10 μM) for 24 h. Total RNA was extracted and reverse transcribed to cDNA using random primers. Quantitative PCR was performed with gene specific primers and probes for *JAK1, STAT1 and OAS3* respectively. The relative levels of *JAK1, STAT1 and OAS3* after normalization to GAPDH (endogenous control) was plotted. The relative levels of *JAK1, STAT1 and OAS3* were calculated using the $2^{-\Delta\Delta Ct}$ (Livak) method. These results are presented as mean and standard deviations of three independent experiments each performed in triplicate wells; *JAK1* (*p*-value ≤ 0.0001), *STAT1* (*p*-value ≤ 0.03) and *OAS3* (*p*-value ≤ 0.05)

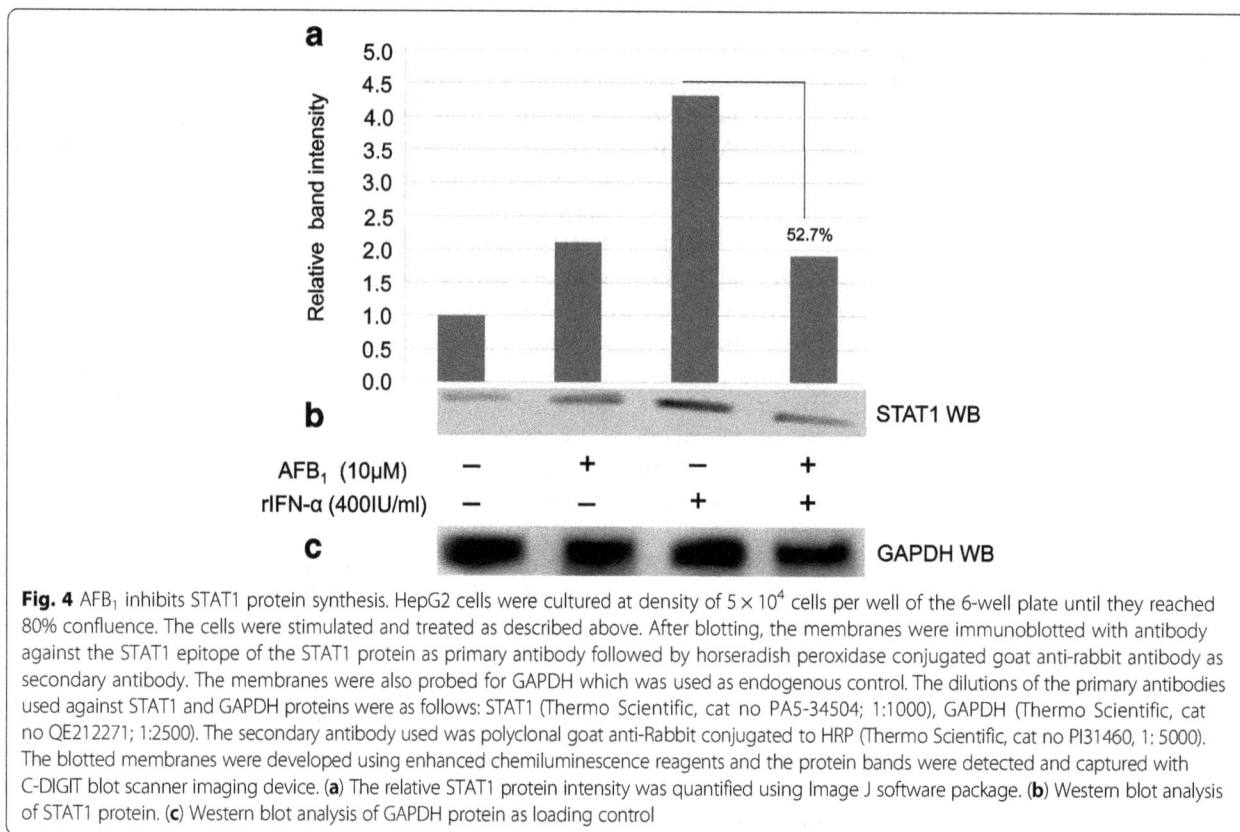

Fig. 4 AFB$_1$ inhibits STAT1 protein synthesis. HepG2 cells were cultured at density of 5×10^4 cells per well of the 6-well plate until they reached 80% confluence. The cells were stimulated and treated as described above. After blotting, the membranes were immunoblotted with antibody against the STAT1 epitope of the STAT1 protein as primary antibody followed by horseradish peroxidase conjugated goat anti-rabbit antibody as secondary antibody. The membranes were also probed for GAPDH which was used as endogenous control. The dilutions of the primary antibodies used against STAT1 and GAPDH proteins were as follows: STAT1 (Thermo Scientific, cat no PA5-34504; 1:1000), GAPDH (Thermo Scientific, cat no QE212271; 1:2500). The secondary antibody used was polyclonal goat anti-Rabbit conjugated to HRP (Thermo Scientific, cat no PI31460, 1: 5000). The blotted membranes were developed using enhanced chemiluminescence reagents and the protein bands were detected and captured with C-DIGIT blot scanner imaging device. (**a**) The relative STAT1 protein intensity was quantified using Image J software package. (**b**) Western blot analysis of STAT1 protein. (**c**) Western blot analysis of GAPDH protein as loading control

suppressor gene p53 [20, 21]. This mutation leads to the inhibition of the p53 mediated transcription and underlines the mechanism by which AFB$_1$ causes HCC [22]. It must be stated however that, the mechanism by which AFB$_1$ causes HCC may not be limited to p53 mutation alone and that AFB$_1$ may also induce cancers by deregulating other anticancer signalling pathways. For example Ubagai et al. [23] demonstrated that AFB$_1$ may also induce tumourigenesis by deregulating the insulin-like growth factor 1 receptor (IGF-IR) signalling pathway suggesting that AFB$_1$ may also induce tumourigenesis by deregulating other anticancer pathways such as the type I IFN signalling pathway. In this study we tested the hypothesis that AFB$_1$ would suppress/inhibit the type I IFN signalling pathway and thus provide another mechanism by which AFB$_1$ may cause cancer. Findings from the current study in which AFB$_1$ was shown to inhibit the type 1 IFN response pathway by targeting the key signalling elements are consistent with that of Jiang et al. [24] who reported that AFB$_1$ inhibited the mRNA expression levels of IL-2, IL-4, IL-6, IL-10, IL-17, IFN-γ and TNF-α in the small intestines of broilers treated with AFB$_1$. Moreover, AFB$_1$ has also been reported to inhibit mRNA and protein expression levels of IL-4, IL-6, IL-10 in the peritoneal macrophages and splenic lymphocyte cell lines [25, 26] and STAT5A gene mRNA expression levels in bovine mammary epithelial cells

[27]. One way by which the type I IFN signalling response exerts its anti-cancer and antiviral response is through the activation of the JAK-STAT-ISRE arm of the pathway. One component of the JAK-STAT-ISRE signalling pathway considered to have tumour suppressor function is STAT1 [28]. When activated, STAT1 suppresses tumour development by inducing apoptosis [29] and also inhibit tumour angiogenesis [30]. Therefore the suppression of STAT1 by AFB$_1$ at the both transcription and translational levels as demonstrated in the current study will impair the ability of STAT1 in orchestrating the expression of myriad of genes which are required to promote apoptosis, inhibit cell proliferation and angiogenesis in response to AFB$_1$.

The activation of the JAK-STAT-ISRE arm of the type I IFN signalling pathway results in the activation of the so called interferon responsive elements including the OAS3, PKR, Mx etc as reviewed in Randall and Goodbourn [18]. The OAS3 pathway when activated leads to the establishment of antiviral state by inhibiting protein synthesis which culminates in the destruction of both viruses and infected cells [31, 32]. The OAS3 has also been reported to play a role in inhibiting tumour development by inducing apoptosis and anti-proliferative responses [33, 34]. The activation of the JAK-STAT-ISRE signalling pathway starts upon the phosphorylation and activation of JAK1 and TYK2 when the correct ligands

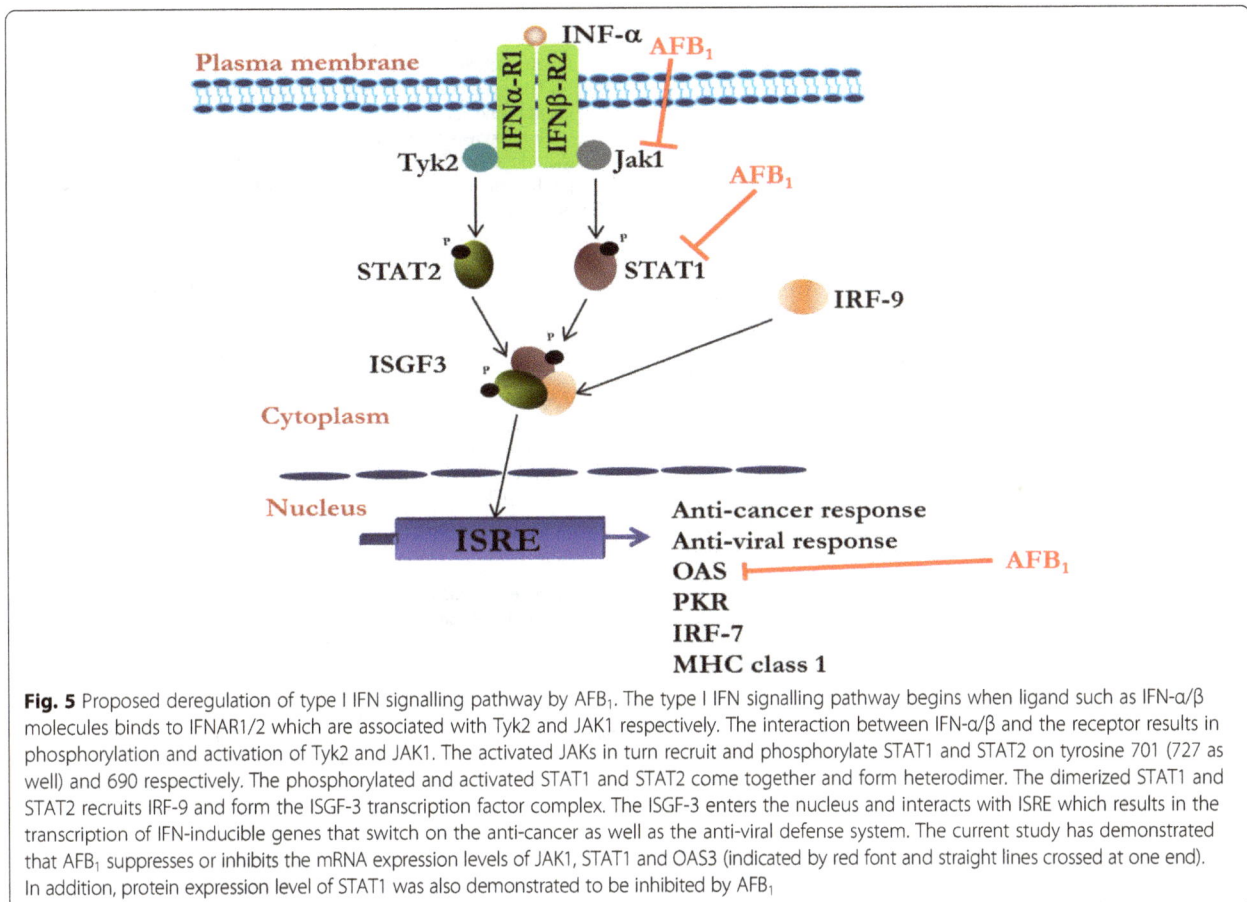

Fig. 5 Proposed deregulation of type I IFN signalling pathway by AFB_1. The type I IFN signalling pathway begins when ligand such as IFN-α/β molecules binds to IFNAR1/2 which are associated with Tyk2 and JAK1 respectively. The interaction between IFN-α/β and the receptor results in phosphorylation and activation of Tyk2 and JAK1. The activated JAKs in turn recruit and phosphorylate STAT1 and STAT2 on tyrosine 701 (727 as well) and 690 respectively. The phosphorylated and activated STAT1 and STAT2 come together and form heterodimer. The dimerized STAT1 and STAT2 recruits IRF-9 and form the ISGF-3 transcription factor complex. The ISGF-3 enters the nucleus and interacts with ISRE which results in the transcription of IFN-inducible genes that switch on the anti-cancer as well as the anti-viral defense system. The current study has demonstrated that AFB_1 suppresses or inhibits the mRNA expression levels of JAK1, STAT1 and OAS3 (indicated by red font and straight lines crossed at one end). In addition, protein expression level of STAT1 was also demonstrated to be inhibited by AFB_1

bind to the IFNAR (Fig. 5). The activated JAK1 and TYK2 in turn phosphorylate STAT1 and STAT2 setting in motion a cascade of events which finally initiates the transcription of IFN-inducible genes switching on the anti-cancer and anti-viral effects as reviewed in Randall and Goodbourn [18]. Therefore, any stimulus which deregulates the expression of either JAK1 or TYK2 could potentially deregulate the entire type I IFN response signalling pathway and thereby weaken the immune system and thus predispose individuals to infections and or cancer.

Taken together, the current study has revealed for the first time the inhibition of the type I IFN response pathway by AFB_1 via the inhibition of the transcripts of *JAK1, STAT1* and *OAS3* and also inhibit the protein accumulation of STAT1. The findings of the current study could be another mechanism by which AFB_1 may cause HCC (Fig. 5).

Conclusions

In conclusion the current study has shown that AFB_1 down-regulated the type I IFN response pathway by significantly inhibiting the key signalling elements such as *JAK1, STAT1 and OAS3* and also the STAT1

protein. Findings from this study reveals the negative effects of AFB_1 on the health of people who consume AFB_1 contaminated food as evidenced by its ability to inhibit and or deregulate the innate immune response. In view of this it is recommended that public education is intensified in Ghana and other developing nations of the world where AFB_1 contaminated food form a greater portion of the diets so as to reduce HCC and its associated deaths.

Abbreviations

AFB_1: Aflatoxin B_1; AIDS: Acquired immunodeficiency syndrome; CYP450: Cytochrome p450; DMEM: Dulbecco's modified eagles' medium; EDTA: Ethylenediaminetetraacetic acid; FBS: Foetal bovine serum; GAPDH: Glyceraldehyde 3-phosphate dehydrogenase; HBV: Hepatitis B virus; HCC: Hepatocellular carcinoma; HCV: Hepatitis C virus; HEPES: (4-(2-hydroxyethyl)-1-piperazineethanesulfonic acid; IARC: International agency for research on cancer; IFN: Interferon; IFN-α: Interferon-alpha; IFN-β: Interferon beta; IGF-IR: Insulin-like growth factor 1 receptor; IL: Interleukin; IRF-9: Interferon regulatory factor 9; ISGF-3: Interferon stimulated gene factor 3; JAK1: Janus activated kinase 1; MEM: Minimum essential medium; OAS3: Oligo adenylate synthetase 3; PBL: Peska Biomedical Laboratories; ppb: Part per billion; PVDF: Polyvinylidene difluoride; SDS-PAGE: Sodium dodecyl sulfate polyacrylamide gel electrophoresis; STAT1: Signal transducer and activator of transcription 1; TNF-α: Tumour necrosis factor-alpha

Acknowledgments

The authors sincerely thank the Leverhulme-Royal Society Africa Award II Scheme for making funds available for this work. The authors also thank

Professor Ellis Owusu-Dabo, Dr. Augustina Annan and the entire staff at the Kumasi Centre for Collaborative Research (KCCR) for their technical support during the RT-qPCR work. The authors also thank everyone who contributed to this work in one way or the other.

Funding

This work was supported with funds from the Leverhulme-Royal Society Africa Award II grant won by both Professor David Blackbourn and Dr. Mohamed Mutocheluh.

Authors' contributions

MM and DJB conceived the idea and designed the experiments. DJB provided the cell lines, and the plasmids used in the study. PWN and MM performed the experiments, analyzed the data and wrote the manuscript. All authors read and approved the final manuscript.

Competing interest

The authors declare that they have no competing interests.

Author details

[1]Department of Clinical Microbiology, School of Medical Sciences, Kwame Nkrumah University of Science and Technology, Kumasi, Ghana. [2]Department of Microbial and Cellular Sciences, School of Biosciences and Medicine, University of Surrey, Surrey GU2 7XH, UK.

References

1. Bekisz J, et al. Anti-proliferative properties of type I and type II Interferon. Pharmaceuticals. 2010;3:994–1015.
2. Aziz TA, Aziz MA, et al. Interferon-alpha gene therapy prevents aflatoxin and carbon tetrachloride promoted hepatic carcinogenesis in rats. Int J Mol Med. 2005;15(1):21–6.
3. Sudakin DL. Dietary aflatoxin exposure and chemoprevention of cancer: a clinical review. J Toxicol Clin Toxicol. 2003;41:195–204.
4. Wild CP, Gong YY. Mycotoxins and human disease: a largely ignored global health issue. Carcinogenesis. 2010;31:71–82.
5. IARC. In: Parkin DM, editor. Cancer Incidence in five continents. IARC scientific publications, vol. VIII (No. 155). Lyon: IARC Press; 2002.
6. Awuah RT, Kpodo KA. High incidence of Aspergillus flavus and aflatoxins in stored groundnut in Ghana and the use of a microbial assay to assess the inhibitory effects of plant extracts on aflatoxin synthesis. Mycopathologia. 1996;134(2):109–14.
7. Kpodo KA, Thrane U, Hald B. Fusaria and fumonisins in maize from Ghana and their co-occurence with aflatoxins. Int J Food Microbiol. 2000;61:147–57.
8. Oyelami OA, et al. Aflatoxins in the autopsy brain tissue of children in Nigeria. Mycopathologia. 1996;132:35–8.
9. Kumi J, et al. Aflatoxins and fumonisins contamination of home-made food (Weanimix) from cereal-legume blends for children. Ghana Med J. 2014; 48(3):121–6.
10. Ladep NG, et al. Problem of hepatocellular carcinoma in West Africa. World J Hepatol. 2014;6(11):783–92.
11. Jemal A, et al. Global cancer statistics. CA Cancer J Clin. 2011;61:69.
12. Groopman JD, Kensler TW, Wild CP. Protective interventions to prevent aflatoxin-induced carcinogenesis in developing countries. Annu Rev Public Health. 2008;29:187–203.
13. Liu Y, Wu F. Global burden of aflatoxin-induced hepatocellular carcinoma: a risk assessment. Environ Health Perspect. 2010;118:818–24.
14. Wu F, Khlangwiset P. Health economic impacts and cost-effectiveness of aflatoxin reduction strategies in Africa: case studies in biocontrol and postharvest interventions. Food Addit Contam Part A. 2010;27:496.
15. Allain JP, et al. The risk of hepatitis B virus infection by transfusion in Kumasi, Ghana. Blood. 2003;101(6):2419–25.
16. Mutocheluh M, et al. Kaposi's sarcoma-associated herpesvirus viral interferon regulatory factor-2 inhibits type 1 interferon signalling by targeting interferon-stimulated gene factor-3. J Gen Virol. 2011;92(Pt 10):2394–8.
17. Livak KJ, Schmittgen TD. Analysis of relative gene expression data using real-time quantitative PCR and the $2 - \Delta\Delta Ct$ method. Methods. 2001;25:402–8.
18. Randall RE, Goodbourn S. Interferons and viruses: an interplay between induction, signalling, antiviral responses and virus countermeasures. J Gen Virol. 2008;89(Pt 1):1–47.
19. Rasooly R, Hernlem B, Friedman M. Low levels of aflatoxin B1, ricin, and milk enhance recombinant protein production in mammalian cells. PLoS One. 2013;8(8):e71682.
20. Aguilar F, Hussain SP, Cerutti P. Aflatoxin B1 induces the transversion of $G \rightarrow T$ in codon 249 of the p53 tumor suppressor gene in human hepatocytes. Proc Natl Acad Sci U S A. 1993;90:8586–90.
21. Hsu IC, et al. Mutational hotspot in the p53 gene in human hepatocellular carcinomas. Nature. 1991;350:427–8.
22. Martin J, Dufour JF. Tumor suppressor and hepatocellular carcinoma. World J Gastroenterol. 2008;14:1720–33.
23. Ubagai T, et al. Aflatoxin B1 modulates the insulin-like growth factor-2 dependent signalling axis. Toxicol In Vitro. 2010;24:783–9.
24. Jiang M, et al. Effects of aflatoxin B1 on T-cell subsets and mRNA expression of cytokines in the intestine of broilers. Int J Mol Sci. 2015;16:6945–59.
25. Bruneau JC, et al. Aflatoxins B1, B2 and G1 modulate cytokine secretion and cell surface marker expression in J774A. 1 murine macrophages. Toxicol In Vitro. 2012;26:686–93.
26. Marin D, et al. Changes in performance, blood parameters, humoral and cellular immune responses in weanling piglets exposed to low doses of aflatoxin. J Anim Sci. 2002;80:1250–7.
27. Forouharmehr A, Harkinezhad T, Qasemi-Panahi B. Evaluation of STAT5A gene expression in aflatoxin B1 treated bovine mammary epithelial cells. Adv Pharm Bull. 2013;3(2):461–4.
28. Dunn GP, Koebel CM, Schreiber RD. Interferons, immunity and cancer immunoediting. Nat Rev Immunol. 2006;6:836–48.
29. Khodarev NN, Roizman B, Weichselbaum RR. Molecular pathways: interferon/stat1 pathway: role in the tumor resistance to genotoxic stress and aggressive growth. Clin Cancer Res. 2012;18(11):3015–21.
30. Pensa S, et al. STAT1 and STAT3 in tumorigenesis: two sides of the same coin. In: Stephanou A, editor. JAK-STAT pathway in disease. Austin: Landes Bioscience; 2008. p. 100–21.
31. Muller U, et al. Functional role of type I and type II interferons in antiviral defense. Science. 1994;264:1918–21.
32. Sen GC. Viruses and interferons. Annu Rev Microbiol. 2001;55:255–81.
33. Silverman RH, et al. Control of the ppp(a2'p)nA system in HeLa cells. Effects of interferon and virus infection. Eur J Biochem. 1982;124:131–8.
34. Stark GR, et al. How cells respond to interferons. Annu Rev Biochem. 1998;67:227–64.

15

Non-pulmonary cancer risk following tuberculosis

Ruta Everatt[1][*] [iD], Irena Kuzmickiene[1], Edita Davidaviciene[2] and Saulius Cicenas[3,4]

Abstract

Background: Lithuania remains one of the highest tuberculosis burden countries in Europe. Epidemiological studies have long pointed to infections as important factors of cancer aetiology, but the association between tuberculosis and the risk of non-pulmonary cancers has rarely been tested and results have been inconsistent. The aim of this population-based cohort study was to examine the risk of cancer among patients diagnosed with tuberculosis using data from Lithuanian Tuberculosis, Cancer and Resident's Registries.

Methods: The study cohort included 21,986 tuberculosis patients yielding 1583 cancers diagnosed during follow-up (1998–2012). Standardized incidence ratios (SIRs) and 95% confidence intervals (95% CIs) were calculated to compare the incidence of cancer among cohort participants with the general population for overall, non-pulmonary, site-specific cancers, as well as for subgroups of smoking-related, alcohol-related, hormone-related and haematological cancers.

Results: The SIRs of all cancers combined were 1.89, 95% CI: 1.79–2.00 in men and 1.34, 95% CI: 1.19–1.50 in women. Risk was increased 3-fold within the first year following diagnosis; it decreased during later years, although remained significantly elevated for ≥5 years. Elevated long-term increased risks persisted for non-pulmonary cancers overall, and for cancers of mouth and pharynx, oesophagus, stomach, larynx, cervix uteri and leukaemias. Tuberculosis was associated with a decreased risk of melanoma. Increased risks were observed for smoking-related cancers in men (SIR 1.95, 95% CI: 1.79–2.13) and women (SIR 1.46, 95% CI: 1.22–1.73), alcohol-related cancers in men (SIR 2.40; 95% CI: 2.14–2.68) and haematological cancers in men (SIR 1.73, 95% CI: 1.33–2.23). The risk of hormone-related cancers was 18% lower (SIR = 0.82, 95% CI: 0.66–0.997) among women, the inverse association was weaker among men (SIR = 0.95, 95% CI: 0.84–1.07).

Conclusions: The risk of total and several non-pulmonary cancers was elevated in a cohort of tuberculosis patients. The recommendation for the awareness of this association among physicians is warranted. Analysis suggests a reduction in risk of hormone-related cancers and melanoma.

Keywords: Non-pulmonary cancers, Risk factors, Tuberculosis, Infection, Retrospective cohort study, Lithuania

Background

The latest World Health Organization (WHO) global tuberculosis report shows 10.4 million new tuberculosis cases and 1.4 million deaths due to tuberculosis worldwide in 2015 [1]. With 1600 new cases (56 cases per 100,000 population) in 2015 Lithuania remains among the countries with the highest incidence of tuberculosis in Europe, although due to recent decrease in rates it is no longer in the WHO's list of high tuberculosis burden countries [1]. The incidence of cancer of several types in Lithuania is among the highest in the world [2].

In addition to smoking or environmental factors, a growing number of bacterial and parasitic infections have been associated with development of cancer [3]. Former analyses observed an increased risk of lung cancer in tuberculosis cohorts, although conclusions with regards to confounding effects of smoking were inconsistent [4–7]. Recently the association between

* Correspondence: ruta.everatt@nvi.lt
[1]Laboratory of Cancer Epidemiology, National Cancer Institute, Baublio g. 3B, LT-08406 Vilnius, Lithuania
Full list of author information is available at the end of the article

tuberculosis infection and certain non-pulmonary malignancies (multiple myeloma [8]; myeloid leukaemia [4], leukaemia [9], Non-Hodgkin lymphoma [4, 10, 11], Hodgkin lymphoma [11, 12], melanoma [13], as well as oesophageal [4, 9], kidney and bladder [8, 9], liver [4, 9] and other cancers [8, 9]) has been reported; however, the evidence remains inconclusive due to the low incidence of cancer following tuberculosis, small sample size or short follow-up. Previous studies led to the suggestion that inflammation caused by *Mycobacterium tuberculosis* infection, could induce genetic damage promoting carcinogenesis [14]. Prior tuberculosis might also indicate the immune deficiency and increased risk for cancer as a result. In addition, chronic immune stimulation and certain infectious diseases have been shown to have a protective effect against cancer, although studies have been inconsistent [11, 15, 16]. Detailed investigation of association between tuberculosis and cancer is important for elucidating the role of this chronic infection in occurrence of cancer as well as for developing an effective cancer prevention strategy.

In this analysis, we aimed to investigate association between tuberculosis infection and risk of overall and site-specific non-pulmonary cancer using a population-based national cohort data.

Methods

Study population

The study was performed using new cases of tuberculosis diagnosed from January 1, 1998 to December 31, 2012; they were identified at the Lithuanian Tuberculosis registry, which covers the entire population. For each individual, information on date of birth, sex, date of diagnosis, diagnosis codes according to ICD-10 (International Statistical Classification of Diseases, 10th Revision) was obtained. In all, 30,594 individuals were available for analysis. Since the occurrence of cancer is rare in the youngest age groups, and diagnoses of the disease are less reliable for those in old age [17] only individuals of 25 to 75 years old at tuberculosis diagnosis were included. More detailed information about the study has been published elsewhere [7]. We excluded records due to age (19.8%), cancer other than non-melanoma skin cancer before start of follow-up (4.8%), unknown vital status (3.1%), duplicates or insufficient data (0.4%), and not being a Lithuanian citizen (0.03%). The final number of participants, included in the current analysis, was 21,986. For patients with multiple cancers, each non-melanoma skin cancer diagnosis was considered as an individual event.

Case ascertainment

For each subject, date of entry into cohort was the date of diagnosis of tuberculosis, and date of exit was the date of diagnosis of cancer other than non-melanoma skin

cancer, death, emigration, or 31 December 2012, whichever occurred first. We identified cases of cancer from the Lithuanian Cancer Registry (LCR). The LCR has population-based information available since 1978; data since the year 1988 have been included in 'Cancer Incidence in Five Continents' [18]. Dates of death and emigration were ascertained by linkage to the Lithuanian Residents' Register Service. The linkages were performed using an individual personal identification number. For calculation of Standardized incidence ratios (SIRs), cancer incidence and population data were obtained from the LCR and Lithuanian Department of Statistics.

Data analysis

We calculated SIRs of total and site-specific non-pulmonary cancer in the tuberculosis cohort, based on person-days of 'follow-up'. Expected numbers were obtained by multiplying Lithuanian national cancer incidence rates according to sex-, age- (5-year groups) and calendar period (1998–2002, 2003–2007 and 2008–2012), by corresponding stratum-specific number of person-days of follow-up accrued in the cohort. Then these stratum-specific expected numbers were summed across all strata in the cohort to obtain the expected total number of people with lung cancer in the cohort. We calculated SIRs by dividing the observed number of events by that expected. We calculated 95% confidence intervals (95% CI) for the SIRs assuming a Poisson distribution. Stratified analysis was performed according to the years since tuberculosis diagnosis and sex. SIRs were computed for total, non-pulmonary, tobacco-related [19], alcohol-related [19], haematological, hormone-related [20, 21] and site-specific cancers.

Analyses were performed using SPSS 19. All tests were two-tailed, and P value below 0.05 was considered statistically significant.

Results

A total of 21,986 patients (70.3% male) with tuberculosis were enrolled in the study (Table 1). The mean age at tuberculosis diagnosis was 47.1 years. The percent of smokers was 63.8% among total population, 78.0% among men and 30.2% among women. Among patients with tuberculosis, 59.3% were unemployed and only 6.4% had high school education. We followed the cohort for a total of 136,816 person-years. During the follow-up we observed 1583 cancers. There were 62 persons having two cancers.

Total cancer SIR among tuberculosis patients, compared with the general population was 1.76, 95% CI: 1.67–1.85 (Table 2). When lung cancer was excluded, all-time SIR was 1.41, 95% CI: 1.33–1.50. Short-term and long-term risks of non-pulmonary cancer were

Table 1 Characteristics of cohort members

Factors	n (%)
Total	21,986 (100)
Sex	
Men	15,456 (70.3)
Women	6530 (29.7)
High school education	1401 (6.4)
Smokers	14,023 (63.8)
Heavy alcohol user	7679 (34.9)
Unemployed	13,038 (59.3)
Age at tuberculosis diagnosis, years, mean (SD)	47.1 (12.9)
Follow-up duration, years, mean (SD)	6.2 (4.4)
Total follow-up duration, person-years	136,816
Cancer cases	1583
Respiratory tuberculosis	20,302 (92.3)
Human immunodeficiency virus infection	77 (0.4)

significantly increased, SIR = 2.03, 95% CI: 1.75–2.34 within first 1 year after diagnosis, 1.38, 95% CI: 1.25–1.52 during 1–4 years and 1.29, 95% CI: 1.18–1.41 during ≥5 years of follow-up (Table 2).

Analysis by cancer type revealed high risks of mouth and pharynx, oesophagus, stomach, liver, pancreas, larynx and bladder cancer (Table 2). Tuberculosis was also positively associated with leukaemias, Hodgkin lymphoma, bone, mesothelial & soft tissue as well as "other" cancers. In addition, results revealed reduced risk of melanoma, SIR = 0.48, 95% CI: 0.19–0.96. Risk of most non-pulmonary cancers was significantly increased within the first year. Elevated long-term risks (≥5 years) persisted for cancers of the mouth and pharynx (SIR = 3.24, 95% CI: 2.36–4.33), oesophagus (SIR = 3.57, 95% CI: 2.33–5.23), stomach (SIR = 1.67, 95% CI: 1.22–2.23), larynx (SIR = 1.96, 95% CI: 1.14–3.14), cervix uteri (SIR = 2.73, 95% CI: 1.77–4.03), leukaemias (SIR = 1.90, 95% CI: 1.16–2.93) and for "other" cancers (SIR = 1.50, 95% CI: 1.04–2.10).

The SIRs of total and most site-specific cancers were higher in men than in women (Table 3). Among men with tuberculosis SIR's were substantially increased for mouth and pharynx, oesophagus, stomach, liver, larynx, bladder, bone, mesothelial and soft tissue cancer, Hodgkin lymphoma, leukaemias and "other" cancer. In contrast, there was reduced incidence of prostate cancer, SIR 0.88, 95% CI: 0.76–1.02. Women were at increased risk of cancer of mouth and pharynx, larynx and cervix uteri, and at reduced risk of cancer of colon, SIR 0.39, 95% CI: 0.13–0.92. High risks of tobacco-related cancers were observed among men (SIR = 1.95, 95% CI: 1.79–2.13) and women (SIR = 1.46, 95% CI: 1.22–1.73). Alcohol-related cancers showed an increased SIR of

2.40, 95% CI: 2.14–2.68 among men, whereas among women there was no increase in risk. An elevated SIR of haematological cancers was also seen for men (SIR = 1.73, 95% CI: 1.33–2.23), it showed a not statistically significant increase in women (SIR = 1.48, 95% CI: 0.93–2.24). The risk of hormone-related cancers was 18% lower (SIR = 0.82, 95% CI: 0.66–0.997) among women, the inverse association was weaker among men (SIR = 0.95, 95% CI: 0.84–1.07).

Discussion

This study, based on a large retrospective cohort, has found a higher than expected risk of cancers of most types in men and women with tuberculosis. Increased risks of tobacco-related cancers, alcohol-related cancers and haematological cancers were observed. The risk of hormone-related cancers and melanoma was lower. Risk remained increased for ≥5 years for most smoking- and alcohol-related cancers, cancer of cervix uteri and leukaemias.

Our data on the 1.8-fold increased risk of overall cancer and 1.4-fold increased risk of non-pulmonary cancer among tuberculosis patients are in line with results from previous studies and reviews [4, 9, 22, 23]. In a Danish nationwide cohort study, comparing cancer risk in tuberculosis patients and the general population, the SIR for all cancers was 1.52, 95% CI: 1.45–1.59, whereas for non-pulmonary cancer it was 1.29, 95% CI: 1.22–1.36 [4]. Tuberculosis infection was also associated with increased long-term risk of tobacco-related and haematological malignancies. The incidence of cancer was also increased in the Taiwan Latent Tuberculosis Infection Cohort [8] and in the Estonian population-based cohort where the standardized mortality ratio for all cancers was 2.85, 95% CI: 2.17–3.68 for men and 3.80, 95% CI: 2.22–6.09 for women [22]. Another population-based study in Taiwan found that after a tuberculosis diagnosis the risk was 2.1-fold for total cancer and 1.7-fold for non-pulmonary cancer [9].

Several studies have reported an increased risk of Hodgkin or non-Hodgkin lymphoma in individuals with a history of tuberculosis [9–12]. In addition, significantly elevated long-term risks for leukaemia were observed [4, 9]. Similarly, the elevated SIRs for Hodgkin lymphoma as well as leukaemia were found in our study. Tuberculosis was associated with markedly increased long-term risk of cervical cancer in our study. Our analysis also revealed reduced risk of melanoma among patients with tuberculosis, in contrast with Taiwanese study results, where melanoma risk among men was significantly increased, particularly during <1 year after tuberculosis diagnosis [9]. Our data are in agreement with case-control study performed by Kölmel KF et al. in six European countries

Table 2 Cancer incidence in patients with tuberculosis according to time since tuberculosis diagnosis

Type of cancer	ICD-O	Time since tuberculosis diagnosis											
		<1 year			1–4 years			≥5 years			Total		
		Exp	Obs	SIR (95% CI)	Exp	Obs	SIR (95% CI)	Exp	Obs	SIR (95% CI)	Exp	Obs	SIR (95% CI)
All but NMS	C00–96, excl. C44	107.7	347	3.22 (2.89–3.58)	377.0	625	1.74 (1.60–1.88)	450.5	611	1.36 (1.25–1.47)	935.2	1583	1.76 (1.67–1.85)
All but NMS & lung	C00–96, excl. C44, C33, C34	91.6	186	2.03 (1.75–2.34)	310.9	429	1.38 (1.25–1.52)	379.6	490	1.29 (1.18–1.41)	782.1	1105	1.41 (1.33–1.50)
Mouth, pharynx	C01–14	4.3	20	4.65 (2.84–7.18)	13.8	57	4.27 (3.24–5.54)	13.9	45	3.24 (2.36–4.33)	32.0	122	3.92 (3.25–4.68)
Oesophagus	C15	2.1	9	4.28 (1.96–8.13)	7.0	28	4.22 (2.80–6.10)	7.3	26	3.57 (2.33–5.23)	16.4	63	3.99 (3.07–5.11)
Stomach	C16	7.6	16	2.11 (1.21–3.44)	24.9	30	1.28 (0.86–1.83)	27.0	45	1.67 (1.22–2.23)	59.4	91	1.60 (1.29–1.96)
Colon	C18	4.9	2	0.41 (0.05–1.47)	17.4	20	1.21 (0.74–1.87)	22.3	18	0.81 (0.48–1.27)	44.7	40	0.93 (0.67–1.27)
Rectum	C19–21	4.8	6	1.25 (0.46–2.75)	16.7	14	0.89 (0.49–1.48)	20.2	23	1.14 (0.72–1.71)	41.7	43	1.08 (0.78–1.45)
Liver	C22	1.2	3	2.47 (0.51–7.25)	4.3	9	2.20 (1.01–4.19)	5.5	9	1.63 (0.74–3.09)	11.1	21	1.98 (1.23–3.03)
Pancreas	C25	3.3	10	3.00 (1.44–5.52)	11.3	16	1.50 (0.86–2.43)	13.2	16	1.21 (0.69–1.97)	27.8	42	1.57 (1.13–2.12)
Larynx	C32	2.7	14	5.17 (2.82–8.67)	8.7	22	2.67 (1.67–4.04)	8.7	17	1.96 (1.14–3.14)	20.0	53	2.74 (2.05–3.59)
Bone, mesothelial & soft tissue	C40–41, C45, C47, C49	0.9	4	4.43 (1.21–11.40)	2.9	4	1.44 (0.39–3.68)	3.1	6	1.97 (0.72–4.28)	6.8	14	2.11 (1.15–3.54)
Melanoma	C43	1.7	1	0.58 (0.02–3.22)	6.0	3	0.51 (0.11–1.50)	7.3	3	0.41 (0.08–1.20)	15.0	7	0.48 (0.19–0.96)
Breast[a]	C50	5.7	3	0.53 (0.11–1.55)	20.3	15	0.74 (0.41–1.22)	25.9	32	1.21 (0.83–1.70)	51.9	50	0.96 (0.72–1.27)
Cervix uteri	C53	2.4	6	2.51 (0.92–5.44)	8.2	20	2.43 (1.48–3.75)	9.2	25	2.73 (1.77–4.03)	19.7	51	2.60 (1.93–3.42)
Corpus uteri	C54, C55	2.1	5	2.36 (0.77–5.50)	7.5	2	0.26 (0.03–0.95)	10.3	6	0.58 (0.21–1.27)	19.9	13	0.66 (0.35–1.13)
Ovary	C56	1.7	5	2.95 (0.96–6.86)	5.8	2	0.34 (0.04–1.23)	7.4	9	1.22 (0.56–2.32)	14.9	16	1.08 (0.62–1.76)
Prostate	C61	20.9	16	0.76 (0.44–1.24)	84.0	66	0.83 (0.64–1.05)	114.2	102	0.89 (0.73–1.08)	219.2	184	0.88 (0.76–1.02)
Kidney	C64	5.6	12	2.13 (1.10–3.72)	19.0	20	1.10 (0.67–1.70)	21.2	14	0.66 (0.36–1.11)	45.9	46	1.04 (0.76–1.38)
Bladder	C67	3.5	14	3.95 (2.16–6.62)	11.7	19	1.77 (1.06–2.76)	13.3	15	1.13 (0.63–1.87)	28.5	48	1.79 (1.32–2.37)
Brain, CNS	C70–72	2.1	3	1.45 (0.30–4.26)	6.8	9	1.36 (0.62–2.59)	7.3	5	0.69 (0.22–1.60)	16.1	17	1.08 (0.63–1.73)
Thyroid	C73	1.8	1	0.57 (0.01–3.15)	6.3	2	0.32 (0.04–1.16)	7.6	7	0.92 (0.37–1.90)	15.6	10	0.65 (0.31–1.19)
HL	C81	0.5	2	4.13 (0.50–14.90)	1.4	4	2.83 (0.77–7.25)	1.2	2	1.74 (0.21–6.30)	3.1	8	2.65 (1.14–5.22)
NHL & other LHT	C82–85, C88, C90, C96	3.0	8	2.71 (1.17–5.34)	10.6	15	1.46 (0.82–2.41)	13.2	11	0.84 (0.42–1.49)	26.7	34	1.31 (0.91–1.84)
Leukaemias	C91–95	2.6	3	1.16 (0.24–3.39)	8.8	18	2.14 (1.27–3.38)	10.6	20	1.90 (1.16–2.93)	22.0	41	1.94 (1.39–2.63)
Other		6.0	23	3.84 (2.43–5.76)	19.5	34	1.75 (1.21–2.44)	22.7	34	1.50 (1.04–2.10)	48.1	91	1.79 (1.43–2.21)

Exp expected cases, *Obs* observed cases, *SIR* standardized incidence ratio, *CI* confidence interval, *NMS* non-melanoma skin, *HL* Hodgkin lymphoma, *NHL* Non-Hodgkin lymphoma, *LHT* lympho-, haematopoietic tissue
[a]in women only, in men $n = 0$

and Israel, where significantly lower Odds ratios of melanoma were found for pulmonary tuberculosis, as well as other infections and BCG vaccination [13].

The mechanism underlying the increase of the long-term risk of cancer following tuberculosis is still not clear. Certain infectious episodes including tuberculosis may potentially trigger the development of Hodgkin lymphoma [12]. Previous studies have also supported an underlying immune deficiency many years prior to cancer diagnosis as a primary phenomenon for haematological cancers [12, 24]. Tuberculosis may induce a prolonged inflammatory response hence, inflammation may explain the increased long-term cancer risk. Occurrence of cervical cancer after tuberculosis has previously been reported rarely. There is a possibility that patients with human papilloma virus infection have a higher chance to

encounter tuberculosis. In addition, it has been suggested that the *Mycobacterium tuberculosis* infection mediates down regulation of dendritic cells function and thereby facilitates the suppression of the host's immunity against infectious pathogens and cervical cancer [25]. It has also been suggested that diverse microbial stimuli induce a defence against cancer: both vaccinations and previous episodes of having a severe infectious disease may induce a protective mechanism, possibly an infection-related Th1-cell activation that prevents the development of melanoma [13, 15]. The long-term increased risk may also be due to certain lifestyle factors, such as smoking or alcohol abuse that are strong risk factors for both tuberculosis and cancer [7, 14, 26–31]. E.g., most people with tuberculosis were tobacco smokers (64%) or heavy alcohol users (35%) in our study

Table 3 Cancer incidence in patients with tuberculosis according to type, sex and aetiology

Type of cancer	ICD-O	Men			Women		
		Exp	Obs	SIR (95% CI)	Exp	Obs	SIR (95% CI)
All but NMS	C00–96, excl. C44	710.6	1285	1.89 (1.79–2.00)	224.7	298	1.34 (1.19–1.50)
All but NMS & lung	C00–96, excl. C44, C33–34	567.4	850	1.50 (1.40–1.60)	214.6	255	1.19 (1.05–1.34)
Mouth, pharynx	C01–14	30.0	116	3.98 (3.28–4.77)	2.0	6	3.05 (1.12–6.64)
Oesophagus	C15	15.5	60	4.01 (3.06–5.16)	0.8	3	3.72 (0.77–10.90)
Stomach	C16	47.8	75	1.65 (1.30–2.07)	11.7	16	1.38 (0.79–2.24)
Colon	C18	31.8	35	1.16 (0.81–1.62)	12.9	5	0.39 (0.13–0.92)
Rectum	C19–21	31.8	37	1.23 (0.87–1.70)	10.0	6	0.61 (0.22–1.32)
Liver	C22	9.0	19	2.23 (1.34–3.48)	2.1	2	0.98 (0.12–3.52)
Pancreas	C25	21.6	33	1.60 (1.10–2.25)	6.2	9	1.47 (0.67–2.79)
Larynx	C32	19.7	49	2.58 (1.91–3.42)	0.4	4	10.88 (2.95–27.7)
Bone, mesothelial & soft tissue	C40–41, C45, C47, C49	5.0	11	2.29 (1.14–4.09)	1.8	3	1.64 (0.34–4.82)
Melanoma	C43	8.9	4	0.46 (0.13–1.19)	6.1	3	0.50 (0.10–1.45)
Breast	C50		-		51.9	50	0.96 (0.72–1.27)
Cervix uteri	C53		-		19.7	51	2.60 (1.93–3.42)
Corpus uteri	C54, C55		-		19.9	13	0.66 (0.35–1.13)
Ovary	C56		-		14.9	16	1.08 (0.62–1.76)
Prostate	C61	219.2	184	0.88 (0.76–1.02)	-		
Kidney	C64	36.8	34	0.96 (0.67–1.34)	9.1	12	1.34 (0.69–2.33)
Bladder	C67	25.6	44	1.83 (1.33–2.46)	2.9	4	1.39 (0.38–3.57)
Brain, CNS	C70–72	11.3	15	1.37 (0.76–2.25)	4.8	2	0.42 (0.05–1.52)
Thyroid	C73	4.8	2	0.43 (0.05–1.55)	10.9	8	0.74 (0.32–1.47)
HL	C81	2.0	6	2.98 (1.09–6.49)	1.0	2	1.98 (0.24–7.15)
NHL & other LHT	C82–85, C88, C90, C96	18.7	22	1.23 (0.77–1.86)	8.0	12	1.51 (0.78–2.64)
Leukaemias	C91–95	16.0	33	2.17 (1.49–3.05)	6.0	8	1.35 (0.58–2.66)
Other		35.4	71	2.00 (1.57–2.53)	12.7	20	1.58 (0.96–2.43)
Cancers by aetiology							
Alcohol-related	C01–15, C18–22, C32, C50	131.7	316	2.40 (2.14–2.68)	79.7	76	0.95 (0.75–1.19)
Smoking-related	C01–16, C18–22, C25, C30–32, C34, C53, C56, C64–68	257.0	502	1.95 (1.79–2.13)	91.8	134	1.46 (1.22–1.73)
Haematological	C81–85, C88, C90–96	35.2	61	1.73 (1.33–2.23)	14.9	22	1.48 (0.93–2.24)
Hormone-related	C18–21, C50, C54–56, C61, C62, C73	276.8	263	0.95 (0.84–1.07)	119.8	98	0.82 (0.66–0.997)

Exp expected cases, *Obs* observed cases, *SIR* standardized incidence ratio, *CI* confidence interval, *NMS* non-melanoma skin, *HL* Hodgkin lymphoma, *NHL* Non-Hodgkin lymphoma, *LHT* lympho-, haematopoietic tissue

and we observed elevated all-term SIRs for smoking- or alcohol-related cancers, thus it is plausible that tobacco smoking and alcohol intake are important shared risk factors. Finally, malnutrition is a risk factor for tuberculosis and low body mass index (BMI) is prevalent in tuberculosis patients [32, 33]. There is substantial evidence that obesity increases the risks of breast, endometrial, ovarian cancer, malignant melanoma as well as some other cancers; its influence is most likely mediated through hormonal mechanisms [20]. Low body weight

could possibly explain a reduced risk of hormone-related cancers or melanoma in the present study.

The strengths of our study include the use of nation-wide population-based registers and the cohort setting which reduced selection bias at baseline. The study also has limitations. There was no appropriate control group to compare the incidence of cancer. It is possible, that patients with tuberculosis differ from the general population with respect to lifestyle factors, like use of tobacco or alcohol. As these factors have been found to be risk factors for various cancer types, confounding by them is likely [27, 28, 34]. In addition, it is possible that the study cohort included individuals with cancer, because tumours may have been interpreted as tuberculosis lesion prior to cancer diagnosis. There is also a potential for bias due to reverse causality, if occult cancer caused a weakening of immunity and malnutrition, resulting in *Mycobacterium tuberculosis* infection or reactivation [35]. Thus, tuberculosis may become clinically apparent earlier than cancer, even though cancer preceded tuberculosis reactivation. Bias from closer medical surveillance received by individuals with tuberculosis than healthy individuals is likely to have had an effect, especially within the first year. However, a reduced risk for melanoma, colon, breast, prostate and thyroid cancer suggests that reverse causality or higher diagnostic activity are unlikely to play major role.

Conclusions

The overall and non-pulmonary cancer risk was elevated in a cohort of tuberculosis patients in relation to the general Lithuanian population. High risks were observed for smoking- and alcohol-related cancers, haematological cancers and cancer of cervix uteri. In addition, we found reduced risk for hormone-related cancers and melanoma. This retrospective study provides suggestion that tuberculosis may be associated with a risk of some non-pulmonary cancers; however, the possibility of confounding effects cannot be completely ruled out. Further studies are needed to determine the role of potential underlying mechanisms in non-pulmonary cancer development among tuberculosis patients. The recommendation for the awareness of this association among physicians remains warranted.

Abbreviations
95% CI: 95% Confidence Interval; BMI: Body mass index; ICD-10: International Statistical Classification of Diseases, 10th Revision; LCR: Lithuanian Cancer Registry; SIR: Standardized incidence ratio; WHO: World Health Organization

Acknowledgements
The authors wish to thank the Lithuanian Tuberculosis Registry, the Lithuanian Cancer Registry and the Lithuanian Residents' Register Service for making data available.

Funding
This research did not receive any specific grant from funding agencies in the public, commercial, or not-for-profit sectors.

Authors' contributions
The study was designed and coordinated by RE and ED. Data acquisition and cleaning was performed by IK, ED, RE. IK and RE prepared the final database, analyzed and interpreted the data and prepared the manuscript. SC contributed to the initial study idea, study design, critically revised the article. All authors read and approved the final manuscript.

Competing interests
The authors declare that they have no competing interests.

Author details
¹Laboratory of Cancer Epidemiology, National Cancer Institute, Baublio g. 3B, LT-08406 Vilnius, Lithuania. ²Vilnius University Hospital Santaros Klinikos, P. Sirvio g. 5, LT-10214 Vilnius, Lithuania. ³Department of Thoracic Surgery and Oncology, National Cancer Institute, Santariskiu g. 1, LT-08660 Vilnius, Lithuania. ⁴Faculty of Medicine, Vilnius University, M. K. Ciurlionio g. 21, LT-03101 Vilnius, Lithuania.

References
1. World Health Organization. Global tuberculosis report 2016. World Health Organization, 2016. http://www.who.int/tb/publications/global_report/en/ (accessed 7 Nov 2016).
2. Ferlay J, Soerjomataram I, Dikshit R, Eser S, Mathers C, Rebelo M, et al. Cancer incidence and mortality worldwide: sources, methods and major patterns in GLOBOCAN 2012. Int J Cancer. 2015;136(5):E359–86. doi:10.1002/ijc.29210.
3. Samaras V, Rafailidis PI, Mourtzoukou EG, Peppas G, Falagas ME. Chronic bacterial and parasitic infections and cancer: a review. J Infect Dev Ctries. 2010;4(5):267–81.
4. Simonsen DF, Farkas DK, Søgaard M, Horsburgh CR, Sørensen HT, Thomsen RW. Tuberculosis and risk of cancer: a Danish nationwide cohort study. Int J Tuberc Lung Dis. 2014;18(10):1211–9.
5. Hong S, Mok Y, Jeon C, Jee SH, Samet JM. Tuberculosis, smoking and risk for lung cancer incidence and mortality. Int J Cancer. 2016;139(11):2447–55.
6. Brenner DR, McLaughlin JR, Hung RJ. Previous lung diseases and lung cancer risk: a systematic review and meta-analysis. PLoS One. 2011;6(3):e1747. doi:10.1371/journal.pone.0017479.9.
7. Everatt R, Kuzmickiene I, Davidaviciene E, Cicenas S. Incidence of lung cancer among patients with tuberculosis: a nationwide cohort study in Lithuania. Int J Tuberc Lung Dis. 2016;20(6):757–63.
8. Su VY, Yen YF, Pan SW, Chuang PH, Feng JY, Chou KT, et al. Latent tuberculosis infection and the risk of subsequent cancer. Medicine. 2016;95(4):e2352. doi:10.1097/MD.0000000000002352.
9. Kuo SC, Hu YW, Liu CJ, Lee YT, Chen YT, Chen TL, et al. Association between tuberculosis infections and non-pulmonary malignancies: a nationwide population-based study. Br J Cancer. 2013;109:229–34.
10. Askling J, Ekbom A. Risk of non-Hodgkin's lymphoma following tuberculosis. Br J Cancer. 2001;84(1):113–5.
11. Tavani A, La Vecchia C, Franceschi S, Serraino D, Carbone A. Medical history and risk of Hodgkin's and non-Hodgkin's lymphomas. Eur J Cancer Prev. 2000;9(1):59–64.
12. Kristinsson SY, Gao Y, Björkholm M, Lund SH, Sjöberg J, Caporaso N, et al. Hodgkin lymphoma risk following infectious and chronic inflammatory diseases: a large population-based case-control study from Sweden. Int J Hematol. 2015;101(6):563–8.
13. Kölmel KF, Pfahlberg A, Mastrangelo G, Niin M, Botev IN, Seebacher C, et al. Infections and melanoma risk: results of a multicentre EORTC case-control study. European Organization for Research and Treatment of Cancer. Melanoma res. 1999;9(5):511–9.
14. Schottenfeld D, Beebe-Dimmer J. Chronic inflammation: a common and important factor in the pathogenesis of neoplasia. CA Cancer J Clin. 2006;56(2):69–83.
15. Krone B, Kölmel KF, Grange JM, Mastrangelo G, Henz BM, Botev IN, et al. Impact of vaccinations and infectious diseases on the risk of melanoma - evaluation of an EORTC case-control study. Eur J Cancer. 2003;39(16):2372–8.
16. Holla S, Ghorpade DS, Singh V, Bansal K, Balaji KN. Mycobacterium bovis BCG promotes tumor cell survival from tumor necrosis factor-α-induced apoptosis. Mol Cancer. 2014;13:210. doi:10.1186/1476-4598-13-210.
17. Fallah M, Kharazmi E. Correction for under-ascertainment in cancer cases in the very elderly (aged 75+): external reference method. Cancer Causes Control. 2008;19(7):739–49.

18. Forman D, Bray F, Brewster DH, Gombe Mbalawa C, Kohler B, Piñeros M, et al., editors. Cancer incidence in five continents. Vol. X. IARC scientific publication no. 164. Lyon: International Agency for Research on Cancer; 2014.
19. International agency for research on cancer (IARC). IARC monographs on the evaluation of carcinogenic risks to humans. A review of human carcinogens: personal habits and indoor combustions, vol. Volume 100E. Lyon: IARC; 2012.
20. Stewart BW, Wild CP, editors. World cancer report 2014. Lyon: IARC; 2014.
21. Zadnik V, Krajc M. Epidemiological trends of hormone-related cancers in Slovenia. Arh Hig Rada Toksikol. 2016;67:83–92.
22. Blöndal K, Rahu K, Altraja A, Viiklepp P, Rahu M. Overall and cause-specific mortality among patients with tuberculosis and multidrug-resistant tuberculosis. Int J Tuberc Lung Dis. 2013;17(7):961–8.
23. Falagas ME, Kouranos VD, Athanassa Z, Kopterides P. Tuberculosis and malignancy. Q J med. 2010;103:461–87.
24. Mbulaiteye SM, Biggar RJ, Goedert JJ, Engels EA. Immune deficiency and risk for malignancy among persons with AIDS. J Acquir Immune Defic Syndr. 2003;32:527–33.
25. Manickam A, Sivanandham M. Mycobacterium bovis BCG and purified protein derivative-induced reduction in the CD80 expression and the antigen up-take function of dendritic cells from patients with cervical cancer. Eur J Obstet Gynecol Reprod Biol. 2011;159(2):413–7.
26. Rehm J, Samokhvalov AV, Neuman MG, Room R, Parry C, Lönnroth K, et al. The association between alcohol use, alcohol use disorders and tuberculosis (TB). A systematic review. BMC Public Health. 2009;9:450. doi:10.1186/1471-2458-9-450.
27. Everatt R, Kuzmickienė I, Virvičiūtė D, Tamošiūnas A. Cigarette smoking, educational level and total and site-specific cancer: a cohort study in men in Lithuania. Eur J Cancer Prev. 2014;23(6):579–86.
28. Everatt R, Tamosiunas A, Virviciute D, Kuzmickiene I, Reklaitiene R. Consumption of alcohol and risk of cancer among men: a 30 year cohort study in Lithuania. Eur J Epidemiol. 2013;28(5):383–92.
29. Waitt CJ, Squire SB. A systematic review of risk factors for death in adults during and after tuberculosis treatment. Int J Tuberc Lung Dis. 2011;5:871–85.
30. Cogliano VJ, Baan R, Straif K, Grosse Y, Lauby-Secretan B, El Ghissassi F, et al. Preventable exposures associated with human cancers. J Natl Cancer Inst. 2011;103(24):1827–39.
31. Marais BJ, Lönnroth K, Lawn SD, Migliori GB, Mwaba P, Glaziou P, et al. Tuberculosis comorbidity with communicable and non-communicable diseases: integrating health services and control efforts. Lancet Infect Dis. 2013;13(5):436–48.
32. Kumari P, Meena LS. Factors affecting susceptibility to Mycobacterium tuberculosis: a close view of immunological defence mechanism. Appl Biochem Biotechnol. 2014;174(8):2663–73.
33. Hayashi S, Takeuchi M, Hatsuda K, Ogata K, Kurata M, Nakayama T, et al. The impact of nutrition and glucose intolerance on the development of tuberculosis in Japan. Int J Tuberc Lung Dis. 2014;18(1):84–8.
34. McKenzie F, Biessy C, Ferrari P, Freisling H, Rinaldi S, Chajès V, et al. Healthy lifestyle and risk of cancer in the European prospective investigation into cancer and nutrition cohort study. Medicine (Baltimore). 2016;95(16):e2850. doi:10.1097/MD.0000000000002850.
35. Vento S, Lanzafame M. Tuberculosis and cancer: a complex and dangerous liaison. Lancet Oncol. 2011;12(6):520–2.

16

Estimation of the overall burden of cancers, precancerous lesions, and genital warts attributable to 9-valent HPV vaccine types in women and men in Europe

Susanne Hartwig[1]* [iD], Jean Lacau St Guily[2], Géraldine Dominiak-Felden[1], Laia Alemany[3] and Silvia de Sanjosé[3,4]

Abstract

Background: In addition to cervical cancer, human papillomavirus (HPV) is responsible for a significant proportion of cancers and precancerous lesions of the vulva, vagina, anus, penis, head and neck, as well as genital warts. We estimated the annual number of new cases of these diseases attributable to 9-valent HPV vaccine types in women and men in Europe.

Methods: The annual number of new cancers of the cervix, vulva, vagina, anus, penis, and selected head and neck sites in the population of the European Medicines Agency territory was estimated based on age-specific incidence rates extracted from Cancer Incidence in 5 Continents, Volume X and Eurostat population data for 2015. The annual number of new cancers attributable to 9-valent HPV vaccine types was estimated by applying the HPV attributable fraction from reference publications based on a large European multicenter study. For non-cervical cancers, HPV attributable fractions were based on oncogenically-active HPV infections only (i.e., detection of HPV DNA and either mRNA and/or p16 positivity). For precancerous lesions of the cervix, vulva, vagina, and anus, and for genital warts, previously published estimations were updated for the 2015 population.

Results: The annual number of new cancers attributable to 9-valent HPV vaccine types was estimated at 47,992 (95% bound: 39,785-58,511). Cervical cancer showed the highest burden (31,130 cases), followed by head and neck cancer (6,786 cases), anal cancer (6,137 cases), vulvar cancer (1,466 cases), vaginal cancer (1,360 cases), and penile cancer (1,113 cases). About 81% were estimated to occur in women and 19% in men. The annual number of new precancerous lesions (CIN2+, VIN2/3, VaIN2/3, and AIN2/3) and genital warts attributable to 9-valent HPV vaccine types was estimated at 232,103 to 442,347 and 680,344 to 844,391, respectively.

Conclusions: The burden of cancers associated with 9-valent HPV vaccine types in Europe is substantial in both sexes. Head and neck cancers constitute a heavy burden, particularly in men. Overall, about 90% of HPV-related cancers, 80% of precancerous lesions, and 90% of genital warts are expected to be attributable to 9-valent HPV vaccine types each year, demonstrating the important preventive potential of the 9-valent HPV vaccine in Europe.

Keywords: Human papillomavirus, Burden of disease, Cancer, Precancerous lesions, Genital warts, Head and neck

Background

Human papillomavirus (HPV) infections are the most common sexually transmitted infections, with more than 40 HPV types that can be transmitted through direct sexual contact, of which about a dozen are classified as high-risk types. Persistent infection with high-risk HPV types can cause cellular changes that may progress to cancer or precancerous lesions of the cervix, vagina, vulva, anus, penis, and head and neck. On the other hand, low-risk types can cause genital warts and recurrent respiratory papillomatosis (RRP), but cause cancer very rarely [1]. Indeed, the high-risk HPV types 16, 18, 31, 33, 45, 52, and 58 are responsible for about 90% of cervical cancers worldwide, whereas HPV6 and 11 are low-risk types for cancer

* Correspondence: susanne.hartwig@merck.com
[1]Department of Epidemiology, Sanofi Pasteur MSD, 162 avenue Jean Jaurès, Lyon, France

but are responsible for about 90% of warts on or around the genitals, anus, mouth, and throat (RRP) [2].

The quadrivalent HPV vaccine, Gardasil®/Silgard® (Sanofi Pasteur MSD/Merck Sharp & Dohme), protects against infection with HPV16, 18, 6, and 11, and was licensed in Europe in 2006. It was followed in 2007 by the bivalent HPV vaccine, Cervarix® (GlaxoSmithKline Biologicals), which protects against infection with HPV16 and 18. Both vaccines have reassuring safety profiles, as demonstrated in clinical trials and several large post-licensure studies [3], and they provide a high level of protection against HPV16- and 18-attributable lesions.

In 2015, the 9-valent HPV vaccine, Gardasil9 (Sanofi Pasteur MSD/Merck Sharp & Dohme), was licensed in Europe for the prevention of cancers and precancerous lesions of the cervix, vulva, vagina, and anus, as well as genital warts caused by HPV6, 11, 16, 18, 31, 33, 45, 52, and 58 [4]. This vaccine protects against five high-risk HPV types not included in first-generation HPV vaccines (HPV31, 33, 45, 52, and 58) [1].

We recently published an estimation of the annual burden of cancers and precancerous lesions of the cervix, vulva, vagina, and anus, and of genital warts attributable to 9-valent HPV vaccine types in Europe in 2013, and compared it to the estimated annual burden of the same lesions attributable to quadrivalent HPV vaccine types [5]. Recently, two new papers [6, 7] based on a large European multicenter study have published information on HPV type distribution and HPV attributable fractions in head and neck and penile cancers, which gave us the opportunity to provide robust estimates on the contribution of 9-valent HPV vaccine types at these sites as well. Therefore, in order to provide a more exhaustive overview of the preventive potential of the 9-valent HPV vaccine, we have updated our previous estimates to 2015. These new estimates include the annual number of new cancers of the cervix, vulva, vagina, anus, penis, and head and neck; the annual number of new precancerous lesions of the cervix, vulva, vagina, and anus; and the annual number of genital warts cases attributable to 9-valent HPV vaccine types, including the low-risk types HPV6 and 11, in Europe in 2015.

Methods

Estimation of the annual number of new HPV-related cancers in Europe

The present evaluation was based on cancer incidence data from Cancer Incidence in Five Continents (CI5) Volume X, which were collected from 2003 through 2007. The CI5 database is available on the website of the International Agency for Research on Cancer (IARC) [8] and contains worldwide data on cancer incidence rates classified by International Classification of Diseases 10th

Revision (ICD-10) codes. These data are obtained from regional or national registries, depending on the country, but to be included in CI5 these registries must meet the IARC's quality criteria, i.e., they must have reliable cancer registry data. We compiled data on 32 countries: 31 countries covered by the European Medicines Agency (EMA, Austria, Belgium, Bulgaria, Croatia, Cyprus, the Czech Republic, Denmark, Estonia, Finland, France, Germany, Greece, Hungary, Iceland, Ireland, Italy, Latvia, Liechtenstein, Lithuania, Luxemburg, Malta, the Netherlands, Norway, Poland, Portugal, Romania, Slovenia, Slovakia, Spain, Sweden, and the United Kingdom) and one not covered by the EMA (Switzerland).

The information in CI5 Volume X was obtained from national cancer registries for Belgium, Bulgaria, Croatia, Cyprus, the Czech Republic, Denmark, Estonia, Finland, Iceland, Ireland, Latvia, Lithuania, Malta, the Netherlands, Norway, Slovenia, Slovakia, and Sweden; and from regional cancer registries for Austria, France, Germany, Italy, Poland, Portugal, Spain, Switzerland, and the United Kingdom. To ensure that national populations were adequately represented in countries where only regional cancer registries exist, we assessed the geographical coverage and distribution of these registries.

Five of the 32 countries selected did not have data available in CI5 Volume X: Greece, Hungary, Liechtenstein, Luxemburg, and Romania. Because of its very low population size, we excluded Lichtenstein from our analysis. For the remaining four countries, we extrapolated age-specific average cancer incidence rates from neighboring countries, or from cancer registries in the same area as the countries selected. The choice of countries used for extrapolation was the same as that used for Globocan [9]. Thus, for Greece data from Bulgaria, Cyprus, and Central Serbia were used; for Hungary data from Austria, Croatia, Central Serbia, Slovakia, and Slovenia were used; for Luxemburg data from French and German cancer registries were used; and for Romania data from Bulgaria, Slovakia, and one regional registry in Romania were used. In conclusion, our results refer to a geographical region of 31 European countries.

The incidence of cancer of the cervix (ICD-10 code C53), vulva (C51), vagina (C52), anus (C21), penis (C60), and selected head and neck cancers that are known to be at least partially related to HPV [6]: oral cavity cancers (C02-06), nasopharyngeal cancers (C11), oropharyngeal cancers (C01, C09, C10), hypopharyngeal cancers (C12-13), unspecified pharyngeal cancers (C14), and laryngeal cancers (C32) [6] was derived from CI5 Volume X. Based on these data, we estimated the mean annual number of new cancers at these sites in 2015 in the 31 selected countries by extrapolating the sex- and age-specific cancer incidence data [10] to the population of each country, using 2015 Eurostat population data [11]. Calculations were performed as follows:

$$Total\ nb\ of\ new\ cases = \frac{\sum_{Countries}\left\{\sum_{age=0}^{85+}\left(AIR\ in\ male * population + \sum_{type\ of\ cancer}\left(AIR\ in\ female * population\right)\right)\right\}}{100,000}$$

where AIR is the age- and sex-specific annual incidence rate, and population is the age- and sex-specific population of a given country. The estimated number of new cancers at these sites in all the selected countries were then summed to obtain the overall European burden of these cancers.

Estimation of the annual number of new cancers attributable to all HPV types and to 9-valent HPV vaccine types in Europe

The number of new cancers attributable to all HPV types and to 9-valent HPV vaccine types (HPV6, 11, 16, 18, 31, 33, 45, 52, and 58) was estimated by applying the corresponding cancer site-specific HPV attributable fraction. For cervical cancers, the HPV attributable fraction was considered to be 100%, as it is generally accepted that HPV infection is necessary for the development of cervical cancer [12]. However, for all other cancer sites, the fraction attributable to all HPV types and to 9-valent HPV vaccine types was based on the prevalence of oncogenically-active HPV infections (i.e., detection of HPV DNA and either mRNA and/or p16 positivity), which was taken from reference publications based on a large European multicenter study (Table 1). These publications

contain the most relevant cancer site-specific data published to-date [6, 7, 13–16] and covered all our selected sites. European data on oncogenically-active HPV infections were not directly available in these publications; they were obtained from the authors, who are also co-authors of the present study (LA and SdS). To avoid overestimating the contribution of individual HPV types due to multiple infections, the contribution of individual HPV types to multiple infections was calculated under a weighting attribution, proportional to the prevalence of each individual HPV type in single infections. We always used European-specific crude data and the same contribution estimates were used for both sexes.

Estimation of the annual number of new precancerous lesions and genital warts cases attributable to all HPV types and to 9-valent HPV vaccine types in Europe

The methodology used to estimate the annual number of new precancerous lesions of the cervix, vulva, vagina, and anus, as well as genital warts was comprehensively described in our previous work [5]. In the present paper we updated this estimate, as well as the fraction attributable to all HPV types and 9-valent HPV vaccine types for the 2015 population [11].

Table 1 Fraction of cancers attributable to all HPV types and to 9-valent HPV vaccine types[a] by cancer site

Cancer site	ICD-10 code	Fraction attributable to all HPV types % [95% CI][b]	Fraction attributable to 4-valent HPV vaccine types (6/11/16/18) % [95% CI][b]	Fraction attributable to 9-valent HPV vaccine types (6/11/16/18/31/33/45/52/58) % [95% CI][b]	Reference
Cervix	C53	100[c]	72.9 [71.0-74.8]	89.1 [87.7-90.4]	[13]
Vulva	C51	15.9 [13.5-18.4]	84.4 [77.3-90.0]	94.3 [89.1-97.5]	[14]
Vagina	C52	70.2 [62.2-77.4]	72.6 [63.1-80.9]	87.1 [78.8-92.6]	[16]
Anus	C21	87.1 [81.0-91.8]	91.5 [85.7-95.6]	94.4 [89.2-97.5]	[15]
Penis	C60	29.0 [24.7-33.7]	78.9 [70.6-85.9]	90.7 [84.1-95.3]	[7]
Oral cavity	C02-06	3.7 [2.4-5.6]	90.9 [70.8-98.9]	90.9 [70.8-98.9]	[6]
Nasopharynx	C11	10.8 [3.0-25.4]	75.0 [19.4-99.4]	75.0 [19.4-99.4]	[6]
Oropharynx	C01, C09, C10	19.9 [17.2-22.8]	93.8 [88.8-97.0]	97.5 [93.7-99.3]	[6]
Hypopharynx	C12-13	2.4 [0.3-8.4]	50.0 [1.3-98.7]	100 [15.8-100]	[6]
Pharynx	C14	25.0 [10.7-44.9]	85.7 [42.1-99.6]	85.7 [42.1-99.6]	[6]
Larynx	C32	2.4 [1.2-4.1]	66.7 [34.9-90.1]	91.7 [61.5-99.8]	[6]

CI confidence interval, HPV human papillomavirus, ICD-10 International Classification of Diseases, 10th Revision, CI confidence interval
[a]Adjusted for multiple infections; [b]Except for cervical cancer, prevalence is based on oncogenically-active HPV infections only (i.e., HPV DNA detection plus either E6*I mRNA expression or p16 overexpression). [c]HPV is the necessary cause for cervical cancer [12]

Results

Estimated annual number of new cancers attributable to all HPV types and to 9-valent HPV vaccine types in Europe (Table 2, Additional file 1)

Cervical cancer

The estimated annual number of new cervical cancers in 2015 was 34,939 (95% bound: 32,863-37,032) in the 31selected European countries combined. Applying our overall HPV attributable fraction of 100%, all of these cases are believed to be HPV-related. The fraction of cases attributable to 9-valent HPV vaccine types was 89.1% (95% CI: 87.7-90.4). Accordingly, a total of 31,130 (95% bound: 28,800-33,495) cases were estimated to be attributable to these types.

Vulvar cancer

The estimated annual number of new vulvar cancers was 9,776 (95% bound: 8,727-10,841). Given an overall HPV attributable fraction of 15.9% (95% CI: 13.5-18.4) [14], 1,554 (95% bound: 1,135-2,044) cases were estimated to be attributable to all HPV types. In our reference publication, the fraction of these cases attributable to 9-valent HPV vaccine types was estimated at 94.3% (95% CI: 89.1-97.5) [14]. Thus 1,466 (95% bound: 1,008-1,994) cases were estimated to be attributable to these types.

Vaginal cancer

The estimated annual number of new vaginal cancers was 2,224 (95% bound: 1,723-2,744). Of these cases, 1,562 (95% bound: 1,058-2,134) were estimated to be attributable to all HPV types, assuming an overall HPV attributable fraction of 70.2% (95% CI: 62.2-77.4) [16]. The fraction of these cases attributable to 9-valent HPV vaccine types in our reference publication was 87.1% (95% CI: 78.8-92.6). Applying this value, 1,360 (95% bound: 827–1,980) cases were estimated to be attributable to these types.

Anal cancer

The estimated annual number of new anal cancers was 4,663 (95% bound: 3,968-5,375) among women and 2,801 (95% bound: 2,260-3,359) among men in Europe. Given an overall HPV attributable fraction of 87.1% (95% CI: 81.0-91.8) [15], 4,062 cases (95% bound: 3,203-4,940) in women and 2,440 cases (95% bound: 1,822-3,088) in men were estimated to be attributable to all HPV types. The fraction of these cases attributable to 9-valent HPV vaccine types in our reference publication was 94.4% (95% CI: 89.2-97.5). After applying this value, 3,834 (95% bound: 2,851-4,818) cases in women and 2,303 (95% bound: 1,621-3,012) cases in men were estimated to be attributable to these types.

Table 2 Estimated mean annual number of new HPV-attributable cancer cases in women and men in Europe

Cancer site	New cancers N, (95% bound)	New cancers attributable to all HPV types N, (95% bound)[a]	New cancers attributable to 9-valent HPV vaccine types (6/11/16/18/31/33/45/52/58) N, (95% bound)[a]
Cervical cancer	34,939 (32,863 – 37,032)	34,939 (32,863 – 37,032)	31,130 (28,800 – 33,495)
Vulvar cancer	9,776 (8,727 – 10,841)	1,554 (1,135 – 2,044)	1,466 (1,008 – 1,994)
Vaginal cancer	2,224 (1,723 – 2,744)	1,562 (1,058 – 2,134)	1,360 (827 – 1,980)
Anal cancer (F)	4,663 (3,968 – 5,375)	4,062 (3,203 – 4,940)	3,834 (2,851 – 4,818)
Head and neck cancers (F)	18,052 (13,977 – 22,183)	1,396 (728 – 2,592)	1,301 (586 – 2,574)
Total (women)	69,654 (61,754 – 77,609)	43,512 (39,256 – 48,387)	39,091 (34,320 – 44,513)
Anal cancer (M):	2,801 (2,260 – 3,359)	2,440 (1,822 – 3,088)	2,303 (1,621 – 3,012)
Penile cancer	4,231 (3,543 – 4,937)	1,227 (845 – 1,697)	1,113 (707 – 1,619)
Head and neck cancers (M)	81,989 (73,563 – 90,469)	5,834 (3,729 – 9,735)	5,485 (2,923 – 9,680)
Total (men)	89,021 (79,558 – 98,543)	9,501 (6,502 – 14,376)	8,901 (5,348 – 14,168)
Total (both sexes)	158,675 (141,617 – 175,815)	53,013 (45,886 – 62,589)	47,992 (39,785 – 58,511)

HPV human papillomavirus, N number, CI confidence interval, F female, M male
[a]Except for cervical cancer, prevalence is based on oncogenically-active HPV infections only (i.e., HPV DNA detection plus either E6[a]I mRNA expression or p16 overexpression)

Penile cancer

The estimated annual number of new penile cancers was 4,231 (95% bound: 3,543-4,937). Assuming an overall HPV attributable fraction of 29.0% (95% CI: 24.7-33.7) [7], 1,227 (95% bound: 845–1,697) cases were estimated to be attributable to all HPV types. Of these cases, the fraction attributable to 9-valent HPV vaccine types in our reference publication was 90.7% (95% CI: 84.1-95.3); thus 1,113 (95% bound: 707–1,619) cases were estimated to be attributable to these types.

Head and neck cancers

The estimated annual number of new head and neck cancers was 18,052 (95% bound: 13,977-22,183) among women and 81,989 (95% bound: 73,563-90,469) among men. Of these, 1,396 (95% bound: 728–2,592) cancers in women and 5,834 (95% bound: 3,729-9,735) cancers in men were estimated to be attributable to all HPV types, given an overall HPV attributable fraction of 3.7% (95% CI: 2.4-5.6) in oral cavity cancers, 10.8% (95% CI: 3.0-25.4) in nasopharyngeal cancers, 19.9% (95% CI: 17.2-22.8) in oropharyngeal cancers, 2.4% (95% CI: 0.3-8.4) in hypopharyngeal cancers, 25.0% (95% CI: 10.7-44.9) in pharyngeal cancers, and 2.4% (95% CI: 1.2-4.1) in laryngeal cancers. The fraction attributable to 9-valent HPV vaccine types in our reference publication was 90.9% (95% CI: 70.8-98.9), 75.0% (95% CI: 19.4-99.4), 97.5% (95% CI: 93.7-99.3), 100% (95% CI: 15.8-100), 85.7% (95% CI:42.1-99.6) and 91.7% (95% CI: 61.5-99.8) for oral cavity cancers, nasopharyngeal cancers, oropharyngeal cancers, hypopharyngeal cancers, pharyngeal cancers, and laryngeal cancers, respectively. After applying these values, a total of 1,301 (95% bound: 586–2,574) head and neck cancers cases in women and 5,485 (95% bound: 2,923-9,680) in men were estimated to be attributable to 9-valent HPV vaccine types. The most frequent HPV type in head and neck cancers is HPV16, which is most commonly present as a single-type infection, but a small proportion of these cancers contain HPV18, or, even less frequently, HPV31 or 33.

Estimated annual number of new precancerous lesions attributable to all HPV types and 9-valent HPV vaccine types in Europe

Cervical intraepithelial neoplasia grade 2 or worse

Based on the age-specific incidence rates, the estimated annual number of new cervical intraepithelial neoplasia grade 2 or worse (CIN2+) cases in women in Europe ranged between 263,227 and 503,010. Of these cases, 82.3% were estimated to be attributable to 9-valent HPV vaccine types. After applying these values, 216,636 to 413,977 new CIN2+ cases were estimated to be attributable to these types in 2015.

Vulvar intraepithelial neoplasia grades 2 and 3

Based on the age-specific incidence data, the estimated annual number of new vulvar intraepithelial neoplasia grades 2 and 3 (VIN2/3) cases was between 13,997 and 27,773. Of these cases, 86.9% (95% CI: 82.6-90.4) were estimated to be attributable to all HPV types, with 9-valent HPV vaccine types accounting for 94.4% (95% CI: 91.0-96.9) of them. Based on these estimates, 12,164 to 24,135 of the VIN2/3 cases were estimated to be attributable to all HPV types and 11,482 to 22,783 to 9-valent HPV vaccine types.

Vaginal intraepithelial neoplasia grades 2 and 3

Based on age-specific incidence data, the estimated annual number of new vaginal intraepithelial neoplasia grades 2 and 3 (VaIN2/3) cases in women in Europe ranged between 2,596 and 4,751. Of these cases, 95.8% (95% CI: 91.8-98.2) are expected to be attributable to all HPV types, with 9-valent HPV vaccine types accounting for 77.6% (95% CI: 70.6-83.3) of them. Based on these estimates, 2,487 to 4,551 cases were expected to be attributable to all HPV types, and 1,930-3,532 cases to 9-valent HPV vaccine types.

Anal intraepithelial neoplasia grades 2 and 3

Based on the age-standardized rate of 0.58 and 0.43 per 100,000 person-years for anal intraepithelial neoplasia grades 2 and 3 (AIN2/3) in women and men, respectively [17], 1,549 new AIN2/3 cases were estimated to occur each year in women and 1,097 cases in men. Of these cases, 95.3% (95% CI: 84.2-99.4) are believed to be attributable to all HPV types [15]. Applying these values resulted in 1,477 and 1,045 cases attributable to all HPV types in women and men, respectively, of which 81.5% (95% CI: 66.4-91.9) were attributable to 9-valent HPV vaccine types, corresponding to 1,203 cases in women and 852 cases in men (Table 3).

Estimated annual number of new genital warts cases attributable to HPV in Europe

The estimated annual number of new genital warts cases ranged between 379,330 and 510,492 in women, and between 376,608 and 427,720 in men. Assuming that the low-risk 9-valent HPV vaccine types account for 90% of all genital warts cases [18], between 341,397 and 459,443 of these cases in women and between 338,947 and 384,948 of these cases in men were estimated to be attributable to these types (Table 4).

Discussion

To our knowledge, this is the first estimation of the annual number of new cancers, precancerous lesions, and genital warts attributable to 9-valent HPV vaccine types in women and men in Europe (EMA territory plus

Table 3 Estimated annual number of new precancerous lesions in women and men in Europe

Precancerous lesion	New precancerous lesions (range)	New precancerous lesions attributable to all HPV types (range)	New precancerous lesions attributable to 9-valent HPV vaccine types (6/11/16/18/31/33/45/52/58) (range)
CIN 2+	263,227 – 503,010	263,227 – 503,010	216,636 – 413,977
VIN 2/3	13,997 – 27,773	12,164 – 24,135	11,482 – 22,783
VaIN 2/3	2,596 – 4,751	2,487 – 4,551	1,930 – 3,532
AIN 2/3 (F)	1,549	1,477	1,203
AIN 2/3 (M)	1,097	1,045	852
Total (both sexes)	282,466 - 538,180	280,399 - 534,218	232,103 - 442,347

HPV human papillomavirus, *CIN2+* cervical intraepithelial neoplasia grade 2 or worse, *VIN2/3* vulvar intraepithelial neoplasia grades 2 and 3, *VaIN2/3* vaginal intraepithelial neoplasia grades 2 and 3, *AIN2/3* anal intraepithelial neoplasia grades 2 and 3, CIN 2+ includes CIN2/3 and AIS, *N* number, *F* female, *M* male

Switzerland), reflecting the overall burden of disease, including penile and head and neck cancers. Our estimates demonstrate the high disease burden associated with 9-valent HPV vaccine types (HPV6, 11, 16, 18, 31, 33, 45, 52, and 58) (Fig. 1). Among the 53,013 (95% bound: 45,886 to 62,589) new cancers attributable to all HPV types occurring yearly in Europe, 47,992 (95% bound: 39,785-58,511) are expected to be attributable to 9-valent HPV vaccine types, i.e., about 90% (see Table 2). About 81% of these cases (39,091; 95% bound: 34,320 to 44,513) occur in women and 19% (8,901; 95% bound: 5,348 to 14,168) in men. Cervical cancer represents the highest burden (31,130 cases), followed by head and neck cancer (6,786 cases), anal cancer (6,137 cases), vulvar cancer (1,466 cases), vaginal cancer (1,360 cases), and penile cancer (1,113 cases). HPV-attributable head and neck cancers constitute a heavy burden in Europe, particularly in men (1,396 cases in women, 5,834 cases in men). Overall 75–100% of these are associated with 9-valent HPV vaccine types, with HPV16 being the main contributor (50–92% attributable to this type specifically, depending on subsite).

In a previous work we estimated the incremental burden attributable to the five new vaccine types [5]; the relative increase in the number of new cancers attributable to HPV16/18/31/33/45/52/58 compared to HPV16/18 was 19%. In the present work we estimated the burden attributable to all nine HPV types and based our estimates for cancers others than cervical cancer on oncogenically-active fractions only. Also, this is the first estimate of the burden of penile and head and neck cancers. However, the additional benefit of the 9-valent vaccine compared to the quadrivalent or bivalent vaccine would not have essentially changed the earlier estimate of 19%, as head and neck cancers are mainly driven by HPV16.

In addition to cancers, 232,103 to 442,347 new precancerous lesions (CIN2+, VIN2/3, VaIN2/3, and AIN2/3) and 680,344 to 844,391 new genital warts cases (341,397 to 459,443 in women; 338,947 to 384,948 in men) per year are expected to be attributable to 9-valent HPV vaccine types. Precancerous lesions of the penis are known to be largely HPV-related: 89.1% of penile high-grade squamous intraepithelial lesions were estimated to be HPV-related in Europe, with 92% of them attributable to 9-valent HPV vaccine types [7]. However, it was not possible to find a robust data source to evaluate the incidence of penile intraepithelial neoplasia in Europe; therefore the burden associated to this disease could not be evaluated. Similarly, the burden of precancerous lesions of the head and neck could not be estimated, as no screening exists. The burden of RRP, a rare but dreadful condition that is almost exclusively attributable to HPV6 and 11, is also missing, as available incidence data are too scarce to be extrapolated to large populations [19, 20].

Strengths and limitations

All data used to evaluate the burden of HPV-attributable cancers, precancerous lesions, and genital warts were collected during the most recent period before HPV vaccine introduction in Europe. Thus these data reflect the theoretical burden of these diseases when cervical cancer screening was the only method for disease prevention; before any impact of vaccination would be evident.

There are regional differences in the incidence of cervical cancer that are due predominantly to the combination of HPV prevalence (that depend on the cultural environment

Table 4 Estimated annual number of new genital warts cases in women and men in Europe

	N of new annual cases (range)	N of new annual cases attributable to HPV6/11 (range)
Women	379,330 – 510,492	341,397 – 459,443
Men	376,608 – 427,720	338,947 – 384,948
Total (both sexes)	755,937 – 938,212	680,344 – 844,391

HPV human papillomavirus, *N* number

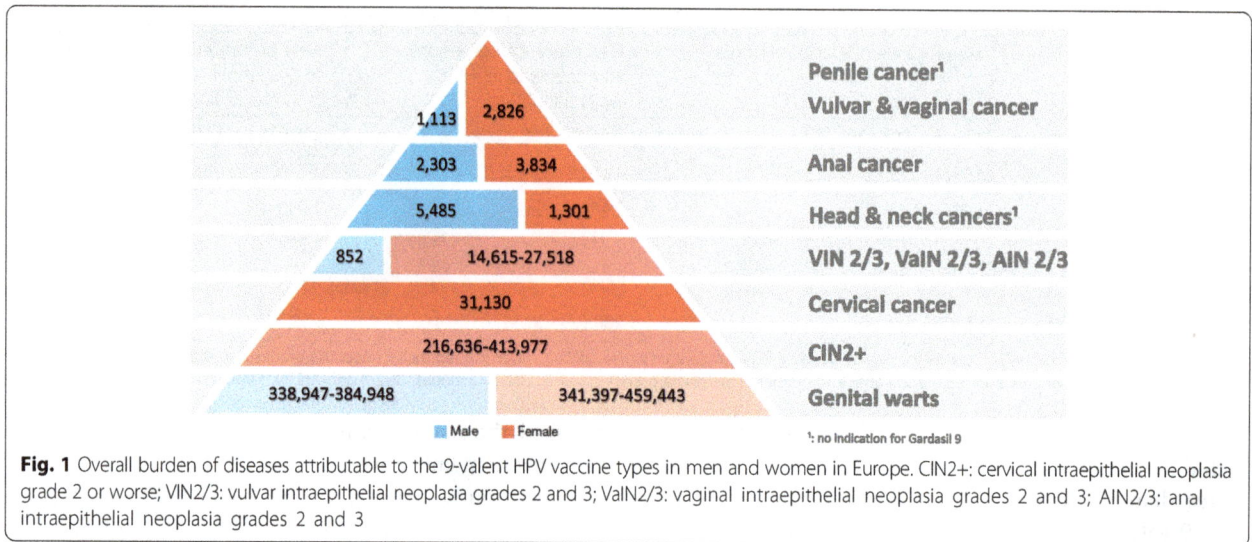

Fig. 1 Overall burden of diseases attributable to the 9-valent HPV vaccine types in men and women in Europe. CIN2+: cervical intraepithelial neoplasia grade 2 or worse; VIN2/3: vulvar intraepithelial neoplasia grades 2 and 3; VaIN2/3: vaginal intraepithelial neoplasia grades 2 and 3; AIN2/3: anal intraepithelial neoplasia grades 2 and 3

and related behavioral pattern) and the presence and effectiveness of population-based screening programs. Within Europe, the highest rates are observed in Eastern Europe, followed by Northern Europe, Southern Europe and Western Europe, where incidence is lowest. Worldwide highest incidence rates are observed in countries with low ranking of the Human Development Index and lowest rates are measured in Western Asia, Australia and the United States [21].

A short-term prediction method was used to estimate the number of new cancer cases in 2015 from the most recent data collected from 2003 to 2007. These estimates presuppose that the incidence rates of the cancers under study remained stable over time. In the case of increasing incidence, as observed for anal cancers and HPV-related head and neck cancers over the last few decades [17, 22–28], this could lead to a slight underestimation of the expected number of cases. The opposite would be true in the case of decreasing incidence.

As mentioned above, the CI5 database contains national cancer incidence rates for 19 European countries. Eight of the countries included in this report had only regional incidence rates available, which were extrapolated to the entire country. Although we assessed the geographical coverage and distribution of these regional registries, other factors could vary and influence regional incidence rates. For the remaining four countries no robust regional or national data were available. We thus extrapolated the mean incidence data from surrounding cancer registries to these countries, but we had no means to check the robustness of this method. Therefore the results for those countries should be interpreted with particular caution.

Our calculations of HPV-attributable cancers other than cervical cancer were based on data provided by a large European multicenter study [6, 7, 13–16], which

contains the most relevant cancer site-specific data published to-date and that provided estimates adjusted for multiple infections, in order not to overestimate the weight of individual HPV types.

Moreover, for cancers other than cervical cancer, the HPV attributable fractions were based on oncogenically-active HPV infections only (i.e., detection of HPV DNA and either mRNA and/or p16 positivity, which are markers of biological activity). Indeed, non-cervical cancers may occur for reasons other than HPV infection; the mere presence of HPV DNA is insufficient to prove causation, as the infection may be transient and not related to the carcinogenic process. This may be particularly true for head and neck cancers, for which tobacco and alcohol are known to be major risk factors. These additional criteria were implemented mainly to avoid overestimating the HPV attributable fraction in non-cervical cancers. Still, we cannot completely rule out the possibility that mRNA or protein was degraded in the paraffin-embedded samples in our reference publication, which could trigger false negativity for biological HPV activity. To evaluate this, we looked at the proportion of oncogenically-active HPV-positive samples with those that were HPV DNA-positive only, and compared it with the proportion observed in a recent meta-analysis on the same topic for head and neck cancers [29]. These proportions were consistent for oropharyngeal cancers (~87% of oncogenically-active HPV-positive cancers in the meta-analysis vs 91% in our reference study). However, this proportion was more heterogeneous for other head and neck cancers: 86% of HPV-related laryngeal cancers were considered to be attributable to HPV based on p16 detection, but this number decreased to 39% when based on mRNA in the meta-analysis (vs 61% in the study we used as reference); 28% of HPV-positive oral cavity cancers were considered to be attributable to

HPV based on p16 detection, but 67% when based on mRNA in the meta-analysis (vs 59% in the reference study). It should also be noted that overall HPV DNA prevalence by subsite in the meta-analysis was higher (41.4% for oropharyngeal cancers, 20.9% for laryngeal cancers, and 17.5 for oral cavity cancers in Europe) than that observed in our reference publication (22.3% for oropharyngeal cancers, 4.8% for laryngeal cancers, and 7.8% for oral cavity cancers). Our estimated annual number of new head and neck cancers attributable to HPV should thus be considered a conservative estimate.

Some regional differences were observed in the prevalence of HPV in head and neck cancers in Europe. For example, the oncogenically-active HPV attributable fraction in oropharyngeal cancer ranged from 9.4% in Southern Europe to 50% in Northern Europe [6]. However, for the purpose of our study it was not possible to apply country-specific data, as the available data did not cover all European countries and small sample sizes would not have provided robust results.

Sex-specific data for HPV prevalence in anal cancer and head and neck cancers were available, but were not used. No sex-specific differences in HPV prevalence were seen in anal cancer (oncogenically-active HPV prevalence was 88.2 (95% CI: 76.1-95.6) in men vs 87.2 (95% CI: 79.4-92.8) in women). Even if some differences in HPV attributable fractions by sex were high in some head and neck subsites, particularly in oropharyngeal cancers (16.9% (95% CI: 14.1-20.0) in men vs 40.2% (95% CI: 31.4-49.4) in women), this was not confirmed by a recent literature review on the topic [30]. According to the analysis of Combes et al., there are regional differences in the sex-specific HPV prevalence of oropharyngeal cancers worldwide and within Europe (male:female HPV prevalence ratio <1 in France, Germany, Italy, and the Czech Republic; male:female ratio ≥1 in the Netherlands, Norway, the United Kingdom, and Sweden). Still, when considering Europe as a whole, and based on 27 studies conducted in 9 countries of the European Union with less than 200 subjects each, the male:female ratio for HPV prevalence in oropharyngeal cancers was 1.0 (0.9-1.1), and the estimated HPV prevalence in oropharyngeal cancers was 40.3 in males and 41.2 in females. In addition, that paper suggested that smoking and heavy drinking may either enhance the carcinogenic effect of HPV or hamper the accurate attribution of oropharyngeal cancers to HPV in men who have both the infection and exhibit the two lifestyle risk factors related to this disease. The sex-specific differences in HPV prevalence in oropharyngeal cancer are mainly a consequence of the vast international variation in male smoking habits. According to these results, and as the difference in the male:female ratio observed in our reference publication may be due to chance (regional representativity of participating countries), we

finally decided to use a single HPV attributable fraction for oropharyngeal cancer for males and females.

Moreover, a declining incidence of HPV-negative oropharyngeal squamous cell carcinoma is currently being observed in the United States that parallels with declines in smoking. In contrast, increasing incidence of HPV-positive OPSCCs perhaps arises from increased oral sex and oral HPV exposure over calendar time. Indeed, prevalence of genital herpes simplex virus 1 (HSV1), HSV2, and genital warts have increased among recent birth cohorts in the United States, accepted surrogates for oral sex, risky sexual behavior, and HPV exposure, respectively. The predominant rise in OPSCC incidence among the young is also consistent with changing HPV exposure among recent birth cohorts. However, the reasons for pronounced increases among men remain unexplained [31]. Therefore it is critical to understand if there is an underlying epidemic of HPV-positive head and neck cancers related to changes in sexual habits, because this could change all our forecasts of the HPV- related epidemiology of head and neck cancer.

A further limitation is represented by the fact that only one-digit ICD codes are available in the CI5 database, meaning that some of the head and neck cancer subsites could not be correctly assigned. For example C.5.1 (soft palate), C.5.2 (uvula) were classified as oral cancers and C.14.2 (Waldeyers ring) as pharyngeal cancers, but anatomically they all belong to the oropharynx.

The method used to calculate the estimated annual number of new precancerous lesions also has some limitations that were described in our previous estimation of HPV-related burden of disease [5].

To our knowledge, the data that we used for our estimation of cancers, precancerous lesions, and genital warts are the most robust data available in Europe todate. However, the results of this evaluation have to be considered with caution, as several extrapolations and assumptions were used. Future studies are necessary; mainly to further evaluate the HPV attributable fraction of head and neck cancers and the real burden of precancerous lesions of the vulva, vagina, and anus, for which no systematic screening is performed. Additionally, incidence data are completely lacking for precancerous lesions of the penis and in the head and neck area and are very scarce for RRP.

Conclusions

The burden of cancers attributable to 9-valent HPV vaccine types in Europe is substantial, both in women and men. Overall, 53,013 (95% bound: 48,160-67,171) HPV-attributable cancers were estimated to occur every year in Europe, of which more than 90%, (47,992 (95% bound: 39,785-58,511)) were estimated to be attributable to 9-valent HPV vaccine HPV types. When considering head and neck cancers in addition to anogenital cancers, about 19% of all HPV-attributable cancers are expected to occur in men, and most of these cancers are attributable to 9-valent HPV vaccine types. In addition to cancers, 232,103 to 442,347 new cases of precancerous lesions (CIN2/3, adenocarcinoma *in situ*, VIN2/3, VaIN2/3, and AIN2/3) and 680,344 to 844,391 new genital warts cases (341,397 to 459,443 in women, 338,947 to 384,948 in men) are expected to be attributable to the 9-valent HPV vaccine types each year. This data demonstrates the important preventive potential of the new 9-valent HPV vaccine in Europe.

Abbreviations
AIN2/3: Anal intraepithelial neoplasia grades 2 and 3; CI: Confidence interval; CI5: Cancer incidence in five continents; CIN2+: Cervical intraepithelial neoplasia grade 2 or worse; EMA: European Medicines Agency; HPV: Human papillomavirus; IARC: International Agency for Research on Cancer; ICD-10: International classification of diseases 10th revision; RRP: Recurrent respiratory papillomatosis; VaIN2/3: Vaginal intraepithelial neoplasia grades 2 and 3; VIN2/3: Vulvar intraepithelial neoplasia grades 2 and 3

Acknowledgements
We would like to thank Xavier Cornen for his great work on data extraction and analysis, Lamia Lafi and Remy Sirope for assistance in the preparation of the graphs, and Trudy Perdrix-Thoma for editorial assistance.

Funding
The work was funded by Sanofi Pasteur MSD.

Authors' contributions
SH contributed to the study design, literature research, data analysis, interpretation of findings, and drafting of the manuscript. JLSG contributed to the interpretation of findings. GDF contributed to the study design and interpretation of findings. LA and SDS contributed to data collection and interpretation of findings. All authors critically reviewed the manuscript and approved the final version.

Competing interests
SH and GDF are employees of Sanofi Pasteur MSD; JLSG is a member if a SPMSD board on HPV Boy's Vaccination and received occasional travel grants to attend scientific meetings from SPMSD; LA received occasional travel grants to attend scientific meetings from MSD and Sanofi Pasteur MSD; SDS received travel grants from MSD, GSK, and Qiagen and unrestricted research grants through ICO from Merck & Co. Inc. and Glaxo Smith Kline.

Author details
[1]Department of Epidemiology, Sanofi Pasteur MSD, 162 avenue Jean Jaurès, Lyon, France. [2]Department of Otolaryngology-Head and Neck Surgery, Tenon Hospital – Assistance Publique-Hopitaux de Paris (AP-HP) and Sorbonne University-Paris 6, Pierre-et-Marie Curie University Cancerology Institute, 4 rue de la Chine, 75020 Paris, France. [3]Cancer Epidemiology Research Program, Institut Català d'Oncologia (ICO)-IDIBELL, L'Hospitalet de Llobregat, Catalonia, Spain. [4]CIBER Epidemiologia y Salud Pública, Barcelona, Spain.

References
1.   Joura EA, Giuliano AR, Iversen OE, Bouchard C, Mao C, Mehlsen J, et al. A 9-valent HPV vaccine against infection and intraepithelial neoplasia in women. N Engl J Med. 2015;372:711–23.
2.   National Institutes of Health, National Cancer Institute. Gardasil 9 Vaccine Protects against Additional HPV Types. https://www.cancer.gov/types/cervical/research/gardasil9-prevents-more-HPV-types. Accessed 30 Nov 2016.
3.   Vichnin M, Bonanni P, Klein NP, Garland SM, Block SL, Kjaer SK, et al. An overview of quadrivalent human papillomavirus vaccine safety: 2006 to 2015. Pediatr Infect Dis J. 2015;34:983–91.
4.   European Medicines Agency. Annexe I. Summary of Product Characteristics. http://www.ema.europa.eu/docs/en_GB/document_library/EPAR_-_Product_Information/human/003852/WC500189111.pdf. Accessed 30 Nov 2016.
5.   Hartwig S, Baldauf JJ, Dominiak-Felden G, Simondon F, Alemany L, de Sanjose S, et al. Estimation of the epidemiological burden of HPV-related anogenital cancers, precancerous lesions, and genital warts in women and men in Europe: potential additional benefit of a nine-valent second generation HPV vaccine compared to first generation HPV vaccines. Papillomavirus Res. 2015;1:90–100.
6.   Castellsague X, Alemany L, Quer M, Halec G, Quiros B, Tous S, et al. HPV involvement in head and neck cancers: comprehensive assessment of biomarkers in 3680 patients. J Natl Cancer Inst. 2016;108:djv403.
7.   Alemany L, Cubilla A, Halec G, Kasamatsu E, Quiros B, Masferrer E, et al. Role of human papillomavirus in penile carcinomas worldwide. Eur Urol. 2016;69:953–61.
8.   International Agency for Research on Cancer. www.iarc.fr. Accessed 30 Nov 2016.
9.   IARC. Globocan 2012: Estimated cancer incidence, mortality and prevalence worldwide in 2012. Data sources and methods. http://globocan.iarc.fr/Pages/DataSource_and_methods.aspx. Accessed 30 Nov 2016.
10. Forman D, Bray F, Brewster DH, Gombe Mbalawa C, Kohler B, Piñeros M, et al. Cancer incidence in five continents, vol. X. Lyon: IARC; 2013.
11. European Commission: Eurostat homepage. http://ec.europa.eu/eurostat/data/database. Accessed 30 Nov.
12. Walboomers JM, Jacobs MV, Manos MM, Bosch FX, Kummer JA, Shah KV, et al. Human papillomavirus is a necessary cause of invasive cervical cancer worldwide. J Pathol. 1999;189:12–9.
13. de Sanjosé S, Quint WG, Alemany L, Geraets DT, Klaustermeier JE, Lloveras B, et al. Human papillomavirus genotype attribution in invasive cervical cancer: a retrospective cross-sectional worldwide study. Lancet Oncol. 2010;11:1048–56.
14. de Sanjosé S, Alemany L, Ordi J, Tous S, Alejo M, Bigby SM, et al. Worldwide human papillomavirus genotype attribution in over 2000 cases of intraepithelial and invasive lesions of the vulva. Eur J Cancer. 2013;49:3450–61.
15. Alemany L, Saunier M, Alvarado-Cabrero I, Quiros B, Salmeron J, Shin HR, et al. Human papillomavirus DNA prevalence and type distribution in anal carcinomas worldwide. Int J Cancer. 2015;136:98–107.
16. Alemany L, Saunier M, Tinoco L, Quiros B, Alvarado-Cabrero I, Alejo M, et al. Large contribution of human papillomavirus in vaginal neoplastic lesions: a worldwide study in 597 samples. Eur J Cancer. 2014;50:2846–54.
17. Nielsen A, Munk C, Kjaer SK. Trends in incidence of anal cancer and high-grade anal intraepithelial neoplasia in Denmark, 1978–2008. Int J Cancer. 2012;130:1168–73.
18. European Centers for Disease Prevention and Control. Introduction of HPV vaccines in EU countries - an update. Stockholm: European Centers for Disease Prevention and Control; 2012.
19. Lindeberg H, Elbrond O. Laryngeal papillomas: the epidemiology in a Danish subpopulation 1965–1984. Clin Otolaryngol Allied Sci. 1990;15:125–31.
20. Silverberg MJ, Thorsen P, Lindeberg H, Grant LA, Shah KV. Condyloma in pregnancy is strongly predictive of juvenile-onset recurrent respiratory papillomatosis. Obstet Gynecol. 2003;101:645–52.
21. Forman D, de MC, Lacey CJ, Soerjomataram I, Lortet-Tieulent J, Bruni L, et al. Global burden of human papillomavirus and related diseases. Vaccine. 2012; 30 Suppl 5:F12–23.
22. Habbous S, Chu KP, Qiu X, La DA, Harland LT, Fadhel E, et al. The changing incidence of human papillomavirus-associated oropharyngeal cancer using multiple imputation from 2000 to 2010 at a Comprehensive Cancer Centre. Cancer Epidemiol. 2013;37:820–9.
23. McCarthy CE, Field JK, Rajlawat BP, Field AE, Marcus MW. Trends and regional variation in the incidence of head and neck cancers in England: 2002 to 2011. Int J Oncol. 2015;47:204–10.

24. Annertz K, Anderson H, Palmer K, Wennerberg J. The increase in incidence of cancer of the tongue in the Nordic countries continues into the twenty-first century. Acta Otolaryngol. 2012;132:552–7.
25. Brewster DH, Bhatti LA. Increasing incidence of squamous cell carcinoma of the anus in Scotland, 1975–2002. Br J Cancer. 2006;95:87–90.
26. Robinson D, Coupland V, Moller H. An analysis of temporal and generational trends in the incidence of anal and other HPV-related cancers in Southeast England. Br J Cancer. 2009;100:527–31.
27. Goldman S, Glimelius B, Nilsson B, Pahlman L. Incidence of anal epidermoid carcinoma in Sweden 1970–1984. Acta Chir Scand. 1989;155:191–7.
28. Van Lieshout A, Pronk A. [Increasing incidence of anal cancer in the Netherlands]. Ned Tijdschr Geneeskd. 2010;154:A1163.
29. Ndiaye C, Mena M, Alemany L, Arbyn M, Castellsague X, Laporte L, et al. HPV DNA, E6/E7 mRNA, and p16INK4a detection in head and neck cancers: a systematic review and meta-analysis. Lancet Oncol. 2014;15:1319–31.
30. Combes JD, Chen AA, Franceschi S. Prevalence of human papillomavirus in cancer of the oropharynx by gender. Cancer Epidemiol Biomarkers Prev. 2014;23:2954–8.
31. Chaturvedi AK, Engels EA, Pfeiffer RM, Hernandez BY, Xiao W, Kim E, et al. Human papillomavirus and rising oropharyngeal cancer incidence in the United States. J Clin Oncol. 2011;29:4294–301.

17

HIV-1 matrix protein p17 and its variants promote human triple negative breast cancer cell aggressiveness

Francesca Caccuri[1]*, Francesca Giordano[2], Ines Barone[2], Pietro Mazzuca[1], Cinzia Giagulli[1], Sebastiano Andò[2], Arnaldo Caruso[1] and Stefania Marsico[2]

Abstract

Background: The introduction of cART has changed the morbidity and mortality patterns affecting HIV-infected (HIV+) individuals. The risk of breast cancer in HIV+ patients has now approached the general population risk. However, breast cancer has a more aggressive clinical course and poorer outcome in HIV+ patients than in general population, without correlation with the CD4 or virus particles count. These findings suggest a likely influence of HIV-1 proteins on breast cancer aggressiveness and progression. The HIV-1 matrix protein (p17) is expressed in different tissues and organs of successfully cART-treated patients and promotes migration of different cells. Variants of p17 (vp17s), characterized by mutations and amino acid insertions, differently from the prototype p17 (refp17), also promote B-cell proliferation and transformation.

Methods: Wound-healing assay, matrigel-based invasion assay, and anchorage-independent proliferation assay were employed to compare the biological activity exerted by refp17 and three different vp17s on the triple-negative human breast cancer cell line MDA-MB 231. Intracellular signaling was investigated by western blot analysis.

Results: Motility and invasiveness increased in cells treated with both refp17 and vp17s compared to untreated cells. The effects of the viral proteins were mediated by binding to the chemokine receptor CXCR2 and activation of the ERK1/2 signaling pathway. However, vp17s promoted MDA-MB 231 cell growth and proliferation in contrast to refp17-treated or not treated cells.

Conclusions: In the context of the emerging role of the microenvironment in promoting and supporting cancer cell growth and metastatic spreading, here we provide the first evidence that exogenous p17 may play a crucial role in sustaining breast cancer cell migration and invasiveness, whereas some p17 variants may also be involved in cancer cell growth and proliferation.

Keywords: HIV-1 matrix protein p17, p17 variants, Breast cancer, Motility, Clonogenicity, ERK1/2 signaling pathway

Background

In the era of cART, a change has emerged in the type of cancers affecting HIV-1-infected (HIV+) patients [1]. The incidence of the three classically AIDS-related cancers (Kaposi's sarcoma, non-Hodgkin lymphoma and cancer of the cervix) is greatly decreased [2], whereas recent clinical studies in the HIV+ population have shown a significant increase of some Non-AIDS Defining Cancers (NADCs) [3, 4]. including breast cancer [5, 6].

Breast cancer is the most frequently diagnosed malignancy in women and the leading cause of cancer death among females in economically developing countries [7]. In early time, the risk of breast cancer in the population with AIDS had been lower than in the general population [8, 9], with small variations in incidence relative to the CD4 count or duration of infection [10]. Today, breast cancer risk in women with AIDS has been increasing and approaching to general population risk [11–14]. More interesting, recent studies have evidenced a more aggressive clinical course, poorer outcome and younger age at diagnosis of breast cancer in the HIV-1 setting compared to general population [15–17]. These findings suggest a

---

* Correspondence: francesca.caccuri@unibs.it
[1]Section of Microbiology, Department of Molecular and Translational Medicine, University of Brescia , Brescia, Italy
Full list of author information is available at the end of the article

likely influence of HIV-1 on breast cancer progression, although the retrovirus does not show any capability to exert a direct tumorigenic effect on this cancer [15].

Numerous studies have shown a direct involvement of viral proteins in carcinogenesis [18–21]. Many viruses encode cytokine homologues that bind to host specific receptors triggering signal transduction cascades and biological responses including activation and proliferation of target cells, thus contributing directly to the cancer associated with viral infection [22]. The HIV-1 matrix protein p17 (p17) is a structural protein with a well-established role in the virus life cycle [23]. It is easily detected in the plasma and tissue specimens of HIV$^+$ patients [24, 25] even in patients under successful cART and in the absence of any in situ viral replication [26, 27]. This is not surprising since latently HIV-1-infected resting T cells are capable of producing HIV-1 proteins without supporting spreading of infection [28]. Moreover, recent data show the capability of Gag-expressing cells to release p17 in the absence of viral protease, following its cellular aspartyl proteases-dependent cleavage from the Gag precursor protein [29]. Overall, these findings indicate that p17 can be produced by cells potentially residing in different tissues and organs, even in the absence of viral replication. Extracellularly, p17 has been found to deregulate the biological activity of different cells that are directly or indirectly involved in AIDS pathogenesis [30–35]. Moreover, we have provided evidence that a p17 variant derived from a Ugandan HIV-1 strain A1 (S75X) triggers an activation of the PI3K/Akt signaling pathway in B-cells, compared to a prototype p17 isolated from clone BH10 of clade B (refp17). As a consequence, the p17 variant S75X was found to increase B-cell proliferation and clonogenicity, providing the first evidence on the existence of p17 natural variants with B-cell transforming activity [36]. More recently, p17 variants (vp17s) endowed with B-cell clonogenic activity, and characterized by amino acid insertions at the C-terminal region of the viral protein, were more frequently detected in plasma of HIV$^+$ patients with than without non-Hodgkin lymphomas (HIV-NHL) [37], focusing our attention on their potential role in lymphomagenesis.

Exogenous p17 binds to CXCR1 and CXCR2 [25, 30], two seven-transmembrane G-protein-coupled receptors for IL-8. Consequently, p17 mimics IL-8 activity on cells expressing these receptors on their surface. Breast cancer cells do express CXCR1 and CXCR2 [38], and increasing evidence indicates that IL-8 plays a critical role in enhancing the invasive and metastatic potential of breast cancer cells [39, 40]. Moreover, targeting IL-8 receptors has proven efficacious in in vivo models of breast cancer, as well as in primary invasive and metastatic breast cancer [41].

All these findings suggest a possible association between p17 and/or its variants expression in tissue microenvironment and breast cancer aggressiveness in HIV$^+$ individuals. The aim of present study was to investigate the biological activity of p17 and its variants on the triple-negative (ER$^-$, PR$^-$ and HER-2$^-$) MDA-MB 231 cells as a model of human breast cancer.

Methods

Cell line and recombinant proteins

The human breast cancer cell line, MDA-MB 231, was obtained from the American Type Culture Collection (ATCC, Manassas, VA, USA) and grown as described. Purified endotoxin (lipopolysaccharide)-free recombinant refp17 (from clone BH10 of clade B isolate) and vp17s (namely NHL-a101, NHL-a102 and NHL-a105 derived from HIV$^+$ patients with NHL) were produced as previously described [31, 37]. The absence of endotoxin contamination (< 0.25 endotoxin U/ml) in the proteins preparation was assessed by Limulus amoebocyte assay (Associates of Cape Cod Inc., East Falmouth, MA, USA).

Wound healing assay

MDA-MB 231 cells were plated into 24-well plates (10^5 cells/well) in complete medium. Confluent monolayers were nutrient starved by growing them for 24 h in medium containing 0.5% FBS and then scratched using a 200 µl pipette tip. After washing, cells were treated or not with 10 ng/ml of refp17 or vp17s in complete medium (10% FBS). When reported, starved MDA-MB 231 cells were pretreated with 2.5 µg/ml of mAb to CXCR1 (mAb 330; R&D, Minneapolis, MN, USA) or to CXCR2 (mAb 331; R&D), or with an isotype-matched mAb (2.5 µg/ml; R&D) for 1 h at 37 °C before proteins stimulation. In some experiments, MDA-MB 231 cells were serum starved for 24 h in the presence or absence of inhibitors of PI3K/Akt (LY294002) (20 µM) (ENZO Life Sciences, Farmingdale, NY, USA), Jak/STAT (AG-490) (20 µM) (Sigma-Aldrich, St. Louis, MO, USA) or MEK/ERK1/2 (PD98059) (10 µM) (Calbiochem, Billerica, MA, USA) signaling pathways. Cell migration was evaluated at different time points using an inverted microscope (DM-IRB microscope system, Leica, Buffalo Grove, IL, USA). Cells were photographed using a CCD camera (Hitachi Inc., Krefeld, Germany). Wound closure was monitored over 12 h. In some experiments, in order to count the cells migrating into the wound area or protruding from the border of the wound, cells were fixed before wound closure and stained with Comassie brilliant blue.

Invasion assay

Cell invasion assay was carried out by the Matrigel-coated transwell system as previously described [42]. Polycarbonate transwell filters (8 µm pore size, Corning, Tewksbury, MA, USA) were coated with 50 µg of Cultrex® basement membrane extract (BME; 10 mg/ml; Trevigen, Gaithersburg, MD, USA) diluted in a total volume of 150 µl of serum-free medium. Then the trans-wells were placed in a 24 well/plate. Cells were seeded into the coated filter at a concentration of 10^4 cells/well. Six hundred µl of medium containing or not 200 ng/ml of refp17 or vp17s were added into the lower chamber. The plate was incubated at 37 °C and after 48 h of incubation, cells that had crossed the filter were fixed, stained with Coomassie brilliant blue and counted. The percentage of invasion was calculated as follow: number of cells invading through Matrigel coated membrane/total number of seeded cells × 100.

Western blot analysis

MDA-MB 231 cells were nutrient starved for 24 h and treated for 30 min with refp17 or vp17s at concentrations ranging from 50 to 200 ng/ml. When indicated, MDA-MB 231 cells were nutrient starved for 24 h in the presence or absence of PD98059 (10 µM) to inhibit the MEK/ERK1/2 signaling pathway. Cells were then lysed in 200 µl of lysis buffer [50 mM HEPES (pH 7.5), 150 mM NaCl, 1.5 mM $MgCl_2$, 1 mM EGTA, 10% glycerol, 1% Triton X-100, protease inhibitors (Sigma-Aldrich)]. Equal amounts of total proteins were resolved on a 11% SDS-polyacrylamide gel and then blotted onto a nitrocellulose membrane. The blots were incubated overnight at 4 °C with rabbit polyclonal antibodies to pAkt (Ser473), Akt (Cell Signaling, Danvers, MA, USA), pSTAT3 (Tyr705), STAT3 (Cell Signaling), ERK1/2 (Santa Cruz Biotechnology, Inc., Santa Cruz, CA) or a mouse monoclonal antibody to pERK (Thr202, Tyr204) (Santa Cruz Biotechnology, Inc.). The antigen-antibody complex was detected by incubation of the membranes for 1 h at room temperature with peroxidase-conjugated goat anti-rabbit IgG or goat anti-mouse IgG (Thermo Scientific, Waltham, MA, USA) and revealed using the Enhanced Chemiluminescence System (ECL System, Santa Cruz Biotechnology, Inc.).

MTT assays

Cell viability was evaluated with the MTT assay (Sigma-Aldrich). MDA-MB 231 cells were seeded in 24-well plates at a density of 2×10^4/well and then treated with refp17 or vp17s, at the indicated concentrations, in phenol red-free medium containing 5% cs-FBS. Forty-eight h after the beginning of proteins stimulation, 100 µl of the MTT stock solution (2 mg/ml) were added to each well and the plate was incubated for 2 h at 37 °C. The medium was then removed and cell lysis was carried out by adding 500 µl of DMSO (Sigma-Aldrich) and shaking the plates for 15 min on an orbital shaker. The absorbance was measured at 570 nm using the Beckman Coulter Spectrophotometer (Brea, CA, USA).

Soft agar anchorage-independent growth assay

MDA-MB 231 cells (3×10^4/well) were plated in 12-well plates in 2 ml of phenol red-free medium containing 0.35% Sea-Plaque agarose (Lonza, Amboise, France) and 5% cs-FBS, over a 0.7% agarose base. One day after plating, medium containing or not viral proteins was added to the top of the layer and replaced every 4 days. After

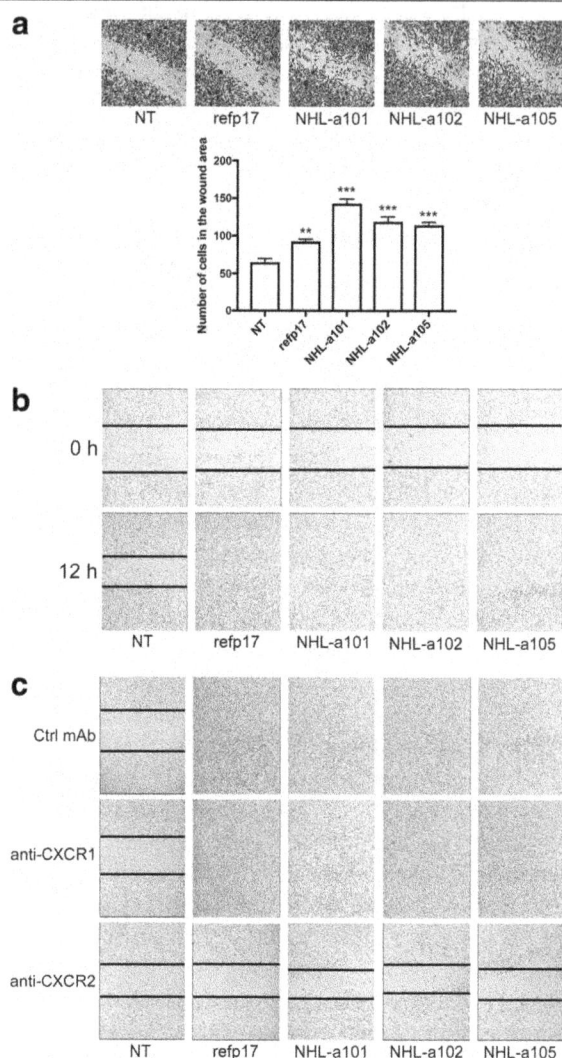

Fig. 1 Refp17 and vp17s promote breast cancer cells migration. In the wound-healing assay, confluent MDA-MB 231 cell monolayers were serum starved for 24 h and then scratched using a 200 µl pipette tip. Cells were cultured in complete medium either unsupplemented or containing 10 ng/ml of refp17 or vp17s. **a** After 6 h of culture cells were fixed and stained with Coomassie brilliant blue. The cells migrated into the wound area were counted. **b** The percentage of wound healing was observed over a period of 12 h. **c** Wound healing assay was performed pretreating MDA-MB 231 cells for 1 h with a neutralizing mAb to CXCR1 (2.5 µg/ml), CXCR2 (2.5 µg/ml), or with an isotype-matched mAb (Ctrl mAb; 2.5 µg/ml). Images are representative of three independent experiments with similar results (original magnification 10×). Statistical analysis was performed by one-way ANOVA and the Bonferroni's post–test was used to compare data (** $p < 0.01$, *** $p < 0.001$)

15 days, 300 μl of MTT (Sigma-Aldrich) were added to each well and allowed to incubate for 4 h at 37 °C. Plates were then placed overnight at 4 °C, and colonies >50 μm diameter were counted.

Statistics

Data obtained from multiple independent experiments are expressed as the mean ± standard deviations (SDs). The data were analyzed for statistical significance by one-way or two-way ANOVA, when appropriate. Bonferroni's post-test was used to compare data. Differences were considered significant at a P value of <0.05. Statistical tests were performed using Prism 5 software (GraphPad).

Results

Refp17 and its variants increase MDA-MB 231 cell migration

The ability of refp17 and vp17s to promote the migratory activity of MDA-MB 231 cells was assessed by wound healing assay. This method allows us to investigate the ability of viral proteins to modulate cell migration by sealing a confluent cell monolayer after mechanical injury. MDA-MB 231 cells were grown into 24-well plates and starved for 24 h. Confluent monolayers were scratched with a pipette tip and the percentage of wound healing was observed over a period of 12 h. The number of MDA-MB 231 cells in the wound area increased more quickly (Fig. 1a) and the wound area decreased more rapidly (Fig. 1b) in refp17- and vp17s-treated cells as compared to control cells. As shown in

Fig. 1b, not treated (NT) MDA-MB 231 cells reached approximately 53% healing (range from 48 to 58%) after 12 h of culture, whereas at the same time cells treated with refp17 or with its variants NHL-a101, NHL-a102 or NHL-a105 reached 100% healing, showing a strong improvement in wound repair ability. To clarify the involvement of the known p17 receptors CXCR1 and CXCR2 in viral proteins-induced MDA-MB 231 cell motility, monolayers were pretreated for 1 h with 2.5 μg/ml of neutralizing mAb to CXCR1, CXCR2, or with 2.5 μg/ml of an isotype-matched mAb (Ctrl mAb). Immediately after pretreatment, confluent monolayers were scratched with a pipette tip and cultured for 12 h with or without 10 ng/ml of refp17, NHL-a101, NHL-a102 or NHL-a105. As shown in Fig. 1c, MDA-MB 231 cells pretreated with the isotype-matched mAb and then treated with viral proteins reached 100% of wound healing after 12 h of culture. Similar results were obtained when cells were pretreated with the neutralizing mAb to CXCR1, whereas pretreatment of cells with the neutralizing mAb to CXCR2 strongly inhibited cell migration promoted by all viral proteins. This finding suggests that refp17 and vp17s utilize CXCR2 to trigger breast cancer cell motility.

Both refp17 and vp17s promote breast cancer cell invasion

The metastatic potential of tumor cells is largely dependent on their ability to degrade and migrate through the extracellular matrix. Therefore we also evaluated the effect of refp17 and vp17s on the migratory capacity of

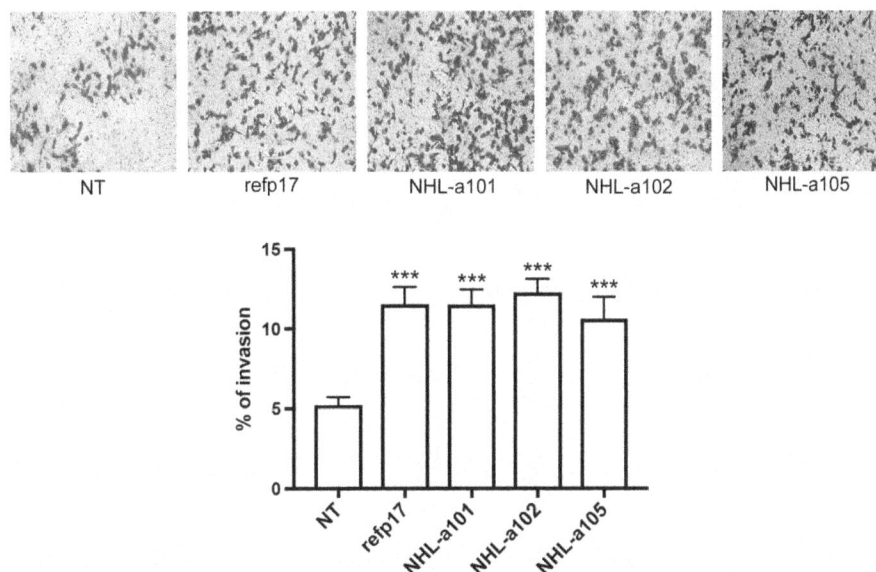

Fig. 2 Refp17 and vp17s increase breast cancer cell invasion. Cell invasion assay was performed by matrigel-coated transwell system. Cells were resuspended in a serum-free medium and seeded in the upper chamber. Medium supplemented with 200 ng/ml of refp17 or vp17s was used as chemoattractant factor in the lower chamber. After 48 h of culture, migrated cells were stained, photographed and counted (original magnification 10×). Data represent the average of three independent experiments performed in triplicate. Images are representative of three independent experiments with similar results. Statistical analysis was performed by one-way ANOVA, and the Bonferroni post-test was used to compare data (*** $P < 0.001$)

breast cancer cells using the Matrigel-based invasion assay. As shown in Fig. 2 (upper panel), invasion of MDA-MB 231 cells strongly increased upon viral proteins stimulation as compared to NT cells. Quantitative analysis showed that only 5.2% of NT cells were able to invade the matrigel and the filter compared to 11.7, 11.5, 12.2 and 10.6% of cells stimulated with refp17, NHL-a101, NHL-a102 and NHL-a105, respectively (Fig. 2, lower panel). This result suggests that MDA-MB 231 cells treated with refp17 and vp17s have a much higher invasive potential than control cells.

Both refp17 and vp17s promote breast cancer cell migration through modulation of the ERK1/2 signaling pathway

Western blot analyses were performed to determine whether refp17 and vp17s effects on MDA-MB 231 cells were mediated by modulation of signaling pathways usually involving tumor cell motility and invasion. We investigate the ability of refp17 and its variants to modify the phosphorylation status of Akt, STAT3 and ERK1/2 of MDA-MB 231 cells. As shown in Fig. 3, breast cancer cells stimulated with refp17 or vp17s showed a significant activation of ERK1/2 compared to NT cells, as evidenced by up-regulation of phosphorylated ERK1/2. On the other hand, all viral proteins did not exert any effect on the phosphorylation status of STAT3, indicating that this pathway is not involved in refp17 and vp17s activity on MDA-MB 231 cells. Surprisingly, inhibition of Akt activation occurred upon stimulation of tumor cells with both refp17 and vp17s. Altogether, our findings are consistent with a potential link between increase of migration and invasion of refp17 and its variants and modulation of ERK1/2 and Akt pathways.

Refp17 and vp17s breast cancer cells promoting activity is specifically mediated by ERK1/2

To investigate further whether ERK1/2 pathway plays a role in refp17- and vp17s-induced migration activity, MDA-MB 231 cells were serum-starved for 24 h in the presence or absence of an optimal concentration of the inhibitors of PI3K/Akt (LY294002; 20 μM), Jak/STAT (AG-490; 20 μM) and MEK/ERK (PD98059; 10 μM). Then, confluent cell monolayers were scratched and incubated with the viral proteins for 6 h at 37 °C. As shown in Fig. 4a, cell migration in refp17- and vp17s-stimulated MDA-MB

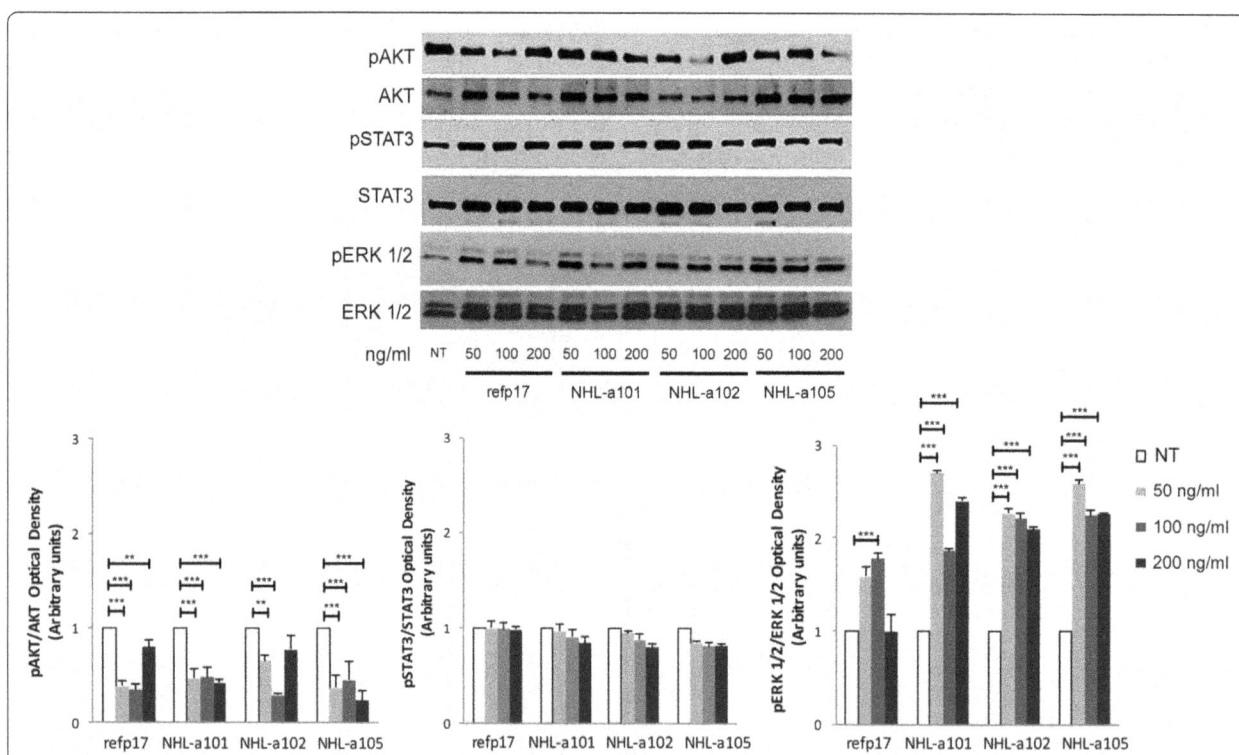

Fig. 3 Effects of refp17 and vp17s on Akt, STAT3 and ERK1/2 activity in MDA-MB 231 cells. Cells were treated or not (NT) for 30 min with 50, 100 and 200 ng/ml of refp17 or vp17s and then lysed. Equal amounts of total cellular extracts were analyzed for expression of pAkt, Akt, pSTAT3, STAT3, pERK1/2 or ERK1/2 by western blot analysis using mAbs to pAkt (Ser473), Akt, pSTAT3 (Tyr705), STAT3, pERK1/2 (Thr202, Tyr204) or ERK1/2 as specific reagents. Phosphorylation of Akt, STAT3 and ERK1/2 was verified by densiometric analysis and plotting of the pAkt/Akt, pSTAT3/STAT3 and pERK1/2/ERK1/2. Upper panel, Blots from one representative experiment of three with similar results are shown. Lower panel, Values reported for Akt, STAT3 and ERK1/2 are the mean ± SD of three independent experiments. Statistical analysis was performed by one-way ANOVA, and the Bonferroni post-test was used to compare data (** $p < 0.01$, *** $p < 0.001$).

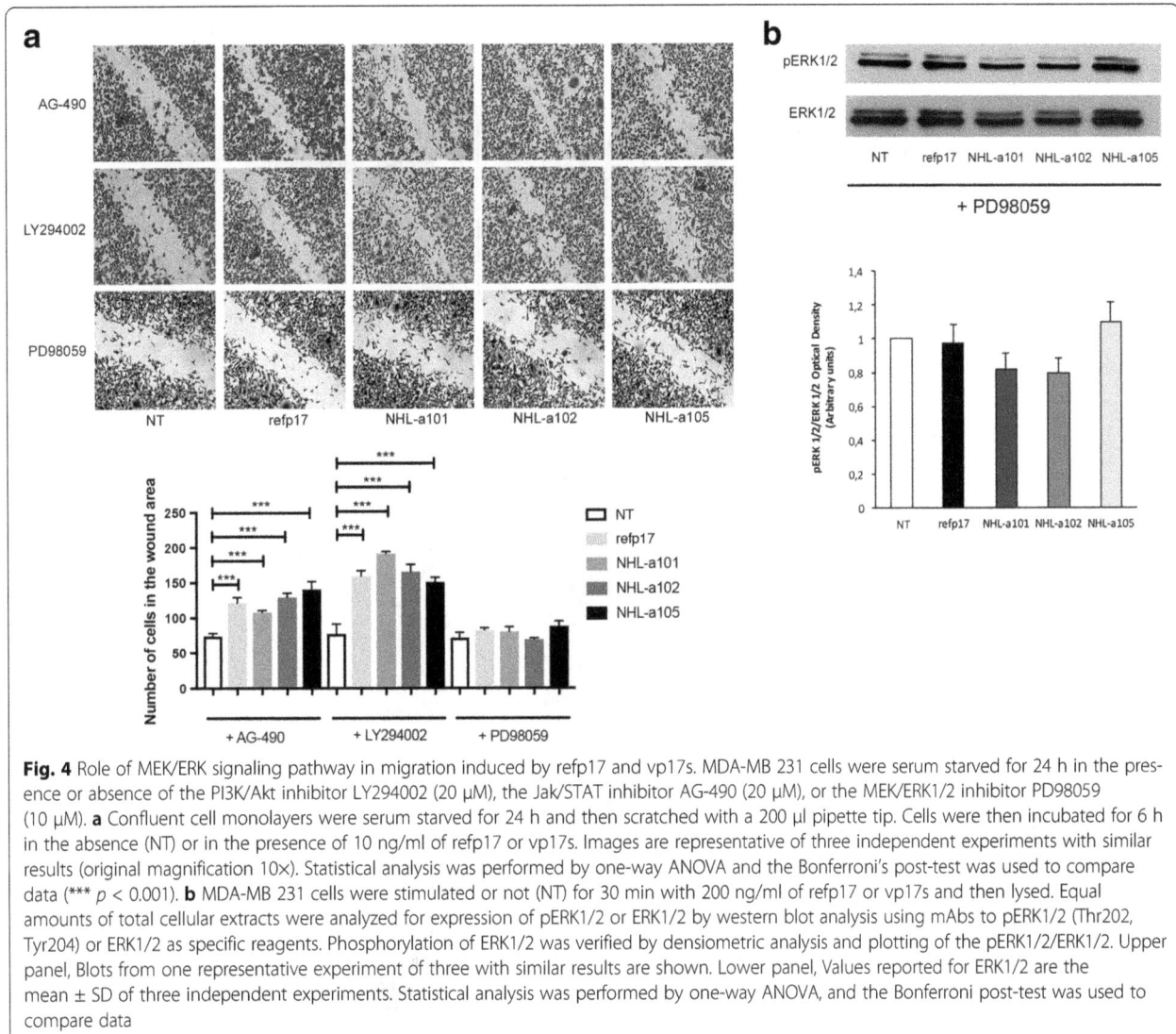

Fig. 4 Role of MEK/ERK signaling pathway in migration induced by refp17 and vp17s. MDA-MB 231 cells were serum starved for 24 h in the presence or absence of the PI3K/Akt inhibitor LY294002 (20 μM), the Jak/STAT inhibitor AG-490 (20 μM), or the MEK/ERK1/2 inhibitor PD98059 (10 μM). **a** Confluent cell monolayers were serum starved for 24 h and then scratched with a 200 μl pipette tip. Cells were then incubated for 6 h in the absence (NT) or in the presence of 10 ng/ml of refp17 or vp17s. Images are representative of three independent experiments with similar results (original magnification 10×). Statistical analysis was performed by one-way ANOVA and the Bonferroni's post-test was used to compare data (*** $p < 0.001$). **b** MDA-MB 231 cells were stimulated or not (NT) for 30 min with 200 ng/ml of refp17 or vp17s and then lysed. Equal amounts of total cellular extracts were analyzed for expression of pERK1/2 or ERK1/2 by western blot analysis using mAbs to pERK1/2 (Thr202, Tyr204) or ERK1/2 as specific reagents. Phosphorylation of ERK1/2 was verified by densiometric analysis and plotting of the pERK1/2/ERK1/2. Upper panel, Blots from one representative experiment of three with similar results are shown. Lower panel, Values reported for ERK1/2 are the mean ± SD of three independent experiments. Statistical analysis was performed by one-way ANOVA, and the Bonferroni post-test was used to compare data

231 cells was significantly inhibited by PD98059. At the same time, the viral proteins activity on MDA-MB 231 cell migration was not affected by LY294002 and AG-490. To confirm this evidence, we analyzed cells lysates of cells pretreated with PD98059 and then stimulated for 30 min with the viral proteins. As shown in Fig. 4b the activation of ERK1/2, previously observed upon viral proteins stimulation, was completely abolished in cells pretreated with the MEK/ERK inhibitor. Our results suggest that MEK/ERK1/2 pathway is required and critical for refp17 and vp17s-induced MDA-MB 231 cell migration.

Vp17s, but not refp17, promote cancer anchorage-independent growth

The effect of refp17 and vp17s on cell viability, was assessed by MTT assay. As shown in Fig. 5a, the treatment with the viral proteins for 48 h did not induced any toxic effect on MDA-MB 231 cells at any tested dose. The viral proteins were then investigated for their ability to enhance clonogenic activity of MDA-MB 231 cells. As shown in Fig. 5b, the vp17s NHL-a101, NHL-a102 and NHL-a105, at concentration ranging from 50 to 200 ng/ml, significantly increased the number of breast cancer cell colonies in soft agar, compared with NT cells. By contrast, refp17 significantly inhibited the colony-forming ability of breast cancer cells compared to NT cultures. These data indicate that the viral proteins treatment is not toxic for the MDA-MB 231 cells and, in agreement with previous results [36], underline the opposite effects of refp17 and vp17s in modulating MDA-MB 231 cell growth and clonogenicity.

Discussion

The epidemiology of breast cancer in HIV+ women is rapidly changing. In the era of cART, the breast cancer

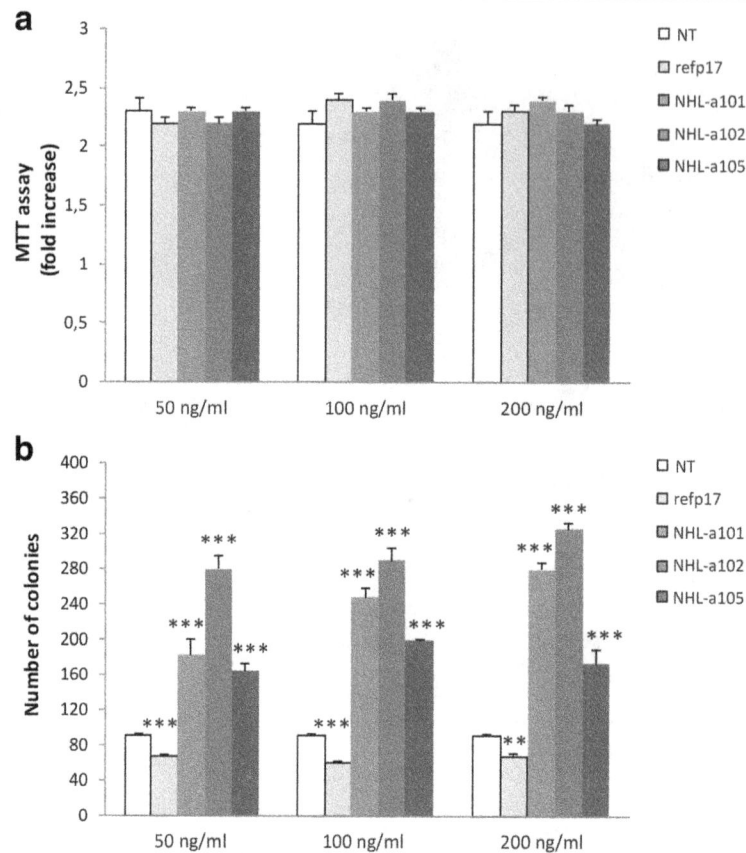

Fig. 5 Effects of refp17 and vp17s on viability and colony-forming capacity of MDA-MB 231 cells. **a** MTT assay was used to determine the viability of MDA-MB 231 cells treated or not for 48 h with refp17 or vp17s as indicated. Data represent the average of three independent experiments performed in triplicate. Statistical analysis was performed by one-way ANOVA, and the Bonferroni post-test was used to compare data. **b** The effect of refp17 and vp17s on breast cancer cells clonogenicity was analyzed by soft agar assay. Cells were plated in six-well plate and, after two days, the medium was replaced using fresh medium with various concentration of refp17 or vp17s (range from 50 to 200 ng/ml). Not treated cells (NT) were used as a negative control. Data represent the average number of colonies ± SD from three independent experiments performed in triplicate. The statistical significance between control and treated cultures was calculated using two-way ANOVA, and the Bonferroni post-test was used to compare data (** $p < 0.01$, *** $p < 0.001$)

incidence in HIV$^+$ women approaches the general female population [11–14] but a younger median age is observed in HIV$^+$ women compared to general population at the time of breast cancer diagnosis [17]. Furthermore, recent studies highlight a strong relationship between HIV-1 infection and stage of breast cancer at diagnosis: more HIV$^+$ women show an advanced tumor stage than general population [17], and this occurs in the absence of any association with viral load or CD4$^+$ T cell count [13, 14]. These findings show that different factors from immunodeficiency are likely candidates to contribute to breast cancer pathogenesis in HIV$^+$ patients and point to the importance of further research into breast cancer in the HIV-1 setting. A key role of HIV-1 proteins is emerging in different pathologies, including cancer [43] so that it is likely to hypothesize their contribution to breast cancer aggressiveness and spreading.

Recent studies highlighted a key role of p17 in lymphoma development [44]. In particular, p17 expression in

different tissues and organs and its known capability of promoting angiogenesis and lymphangiogenesis by activating an autophagy-based pathway [45] has been linked to processes of tumor growth and metastasis [43]. Moreover, vp17s endowed with a potent B-cell growth promoting and transforming activity have been detected in plasma and PBMCs of HIV$^+$ patients with NHL [37, 46].

Data presented in this study show that both refp17 and some vp17s isolated from plasma of HIV$^+$ patients with NHL strongly enhance MDA-MB 231 cell migration and invasiveness. The most aggressive breast cancer cell behavior was mediated by MAPK pathway activation following viral proteins interaction with CXCR2. In fact, the phosphorylation status of ERK1/2 increased in MDA-MB 231 cells treated with either refp17 or vp17s, whereas the specific ERK-dependent pathway inhibitor PD98059, targeting the upstream kinase MEK1, strongly impaired the p17-driven cell migratory activity. Our data are in agreement with previous studies showing that activation of the ERK1/2 pathway promotes cell motility [47] and invasiveness [48]. In addition, they show a quite similar biological activity between refp17 and vp17s with IL-8 in promoting MDA-MB 231 cell invasiveness. In fact, also IL-8 exerts its activity on the triple negative cancer cell line by activating the MEK/ERK signaling pathway following its interaction with CXCR1 and CXCR2 [49].

The one striking difference between refp17 and vp17s resides in the clonogenic activity exerted on MDA-MB 231 by vp17s only. In previous reports, a marked activation of the Akt signaling pathway was found to be promoted by vp17s – but not by refp17 – on B-cell lymphoma cells [36, 37]. In this study, both refp17 and vp17s showed a dramatic down-modulation of the Akt signaling pathway in MDA-MB 231 cells. At the same time, refp17 and vp17s did not show any STAT3 activation but all were effective in activating ERK1/2 compared to untreated cells. This suggests the presence of unidentified mechanisms at work for vp17s in promoting breast cancer cell clonogenicity. It is worth noting that all vp17s endowed with B-cell and breast cancer cell clonogenic activity are misfolded, compared to refp17 [37, 50]. Therefore, it is likely to hypothesize the presence of a specific epitope(s) involved in tumor cell clonogenic activity, which is exposed in vp17s and masked in refp17, and possibly binding to an alternate receptor(s). Further studies are needed to address this crucial question. Interestingly, although misfolded, vp17s were found to exert a refp17-like angiogenic and lymphangiogenic activity in vitro and in vivo [36, 45, 51]. Collectively, all this evidence corroborates the hypothesis that vp17s, because of their peculiar biological properties on both breast cancer cells and endothelial cells, are the most favorable microenvironmental proteins to promote breast cancer aggressiveness and spreading in HIV$^+$ patients.

Conclusion

Although limited to one single cell line here we provide the first evidence that refp17 and vp17s may play a key role in promoting human breast cancer cell migration and invasion, whereas vp17s may also affect breast cancer cell growth and transformation. Therefore, targeting p17 by specific neutralizing antibodies [52] or drugs [53] may be beneficial for treatment and better prognosis of breast cancer in the HIV-1 setting.

Abbreviations

AIDS: Acquired immunodeficiency syndrome; Akt: Serine/threonine protein kinase; cART: Combined antiretroviral therapy; cs-FBS: Charcoal stripped-fetal bovine serum; CXCR1-2: C-X-C motif chemokine receptor 1-2; DMSO: Dimethyl sulfoxide; EGTA: Ethylene glycol-bis(β-aminoethyl ether)-N,N,N',N'-tetraacetic acid; ER: Estrogen receptor; ERK: Extracellular signal-regulated kinase; FBS: Fetal bovine serum; Gag: Group-specific antigen; HEPES: 4-(2-hydroxyethyl)-1-piperazineethanesulfonic acid; HER2: Human epidermal growth factor receptor; HIV-1: Human immune deficiency virus type 1; IL-8: Interleukin-8; Jak: Janus kinase; mAb: Monoclonal antibody; MAPK: Mitogen-activated protein kinases; MTT: 3-(4,5-dimethylthiazol-2-yl)-2,5-diphenyltetrazolium; PI3K: Phosphatidylinositol-4,5-bisphosphate 3-kinase; PR: Progesterone receptor; STAT: Signal transducer and activator of transcription

Acknowledgements
The authors wish to thank Marta Comini and Sara Roversi for excellent technical assistance.

Funding
Not applicable.

Authors' contributions
AC, SA, SM designed and supervised the experiments. FC, SA, AC and SM wrote the manuscript. FC and PM performed wound healing assays. FG performed the MTT assay. FG and IB performed western blot analyses. PM prepared and purified the recombinant proteins. CG performed the soft agar assay. AC and SM analyzed and interpreted the data. All authors read and approved the final manuscript.

Competing interests
The authors declare that they have no competing interests.

Author details
[1]Section of Microbiology, Department of Molecular and Translational Medicine, University of Brescia , Brescia, Italy. [2]Department of Pharmacy, Health and Nutritional Sciences, University of Calabria, Arcavacata di Rende, Italy.

References

1. Pantanowitz L, Dezube BJ. Evolving spectrum and incidence of non-AIDS-defining malignancies. Curr Opin HIV AIDS. 2009;4:27–34.
2. Crum-Cianflone N, Hullsiek KH, Marconi V, Weintrob A, Ganesan A, Barthel RV, Fraser S, Agan BK, Wegner S. Trends in the incidence of cancers among HIV-infected persons and the impact of antiretroviral therapy: a 20-year cohort study. AIDS. 2009;23:41–50.
3. Engels EA, Biggar RJ, Hall HI, Cross H, Crutchfield A, Finch JL, Grigg R, Hylton T, Pawlish KS, McNeel TS, et al. Cancer risk in people infected with human immunodeficiency virus in the United States. Int J Cancer. 2008;123:187–94.
4. Engels EA. Non-AIDS-defining malignancies in HIV-infected persons: etiologic puzzles, epidemiologic perils, prevention opportunities. AIDS. 2009;23:875–85.
5. Shiels MS, Pfeiffer RM, Gail MH, Hall HI, Li J, Chaturvedi AK, Bhatia K, Uldrick TS, Yarchoan R, Goedert JJ, et al. Cancer burden in the HIV-infected population in the United States. J Natl Cancer Inst. 2011;103:753–62.
6. Kiertiburanakul S, Likhitpongwit S, Ratanasiri S, Sungkanuparph S. Malignancies in HIV-infected Thai patients. HIV Med. 2007;8:322–3.
7. Jemal A, Bray F, Center MM, Ferlay J, Ward E, Forman D. Global cancer statistics. CA Cancer J Clin. 2011;61:69–90.
8. Frisch M, Biggar RJ, Engels EA, Goedert JJ. Association of cancer with AIDS-related immunosuppression in adults. JAMA. 2001;285:1736–45.
9. Goedert JJ, Cote TR, Virgo P, Scoppa SM, Kingma DW, Gail MH, Jaffe ES, Biggar RJ. Spectrum of AIDS-associated malignant disorders. Lancet. 1998;351:1833–9.
10. Goedert JJ, Schairer C, McNeel TS, Hessol NA, Rabkin CS, Engels EA. Risk of breast, ovary, and uterine corpus cancers among 85,268 women with AIDS. Br J Cancer. 2006;95:642–8.
11. Patel P, Hanson DL, Sullivan PS, Patel P, Hanson DL, Sullivan PS, Novak RM, Moorman AC, Tong TC, Holmberg SD, Brooks JT, Adult and Adolescent Spectrum of Disease Project and HIV Outpatient Study Investigators.

Incidence of types of cancer among HIV infected persons compared with the general population in the United States, 1992-2003. Ann Intern Med. 2008;148:728–36.

12. Spano JP, Lanoy E, Mounier N, Katlama C, Costagliola D, Heard I. Breast cancer among HIV infected individuals from the ONCOVIH study, in France: therapeutic implications. Eur J Cancer. 2012;48:3335–41.

13. Cubasch H, Joffe M, Hanisch R, Schuz J, Neugut AI, Karstaedt A, Broeze N, van den Berg E, McCormack V, Jacobson JS. Breast cancer characteristics and HIV among 1,092 women in Soweto, South Africa. Breast Cancer Res Treat. 2013;140:177–86.

14. Shaaban HS, Modi Y, Guron G. Is there an association between human immunodeficiency virus infection and breast cancer? Med Oncol. 2012;29:446–7.

15. Voutsadakis IA, Silverman LR. Breast cancer in HIV-positive women: a report of four cases and review of the literature. Cancer Invest. 2002;20:452–7.

16. Gomez A, Montero AJ, Hurley J. Clinical outcomes in breast cancer patients with HIV/AIDS: a retrospective study. Breast Cancer Res Treat. 2015;149:781–8.

17. Pantanowitz L, Connolly JL. Pathology of the breast associated with HIV/AIDS. Breast J. 2002;8:234–43.

18. Dawson CW, Laverick L, Morris MA, Tramoutanis G, Young LS. Epstein–Barr virus-encoded LMP1 regulates epithelial cell motility and invasion via the ERK-MAPK pathway. J Virol. 2008;82:3654–64.

19. Mesri EA, Feitelson MA, Munger K. Human viral oncogenesis: a cancer hallmarks analysis. Cell Host Microbe. 2014;15:266–82.

20. Yoshida T, Hanada T, Tokuhisa T, Kosai K, Sata M, Kohara M, Yoshimura A. Activation of STAT3 by the hepatitis C virus core protein leads to cellular transformation. J Exp Med. 2002;196:641–53.

21. Ringelhan M, Protzer U. Oncogenic potential of hepatitis B virus encoded proteins. Curr Opin Virol. 2015;14:109–15.

22. Alcami A. Viral mimicry of cytokines, chemokines and their receptors. Nat Rev Immunol. 2003;3:36–50.

23. Fiorentini S, Marini E, Caracciolo S, Caruso A. Functions of the HIV-1 matrix protein p17. New Microbiol. 2006;29:1–10.

24. Fiorentini S, Riboldi E, Facchetti F, Avolio M, Fabbri M, Tosti G, Becker PD, Guzman CA, Sozzani S, Caruso A. HIV-1 matrix protein p17 induces human plasmacytoid dendritic cells to acquire a migratory immature cell phenotype. Proc Natl Acad Sci U S A. 2008;105:3867–72.

25. Caccuri F, Giagulli C, Bugatti A, Benetti A, Alessandri G, Ribatti D, Marsico S, Apostoli P, Slevin MA, Rusnati M, et al. HIV-1 matrix protein p17 promotes angiogenesis via chemokine receptors CXCR1 and CXCR2. Proc Natl Acad Sci U S A. 2012;109:14580–5.

26. Popovic M, Tenner-Racz K, Pelser C, Stellbrink HJ, van Lunzen J, Lewis G, Kalyaraman VS, Gallo RC, Racz P. Persistence of HIV-1 structural proteins and glycoproteins in lymph nodes of patients under highly active antiretroviral therapy. Proc Natl Acad Sci U S A. 2005;102:14807–12.

27. Dolcetti R, Gloghini A, Caruso A, Carbone A. A lymphomagenic role for HIV beyond immune suppression? Blood. 2016;127:1403–9.

28. Pace MJ, Graf EH, Agosto LM, Mexas AM, Male F, Brady T, Bushman FD, O'Doherty U. Directly infected resting CD4+ T cells can produce gag without spreading infection in a model of HIV latency. PLoS Pathog. 2012;8:e1002818.

29. Caccuri F, Iaria ML, Campilongo F, Varney K, Rossi A, Mitola S, Schiarea S, Bugatti A, Mazzuca P, Giagulli C, et al. Cellular aspartyl proteases promote the unconventional secretion of biologically active HIV-1 matrix protein p17. Sci Rep. 2016;6:38027.

30. Giagulli C, Magiera AK, Bugatti A, Caccuri F, Marsico S, Rusnati M, Vermi W, Fiorentini S, Caruso A. HIV-1 matrix protein p17 binds to the IL-8 receptor CXCR1 and shows IL-8-like chemokine activity on monocytes through rho/ROCK activation. Blood. 2012;119:2274–83.

31. De Francesco MA, Baronio M, Fiorentini S, Signorini C, Bonfanti C, Poiesi C, Popovic M, Grassi M, Garrafa E, Bozzo L, et al. HIV-1 matrix protein p17 increases the production of proinflammatory cytokines and counteracts IL-4 activity by binding to a cellular receptor. Proc Natl Acad Sci U S A. 2002;99:9972–7.

32. Vitale M, Caruso A, De Francesco MA, Rodella L, Bozzo L, Garrafa E, Grassi M, Gobbi G, Cacchioli A, Fiorentini S. HIV-1 matrix protein p17 enhances the proliferative activity of natural killer cells and increases their ability to secrete proinflammatory cytokines. Br J Haematol. 2003;120:337–43.

33. Marini E, Tiberio L, Caracciolo S, Tosti G, Guzman CA, Schiaffonati L, Fiorentini S, Caruso A. HIV-1 matrix protein p17 binds to monocytes and selectively stimulates MCP-1 secretion: role of transcriptional factor AP-1. Cell Microbiol. 2008;10:655–66.

34. Caccuri F, Rueckert C, Giagulli C, Schulze K, Basta D, Zicari S, Marsico S, Cervi E, Fiorentini S, Slevin M, et al. HIV-1 matrix protein p17 promotes

35. Fiorentini S, Giagulli C, Caccuri F, Magiera AK, Caruso A. HIV-1 matrix protein p17: a candidate antigen for therapeutic vaccines against AIDS. Pharmacol Ther. 2010;128:433–44.

36. Giagulli C, Marsico S, Magiera AK, Bruno R, Caccuri F, Barone I, Fiorentini S, Andò S, Caruso A. Opposite effects of HIV-1 p17 variants on PTEN activation and cell growth in B cells. PLoS One. 2011;6:e17831.

37. Dolcetti R, Giagulli C, He W, Selleri M, Caccuri F, Eyzaguirre LM, Mazzuca P, Corbellini S, Campilongo F, Marsico S, et al. Role of HIV-1 matrix protein p17 variants in lymphoma pathogenesis. Proc Natl Acad Sci U S A. 2015;112:14331–6.

38. Miller LJ, Kurtzman SH, Wang Y, Anderson KH, Lindquist RR, Kreutzer DL. Expression of interleukin-8 receptors on tumor cells and vascular endothelial cells in human breast cancer tissue. Anticancer Res. 1998;18:77–81.

39. Singh JK, Simoes B, Howell SJ, Farnie G, Clarke RB. Recent advances reveal IL-8 signaling as a potential key targeting breast cancer stem cells. Breast Cancer Res. 2013;15:210.

40. Wu K, Katiyar S, Li A, Liu M, Ju X, Popov VM, Jiao X, Lisanti MP, Casola A, Prestell RG. Dachshund inhibits oncogene-induced breast cancer cellular migration and invasion through suppression of interleukin-8. Proc Natl Acad Sci U S A. 2008;105:6924–9.

41. Ginestier C, Kiu S, Diebel ME, Korkaya H, Luo M, Brown M, Wicinski J, Cabaud O, Charafe-Jauffret E, Bimbaum D, et al. CXCR1 blockade selectively targets human breast cancer cells in vitro and in xenografts. J Clin Invest. 2010;120:485–97.

42. Caccuri F, Ronca R, Laimbacher AS, Berenzi A, Steimberg N, Campilongo F, Mazzuca P, Giacomini A, Mazzoleni G, Benetti A, et al. U94 of human herpesvirus 6 down-modulates Src, promotes a partial mesenchymal-to-epithelial transition and inhibits tumor cell growth, invasion and metastasis. Oncotarget. 2017; 10.18632/oncotarget.17817.

43. Carroll VA, Lafferty MK, Marchionni L, Bryant JL, Gallo RC, Garzino-Demo A. Expression of HIV-1 matrix protein p17 and association with B-cell lymphoma in HIV-1 transgenic mice. Proc Natl Acad Sci U S A. 2016;113:13168–73.

44. Mazzuca P, Marsico S, Schulze K, Mitola S, Pils MC, Giagulli C, Guzman CA, Caruso A, Caccuri F. Role of autophagy in the HIV-1 matrix protein p17-driven lymphangiogenesis. J Virol. 2017; 10.1128/JVI.00801-17.

45. Mazzuca P, Caruso A, Caccuri F. HIV-1 infection, microenvironment and endothelial cell dysfunction. New Microbiol. 2016;39:163–73.

46. Selleri M, Dolcetti R, Caccuri F, Giombini E, Rozera G, Abbate I, Mammone A, Zanussi S, Martorelli D, Fiorentini S, et al. In-depth analysis of compartimentalization of HIV-1 matrix protein p17 in PBMC and plasma. New Microbiol. 2017;40:58–61.

47. Joslin EJ, Opresko LK, Wells A, Wiley HS, Lauffenburger DA. EGF-receptor-mediated mammary epithelial cell migration is driven by sustained ERK signalling from autocrine stimulation. J Cell Sci. 2007;120:3688–99.

48. Price DJ, Avraham S, Feuerstein J, Fu Y, Avraham HK. The invasive phenotype in HMT-3522 cells requires increased EGF receptor signaling through both PI 3-kinase and ERK 1,2 pathways. Cell Commun Adhes. 2002;9:87–102.

49. Kim S, Lee J, Jeon M, Lee JE, Nam SJ. MEK-dependent IL-8 induction regulates the invasiveness of triple-negative breast cancer cells. Tumor Biol. 2016;37:4991–9.

50. Caccuri F, Giagulli C, Reichelt J, Martorelli D, Marsico S, Bugatti A, Barone I, Rusnati M, Guzman CA, Dolcetti R, et al. Simian immunodeficiency virus and human immunodeficiency virus type 1 matrix proteins specify different capabilities to modulate B cell growth. J Virol. 2014;88:5706–17.

51. Basta D, Latinovic O, Lafferty MK, Sun L, Bryant J, Lu W, Caccuri F, Caruso A, Gallo RC, Garzino-Demo A. Angiogenic, lymphangiogenic and adipogenic effects of HIV-1 matrix protein p17. Pathog Dis. 2015;73:ftv062.

52. Iaria ML, Fiorentini S, Focà E, Zicari S, Giagulli C, Caccuri F, Francisci D, Di Perri G, Castelli F, Baldelli F, et al. Synthetic HIV-1 matrix protein p17-based AT20-KLH therapeutic immunization in HIV-1-infected patients receiving antiretroviral treatment: a phase I safety and immunogenicity study. Vaccine. 2014;32:1072–8.

53. Haffar O, Dubrovsky L, Lowe R, Berro R, Kashanchi F, Godden J, Vanpouille C, Rajorath J, Bukrinsky M. Oxadiazols: a new class of rationally designed anti-human immunodeficiency virus compounds targeting the nuclear localization signal of the viral matrix protein. J Virol. 2005;79:13028–36.

18

Clinico-pathological features of oropharyngeal squamous cell carcinomas in Malaysia with reference to HPV infection

Lee Fah Yap[1,2], Sook Ling Lai[1], Anthony Rhodes[3], Hans Prakash Sathasivam[4,5], Maizaton Atmadini Abdullah[6], Kin-Choo Pua[7], Pathmanathan Rajadurai[8], Phaik-Leng Cheah[9], Selvam Thavaraj[10], Max Robinson[4] and Ian C. Paterson[1,2]* [iD]

Abstract

Background: The incidence of oropharyngeal squamous cell carcinoma (OPSCC) has been rising in Western countries and this has been attributed to human papillomavirus (HPV) infection. p16 expression is a marker for HPV infection and p16 positive OPSCC is now recognized as a separate disease entity. There are only limited data available regarding HPV-related OPSCC in Asian countries and no data from Malaysia.

Methods: We identified 60 Malaysian patients with OPSCC over a 12-year period (2004–2015) from four different hospitals in two major cities, Kuala Lumpur and Penang. The detection of HPV was carried out using p16 immunohistochemistry and high risk HPV DNA in situ hybridisation.

Results: Overall, 15 (25%) tumours were p16 positive by immunohistochemistry, 10 of which were also positive for high risk HPV DNA by in situ hybridisation. By comparison, a matched cohort of UK patients had a p16 positive rate of 49%. However, between 2009 and 2015, where cases were available from all four hospitals, 13 of 37 (35%) cases were p16 positive. In our Malaysian cohort, 53% of patients were of Chinese ethnicity and 80% of the p16 positive cases were found in these patients; no Indian patients had p16 positive disease, despite representing 35% of the total cohort.

Conclusion: The proportion of OPSCCs associated with HPV in Malaysia appears to be lower than in European and American cohorts and could possibly be more prevalent amongst Malaysians of Chinese ethnicity. Further, our data suggests that the burden of HPV-related OPSCC could be increasing in Malaysia. Larger cross-sectional studies of Malaysian patients are required to determine the public health implications of these preliminary findings.

Keywords: Oropharyngeal, Squamous cell carcinoma, p16, Human papillomavirus, Malaysia

Background

The profile of head and neck squamous cell carcinoma (SCC) has changed over the past few decades with increased rates of oropharyngeal SCC (OPSCC) having been documented in Europe and the USA [1]. Although risk factors such as tobacco and alcohol consumption are still important for the development of OPSCC, it has become apparent that oncogenic human papillomavirus (HPV) is also an important aetiological agent [2]. HPV is thought to account for the relatively recent increase in OPSCC, with data from Sweden and the USA indicating that 70–80% of OPSCC are HPV positive [3, 4]. Patients with HPV positive tumours are typically non-smokers and have a low consumption of alcohol. Sexual behaviour, such as early age of sexual debut and increasing numbers of sex partners appears to correlate with HPV-related OPSCC [5, 6]. Furthermore, HPV-related OPSCC patients have better survival rates than those with HPV negative tumours [6–12].

p16 immunohistochemistry is used clinically as a surrogate marker for oncogenic HPV infection in OPSCCs and in 2017 UICC and AJCC TNM8 classification assigned p16 positive OPSCC a separate staging system

* Correspondence: ipaterson@um.edu.my
[1]Faculty of Dentistry, University of Malaya, Kuala Lumpur, Malaysia
[2]Oral Cancer Research and Coordinating Centre, Faculty of Dentistry, University of Malaya, Kuala Lumpur, Malaysia
Full list of author information is available at the end of the article

[13]. In developed countries, routine testing for p16 is now recommended for all patients with OPSCC as well as those with metastatic SCC of unknown primary in the head and neck region [14, 15].

At this point in time, there is a lack of accurate epidemiological and clinico-pathological data on the burden of HPV-related OPSCC in Malaysia, as reported by the HPV Information Centre [16]. Two previous studies on HPV-related HNSCCs in Malaysian patients were performed on mostly oral SCC specimens and as such are not representative of the burden of HPV-related OPSCC in Malaysia [17, 18]. Therefore, the aim of this study was to measure the proportion of Malaysian patients with p16 positive OPSCC and to examine the clinico-pathological features.

Methods

Patients and specimens

To ensure that the cohort was representative of the Malaysian population and to limit bias, cases were obtained from four different hospitals in two major cities. Cases were identified by searching pathology databases for SCCs coded as oropharynx, tonsil and soft palate. The patients were identified over a 12-year period (2004–2015). Formalin-fixed paraffin-embedded (FFPE) tissue blocks were obtained from the relevant pathology tissue archives and clinico-pathological information were obtained from clinical databases and review of medical records. All patient information was anonymised. This study had ethical approval from the relevant institutional medical research and ethics boards (Reference Numbers: NMRR-12-13,577; UMMC 20164–2341; SDMC 201211.3).

A matched UK cohort of patients was identified from an existing database at Newcastle-upon-Tyne Hospitals NHS Foundation Trust. Cases were matched by year of diagnosis, age at diagnosis (±10 years) and sex. Results for p16 immunohistochemistry staining were obtained from patient records. The study had favourable ethical opinion from the National Research Ethics Service Committee North East, Sunderland (REC reference: 11/NE/0118).

HPV testing

p16 immunohistochemistry

p16 immunohistochemistry (IHC) was performed using a proprietary kit (CINtec Histology, Roche mtm laboratories AG, Germany) on a Ventana Benchmark Autostainer (Ventana Medical Systems Inc., USA). Normal tonsil was used as a negative control and OPSCC with high p16 expression was used as a positive control. p16 staining was assessed as positive when there was strong and diffuse nuclear and cytoplasmic staining present in greater than 70% of the malignant cells [19, 20].

High risk HPV DNA in situ hybridisation

HR- HPV DNA in-situ hybridisation (HR-HPV ISH) was carried out using proprietary reagents (Inform HPV III Family 16 Probe (B), Ventana Medical Systems Inc., USA) on a Benchmark Autostainer (Ventana Medical Systems Inc., USA). The Inform HPV III Family 16 Probe (B) detects high risk genotypes HPV-16, – 18, – 31, – 33, – 35, – 39, – 45, – 51, – 52, – 56, – 58 and – 66. Three control samples were used: FFPE CaSki cells (HPV-16 positive; 200–400 copies per cell), HeLa cells (HPV-18 positive; 10–50 copies per cell) and C-33A (HPV negative; Ventana Medical Systems Inc., USA). The HR- HPV ISH test was scored as positive if there was any blue reaction product that co-localised with the malignant cells [21].

Statistical analysis

Statistical analysis was performed using SPSS for Windows (version 21.0; SPSS Inc., USA). p16 positive and negative cases and patient characteristics were compared using independent t tests and Pearson's Chi Square test. Results were considered significant at the 5% level ($p < 0.05$).

Results

HPV status of OPSCCs

We tested OPSCCs from 60 patients identified from four hospitals. 15 (25%) cases showed p16 expression, but only 10 of the p16 positive tumours (67%) showed evidence of high risk HPV DNA by in situ hybridisation (Table 1; Fig. 1). To make a more representative comparison, we identified samples collected from all four hospitals within the same period of time. A total of 37 samples were collected between 2009 and 2015 and 35% (13 of 37) of these cases were p16 positive.

Clinico-pathological profile of patients

Complete demographic data were available for 54 patients; the age and sex for six of the patients were not available. The clinico-pathological profiles of the patients are shown in Table 2. The mean age of patients was 65.44 years (± 12.16) at diagnosis and ranged from 36 to 93 years-old. There was no statistically significant difference in age between patients who had p16 negative and p16 positive OPSCC ($p = 0.214$). However, the two youngest (36 and 41 years of age) patients in the cohort had p16 positive disease. The overall male to female ratio was 2.4:1 and the ratio was similar in p16 negative cases (2.7:1), however, the ratio was lower in p16 positive cases (1.6:1). Most patients in the cohort were of Chinese ethnicity (53.3%) followed by Indians (35.0%). All the Indian patients had p16 negative disease, whilst 80% of the HPV positive cases were Chinese; this finding was statistically significant ($p = 0.004$). Overall, most of the

Table 1 Demographics of Malaysian patients with p16 positive OPSCC

Case	Year of diagnosis	Age	Sex	Ethnicity	p16 IHC	HR-HPV ISH
1	2005	NK	NK	Malay	+	–
2	2006	88	F	Chinese	+	+
3	2009	41	F	Chinese	+	–
4	2010	64	F	Chinese	+	+
5	2012	56	M	Chinese	+	–
6	2012	56	M	Chinese	+	+
7	2012	67	F	Chinese	+	+
8	2013	NK	NK	Chinese	+	+
9	2013	74	M	Malay	+	+
10	2013	36	M	Malay	+	+
11	2013	53	M	Chinese	+	+
12	2013	70	M	Chinese	+	–
13	2014	72	M	Chinese	+	–
14	2014	72	F	Chinese	+	+
15	2015	54	M	Chinese	+	+

OPSCC were classified as moderately differentiated SCC (40%) and this was similar for p16 negative cases (47%). By contrast, the majority of p16 positive cases (60%) were poorly differentiated SCC, which was statistically significant ($p = 0.016$).

Comparison with a matched UK cohort

A UK cohort of patients with OPSCC was used as a comparator. The Malaysian patients were matched with UK patients by year of diagnosis, age at diagnosis (±10 years) and sex. Fifty-one patients could be matched between the cohorts; six Malaysian patients had incomplete demographic data and three had data that could not be matched with a UK counterpart. The matched UK patients had a p16 positive rate of 49%, which was double that of the Malaysian patients (24%).

Discussion

In previous years, SCCs of the oral cavity and oropharynx were often grouped together and thought of as being a single disease entity [22]. However, this has changed in recent years due to the recognition of HPV as a major aetio-pathogenic agent in a subset of OPSCC. HPV positive OPSCC is now recognised as a clinico-pathologically unique form of HNSCC with distinct demographic, clinical and morphological features, as well as being associated with improved clinical outcomes [7, 23–26]. These findings have prompted the changes to oropharyngeal tumours in the 2017 edition of the WHO Classification of Head and Neck Tumours. The new edition has divided tumours of the oral cavity and oropharynx into different chapters and has also sub-classified OPSCC according to HPV status [27]. Furthermore, the UICC and AJCC have recently recommended new clinical and pathological

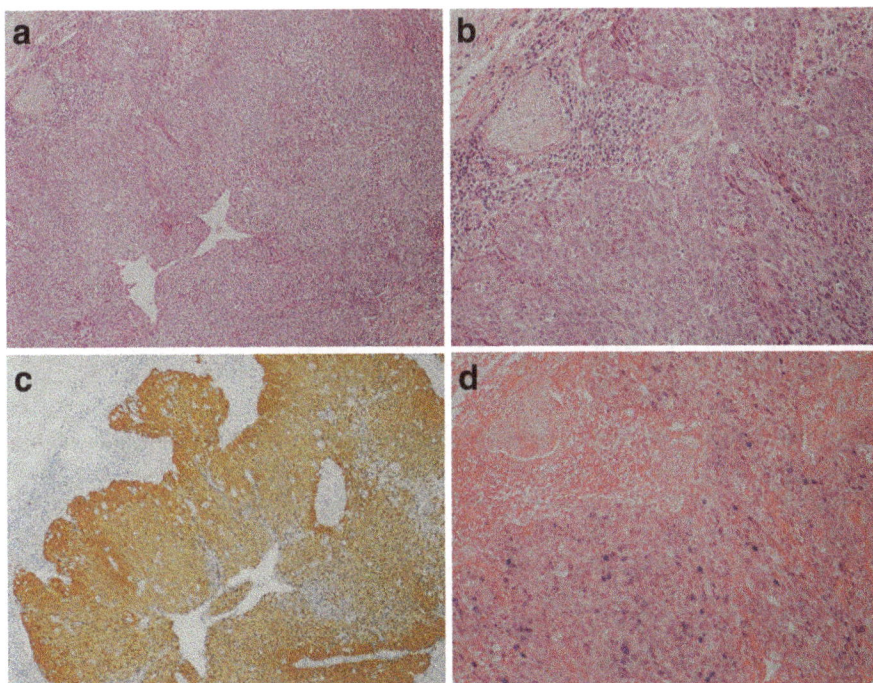

Fig. 1 HPV-related oropharyngeal squamous cell carcinoma (**a** & **b**; H&E stain) showing high levels of p16 expression by immunohistochemistry (**c**) and evidence of high risk HPV DNA by in situ hybridisation (**d**)

Table 2 Clinico-pathological characteristics of Malaysian patients with OPSCC

	All patients (n = 60; 100%)	p16 negative (n = 45; 75%)	p16 positive (n = 15; 25%)	p-value
Age at diagnosis (years; n = 54)				
Mean (±SD)	65.44 (±12.16)	66.61 (±11.36)	61.77 (±14.28)	[a]0.214
Sex (n = 54)				
Male	38 (70.4%)	30 (73.2%)	8 (61.5%)	[b]0.493
Female	16 (29.6%)	11 (26.8%)	5 (38.5%)	
Ethnicity (n = 60)				
Malay	7 (11.7%)	4 (8.9%)	3 (20%)	[b]0.004
Chinese	32 (53.3%)	20 (44.4%)	12 (80%)	
Indian	21 (35.0%)	21 (46.7%)	0 (0%)	
Broder's grade (n = 60)				
WD	16 (26.7%)	13 (28.9%)	3 (20.0%)	[b]0.016
MD	24 (40.0%)	21 (46.7%)	3 (20.0%)	
PD	17 (28.3%)	8 (17.8%)	9 (60.0%)	
Others	3 (5.0%)	3 (6.7%)	0 (0%)	

[a]Independent sample's t-test
[b]Pearson's Chi-Square test
WD Well differentiated, *MD* Moderately differentiated, *PD* Poorly differentiated

staging systems for p16 positive OPSCC, which reflects the improved prognosis of the disease [13, 28].

The prevalence of p16 positive OPSCC in the Malaysian cohort was half that of a matched UK cohort (25% vs. 49%). The matched UK cohort was representative of a larger (n = 1529) multicentre prevalence study carried out in the UK demonstrating that OPSCC had a p16 positive rate of 54% [29]. Higher rates have also been reported elsewhere in Europe and America (35% vs 80%) [1]. A recent meta-analysis looking at the burden of HPV related head and neck cancers in the Asia Pacific region reported an overall prevalence of 40.53% for oropharyngeal cancers [30]. However, there were considerable differences in the rates between regions and countries; the region with the highest prevalence was Oceania (49.32%) and the country with the lowest prevalence was China (9.50%) [30]. Our findings taken for cases diagnosed between 2009 and 2015 (35%) are comparable to the reported rates in East and South Asian regions (25.8 and 38.7% respectively) and Singapore (42%) [31]. In the present study, 80% of the p16 positive cases were from patients of Chinese ethnicity, whilst all the Indian patients had p16 negative OPSCC. This finding could be particularly relevant because according to the 2010 Population and Housing Census of Malaysia, the Chinese account for only 24.6% of the total population [32]. Although this potentially alarming finding needs to be confirmed in a larger cohort, further research specifically into risk factors that predispose to

HPV infection in the oropharynx are warranted in different populations.

Most epidemiological and clinical studies have indicated that patients with HPV positive OPSCC are relatively younger than patients with HPV negative disease [6, 30, 33–35], although our findings do concur with those studies with the mean age of HPV positive patients being slightly lower than the mean age of HPV negative patients, the finding was not statistically significant. According to the recent meta-analysis by Shaikh et al. [30], the prevalence of HPV associated head and neck cancer is higher amongst males, however the studies involved in the meta-analysis involved small study samples as well as unequal gender distributions [30]. The findings from our study are also similar with the findings of the meta-analysis with a slight male predilection.

The recent WHO 2017 edition has discouraged histologic grading of HPV positive OPSCC as there is insufficient evidence to correlate histopathological grading with clinical behaviour and outcomes [27]. All the cases in our study were diagnosed well before the release of the new WHO guideline and were based on previous guidelines that grouped oropharyngeal SCCs with oral cavity SCCs. The majority of HPV positive cases were graded as being poorly differentiated SCCs (70%). This "high grade" histopathologic category was probably based on the non-keratinized, immature and basaloid appearance of the tumour cells. However, such grading may not be accurate as HPV positive OPSCCs mostly arise from the epithelial lining of the tonsillar crypts and therefore retain the non-keratinizing and basaloid appearance of this epithelium.

The disparity between p16 positive rates (25%) and the detection of HR-HPV DNA (17%) is a consequence of the low sensitivity of HR-HPV DNA in situ hybridisation, which has been reported previously [36]. The relatively high rate of p16 positive, high risk HPV DNA ISH negative cases (5 of 15) is likely to reflect pre-analytical variables related to tissue fixation, processing and storage conditions. The HPV tests were conducted in an ISO15189:2012 accredited UK pathology laboratory, where such cases represent around 10% of OPSCCs tested [21]. The use of polymerase chain reaction and RNA-based in situ hybridisation has been shown to increase the detection rates and mitigate against false negative results [37].

Conclusion

The results from this study suggest that the occurrence of HPV-related OPSCC in Malaysia may not be as high as those reported in developed nations such as the UK and the USA, but the proportion of OPSCCs that are HPV positive appears to be increasing, particularly in patients of Chinese ethnicity. Further studies will be required to determine how these observations might impact upon Malaysian communities and the national healthcare system in the future.

Abbreviations
HPV: Human papillomavirus; ISH: In-situ hybridisation; OPSCC: Oropharyngeal squamous cell carcinoma; SCC: Squamous cell carcinoma

Acknowledgments
The authors would like thank the Director General of Health of Malaysia for his permission to publish this article.

Funding
This study was supported in part by a High Impact Research Grant (UM.C/625/1/HIR/MOHE/DENT/22) from the University of Malaya awarded to ICP and LFY. The funding body had no role in the design of the study or the analysis of the data.

Authors' contributions
LFY, MR and ICP conceived the study. MAA, KCP, PR and PLC identified suitable cases, provided samples and clinical details. MR and ST performed and analysed the immunohistochemistry and in-situ hybridisation. SLL participated in study design and undertook data collection. HPS undertook data collection and performed statistical analysis. LFY, HPS, MR and ICP drafted the manuscript. All authors approved the final manuscript.

Competing interests
The authors declare that they have no competing interests.

Author details
[1]Faculty of Dentistry, University of Malaya, Kuala Lumpur, Malaysia. [2]Oral Cancer Research and Coordinating Centre, Faculty of Dentistry, University of Malaya, Kuala Lumpur, Malaysia. [3]School of Medicine, Taylor's University, Subang Jaya, Selangor, Malaysia. [4]Centre for Oral Health Research, Newcastle University, Newcastle-upon-Tyne, UK. [5]Ministry of Health, Kuala Lumpur, Malaysia. [6]Faculty of Medicine and Health Sciences, University Putra Malaysia, Serdang, Malaysia. [7]Penang General Hospital, Penang, Malaysia. [8]Subang Jaya Medical Centre, Subang Jaya, Selangor, Malaysia. [9]Faculty of Medicine, University of Malaya, Kuala Lumpur, Malaysia. [10]Head and Neck Pathology, Dental Institute, King's College London, London, UK.

References
1. Mehanna H, Beech T, Nicholson T, El-Hariry I, McConkey C, Paleri V, et al. Prevalence of human papillomavirus in oropharyngeal and nonoropharyngeal head and neck cancer–systematic review and meta-analysis of trends by time and region. Head Neck. 2013;35:747–55.
2. Leemans CR, Braakhuis BJM, Brakenhoff RH. The molecular biology of head and neck cancer. Nat Rev Cancer Nature Publishing Group. 2011;11:9–22.
3. Nasman A, Attner P, Hammarstedt L, Du J, Eriksson M, Giraud G, et al. Incidence of human papillomavirus (HPV) positive tonsillar carcinoma in Stockholm, Sweden: an epidemic of viral-induced carcinoma? Int J Cancer. 2009;125:362–6.
4. Chaturvedi AK, Engels EA, Pfeiffer RM, Hernandez BY, Xiao W, Kim E, et al. Human papillomavirus and rising oropharyngeal cancer incidence in the United States. J Clin Oncol. 2011;29:4294–301.
5. D'Souza G, Kreimer AR, Viscidi R, Pawlita M, Fakhry C, KOch WM, et al. Case-control study of human papillomavirus and Oropharyngeal Cancer. N Engl J Med. 2007;356:1944–56.
6. Gillison ML, D'Souza G, Westra W, Sugar E, Xiao W, Begum S, et al. Distinct risk factor profiles for human papillomavirus type 16-positive and human papillomavirus type 16-negative head and neck cancers. J Natl Cancer Inst. 2008;100:407–20.
7. Ang KK, Harris J, Wheeler R, Weber R, Rosenthal DI, Nguyen-Tan PF, et al. Human papillomavirus and survival of patients with oropharyngeal cancer. N Engl J Med. 2010;363:24–35.
8. Chaturvedi AK, Engels EA, Anderson WF, Gillison ML. Incidence trends for human papillomavirus-related and -unrelated oral squamous cell carcinomas in the United States. J Clin Oncol. 2008;26:612–9.
9. Marur S, D'Souza G, Westra WH, Forastiere AA. HPV-associated head and neck cancer: a virus-related cancer epidemic. Lancet Oncol Elsevier Ltd. 2010;11:781–9.
10. Mellin H, Friesland S, Lewensohn R, Dalianis T, Munck-Wikland E. Human papillomavirus (HPV) DNA in tonsillar cancer: clinical correlates, risk of relapse, and survival. Int J Cancer. 2000;89:300–4.
11. O'Rorke MA, Ellison MV, Murray LJ, Moran M, James J, Anderson LA. Human papillomavirus related head and neck cancer survival: a systematic review and meta-analysis. Oral Oncol. 2012;48:1191–201.
12. Sturgis EM, Cinciripini PM. Trends in head and neck cancer incidence in relation to smoking prevalence: an emerging epidemic of human papillomavirus-associated cancers? Cancer. 2007;110:1429–35.
13. Huang SH, O'Sullivan B. Overview of the 8th edition TNM classification for head and neck Cancer. Curr treat Options Oncol. 2017;18:40.
14. Paleri V, Roland N. Head and neck Cancer: UK multidisciplinary management guidelines. 5th edition. J Laryngol Otol. 5th ed. London: British Association of Otorhinolaryngology, head and neck Surgery; 2016;130:S3–224.
15. Helliwell T, Woolgar J. Dataset for histopathology reporting of mucosal malignancies of the oral cavity. In: Stand. Datasets report. Cancers. London: the Royal College of Pathologists; 2013.
16. Bruni L, Barrionuevo-Rosas L, Albero G, Serrano B, Mena M, Gómez D, et al. Human papillomavirus and related diseases in Malaysia. Summary report. ICO Inf. Cent. HPV Cancer (HPV Inf. Centre). 2017.
17. Saini R, Tang T-H, Zain RB, Cheong SC, Musa KI, Saini D, et al. Significant association of high-risk human papillomavirus (HPV) but not of p53 polymorphisms with oral squamous cell carcinomas in Malaysia. J Cancer Res Clin Oncol Germany. 2011;137:311–20.
18. Lim KP, Hamid S, Lau S-H, Teo S-H, Cheong SC. HPV infection and the alterations of the pRB pathway in oral carcinogenesis. Oncol Rep Greece. 2007;17:1321–6.
19. Singhi AD, Westra WH. Comparison of human papillomavirus in situ hybridization and p16 immunohistochemistry in the detection of human papillomavirus-associated head and neck cancer based on a prospective clinical experience. Cancer. 2010;116:2166–73.
20. Jordan RC, Lingen MW, Perez-Ordonez B, He X, Pickard R, Koluder M, et al. Validation of methods for Oropharyngeal Cancer HPV status determination in US cooperative group trials. Am J Surg Pathol. 2012;36:945–54.
21. Thavaraj S, Stokes A, Guerra E, Bible J, Halligan E, Long A, et al. Evaluation of human papillomavirus testing for squamous cell carcinoma of the tonsil in clinical practice. J Clin Pathol. 2011;64:308–12.
22. Barnes L, Eveson JW, Reichart P, Sidransky D. Pathology and genetics of head and neck Tumours. First edit. Lyon. France: World Health Organization, IARC; 2005.
23. Westra WH. The changing face of head and neck Cancer in the 21st century: the impact of HPV on the epidemiology and pathology of oral Cancer. Head Neck Pathol New York: Humana Press Inc. 2009;3:78–81.
24. Gondim DD, Haynes W, Wang X, Chernock RD, El-Mofty SK, Lewis JSJ. Histologic typing in Oropharyngeal squamous cell carcinoma: a 4-year prospective practice study with p16 and high-risk HPV mRNA testing correlation. Am J Surg Pathol United States. 2016;40:1117–24.
25. Gillison ML, Chaturvedi AK, Anderson WF, Fakhry C. Epidemiology of human papillomavirus-positive head and neck squamous cell carcinoma. J Clin Oncol United States. 2015;33:3235–42.
26. Hayes DN, Van Waes C, Seiwert TY. Genetic landscape of human papillomavirus-associated head and neck Cancer and comparison to tobacco-related tumors. J Clin Oncol United States. 2015;33:3227–34.

27. El-Naggar A, Chan J, Grandis J, Takata T, Slootweg P, editors. WHO classification of head and neck Tumours. 4th ed. WHO/IARC classification of Tumours; 2017.

28. Brierley J, Gospodarowicz M, Wittekind C. UICC International Union against Cancer TNM classification of malignant Tumours 8th edition. 8th Editio. Wiley-Blackwell; 2017.

29. Schache AG, Powell NG, Cuschieri KS, Robinson M, Leary S, Mehanna H, et al. HPV-related oropharynx cancer in the United Kingdom: an evolution in the understanding of disease etiology. Cancer Res United States. 2016;76: 6598–606.

30. Shaikh MH, McMillan NA, Johnson NW. HPV-associated head and neck cancers in the Asia Pacific: a critical literature review & meta-analysis. Cancer Epidemiol. 2015;39:923–38.

31. Tan LSY, Fredrik P, Ker L, Yu FG, Wang DY, Goh BC, et al. High-risk HPV genotypes and P16INK4a expression in a cohort of head and neck squamous cell carcinoma patients in Singapore. Oncotarget. 2016;7:86730–9.

32. 2010 Population and Housing Census of Malaysia. Malaysian department of Statistics; 2011.

33. Ryerson AB, Peters ES, Coughlin SS, Chen VW, Gillison ML, Reichman ME, et al. Burden of potentially human papillomavirus-associated cancers of the oropharynx and oral cavity in the US, 1998-2003. Cancer. 2008;113:2901–9.

34. Llewellyn CD, Johnson NW, Warnakulasuriya KA. Risk factors for squamous cell carcinoma of the oral cavity in young people–a comprehensive literature review. Oral Oncol England. 2001;37:401–18.

35. Gillison ML. Human papillomavirus and prognosis of Oropharyngeal squamous cell carcinoma: implications for clinical research in head and neck cancers. J Clin Oncol American Society of Clinical Oncology. 2006;24: 5623–5.

36. Schache AG, Liloglou T, Risk JM, Jones TM, Ma X-J, Wang H, et al. Validation of a novel diagnostic standard in HPV-positive oropharyngeal squamous cell carcinoma. Br J Cancer. 2013;108:1332–9.

37. Robinson M. HPV testing of head and neck Cancer in clinical practice. Recent Results Cancer Res. 2017;206:101–11.

19

Association of Epstein - Barr virus and breast cancer in Eritrea

Ghimja Fessahaye[1,4], Ahmed M. Elhassan[1], Elwaleed M. Elamin[2], Ameera A. M. Adam[3], Anghesom Ghebremedhin[4] and Muntaser E. Ibrahim[1*]

Abstract

Background: The oncogenic potential of Epstein-Barr virus (EBV) in breast cancer is being increasingly recognized. Despite some controversies regarding such role, new evidence is suggesting a culpability of EBV in breast cancer, particularly in Africa where the virus has been originally associated with causation of several solid and hematological malignancies. One example is a report from Sudan implicating EBV as a prime etiologic agent for an aggressive type of breast cancer, where nearly 100% of tumor tissues were shown to carry viral signatures. To get a broader view on such association, other nearby countries should be investigated. The present study aims to determine the prevalence and possible associations of the virus in Eritrean breast cancer patients.

Methods: Detection of EBV genome using primers that target Epstein Barr Encoded RNA (EBER) gene and Latent Membrane Protein-1 (LMP-1) gene sequences was performed by polymerase chain reaction (PCR) on DNA samples extracted from 144 formalin fixed paraffin embedded breast cancer tissues and 63 non-cancerous breast tissue as control group. A subset of PCR positive samples was evaluated for EBER gene expression by in situ hybridization (ISH). Expression of Latent Membrane Protein-2a (LMP2a) was also assessed by immunohistochemistry in a subset of 45 samples.

Results: Based on PCR results, EBV genome signals were detected in a total of 40 samples (27.77%) as compared to controls (p-value = 0. 0031) with a higher sensitivity when using the EBER primers. Five out of the 14 samples stained by EBER-ISH 35.71% were positive for the virus indicating the presence of the viral genome within the tumor cells. Of those stained for IHC 7 (15.55%) were positive for LMP2a showing low viral protein frequency.

Conclusions: Based on these findings it can be concluded that EBV in Eritrea is associated with a smaller subset of tumors, unlike neighboring Sudan, thus pointing to possible differences in population predisposition and diseases epidemiology.

Keywords: Eritrea, Breast cancer, Epstein–Barr virus, Polymerase chain reaction, Immunohistochemistry, *in situ* hybridization

Background

Breast cancer is the most common form of malignancy in women both in developed and the developing countries [1]. In Sub Saharan Africa, although the prevalence is relatively lower compared to that of the western countries, it is characterized by aggressive course and targets more women at a younger age [2]. Breast cancer etiology is not yet entirely known, but its incidence is partially explained by environmental factors including viruses such as Epstein-Barr virus [3]. EBV is closely associated with endemic Burkitt lymphoma in sub-Saharan Africa [4] and more recently reported to be a culprit of breast cancer in Sudan [5]. It is a cosmopolitan γ-herpes virus which infects usually at younger age [6]. Its main target are B lymphocytes but it has a potential to infect epithelial cells as well [7] and is associated with a number of lymphoid and epithelial [8] cancers and thus it is classified as a carcinogenic agent by the International Agency for Research in Cancer [9].

There is conflicting evidence as to the role of EBV in breast cancer [5, 10–25]. The differences are believed to be due to the usage of different techniques, various types

* Correspondence: mibrahim@iend.org
[1]Department of Molecular Biology, Institute of Endemic Diseases, University of Khartoum, Al-Qasr Street, P.O. Box 102, Khartoum, Sudan
Full list of author information is available at the end of the article

of tissue samples, geographical and genetic variation of viral and host genomes, racial and socioeconomic variation of study populations [26–28]. Some authors believe that EBV may play a role in breast cancer oncogenesis not as a primary etiological agent but acts in concert with other co-factors [29]. A meta-analysis study concluded that EBV acts as a cofactor in breast cancer development [30].

In Sudan, where aggressive breast cancer is prevailing, EBV is believed to be associated with this cancer based on viral detection in cancer tissues [5] and on molecular evidence from methylome analysis and expression data published online (bioRxivDoi: 10.1101/03432).

The current study was initiated with the aim of finding out whether EBV is a common etiology of breast cancer in East Africa or whether different countries and populations may present with different pattern.

Methods
Patients and tissues

This study comprises formalin fixed paraffin- embedded (FFPE) cancer biopsies from 144 cases of breast carcinoma retrieved from the Department of Histopathology, National Health Laboratory, Ministry of Health, Eritrea during 2013, 2014. The Department is the only of its kind and receives sample from all hospitals within the country. Noncancerous tissue samples from the same directory (n=63) were used as a controls. Clinical data including age, tumor type, size and involved lymph node were also collected. Eight 10µ thick sections were cut by a sterile microtome blade from each tumor paraffin blocks for subsequent DNA extraction and then amplification. From a subset (n=59) of the study blocks additional 4µm thick sections were cut and put onto positive charged slides (Dako) for the use of immunohistochemistry (IHC) as well as in situ hybridization (ISH) assays.

DNA extraction from FFPE

DNA was extracted from FFPE breast cancer tissues (n=144) and non-cancerous tissues (n= 63) using guanidine chloride for buccal wash method (Black-well laboratory Cambridge, UK) modified to suite for FFPE samples as follows: without dewaxing samples were subject to lyses solution containing 400mMNaCl, 6M guanidine chloride and 300 µl of 7.5% ammonium acetate without proteinase K and heat treated at 98°C for 20 minutes in water bath to reverse formaldehyde modification of the FFPE samples. After cooling10µl (20 mg/ml stock) proteinase K was added and incubated for overnight at 56°C. On day two, second heat treatment was applied by incubating samples at 98 °C for 5 minutes in a water bath. After cooling 10µl proteinase k was added, briefly vertoxed and incubated at 56 °C for overnight. During the whole incubation period samples were put on a shaker at interval for about 30 minutes. Chloroform

was then added, the supernatant was collected, and DNA was precipitated by ethanol, dissolved in 100 µl TE storage buffer. The purity and quality of the extracted DNA was analyzed based on absorbance of the extracted DNA at 260 and 280 nm wavelengths using a spectrophotometer (NanoDrop-1000, Thermo Fisher Scientific, and Wilmington, USA).

PCR amplifications of extracted DNA

Before viral amplification, the DNA quality was checked by amplifying a certain region of the glyceraldehyde-3-phosphate dehydrogenase (GAPDH) gene using primers (forward primer 5'GGCCTCCAAGGAGTAAGAC-C3'and reverse primer: 5'CCCCTCTTCAAGGGGTC-TAC3'). After validation specific regions of the viral genome were amplified by using two primers: Epstein Barr Encoded RNA (EBER) gene (forward primer 5'CCCTAGTGGTTTCGGACACA3' and reverse primer 5'ACTTGCAAATGCTCTAGGCG3') [12] and Latent Membrane Protein-1 (LMP-1) gene (forward primer: 5' CCGAAGAGGTTGAAAACAAA 3' and reverse primer 5'GTGGGGGTCGTCATCATCTC 3') [5]. DNA from EBV-positive nasopharyngeal carcinoma (NPC) was used as a positive control and nuclease-free distilled water was used as a negative control. Electrophoresis of PCR products were done in 2% ethidium bromide-stained agarose gel in TBE buffer at 90 V for 1 h. DNA bands were visualized by a transilluminator (UV doc, England. DNA ladder 100 base pair (bp) (Fermentas-Russia) was used as indicator of band size.

EBER RNA in situ hybridization

In order to localize viral transcript within the tumor cells, 14 samples which were positive by PCR in duplicate assay and which have relatively brighter bands in agarose gel were further tested by ISH technique using PNA ISH detection Kit following the manufacturer's instruction. Briefly, 4 µ thick FFPE tissue sections on positively charges slides (BioGenex, USA) were deparaffinized in xylene, rehydrated in serial graded ethanol washes, digested with proteinase K and then followed by hybridization of EBV- EBER peptide nucleic acid (PNA) Probe/ Fluorescein (Dako) for 90 minutes at 55°C. Detection was accomplished by alkaline phosphatase (AP)-conjugated anti-fluorescein antibodies using nitro blue tetrazolium (NBT)/BromochloroIndoyl phosphate (BCIP) (Dako) as a substrate. Slides were counterstained with hematoxylin (Chem Cruz, Santa Cruz Biotechnology) and mounted with DPX Mountant (Atom Scientific). Positive and negative controls provided by the manufacturer were used. Section from EBV positive nasopharyngeal carcinoma was used as an additional positive control. A case was considered as expressing EBER if the nucleus of a tumor cell stained dark blue or black.

Immunohistochemistry (IHC) test

Sections of 4 μm thick were cut from 45 paraffin blocks of breast cancer using a microtome and put on coated immunoslides and were de-paraffinized in xylene, rehydrated through series of graded alcohol, submitted to heat retrieval in citrate buffer (pH 6.0) for 40 minutes in water bath. After heating, the slides were allowed to cool to room temperature and washed with phosphate buffered saline (PBS). Endogenous peroxidase activity was blocked with 1% hydrogen peroxide in methanol for 5 minutes blocking serum was used for 1hr in order to block nonspecific immunoreactions. Monoclonal antibodies for LMP2a (Santa Cruz Biotechnology) were applied at a dilution of 1:100 on all tissue sections for overnight at 4°C to evaluate the expression of LMP2a. Detection was performed using Santa Cruz biotechnology envision dual link system according to the manufacturer's instruction. After that, slides were visualized using Santa Cruz liquid DAB. Mayer's hematoxylin was used as a counter stain. As a positive control, we used EBV infected nasopharyngeal carcinoma. In negative controls, the primary antibodies were omitted.

Statistical analysis

Data were entered and analyzed using the software Statistical Package for Social Sciences version 20 (SPSS, Inc., Chicago, IL, USA). Proportions were compared for significance using the Fisher exact test to determine whether there was any significant difference between the frequency of EBV in the carcinoma and the noncancerous samples and its relationship with breast cancer. A p- value of ≤ 0.05 was considered indicative of a statistically significant difference.

Results

Clinicopathological features

During this study breast cancer samples were collected from 144 patients mean age of 51.48 years (range, 19 to 91 years). The mean age of the controls with fibroadenoma was 26 years (range). Histological tumor types were: ductal carcinoma 96 (66.66%) (Of which 56 (58.33%) were invasive ductal carcinoma), medullary carcinoma 12 (8.33), lobular carcinoma 2(1.38%) and all other types 34 (23.61%). Lymph node involvement was detected in 35 (24.30%) of all cases (Table 1).

Molecular detection of EBV in breast cancer cases

DNA was successfully extracted from 144 FFPE samples of breast carcinoma patients, and from 63 non- cancerous benign tissues samples. The extracted DNA from FFPE breast cancer tissue was successfully amplified using GAPDH primers indicating good quality DNA for further viral detection assay. Amplification fragments of both LMP1 & EBER were detected using PCR.

Table 1 Clinicopathological features of breast cancer samples (n=144) from Eritrean patients

Feature	Value
Age (years)	
Mean	51.48
Range	19-91
Histology	
Ductal	96 (66.66%)
Lobular	2 (1.38%)
Medullary	12 (8.33%)
Others	34 (23.61%)
Lymph node involvement	45 (31.25%)

One hundred fourty-four formalin fixed paraffin- embedded (FFPE) tissue sections of breast carcinoma retrieved from the Department of Histopathology, National Health Laboratory, Ministry of Health, Eritrea. The age of the patients ranged from 19 to 91 years with a mean age of 51.48 years. The constitution of the types was: duct carcinoma 66.66% (96/144), lobular carcinoma 1.38% (2/144), medullary 8.33% (12/144) and others 23.61% (34/144). Lymph node was involved in 31.25% (45/144)

Combining the two markers a total of 40 (27.77%) of 144 breast cancer samples showed faint bands compared to the band formed by the positive control from a case of nasopharyngeal carcinoma. Repeated trial was done for those samples with faint bands and the result was the same as the first trial. Out of the samples with faint band 33(22.91%) were revealed using EBER and 14 (9.72%) using LMP1. As reviewed by Hou and his team, in three previous studies, the detection potential of EBER was higher than that of LMP1 [30]. Six (9.52%) out of 63 control samples showed very faint bands. Statistically, using EBER marker, association between EBV and breast cancer (P= 0.0031) was observed compared to the control group but the association employing LMP1 marker was not significant (P =0.1563), Fisher's exact test (Table 2).

ISH detection of EBER1 gene transcript

In order to confirm the presence of EBV within the tumor cells, Epstein-Barr virus-encoded RNA-1 (EBER1) *in situ* hybridization technique was used on those cases which were PCR positive in duplicate trials and/or those showing relatively brighter bands on agarose gel electrophoresis and or those which were positive by two markers (n=14). Signal for viral transcripts was observed in 35.71% (5/14) indicated by its nuclear localization in the tumor cells. Figure 1a shows positive staining of a case of poorly differentiated invasive ductal carcinoma exhibiting nuclear positivity indicated by dark staining in malignant cell. Fig 1b is the hematoxyline and eosin staining of the section in Fig 1a). A tissue section from a case of NPC was used as a positive control (Fig. 1c) and as a

Table 2 Detection of EBV genome in breast cancer samples by PCR using EBER and LMP-1 primers

Primer Breast cancer cases		Noncancerous cases	p-Val*
EBER			
Positive	33	4	0.0031*
Negative	111	59	
LMP1			
Positive	14	2	0.1563
Negative	130	61	

Amplification fragments of both EBER and LMP1 of EBV were detected using PCR. A total of 40 (27.77%) of 144 breast cancer samples showed faint bands compared to the band formed by the positive control from a case of nasopharyngeal carcinoma by either of the markers. Of this faint band 33(22.91%) were revealed using EBER and14 (9.72%) using LMP1and 7(4.86%) were positive by both markers. Out of the 63 control samples 6 by both markers. Were positive (9.52%)showed very faint bands. Statistically, using EBER marker, association between EBV and breast cancer (p-0.0031) was observed compared to the control group but the association employing LMP1 marker was not significant (p-0.1563), Fisher's exact test
*P value < 0.05 is considered as significant (Fisher's exact test). Abbreviation: EBER Epstein-Barr virus encoded RNA, LMP1 Latent membrane protein 1

negative control a breast cancer section without the primary antibody was employed.

IHC staining for detection of viral protein (LMP2a)

To assess expression of viral protein, IHC assay using LMP2a antibody was performed on 45 samples and LMP2a was expressed in 15.55% (7/45) of which six (13.33%) were also positive for EBV by PCR.

Discussion

Three detection methods: PCR. ISH and IHC were employed in the determination of EBV association with breast cancer. PCR results indicated the presence of EBV genome in 27.77% (n=144) of breast cancer samples amplified using EBER and LMP1 viral DNA fragments. This finding is in line with a metanalysis study in which about 29.32 % of the patients with breast cancer were infected with the virus [30]. In this study the number of EBV positive samples as well as that of EBV infected cells within positive samples were observed to be quite low as indicated by the faint bands on agarose gel and the scarce infected tumor cells in the ISH stained slides as compared to the positive controls from a case of NPC. PCR amplification was repeated for those samples with faint bands and got similar result. It is reported that as low as 0.00004 EBV genomes per infected cell can be detected using quantitative PCR [20] and Perrigoue and his team define ' EBV positive ' as the majority of tumor cells each to contain at least one copy of EBV DNA [19]. In a similar study low level EBV DNA in about 50% of the study breast cancer samples were detected by PCR [31]. EBV positive tumor infiltrating lymphocytes are believed to give false positive results during PCR assay [23, 32]. To rule out this, EBER-ISH technique which is considered as a gold standard technique for detection of EBV [33] was performed and viral transcripts were detected in 35.71% of the 14 stained samples. Fig. 1a shows

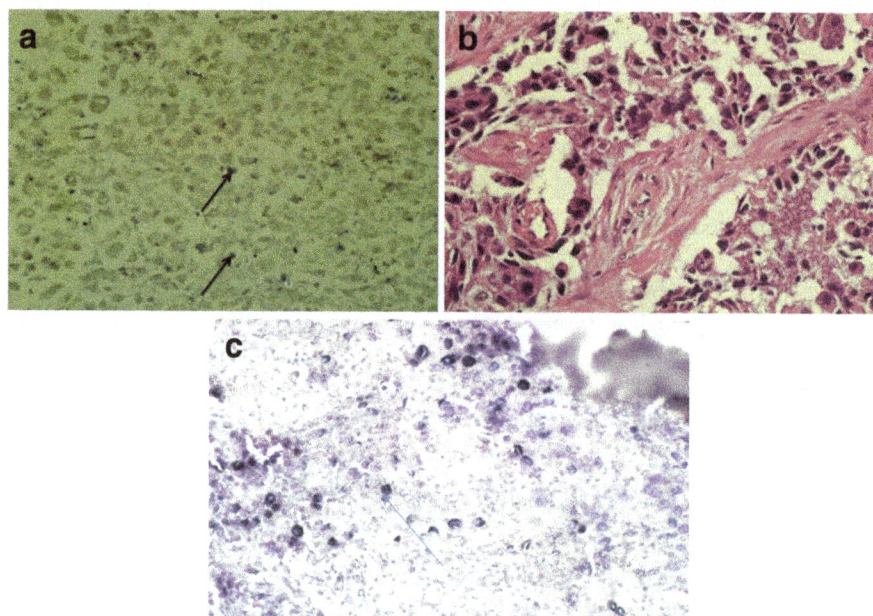

Fig. 1 Detection of EBV in poorly differentiated invasive ductal carcinoma tissue section using EBER-ISH nuclear staining. Epstein-Barr virus-encoded RNA-1 (EBER1) in situ hybridization technique was used on those samples which were relatively more positive by PCR (n = 14) and signal for viral transcripts was observed in 35.71% (5/14). Figure 1**a** shows a case of poorly differentiated invasive ductal carcinoma exhibiting nuclear positivity indicated by dark staining within malignant cells (arrows). (X 40 objective). Figure. 1**b** is the hematoxyline and eosin staining of the image in Fig. 1**a**. (X 40 objective). Figure 1**c** is a positive control from a case of EBV infected nasopharyngeal carcinoma tissue section showing dark nuclear staining (arrows). (X40 objective)

one of the positive slides revealing nuclear localization of the viral transcript within the tumor cells, though compared to the positive control from a case of NPC (Fig. 1c) the viral copies seems quite low.

Of interest here, from epidemiological point of view, the frequency difference in Eritrean cases in comparison to neighboring Sudan where a frequency as high as 100% EBV infection in breast cancer has been reported [5]. This variation may be influenced by factors such as geographical and immunological differences and ethnicity [15, 34]. Lopategui and his team in their study in cases of sinonasal undifferentiated carcinomas comparing populations from two different regions suggested that genetic predisposition or environmental cofactors play an important role in determining the strength of the association of malignancy with EBV [35]. Similar to the present work, low copy number of EBV in breast cancer is also reported in other studies though, latently EBV infected cells contain massive EBER viral transcripts [36, 37] as is the case in NPC in which the frequency is 100%. Magrath and Bhatia suggested that the presence of EBV genome in only a subset of tumor cells indicates that EBV may infect already formed cancer cell implying its absence in neoplastic clone at the time of malignant transformation, but they do not rule out selective loss of viral genome [32]. Kalkan and his team detected EBV genome in a subset of breast cancer tissues and based on their finding and the findings of other studies, concluded that EBV if it has a role in breast cancer it is only in a limited subset of the cases [38]. In our findings not all PCR positive samples were also positive by ISH. The in concordance between the results of these two assays was previously reported. Richardson and his team reviewed 16 studies that used both ISH and PCR to detect EBV in breast cancer tissue and found out that in nine (56%) of the studies PCR positive cases were negative by ISH [28]. Most of our samples which were EBV-ISH positive were poorly differentiated invasive ductal carcinoma which indicates that the virus may probably have a role in complicating existing tumor. It is known that EBV is usually detected in undifferentiated nasopharyngeal carcinoma [4] and its association with highly invasive breast tumors is also reported [12].

LMP2A is over expressed in 15.55% ($n=7$) of the 45 breast cancer samples stained by immunostaining. This indicates low frequency of viral protein expression in breast cancer samples from Eritrea. This protein was observed to be expressed in about half of the samples from NPC and is mainly localized at the tumor invasive front [39].

EBV is one of the most successful pathogens to establish perfect host pathogen equilibrium and lives latently without too much interfering into the health of humans and according to some authors [40, 41] its carcinogenic effect is the outcome of its coordination with other cofactors. Even in its well established association with lymphomas it is mainly detected in immunodeficiency state and is known as a ubiquitous virus which usually causes cancer in immune suppressed individuals [42]. Some authors believe that, pathogenesis of EBV may be of significance only in the presence of environmental carcinogens or pre-existing epithelial damage [32].

Interestingly, EBV genome was also detected in six (9.52%) out of a total 63 controls (fibroadenomas). One sample was also positive by IHC for LMP2a protein and another one was positive by EBER-ISH. The role of EBV in the pathogenesis of fibroadenoma is suggested in a study performed on immunosuppressed individuals [43]. In another study benign breast tissues were positive for EBV DNA [38] and it is reported to infect non- cancerous gastric epithelium such as atrophic gastric mucosa which may progress to cancer [44, 45]. Further study is required for the role of EBV in non-cancerous breast tissues such as fibroadenomas.

In this study, even if the viral genome was detected within tumor epithelial cells and the low copy number was accepted as having a role in pathophysiology of the disease; majority of our test samples were free of the viral genome. The loss of viral genome during tumor development due to 'Hit and run' hypothesis was previously suggested [46] but have doubt as whether this can explain the whole scenario. Thus, in this study, though there seems to be an association of EBV with breast cancer, considering the low number of infected samples and low viral copy number in each infected samples, it is difficult to generalize the viral casual role.

Conclusion

Based on the present finding which showed very low frequency of EBV in breast cancer tumors as well as low viral copy number within positive tumors, it can be concluded that though there could probably be some sort of association between EBV and breast cancer, its role as prime tumor initiator in breast cancer in Eritrea seems less probable. Further studies are required to determine the role of the few infected cells in carcinogenesis as well as tumor progression and the epidemiological cofactors which impact on EBV association with breast cancer in Eritrea.

Abbreviations

EBER: Epstein Barr Encoded RNA; EBV: Epstein-Barr virus; FFPE: Formalin fixed paraffin- embedded; GAPDH: Glyceraldehyde-3-phosphate-dehydrogenase; IARC: International Agent for Research in Cancer; IHC: Immunohistochemistry; ISH: In situ hybridization; LMP-1: Latent Membrane Protein-1; LMP2a: Latent Membrane Protein-2a; NPC: Nasopharyngeal carcinoma; PCR: Polymerase chain reaction

Acknowledgements

The authors express their appreciation to the Department of Histopathology, National Health Laboratory; Department of Surgery, Orotta Referral Hospital; and Keren Referral Hospital, Ministry of Health, Eritrea for granting us permission to collect samples from their respective facilities. We thank Dr. Babikir Ishag Mohamed Fadul, Radiation and Isotope Center, Khartoum, for initially reading the ISH stained slides.

Funding

This study was funded by African Developing Bank (ADB) through the National Commission for Higher Education, Eritrea.

Authors' contributions

GF & MI conceived of the study idea and wrote the manuscript; GF performed laboratory experiments data analysis; AG participated in sample collection and analysis of the 10 years breast cancer data, AME and AAMA analyzed the *In situ* hybridization stained slides and. EME analyzed the immunochemistry stained slides. All authors read and approved the final manuscript.

Authors' information

GF, PhD in molecular biology, Asmara College of Health Sciences, Eritrea. AME, Emeritus professor of pathology, Institute of Endemic Diseases, University of Khartoum, Khartoum, Sudan, EME, Faculty of Medical Laboratory Sciences, Alzaeim Alazhari University, Khartoum, Sudan. AAMA. PhD in Molecular Biology, Department of Molecular Biology, Institute of Endemic Diseases, University of Khartoum, Khartoum, Sudan. AG, Graduate assistant, Asmara College of Health Sciences, MEI, Professor of genetics, Department of molecular biology, Institute of Endemic Diseases, University of Khartoum, Khartoum, Sudan

Competing interests

The authors declare that they have no competing interests.

Author details

[1]Department of Molecular Biology, Institute of Endemic Diseases, University of Khartoum, Al-Qasr Street, P.O. Box 102, Khartoum, Sudan. [2]Faculty of Medical Laboratory Sciences, Alzaeim Alazhari University, Khartoum, Sudan. [3]Faculty of Medical Laboratory Sciences, Department of Histopathology and Cytology, Al Neelain University, Khartoum, Sudan. [4]Asmera College of Health Sciences, Asmara, Eritrea.

References

1. Ferlay J, Soerjomataram I, Ervik M, Dikshit R, Eser S, Mathers C, et al. GLOBOCAN 2012 v1.0 Cancer Incidence and Mortality Worldwide: IARC Cancer Base No. 11. Lyon France: International Agency for Research on Cancer; 2013. Available from: http://globocan.iarc.fr accessed on 10/8/2016.
2. Fregene A, Newman LA. Breast cancer in sub-Saharan Africa: how does it relate to breast cancer in African-American women? Cancer. 2005;103:1540–50.
3. Pogo BG, Holland JF. Possibilities of a viral etiology for human breast cancer. Biol Trace Elem Res. 1997;56:131–42.
4. Tang W, Harmon P, Gulley ML, Mwansambo C, Kazembe PN, Martinson F. Viral Response to Chemotherapy in Endemic Burkitt Lymphoma. Clin Cancer Res. 2010;16(7):2055–64.
5. Yahia ZA, Adam AA, Elgizouli M, Hussein A, Masri MA, Kamal M, Ibrahim ME. Epstein Barr virus: a prime candidate of breast cancer aetiology in Sudanese patients. Infect Agent Cancer. 2014;9:9.
6. Schooley RT. Epstein-Barr Virus (Infectious Mononucleosis). In: Mandell GL, Bennett JE, Dolin R, editors. Mandell, Douglas, and Benett's principles and practice of infectious diseases vol 2. 4th ed. New York, N.Y: Churchill Livingstone; 1995. p. 1364–77.
7. Pegtel DM, Middeldorp J, Thorley-Lawson DA. Epstein-Barr virus infection in ex vivo tonsil epithelial cell cultures of asymptomatic carriers. J Virol. 2004; 78(22):12613–24.
8. Rickinson AB, Kieff E. Epstein-Barr virus. In: Fields BN, Knipe DM, Howley PM, editors. Virology. 3rd ed. New York, N.Y: Raven Press; 1996. p. 2397–446.
9. Epstein-barr IARC. virus and Kaposi's sarcoma herpesvirus/Human herpesvirus 8. IARC Monogr Eval Carcinog Risks Hum. 1997;70:1–492.
10. Labrecque LG, Barnes DM, Fentiman IS, Griffin BE. Epstein-Barr virus in epithelial cell tumors: a breast cancer study. Cancer Res. 1995;55:39–45.
11. Lespagnard L, Cochaux P, Larsimont D, Degeyter M, Velu T, Heimann R. Absence of Epstein-Barr virus in medullary carcinoma of the breast as demonstrated by immunophenotyping in situ hybridization and polymerase chain reaction. Am J Clin Pathol. 1995;103:449–52.
12. Bonnet M, Guinebretiere JM, Kremmer E, Grunewald V, Benhamou E, Contesso G. Detection of Epstein-Barr virus in invasive breast cancers. J Natl Cancer Inst. 1999;91:1376–81.
13. Joab I. Detection of Epstein–Barr virus in invasive breast cancers. J Natl Cancer Inst. 2000;92:656.
14. Angeloni A, Farina A, Gentile G, Capobianchi A, Martino P, Visco V. Epstein-Barr virus and breast cancer: search for antibodies to the novel BFRF1 protein in sera of breast cancer patients. J Natl Cancer Inst. 2001;93:560–1.
15. Fina F, Romain S, Ouafik L, Palmari J, Ayed FB, Benharkat S, et al. Frequency and genome load of Epstein-Barr virus in 509 breast cancers from different geographical areas. Br J Cancer. 2001;84(6):783–90.
16. Murray PG, Young LS. Epstein–Barr virus infection: basis of malignancy and potential for therapy. Exp Rev Mol M Med. 2001;3(28):1–20.
17. Deshpande CG, Badve S, Kidwai N, Longnecker R. Lack of expression of the Epstein-Barr virus (EBV) gene products EBERs EBNA1 LMP1 and LMP2A in breast cancer cells. Lab Investig. 2002;82:1193–9.
18. Hermann K, Niedobitek G. Lack of evidence for an association of Epstein-Barr virus infection with breast carcinoma. Breast Cancer Res. 2003;5:R13–7.
19. Perrigoue JG, den Boon JA, Friedl A, Newton MA, Ahlquist P, Sugden B. Lack of association between EBV and breast carcinoma. Cancer Epidemiol Biomark Prev. 2005;14:809–14.
20. Perkins RS, Sahm K, Marando C, Witmer DD, Pahnke GR, Mitchell M. Analysis of Epstein-Barr virus reservoirs in paired blood and breast carcinoma primary biopsy specimens by real time PCR. Breast Cancer Res. 2006;8: R70.'
21. Joshi D, Quadri M, Gangane N, Joshi R, Gangane N. Association of Epstein Barr Virus Infection (EBV) with Breast Cancer in Rural Indian Women. PLoS One. 2009;4(12):e8180.
22. Lorenzetti MA, De Matteo E, Gass H, Martinez Vazquez P, Lara J, Gonzalez P, et al. Characterization of Epstein Barr Virus Latency Pattern in Argentine Breast Carcinoma. PLoS One. 2010;5(10):e13603.
23. Khan G, Philip PS, Al Ashari M, Houcinat Y, Daoud S. Localization of Epstein-Barr virus to infiltrating lymphocytes in breast carcinomas and not malignant cells. Exp Mol Pathol. 2011;91(1):466–70.
24. Mazouni C, Fina F, Romain S, Ouafik L, Bonnier P, Brandone JM, Martin PM. Epstein-Barr virus as a marker of biological aggressiveness in breast cancer. Br J Cancer. 2011;104(2):332–7.
25. Fadavi P, Rostamian M, Arashkia A, Shafaghi B, Niknam HM. Epstein- barr virus may not be associated with breast cancer in Iranian patients. Oncol Discov. 2013;1:3.
26. Glaser SL, Hsu JL, Gulley ML. Epstein-barr virus and breast cancer: state of the evidence for viral carcinogenesis. Cancer Epidemiol Biomark Prev. 2004; 13(5):688–97.
27. Lorenzetti MA, Gantuz M, Altcheh J, De Matteo E, Chabay PA, Preciado MV. Distinctive Epstein-Barr Virus Variants Associated with Benign and Malignant Pediatric Pathologies: LMP1 Sequence Characterization and Linkage with Other Viral Gene Polymorphisms. J Clin Microbiol. 2012;50(3):609–18.
28. Richardson AK, Currie MJ, Robinson BA, Morrin H, Phung Y, Pearson JF. Cytomegalovirus and Epstein - Barr virus in Breast Cancer. PLoS One. 2015; 10(2):e0118989.
29. Khabaz MN. Association of Epstein-Barr virus infection and breast carcinoma. Arch Med Sci. 2013;9(4):745–51.
30. Huo Q, Zhang N, Yang Q. Epstein-Barr Virus Infection and Sporadic Breast Cancer Risk: A Meta-Analysis. PLoS One. 2012;7(2):e31656.
31. Arbach H, Viglasky V, Lefeu F, Guinebretière JM, Ramirez V, Bride N. Epstein-Barr Virus (EBV) Genome and Expression in Breast Cancer Tissue: Effect of EBV Infection of Breast Cancer Cells on Resistance to Paclitaxel (Taxol). J Virol. 2006;80(2):845–53.
32. Magrath I, Bhatia K. Breast cancer: a new Epstein–Barr virus-associated disease. J Natl Cancer Inst. 1999;91(16):1349–50.

33. Chang KL, Chen YY, Shibata D, Weiss LM. Description of an in situ hybridization methodology for detection of Epstein-Barr virus RNA in paraffin- embedded tissues with a survey of normal and neoplastic tissues. Diagn Mol Pahol. 1992;1:246–55.
34. Thompson MP, Kurzrock R. Epstein-Barr virus and cancer. Clin Cancer Res. 2004;10:803–21.
35. Lopategui JR, Gaffey MJ, Weiss LM. Detection of Epstein-Barr viral RNA in sinonasal undifferentiated carcinoma from Western and Asian patients. Am J Surg Pathol. 1994;18:391–8.
36. TC W, Mann RB, Epstein JL, MacMahon E, Lee WA, Charache P, et al. Abundant expression of EBER1 small nuclear RNA in nasopharyngeal carcinoma. A morphologically distinctive target for detection of Epstein-Barr virus in formalin-fixed paraffin-embedded carcinoma specimens. Am J Pathol. 1991;138:1461–9.
37. Gulley ML. Molecular diagnosis of Epstein-Barr virus related diseases. J Mol Diagn. 2001;3(1):1–10.
38. Kalkan A, Ozdarendeli A, Bulut Y, Yekeler H, Cobanoglu B, Doymaz MZ. Investigation of Epstein-Barr virus DNA in Formalin-Fixed and Paraffin-Embedded Breast Cancer Tissues. Med Princ Pract. 2005;14:268–71.
39. Kong QL, LJ H, Cao JY, Huang YJ, LH X, Liang Y, et al. Epstein-Barr Virus-Encoded LMP2A Induces an Epithelial–Mesenchymal Transition and Increases the Number of Side Population Stem-like Cancer Cells in Nasopharyngeal Carcinoma. PLoS Pathog. 2010;6(6):e1000940–10.
40. Griffin B. Epstein-Barr virus (EBV) and human disease: Facts opinions and problems. Mutat Res. 2000;462:395–405.
41. Crawford DH. Biology and disease associations of Epstein-Barr virus. Philos Trans R Soc Lond. 2001;356:461–73.
42. Raab-Traub N. Pathogenesis of Epstein–Barr virus and its associated malignancies. Semin Virol. 1996;7:315–23.
43. Kleer CG, Tseng MD, Gutsch DE, Rochford RA, Wu Z, Joynt LK, et al. Detection of Epstein-Barr virus in rapidly growing fibroadenomas of the breast in immune suppressed hosts. Mod Pathol. 2002;15(7):759–64.
44. Arikawa J, Tokunaga M, Tashiro Y, Tanaka S, Sato E, Haraguchi K. Epstein-Barr virus-positive multiple early gastric cancers and dysplastic lesions: a case report. Pathol Int. 1997;47:730–4.
45. Yanai H, Takada K, Shimizu N, Mizugaki Y, Tada M, Okita K. Epstein-Barr virus infection in non-carcinomatous gastric epithelium. J Pathol. 1997;183:293–8.
46. Ambinder RF. Gamma herpes viruses and hit and run oncogenesis. Am J Pathol. 2000;156:1–3.

20

Human papillomavirus genome variants and head and neck cancers

Jean-Damien Combes[1]*⦿ and Silvia Franceschi[2]

Abstract

Human papillomaviruses (HPV) cause infections that are responsible for diverse clinical manifestations from benign conditions to invasive cancer. As different HPV types are associated with variable pathogenic potential, minor genetic variations within a given high-risk HPV type might also be associated with distinct oncogenic capacities, through variable ability of persistence or risk of progression to precancer/cancer. Most recent HPV variant studies in the cervix using latest sequencing technology confirmed that minor changes in the HPV genome can have a major influence on carcinogenesis and have revealed key data that help better understand the carcinogenicity of HPV at a molecular level. Here we review the limited number of studies on HPV genome variants in head and neck cancers (HNC) and discuss their implications for cancer research in the light of accumulated knowledge for the cervix. Challenges in transposing HPV variant studies from the lower anogenital to the upper aerodigestive tract are also discussed, highlighting the main gaps of knowledge in the field of HPV-induced HNC. Specifically in the head and neck region, the lack of characterisation of precancerous lesions and the difficulty in sampling normal tissue will challenge the development of accurate studies. Although there is so far no indication that HPV variant research in HNC could directly translate into clinical application, such research is expected to be useful to disentangle unanswered questions in the pathogenesis of HNC. Yet, history of HPV variant research suggests that, to be successful, studies will require large international collaborative efforts.

Keywords: Human papillomavirus, HPV variants, HPV genome, Head and neck cancer, Epidemiology

Background

Human papillomaviruses (HPV) cause infections that are responsible for diverse clinical manifestations from warts (papillomas) to invasive cancer. A dozen high-risk (HR) HPV types are powerful human carcinogens and the primary cause of cancer of the cervix and anogenital tract [1]. In the upper aerodigestive tract, HPV16 is recognized as the cause of a growing proportion of cancer of the oropharynx, particularly in the tonsil and the base of the tongue, although with substantial international variations [2].

It is well established that although all HPV are genetically related, their pathogenic characteristics differ widely [1]. As different HR-HPV types are associated with variable pathogenic potential [3], minor genetic variations within a given HR-HPV type might also be associated with distinct oncogenic capacities, through variable ability of persistence or risk of progression to precancer/cancer [4]. With recent improvement in DNA sequencing technology [5], promising findings were reported on the influence of HPV variants in carcinogenesis in cervical cancer that has been much more extensively studied than head and neck cancer (HNC) [6, 7], opening potential scope for clinical applications.

In the present article, we reviewed the limited number of studies on HPV genome variants in HNC and discussed their implications for cancer research in the light of accumulated knowledge in the cervix. Challenges in transposing HPV variant studies from cervical to HNC are also discussed, highlighting the main gaps of knowledge in the field of HPV-induced HNC.

Terminology

Papillomaviruses are small non-enveloped viruses with circular double-stranded DNA of around 7000–8000 nucleotides infecting skin and mucosa of a variety of mammals, reptiles and birds [1]. Papillomaviruses are highly species-specific and are considered to have coevolved

* Correspondence: CombesJD@iarc.fr
[1]International Agency for Research on Cancer, 150 cours Albert Thomas, 69372 Cedex 08 Lyon, France
Full list of author information is available at the end of the article

with their host since their origin, for hundreds of millions of years. The stability of the double-stranded structure of the genome results in a low mutation rate and it is considered that it takes millions of years for sequential accumulation of genetic changes to become fixed, leading to distinct HPV types [8].

Papillomaviruses are subdivided in genus, species, types and subtypes according to degree of viral genetic variation. Evaluation of differences in the L1 open reading frame DNA sequence is considered sufficient up to type-level classification, as it is accepted that L1 is robust enough to fully determine these subdivisions [9]. Differences of more than 40% between 2 HPV sequences define different "genus" (e.g., *Alphapapillomavirus*, *Betapapillomavirus*), differences of 30–40% define "species" (e.g., *Alphapapillomavirus* 7, *Alphapapillomavirus* 8), and differences of 10–30% define "types" (e.g., human papillomavirus 16 belonging to *Alphapapillomavirus* 9). Of note, the International Committee on Taxonomy of Viruses provides a taxonomic nomenclature only up to the species level [10].

HPV "variants" are smaller genetic variations in the viral DNA sequence within a given HPV type. At the subtype level, the evaluation of the difference in the whole genome sequence is considered necessary [9]. Differences between 1 and 10% define "lineages" (e.g., HPV16_A, HPV16_B) and differences between 0.5 to 1% define "sublineages" (e.g., HPV16_A1, HPV16_A2). The terminology is, however, evolving rapidly following progress in molecular biology and often hampers appropriate comparisons across studies. Previously used HPV variant classification referring to geography (e.g., "African-1", "Asia-American", "European") corresponds to population groups where each lineage is most often found, but, although being practical, the use of this terminology is no longer recommended [9, 11]. Sublineages A1, A2 and A3 correspond to previously termed "European" lineage; lineages B and C to "African-1" and "African-2", respectively, sublineage D1 to "North-American", sublineages D2 and D3 to "Asian-Amercian", and sublineage A4 to "Asian".

At the subtype level, minor genetic variations that do not fit a phylogenetic tree are also characterised (hereinafter referred to as "non-lineage-specific HPV variants") and correspond to more recent mutations. These non-synonymous single nucleotide changes that can appear independently from lineages are characterised by their DNA or amino acid substitution (e.g., HPV16 T350G located on E6 gene corresponds to L83 V amino acid change).

Early studies on HPV variants and cervical cancer

All twelve HR-HPV belong to the *Alphapapillomavirus* genus (species 5, 6, 7 or 9) but widely differ in prevalence (related to evolutionary fitness) and risk of causing

precancer/cancer. In the same manner, intra-type genetic variations might present differential pathogenic properties, through variable capacity to trigger immune response, ability to persist, or risk of progression to precancer/cancer. It is, for instance, conceivable that a minor variation in the E6 or E7 sequence may induce differential propensity of the corresponding protein to bind p53 or pRB and impact the risk of progression to cancer by modifying their capacity to inactivate the corresponding tumour suppressor functions.

Risk associated to HPV variants in cervical carcinogenesis has been studied since the early 1990s [12, 13]. There is a substantial accumulation of data from epidemiologic and mechanistic studies on the influence of various HPV variants in cervical pathogenesis. Historically, HPV variants in the cervix were compared for "European" versus "non-European" HPV lineages ("A" vs. "B/C/D" (sub)lineages following the most recent nomenclature). The "non-European" HPV16 lineages have been generally found to be associated with higher persistence [14, 15] and higher progression to cancer [14–20] compared to "European" lineages, most often in studies from Europe and USA. Another well-studied HPV variant, T350G, is non-lineage-specific and corresponds to a single nucleotide change in the HPV16 E6 gene. HPV16 350G was similarly associated with higher persistence [21–23] and progression to cancer [24–28] compared to HPV16 350 T. Some experimental and mechanistic evidence has partly supported the plausibility of these associations [28–36]. Other studies have also suggested differential risk of glandular vs. squamous cancers associated with specific HPV lineages [20, 37, 38].

However, globally, early studies on HPV variants in the cervix were judged as relatively disappointing. Inadequate sample size probably partly explains the inconsistencies between these studies with regard to the direction of the variants' effect, but also prevented further evaluation of these observations [39–47]. Indeed, functional differences might be attributed not only to the effect of one isolated genetic variation but to specific combinations of amino acid changes. In fact, early studies had already by that time strongly suggested that the observed increased pathogenicity related to some HPV variants could be specific to a population [48–50] because of host-related factors [42, 51–53].

Next-generation sequencing era and studies on HPV variants

With recent development of next-generation methods, their increasing availability and adaptability to large-scale populations, promising findings have emerged on pathogenic effects related to HPV variants in cervical cancer. These greatly improved approaches pave the way for the evaluation of variants in other HPV-associated cancer sites such as cancer of the oropharynx.

Mirabello et al. evaluated the association between HPV16 lineages and risk of precancer/cancer in 3200 women from a US cohort [6], using a whole genome sequencing assay optimized for HPV genome sequencing [5]. This study confirmed the early observation of a higher risk of precancer/cancer associated with B/C/D as a group compared to A lineages. Most importantly, further stratification by sublineage and by specific histologic outcome was possible due to appropriate sample size. In this case-control analysis (controls being HPV16-positive women without cervical intraepithelial neoplasia (CIN) grade 2+ after ≈3 years follow-up), it was shown that the overall association between HPV16 lineage and cervical cancer risk masked strong heterogeneity in pathogenicity according to sub-lineage and disease outcome.

Indeed, it was shown that previously defined "European" variants actually regrouped sublineages with substantially different risks of precancer/cancer. For instance, risk associated with sublineage A4 was markedly higher compared to A1/A2. In the same manner, risk associated with histology outcome showed strong heterogeneity. Odds ratio (OR) of glandular cancer for D2 vs A1/A2 sublineages was 137.3 (95% CI: 37.2–506.9) whereas OR of squamous cancer was 7.6 (95%CI: 1.4–39.8). This finding was corroborated by a comparable study using samples collected worldwide [54]. Although the absolute risk of cervical adenocarcinoma remains low, such a high effect size points to possibilities for a clinical application, given the difficulty to identify glandular lesions by cytology and a poorer prognosis compared to squamous type.

In addition, this study confirmed the early observation that some variants present a higher carcinogenic effect in women whose genetic background corresponds to that of the virus. For instance, Caucasian white women infected with A1/A2 variant were at a higher risk of CIN3+ compared to women of other genetic backgrounds. Similarly, Asian and Hispanic women had increased risk, although non-significant, associated with A4 and D2/D3 sublineages compared with other races/ethnicities. Of note, the magnitude of the effect of associations with genetic backgrounds was relatively low (OR≈1.5).

An important and unexpected finding came from the same collaborative group who analysed more than 5000 HPV16 case control samples worldwide [7]. It was shown that the HPV16 E7 sequence (98 amino acids) leading to cervical cancer is virtually invariant compared to high sequence variability in controls. This finding was confirmed to be consistent across regions and ethnicity. Of note, an earlier study has also suggested that the E7 sequence of HPV type 16 was less variable compared to other high risk types (HPV31) [55]. Although to be confirmed, a strict conservation of E7 could represent a promising highly specific biomarker and may also be important for HPV-associated and for non-cervical cancers.

HPV variant studies and head and neck cancers

HNC includes numerous tumours that generally share strong associations with tobacco and alcohol consumption [56]. HPV16 is generally accepted as a carcinogen in tonsil and base of the tongue, but its implication in other sites such as oral cavity, larynx or even in oropharyngeal tissues outside the Waldeyer's ring is at most a weak one [57, 58]. It is nonetheless conceivable that many non-tonsillar HNC are falsely classified as HPV-positive or are actually misclassified tonsillar or oropharyngeal cancers (OPC), as characterisation of the true site of origin is often difficult due to fast local extension and unclear anatomical boundaries.

HPV-induced OPCs involve both genders, although with higher incidence in men compared to women [59]. This sex-ratio is mainly explained by the higher HPV transmission for vaginal-oral rather than penile-oral sexual intercourse. Saunders et al. recently showed that risk of OPC was higher in women having sex with women compared with heterosexual women, although this association was not found in men having sex with men, in agreement with a higher risk of HPV transmission by vaginal- vs. penile-oral sex [60]. The lower risk of HPV-induced OPC observed in women could also be partly explained by the higher immunity acquired by women due to more frequent exposure to HPV in the genital mucosa and by a still little understood role of the combined exposure to HPV and tobacco that is generally stronger in men than women [59]. As for cervical cancer, the presence of other risk factors and host-characteristics should be considered in HPV variant studies of HNC.

Few studies reporting HPV16 variants in HNC are available (Table 1), including on the distribution of HPV variant lineages [61–67], T350G [61, 66, 68, 69] and other non-lineage-specific variants [61, 66, 67, 70]. These studies resemble early studies of cervical cancer in being mere descriptions of variant prevalence in small populations from North America and Europe. Some of these studies did not present data separately for oropharyngeal and other head and neck sites, and the definition of HPV-induced HNC is variable, using frequently only HPV-DNA detection or p16-positivity. These major limitations prevented us from any interpretation, thus our report regarding those studies remains descriptive.

In an early study on the role of HPV in HNC, Gillison et al. provided data on prevalence of HPV variant lineages, T350G and other non-lineage-specific variants among 52 HPV16-positive HNC from the USA [67]. The observed distribution of HPV variants was judged

Table 1 Studies on HPV16 variants in head and neck cancers

Study	Country	N HPV16 + samples	Seq.	Variant lineage (n)	Non lineage specific variants (n)
Gillison 2000 [67]	USA	52 HNC	E6	39 Eur; 9 Asian; 2 NA; 1 Afr-1	20 T350G 6 A131G
Hoffmann 2004 [70]	DE	21 HNC (5 OPC)	E6/E7		8 T350G (2 in OPC) 7 A131G (1 in OPC)
Badaracco 2007 [62]	IT	13 HNC (5 TC)	L1	9 Eur 2 Af-2; 1 AA	
Agrawal 2008 [61]	USA	14 HNC	E6	13 Eur 1 As	3 T350G
Boscolo Rizzo 2009 [68]	IT	8 HNC (4 OPC)	E6		5 T350G
Blakaj 2012 [65]	USA	43 HNC (28 OPC)	E6	31 Eur 7 AA; 3 Af	
Du 2012 [66]	SW	108 TC	E6	51(/55) EUR	43 T350G 21 A131G
Barbieri 2014 [63]	IT	51 OPC	L1	41 Eur 10 Af	
Hassani 2015 [69]	JP	10 TC	E6		8 T350G (1/3 T350G in tonsillitis)
Betiol 2016 [64]	BR	21 HNC (3 OPC)	E6	12 Eur 9 AA or NA1	

Abbreviations: *HNC* Head and neck cancer, *OPC* Oropharyngeal cancer
Countries: *BR*Brazil, *DE* Germany, *IT* Italia, *JP*, Japan, *SW* Sweden
HPV variant lineages: *EUR* European, *A* Asian, *AA* Asian American, *NA* North American, *Af* African

similar to that in a contemporary study of cervical cancers in North America. In a comprehensive study on oral HPV infection before and after treatment, Agrawal et al. reported HPV variant lineage distribution as well as T350G and T131G in patients diagnosed with HPV-induced HNC in the USA. In the latter study, oral rinses were also collected and E6 sequence identity was compared with the tumour (concordant in 10/11) [61].

Blakaj et al. have evaluated the association between variant lineages and HNC disease stage, hypothesising differential variant distribution in higher TNM and N+ staged tumours [65]. Barbieri et al. have also compared clinical stage according to HPV variant lineages in 51 OPC cases from Italy but failed to detect any association [63]. Unexpectedly in this study, African lineage was detected in 10 out of 51 OPC. In Hassani et al., frequency of T350G was reported in 10 HPV16-positive tonsillar cancer and 3 HPV-positive tonsillitis specimens [69]. The same team had also previously compared distribution of HPV variant lineages and non-lineage-specific variants in Japan, Pakistan and Columbia in oral cavity and oesophageal cancer, but not in OPC [71].

One notable study compared E6 variants A131G (R10G) and T350G in 108 tonsillar and cervical cancers in Swedish patients [66]. In this study, a significantly higher representation of A131G was reported in tonsillar cancer (21/108) compared to cervical samples (2/51) and cervical cancer (0/52). The role of A131G is not clearly established but has been linked to p53 binding and degradation [72]. Of note, among other findings, presence of A131G variant was not associated with disease-free survival and T350G variant was common in tonsillar cancer (45%), cervical cancer (31%) and cervical samples (29%).

Challenges and perspectives in studying HPV variants in head and neck cancers

Critical differences between genital and upper aerodigestive tracts need to be underlined [73, 74], implying specific challenges in research on HPV variants. Cervical cancer is nearly always caused by HPV and, worldwide, it is a much more frequent cancer than HPV-induced HNC [2]. Also importantly, the collection of cervical samples at different steps of carcinogenesis is relatively easy for anatomical reasons and the long going practice of screening around the world. In the cervix, it is thus possible not only to analyse cancer cases but also longitudinal data at the individual level to evaluate the risk of persistent infection or progression to precancer/cancer associated with specific HPV variants.

The major challenge for the head and neck consists in the lack of characterisation of the carcinogenetic steps from normal tissue to cancer. Although few studies have attempted to collect precancerous lesions in non-cancerous patients using cytology from in vivo [75–77] or ex vivo [78] tonsillar brushings, none were successful. There is however a clue that a precancerous state exists, and long before the diagnosis of cancer. Two longitudinal studies evaluating HPV16 serology reported not only a high specificity but most importantly that in OPC cases, HPV16 seropositivity could be detected more than 10 years prior to diagnosis [79, 80]. Yet the suspected precancerous lesions are hardly identifiable most probably because HPV-induced tonsillar cancer is believed to arise from the depth of the crypts and is hence challenging to sample [78].

An additional critical challenge exists when trying to assess whether certain HPV variants show differential risk of persistent infection. Indeed sampling non-cancerous tonsillar or oropharyngeal tissue to detect HPV infection is problematic. All sampling methods are imperfect due to specific limitations [81, 82]: evaluation of frozen or paraffin biopsies suffers from a lack of exhaustiveness; although more representative than a biopsy; oropharyngeal brushing hardly permits sampling inside the crypt; rinse/gargle does not inform on what tissue is evaluated and gargle can be impossible to some patients due to laryngeal spasm in addition to the uncertainty that even a proper gargle can detect an infection inside a crypt. We recently showed that concordance between HPV detection using rinse/gargle, tonsil ex vivo brushing and frozen biopsies is critically low [81, 82]. Accordingly, studies of the natural history of HPV in the oropharynx have not been possible so far.

Yet case-case comparisons including other HPV-induced cancer sites should be informative [11]. The greater predominance of HPV16 in OPC (around 90%) compared to the cervix (50/60%) suggests a different host-viral interaction in the two sites. It is therefore credible that some HPV variants without influence in cervical pathogenesis could play a role in the oropharynx, as specific sublineages are associated with specific histological subtypes [6], some HPV variants could be more prone to infect or to trigger progression to cancer in oropharyngeal compared to cervical tissue. Likewise, although there is no data so far suggesting that HPV variants could have an effect on therapeutic response, an influence is possible, for instance through modification of the tumour microenvironment.

There is so far no indication that HPV variant research in HNC would be directly clinically relevant. However, such research could be useful to disentangle other unanswered questions including HPV genome integration [83–85], the identification of a robust method to determine a truly HPV-driven HNC or those with the best prognosis [58, 86, 87], or a possible distinct pathogenesis in an immunosuppressed population. Of note, the use of complete genome sequencing obviously allows finer definition of persistent vs. cleared infection in longitudinal studies [88] or finer confirmation of the concordance of HPV detection in rinse/gargles with HPV-HNC tissue [61]. Other illustrations of HPV variant studies included evaluation of their influence on HPV serological response [89] or on HPV vaccine efficacy [90]. Regarding non-cancerous HPV-related conditions, such as recurrent papillomatosis or genital warts, yet unanswered questions might also take advantage of HPV variant studies [91–93].

Conclusion

In conclusion, our review suggests that the most recent HPV variant studies in cervical cancer are of importance in planning the evaluation of HPV heterogeneity in other HPV-associated cancer including HNC. HPV variant studies using recent sequencing technology have generated key data that should help better understand the carcinogenicity of HPV at a molecular level. If these successful studies have confirmed that minor changes in the HPV genome can have a major influence on carcinogenesis, they also highlight the crucial need for international collaborative efforts to allow appropriate in depth analyses.

Abbreviations

CI: confidence interval; CIN: Cervical intraepithelial neoplasia; HNC: head and neck cancer; HR-HPV: high-risk human papillomavirus virus; OPC: oropharyngeal cancers

Acknowledgements

Not applicable.

Funding

Not applicable.

Authors' contributions

Both authors have directly participated in the planning and execution of this review, have read and approved the final version.

Competing interests

The authors declare they have no competing interests.

Author details

[1]International Agency for Research on Cancer, 150 cours Albert Thomas, 69372 Cedex 08 Lyon, France. [2]Cancer Epidemiology Unit, CRO Aviano National Cancer Institute IRCCS, Via Franco Gallini 2, 33081 Aviano, PN, Italy.

References

1. IARC. Biological agents. IARC Monogr Eval Carcinog Risks Hum. 2012;100B:1–475. http://monographs.iarc.fr/ENG/Monographs/vol100B/index.php. Accessed 30 December 2017
2. de Martel C, et al. Worldwide burden of cancer attributable to HPV by site, country and HPV type. Int J Cancer. 2017;141(4):664–70.
3. Combes JD, et al. Judging the carcinogenicity of rare human papillomavirus types. Int J Cancer. 2015;136(3):740–2.
4. Bernard HU, Calleja-Macias IE, Dunn ST. Genome variation of human papillomavirus types: phylogenetic and medical implications. Int J Cancer. 2006;118(5):1071–6.
5. Cullen M, et al. Deep sequencing of HPV16 genomes: a new high-throughput tool for exploring the carcinogenicity and natural history of HPV16 infection. Papillomavirus Res. 2015;1:3–11.
6. Mirabello L, et al. HPV16 sublineage associations with histology-specific Cancer risk using HPV whole-genome sequences in 3200 women. J Natl Cancer Inst. 2016;108(9)
7. Mirabello, L., et al., HPV16 E7 Genetic Conservation Is Critical to Carcinogenesis. Cell, 2017. 170(6): p. 1164–1174 e6.
8. Chen Z, et al. Evolutionary dynamics of variant genomes of human papillomavirus types 18, 45, and 97. J Virol. 2009;83(3):1443–55.
9. Burk RD, Harari A, Chen Z. Human papillomavirus genome variants. Virology. 2013;445(1–2):232–43.
10. Bernard HU, et al. Classification of papillomaviruses (PVs) based on 189 PV types and proposal of taxonomic amendments. Virology. 2010;401(1):70–9.

11. Nicolas-Parraga S, et al. HPV16 variants distribution in invasive cancers of the cervix, vulva, vagina, penis, and anus. Cancer Med. 2016;5(10):2909–19.

12. Hecht JL, et al. Genetic characterization of the human papillomavirus (HPV) 18 E2 gene in clinical specimens suggests the presence of a subtype with decreased oncogenic potential. Int J Cancer. 1995;60(3):369–76.

13. Yamada T, et al. Human papillomavirus type 16 variant lineages in United States populations characterized by nucleotide sequence analysis of the E6, L2, and L1 coding segments. J Virol. 1995;69(12):7743–53.

14. Schiffman M, et al. A population-based prospective study of carcinogenic human papillomavirus variant lineages, viral persistence, and cervical neoplasia. Cancer Res. 2010;70(8):3159–69.

15. Villa LL, et al. Molecular variants of human papillomavirus types 16 and 18 preferentially associated with cervical neoplasia. J Gen Virol. 2000;81(Pt 12): 2959–68.

16. Hildesheim A, et al. Human papillomavirus type 16 variants and risk of cervical cancer. J Natl Cancer Inst. 2001;93(4):315–8.

17. Sichero L, et al. High grade cervical lesions are caused preferentially by non-European variants of HPVs 16 and 18. Int J Cancer. 2007;120(8):1763–8.

18. Xi LF, et al. Risk for high-grade cervical intraepithelial neoplasia associated with variants of human papillomavirus types 16 and 18. Cancer Epidemiol Biomark Prev. 2007;16(1):4–10.

19. Zuna RE, et al. Association of HPV16 E6 variants with diagnostic severity in cervical cytology samples of 354 women in a US population. Int J Cancer. 2009;125(11):2609–13.

20. Berumen J, et al. Asian-American variants of human papillomavirus 16 and risk for cervical cancer: a case-control study. J Natl Cancer Inst. 2001;93(17): 1325–30.

21. Londesborough P, et al. Human papillomavirus genotype as a predictor of persistence and development of high-grade lesions in women with minor cervical abnormalities. Int J Cancer. 1996;69(5):364–8.

22. Gheit T, et al. Risks for persistence and progression by human papillomavirus type 16 variant lineages among a population-based sample of Danish women. Cancer Epidemiol Biomark Prev. 2011;20(7):1315–21.

23. Grodzki M, et al. Increased risk for cervical disease progression of French women infected with the human papillomavirus type 16 E6-350G variant. Cancer Epidemiol Biomark Prev. 2006;15(4):820–2.

24. Zehbe I, et al. Human papillomavirus 16 E6 variants are more prevalent in invasive cervical carcinoma than the prototype. Cancer Res. 1998; 58(4):829–33.

25. Andersson S, et al. Uneven distribution of HPV 16 E6 prototype and variant (L83V) oncoprotein in cervical neoplastic lesions. Br J Cancer. 2000;83(3): 307–10.

26. Brady CS, et al. Human papillomavirus type 16 E6 variants in cervical carcinoma: relationship to host genetic factors and clinical parameters. J Gen Virol. 1999;80(Pt 12):3233–40.

27. Lee K, et al. Human papillomavirus 16 E6, L1, L2 and E2 gene variants in cervical lesion progression. Virus Res. 2008;131(1):106–10.

28. Kammer C, et al. Variants of the long control region and the E6 oncogene in European human papillomavirus type 16 isolates: implications for cervical disease. Br J Cancer. 2002;86(2):269–73.

29. Togtema M, et al. The human papillomavirus 16 European-T350G E6 variant can immortalize but not transform keratinocytes in the absence of E7. Virology. 2015;485:274–82.

30. Zehbe I, et al. Human papillomavirus 16 E6 variants differ in their dysregulation of human keratinocyte differentiation and apoptosis. Virology. 2009;383(1):69–77.

31. von Knebel Doeberitz M, et al. Correlation of modified human papilloma virus early gene expression with altered growth properties in C4-1 cervical carcinoma cells. Cancer Res. 1988;48(13):3780–6.

32. Stoppler MC, et al. Natural variants of the human papillomavirus type 16 E6 protein differ in their abilities to alter keratinocyte differentiation and to induce p53 degradation. J Virol. 1996;70(10):6987–93.

33. Casas L, et al. Asian-american variants of human papillomavirus type 16 have extensive mutations in the E2 gene and are highly amplified in cervical carcinomas. Int J Cancer. 1999;83(4):449–55.

34. Matsumoto K, et al. Human papillomavirus type 16 E6 variants and HLA class II alleles among Japanese women with cervical cancer. Int J Cancer. 2003;106(6):919–22.

35. Chakrabarti O, et al. Human papillomavirus type 16 E6 amino acid 83 variants enhance E6-mediated MAPK signaling and differentially regulate

tumorigenesis by notch signaling and oncogenic Ras. J Virol. 2004;78(11): 5934–45.

36. Jackson R, et al. Functional variants of human papillomavirus type 16 demonstrate host genome integration and transcriptional alterations corresponding to their unique cancer epidemiology. BMC Genomics. 2016; 17(1):851.

37. Burk RD, et al. Distribution of human papillomavirus types 16 and 18 variants in squamous cell carcinomas and adenocarcinomas of the cervix. Cancer Res. 2003;63(21):7215–20.

38. Quint KD, et al. HPV genotyping and HPV16 variant analysis in glandular and squamous neoplastic lesions of the uterine cervix. Gynecol Oncol. 2010; 117(2):297–301.

39. Nindl I, et al. Uniform distribution of HPV 16 E6 and E7 variants in patients with normal histology, cervical intra-epithelial neoplasia and cervical cancer. Int J Cancer. 1999;82(2):203–7.

40. Hu X, et al. HPV16 E6 gene variations in invasive cervical squamous cell carcinoma and cancer in situ from Russian patients. Br J Cancer. 2001;84(6):791–5.

41. Cornet I, et al. Human papillomavirus type 16 E6 variants in France and risk of viral persistence. Infect Agent Cancer. 2013;8(1):4.

42. Zehbe I, et al. Human papillomavirus 16 E6 polymorphisms in cervical lesions from different European populations and their correlation with human leukocyte antigen class II haplotypes. Int J Cancer. 2001;94(5):711–6.

43. Chan PK, et al. Human papillomavirus type 16 intratypic variant infection and risk for cervical neoplasia in southern China. J Infect Dis. 2002;186(5): 696–700.

44. Kang S, et al. Polymorphism in the E6 gene of human papillomavirus type 16 in the cervical tissues of Korean women. Int J Gynecol Cancer. 2005;15(1):107–12.

45. Vaeteewoottacharn K, Jearanaikoon P, Ponglikitmongkol M. Co-mutation of HPV16 E6 and E7 genes in Thai squamous cervical carcinomas. Anticancer Res. 2003;23(2C):1927–31.

46. Marongiu L, et al. Human papillomavirus type 16 long control region and E6 variants stratified by cervical disease stage. Infect Genet Evol. 2014;26:8–13.

47. Tu JJ, et al. Molecular variants of human papillomavirus type 16 and risk for cervical neoplasia in South Africa. Int J Gynecol Cancer. 2006;16(2):736–42.

48. Xi LF, et al. Human papillomavirus type 16 and 18 variants: race-related distribution and persistence. J Natl Cancer Inst. 2006;98(15):1045–52.

49. Cornet I, et al. HPV16 genetic variation and the development of cervical cancer worldwide. Br J Cancer. 2013;108(1):240–4.

50. Zehbe I, et al. Risk of cervical cancer and geographical variations of human papillomavirus 16 E6 polymorphisms. Lancet. 1998;352(9138):1441–2.

51. Bontkes HJ, et al. HPV 16 infection and progression of cervical intra-epithelial neoplasia: analysis of HLA polymorphism and HPV 16 E6 sequence variants. Int J Cancer. 1998;78(2):166–71.

52. Zehbe I, et al. Association between human papillomavirus 16 E6 variants and human leukocyte antigen class I polymorphism in cervical cancer of Swedish women. Hum Immunol. 2003;64(5):538–42.

53. van Duin M, et al. Analysis of human papillomavirus type 16 E6 variants in relation to p53 codon 72 polymorphism genotypes in cervical carcinogenesis. J Gen Virol. 2000;81(Pt 2):317–25.

54. Nicolas-Parraga S, et al. Differential HPV16 variant distribution in squamous cell carcinoma, adenocarcinoma and adenosquamous cell carcinoma. Int J Cancer. 2017;140(9):2092–100.

55. Safaeian M, et al. Lack of heterogeneity of HPV16 E7 sequence compared with HPV31 and HPV73 may be related to its unique carcinogenic properties. Arch Virol. 2010;155(3):367–70.

56. IARC. List of Classifications by cancer sites with sufficient or limited evidence in humans, Volumes 1 to 120. 27 October 2017 [cited 2017 08/12/2017]; Available from: http://monographs.iarc.fr/ENG/Classification/Table4.pdf.

57. Combes JD, Franceschi S. Role of human papillomavirus in non-oropharyngeal head and neck cancers. Oral Oncol. 2014;50(5):370–9.

58. Gelwan E, et al. Nonuniform distribution of high-risk human papillomavirus in squamous cell carcinomas of the oropharynx: rethinking the anatomic boundaries of oral and oropharyngeal carcinoma from an oncologic HPV perspective. Am J Surg Pathol. 2017;41(12):1722–8.

59. Combes JD, Chen AA, Franceschi S. Prevalence of human papillomavirus in cancer of the oropharynx by gender. Cancer Epidemiol Biomark Prev. 2014; 23(12):2954–8.

60. Saunders CL, et al. Associations between sexual orientation and overall and

site-specific diagnosis of Cancer: evidence from two National Patient Surveys in England. J Clin Oncol. 2017;35(32):3654–61.

61. Agrawal Y, et al. Oral human papillomavirus infection before and after treatment for human papillomavirus 16-positive and human papillomavirus 16-negative head and neck squamous cell carcinoma. Clin Cancer Res. 2008; 14(21):7143–50.

62. Badaracco G, et al. Molecular analyses and prognostic relevance of HPV in head and neck tumours. Oncol Rep. 2007;17(4):931–9.

63. Barbieri D, et al. Detection of HPV16 African variants and quantitative analysis of viral DNA methylation in oropharyngeal squamous cell carcinomas. J Clin Virol. 2014;60(3):243–9.

64. Betiol JC, et al. Prevalence of human papillomavirus types and variants and p16(INK4a) expression in head and neck squamous cells carcinomas in Sao Paulo, Brazil. Infect Agent Cancer. 2016;11:20.

65. Blakaj, D.G., M.; Chen, Z.; Smith, R.; Prystowsky, M.; Burk, R.; Schlecht, N.; Guha, C.; Kalnicki, S. Characterization of Human Papillomavirus 16 Variants in Head-and-Neck Squamous Cell Carcinoma Patients. ELSEVIER SCIENCE INC, 360 PARK AVE SOUTH, NEW YORK, NY 10010–1710 USA.

66. Du J, et al. Human papillomavirus (HPV) 16 E6 variants in tonsillar cancer in comparison to those in cervical cancer in Stockholm, Sweden. PLoS One. 2012;7(4):e36239.

67. Gillison ML, et al. Evidence for a causal association between human papillomavirus and a subset of head and neck cancers. J Natl Cancer Inst. 2000;92(9):709–20.

68. Boscolo-Rizzo P, et al. HPV-16 E6 L83V variant in squamous cell carcinomas of the upper aerodigestive tract. J Cancer Res Clin Oncol. 2009;135(4):559–66.

69. Hassani S, et al. Molecular pathogenesis of human papillomavirus type 16 in tonsillar squamous cell carcinoma. Anticancer Res. 2015;35(12):6633–8.

70. Hoffmann M, et al. Human papillomavirus type 16 E6 and E7 genotypes in head-and-neck carcinomas. Oral Oncol. 2004;40(5):520–4.

71. Castillo A, et al. Human papillomavirus in upper digestive tract tumors from three countries. World J Gastroenterol. 2011;17(48):5295–304.

72. Zehbe I, et al. Rare human papillomavirus 16 E6 variants reveal significant oncogenic potential. Mol Cancer. 2011;10:77.

73. Berman TA, Schiller JT. Human papillomavirus in cervical cancer and oropharyngeal cancer: one cause, two diseases. Cancer. 2017;123(12):2219–29.

74. Gillison ML, et al. Comparative epidemiology of HPV infection and associated cancers of the head and neck and cervix. Int J Cancer. 2013;

75. Dona MG, et al. Cytology and human papillomavirus testing on cytobrushing samples from patients with head and neck squamous cell carcinoma. Cancer. 2014;120(22):3477–84.

76. Fakhry C, et al. Associations between oral HPV16 infection and cytopathology: evaluation of an oropharyngeal "pap-test equivalent" in high-risk populations. Cancer Prev Res (Phila). 2011;4(9):1378–84.

77. Nordfors C, et al. Human papillomavirus prevalence is high in oral samples of patients with tonsillar and base of tongue cancer. Oral Oncol. 2014;50(5):491–7.

78. Franceschi S, et al. Deep brush-based cytology in tonsils resected for benign diseases. Int J Cancer. 2015;137(12):2994–9.

79. Kreimer AR, et al. Evaluation of human papillomavirus antibodies and risk of subsequent head and neck cancer. J Clin Oncol. 2013;31(21):2708–15.

80. Kreimer AR, et al. Kinetics of the human papillomavirus type 16 E6 antibody response prior to oropharyngeal Cancer. J Natl Cancer Inst. 2017;109(8)

81. Combes JD, et al. Prevalence of human papillomavirus in tonsil brushings and gargles in cancer-free patients: the SPLIT study. Oral Oncol. 2017;66:52–7.

82. Lingen MW. Brush-based cytology screening in the tonsils and cervix: there is a difference! Cancer Prev Res (Phila). 2011;4(9):1350–2.

83. Speel EJ. HPV integration in head and neck squamous cell carcinomas: cause and consequence. Recent Results Cancer Res. 2017;206:57–72.

84. Morgan IM, DiNardo LJ, Windle B. Integration of human papillomavirus genomes in head and neck Cancer: is it time to consider a paradigm shift? Viruses. 2017;9(8)

85. Walline HM, et al. Integration of high-risk human papillomavirus into cellular cancer-related genes in head and neck cancer cell lines. Head Neck. 2017; 39(5):840–52.

86. Laban S, Hoffmann TK. Human papilloma virus immunity in oropharyngeal cancer: time to change the game. Clin Cancer Res. 2017;

87. Wasylyk B, Abecassis J, Jung AC. Identification of clinically relevant HPV-related HNSCC: in p16 should we trust? Oral Oncol. 2013;49(10):e33–7.

88. van der Weele P, Meijer C, King AJ. Whole-genome sequencing and variant analysis of human papillomavirus 16 infections. J Virol. 2017;91(19)

89. Nindl I, et al. Absence of antibody against human papillomavirus type 16 E6 and E7 in patients with cervical cancer is independent of sequence variations. J Infect Dis. 2000;181(5):1764–7.

90. Harari A, et al. Cross-protection of the bivalent human papillomavirus (HPV) vaccine against variants of genetically related high-risk HPV infections. J Infect Dis. 2016;213(6):939–47.

91. Measso do Bonfim C, et al. Differences in transcriptional activity of human papillomavirus type 6 molecular variants in recurrent respiratory papillomatosis. PLoS One. 2015;10(7):e0132325.

92. Flores-Diaz, E., et al., HPV-6 Molecular Variants Association With the Development of Genital Warts in Men: The HIM Study. J Infect Dis, 2017. 215(4): p. 559-565.

93. Flores-Diaz E, et al. HPV-11 variability, persistence and progression to genital warts in men: the HIM study. J Gen Virol. 2017;98(9):2339–42.

21

Survival after cancer diagnosis in a cohort of HIV-positive individuals in Latin America

Valeria I. Fink[1]*, Cathy A. Jenkins[2], Jessica L. Castilho[2], Anna K. Person[2], Bryan E. Shepherd[2], Beatriz Grinsztejn[3], Juliana Netto[3], Brenda Crabtree-Ramirez[4], Claudia P. Cortés[5], Denis Padgett[6], Karu Jayathilake[2], Catherine McGowan[2] and Pedro Cahn[1], on behalf of CCASAnet

Abstract

Background: This study aimed to evaluate trends and predictors of survival after cancer diagnosis in persons living with HIV in the Caribbean, Central, and South America network for HIV epidemiology cohort.

Methods: Demographic, cancer, and HIV-related data from HIV-positive adults diagnosed with cancer ≤ 1 year before or any time after HIV diagnosis from January 1, 2000-June 30, 2015 were retrospectively collected. Cancer cases were classified as AIDS-defining cancers (ADC) and non-AIDS-defining cancers (NADC). The association of mortality with cancer- and HIV-related factors was assessed using Kaplan-Meier curves and Cox proportional hazards models stratified by clinic site and cancer type.

Results: Among 15,869 patients, 783 had an eligible cancer diagnosis; 82% were male and median age at cancer diagnosis was 39 years (interquartile range [IQR]: 32–47). Patients were from Brazil (36.5%), Argentina (19.9%), Chile (19.7%), Mexico (19.3%), and Honduras (4.6%). A total of 564 ADC and 219 NADC were diagnosed. Patients with NADC had similar survival probabilities as those with ADC at one year (81% vs. 79%) but lower survival at five years (60% vs. 69%). In the adjusted analysis, risk of mortality increased with detectable viral load (adjusted hazard ratio [aHR] = 1.63, $p = 0.02$), age (aHR = 1.02 per year, $p = 0.002$) and time between HIV and cancer diagnoses (aHR = 1.03 per year, $p = 0.01$).

Conclusion: ADC remain the most frequent cancers in the region. Overall mortality was related to detectable viral load and age. Longer-term survival was lower after diagnosis of NADC than for ADC, which may be due to factors unrelated to HIV.

Keywords: Cohort studies, HIV, Cancer, Survival, Latin America, AIDS defining cancer, Non AIDS defining cancer

Background

Since the beginning of the epidemic, human immunodeficiency virus (HIV) and cancer have been intimately linked. People living with HIV have an increased cancer risk in comparison to the general population, not only for AIDS-defining cancers (ADC) but also for several non-AIDS-defining cancers (NADC) including Hodgkin lymphoma, anal cancer, lung cancer, liver cancer and certain skin cancers [1–3]. In high-income countries, although ADC were the most prevalent malignancies observed in the early years of the HIV epidemic, NADC increasingly account for cancer morbidity in the era of widespread availability of combined antiretroviral therapy (cART) [4–9]. As life expectancy increases for persons living with HIV, long-term exposure to known cancer risk factors such as oncogenic viruses (hepatitis B and C, Epstein Barr [EBV], and human papillomavirus [HPV]) and tobacco, and aging itself have contributed to an increase in the occurrence of NADC [1, 4–6]. Particularly in resource-rich countries with broad access to cART, causes of death have similarly shifted from AIDS-related conditions to other diseases [10, 11]. Cancer, particularly NADC, has become one of the most important causes of death in HIV-positive adults receiving cART [4, 7, 9, 12].

Several studies from high-income settings have examined predictors of mortality following cancer diagnosis in adults living with HIV. While cART use is associated with improved survival following ADC, it has not been

* Correspondence: valeria.fink@huesped.org.ar
[1]Fundación Huésped, Pasaje Gianantonio 3932, C1202ABB Buenos Aires, Argentina
Full list of author information is available at the end of the article

associated with increased survival following NADC diagnosis [13, 14]. Additionally, CD4 count at cancer diagnosis has been less consistently associated with survival in patients with NADC [13, 15]. Poorer survival following NADC has also been associated with behavioral factors such as intravenous drug use and smoking in HIV cohorts [13, 15]. For some NADC, HIV- positive persons are more likely to be diagnosed at more advanced stage and may be less likely to receive standard chemotherapy compared to their uninfected peers, resulting in worse outcomes [13, 14, 16].

As cART has become increasingly available in Latin America, several studies have shown a growing prevalence of non-AIDS causes of morbidity and mortality, including cancer related deaths [15–20]. However, ADC remain frequent, and were the most common cause of cancer observed in a previous study from the region [20, 21]. Survival after cancer diagnosis has been described for resources-rich settings but there is a paucity of data from low- and middle-income countries, including Latin America, where cancer epidemiology and treatments may differ throughout the region [22–25]. This study aimed to describe cancer frequency and survival among HIV-positive individuals in Latin America. We also aimed to identify HIV clinical factors associated with survival following cancer diagnosis.

Methods

Cohort description and population

The Caribbean, Central and South America Network for HIV Epidemiology (CCASAnet) includes HIV clinical sites from seven countries (Argentina, Brazil, Chile, Haiti, Honduras, Mexico and Peru) and constitutes part of the International Epidemiologic Databases to Evaluate AIDS (IeDEA) [26]. Five sites contributed data to this study – Argentina (Fundación Huésped/Hospital Fernández [FH/HF], Buenos Aires, Argentina); Brazil (Instituto Nacional de Infectologia Evandro Chagas, Fundação Oswaldo Cruz, Rio de Janeiro, Brazil); Chile (Fundación Arriarán [FA], Santiago, Chile); Honduras (Instituto Hondureño de Seguridad Social [IHHS] and Hospital Escuela Universitario [HE], Tegucigalpa, Honduras); and Mexico (Instituto Nacional de Ciencias Médicas y Nutrición Salvador Zubirán [INNSZ], Mexico City, Mexico). HIV-positive individuals aged ≥18 years with at least one cancer diagnosis no more than one year before the date of HIV diagnosis or any time after HIV diagnosis and occurring between January 1, 2000 and June 30, 2015 were included in this study. HIV diagnosis date was considered as the reported date of HIV diagnosis, independently from the cancer diagnosis. Patients were excluded if they had an undetectable viral load at cART initiation, suggesting likely inaccurate cART data. Cancer cases were validated and categorized retrospectively as ADC

(Kaposi sarcoma, non-Hodgkin lymphoma, invasive cervical cancer) or NADC (all other cancers) according to the CDC definition [27].

Data management

Demographic, clinical, and laboratory data were collected at each site, de-identified, and sent to the CCASAnet Data Coordinating Center at Vanderbilt University (VDCC), Nashville, TN, USA, for data harmonization and processing. The data were checked for internal consistency and missing data, and quality assessments, including onsite audits, were performed. Institutional Ethics Review Boards from all sites and Vanderbilt approved the project, waiving the requirement for individual patient informed consent.

Study outcomes

The primary outcome was time from cancer diagnosis to death due to any cause.

Death was ascertained by different means at the different sites. At IHSS/HE-Honduras, death was recorded when field workers were notified by family members after a call due to patients missing a visit. At all other sites, relatives of patients informed staff of the death (unless it occurred, and was already recorded, at the hospital), and in addition, study staff checked government death registry databases at least annually for subjects lost to follow-up for the FIOCRUZ-Brazil, FA-Chile, and INNSZ-Mexico sites. Patients were considered to be lost to follow- up if their vital status was unknown, and they had no clinical visit within the year prior to the database closing date at their site [28]. Closing dates for the databases were February 11, 2014 for FH/HF-Argentina, January 5, 2015 for FIOCRUZ-Brazil, August 11, 2014 for FA-Chile, October 29, 2015 for IHSS/HE-Honduras, and May 14, 2015 for INNSZ-Mexico.

Statistical analysis

Demographic and clinical characteristics at the time of cancer diagnosis were summarized by site using median (Interquartile Range [IQR]) or percent (frequency), as appropriate.

The association of mortality with potential risk factors was assessed using Kaplan-Meier curves (overall, by cancer type, and by clinic site), log-rank tests, and Cox proportional hazard models, stratified (i.e., separate baseline hazards estimated) by site and type of cancer (ADC or NADC). Unadjusted models as well as multivariable models were fit. Additional analyses fit separate models for ADC and NADC. To investigate whether risk factors for mortality differed by type of cancer, separate analyses included type of cancer as a covariate and examined interaction terms between type of cancer and other predictor variables. Covariates included in the Cox models were selected a priori and included age, CD4 count (square root transformed), and plasma HIV-1 RNA level

(VL) dichotomized to detectable versus undetectable using the threshold of 400 copies/mL at the time of cancer diagnosis, sex, timing of the cancer diagnosis relative to cART initiation (before/on vs. after cART initiation), and years from HIV diagnosis to cancer diagnosis. Baseline CD4 count was the closest non-missing value within a window 180 days before to 30 days after the date of cancer diagnosis. Baseline VL was considered the closest non-missing value using a window of 180 days before to 7 days after the date of cancer diagnosis. CD4 was included in models using restricted cubic splines to avoid assuming a linear relationship with the outcome. Missing data were present for CD4 (31%), VL (46%), and years from HIV diagnosis to cancer diagnosis (1.4%). Multiple imputation, using five imputation replications, was used to account for missing data in the multivariable models. All analyses were performed using R statistical software, Version 3.3.0 (https://www.R-project.org). Analysis code is posted at http://biostat.mc.vanderbilt.edu/ArchivedAnalyses.

Results

Among 15,869 eligible adult patients (FH/HF- Argentina: 4912, FIOCRUZ-Brazil: 5807, FA-Chile: 2476, IHSS/HE-Honduras: 1326, INNSZ-Mexico: 1348), 954 (6%) had at least one cancer diagnosis, of which 783 (5%) were eligible for this analysis. Of those patients excluded, 126 were diagnosed with cancer before the year 2000, 23 were diagnosed with cancer on the last day of their follow up, five had inaccurate cART information, 16 had an unknown date of cancer diagnosis, and one had cancer diagnosis at < 18 years old.

Table 1 shows the characteristics of patients with cancer diagnoses overall and by site. In all sites except IHSS/HE-Honduras the majority of the patients were male. Median age at cancer diagnosis was 39 years (IQR 32–47); patients with cancer were older in FIOCRUZ-Brazil and IHSS/HE-Honduras (41 years) and younger in INNSZ-Mexico (34 years). Median time between HIV diagnosis and cancer diagnosis was 1.7 years (IQR 0.2–6.7), ranging from a median of 0.4 years in INNSZ-Mexico to 4.0 years in FIOCRUZ-Brazil. Median time between HIV diagnosis and cART start was 0.5 years (IQR 0.1–3.1), being longer for FIOCRUZ-Brazil (0.6) and FA-Chile (1.0) and shorter for IHSS/HE-Honduras (0.3) and INNSZ-Mexico (0.2). Median CD4 count at cancer diagnosis was 148 cells/μL (IQR 44–364), ranging from 82 cells/μL for patients in FH/HF-Argentina to 190 cells/μL in FIOCRUZ-Brazil. Forty-two percent of the patients were diagnosed with cancer before or concomitant to cART initiation, ranging from 36% in FIOCRUZ-Brazil and IHSS/HE-Honduras to 54% in INNSZ-Mexico. Approximately 4% of patients never started cART. Among the 306 patients on cART at cancer

diagnosis with available viral load, 185 (60%) had an undetectable VL (< 400 copies/ml).

As shown in Table 1, 564 of the 783 (72%) cancer cases were ADC, ranging from 66% in FIOCRUZ-Brazil to 82% in FH/HF-Argentina. Overall, Kaposi sarcoma (KS) was the most frequent cancer (48%), followed by non-Hodgkin lymphoma (19%) and cervical cancer (5%). Among NADC, anal cancer (42 cases, 5%) was the most common cancer followed by skin cancer (37 cases, 5%) and Hodgkin lymphoma (23 cases, 3%).

Table 2 compares characteristics of persons diagnosed with ADC and NADC. ADC were more likely to be diagnosed in males than NADC (86% vs 72%). Patients diagnosed with ADC were younger at cancer diagnosis than those diagnosed with NADC (median 37 vs 45 years), had a more recent HIV diagnosis (median 0.8 vs 5.3 years), had spent less time on cART (median 0.0 vs 3.1 years), had lower CD4 count at cancer diagnosis (median 89 vs 376 cells/μL), and were more likely to have a detectable VL (69% vs 30%). A higher percentage of NADC were diagnosed in the later periods of our study (65% of all NADC were diagnosed after 2008 vs. 52% of all ADC). Specifically, 12% (17 of 137), 29% (60 of 210), 32% (83 of 256), and 33% (59 of 180) of the cancers diagnosed during 2000–2003, 2004–2007, 2008–2011 and 2012–2015, respectively, were NADC.

A total of 231 (30%) patients diagnosed with cancer died of any cause during the follow-up period; the median follow-up after cancer diagnosis was 2.5 years (IQR 0.7–6.1). Overall survival probabilities at 1, 3, and 5 years after diagnosis were 80%, 72%, and 67%, respectively. Survival probabilities for those with ADC and NADC are shown in Fig. 1.

Survival was initially higher for those with NADC than ADC, but at the end of one year it was similar (81% vs 79%), and at three and five years it was lower (67% vs 74% and 60% vs 69%, respectively). Overall survival curves did not statistically differ ($p = 0.18$). Survival after cancer diagnosis differed by site ($p < 0.001$); at five years it was estimated as 79% for INNSZ-Mexico, 78% for FH/HF-Argentina, 67% for FA-Chile, 56% for FIOCRUZ-Brazil and 49% for IHSS/HE-Honduras (Fig. 2).

Table 3 shows results from univariate and multivariable Cox proportional hazard models assessing associations between patient characteristics at cancer diagnosis and mortality, stratified by cancer type and clinic site. In the unadjusted analyses, patients with lower CD4 count tended to have higher hazards of mortality (18% higher for patients with 100 CD4 cells/μl vs 350 cells/μl), but this association became less pronounced after adjusting for other variables ($p = 0.80$). In the adjusted analysis, patients with a detectable VL at cancer diagnosis (≥ 400 copies/mL) had a 63% higher hazard of death than patients with an undetectable VL (95% confidence interval [CI] for

Table 1 Patients' characteristics and cancer type by site

	Argentina N = 156	Brazil N = 286	Chile N = 154	Honduras N = 36	Mexico N = 151	Combined N = 783
Sex (n = 783), % (n)						
Female	12% (19)	23% (67)	9% (14)	53% (19)	14% (21)	18% (140)
Male	88% (137)	77% (219)	91% (140)	47% (17)	86% (130)	82% (643)
Age at cancer diagnosis (n = 783), median (IQR)	38 (33–45)	41 (35–48)	39 (33–49)	41 (30–48)	34 (29–42)	39 (32–47)
Years from HIV diagnosis to cancer diagnosis (n = 772), median (IQR)	1.79 (0.10–5.94)	3.97 (0.25–9.95)	1.88 (0.38–7.05)	1.60 (0.41–4.69)	0.45 (0.06–2.77)	1.67 (0.18–6.74)
Years from cART initiation to cancer diagnosis (n = 749), median (IQR)	0.040 (− 0.080–2.49)	0.53 (− 0.02–5.86)	0.33 (− 0.04–1.93)	0.53 (− 0.04–2.30)	−0.010 (− 0.09–0.93)	0.19 (− 0.06–2.87)
Cancer diagnosis relative to cART initiation (n = 783), % (n)						
Cancer diagnosis after cART initiation	53% (83)	64% (183)	63% (97)	64% (23)	46% (69)	58% (455)
Cancer diagnosis before/at cART initiation/Did not start cART	47% (73)	36% (103)	37% (57)	36% (13)	54% (82)	42% (328)
CD4 count (cells/μL) at cancer diagnosis (n = 537), median (IQR)	82 (14–276)	190 (54–425)	171 (56–388)	176 (90–382)	141 (45–300)	148 (44–364)
HIV-1 RNA at cancer diagnosis ($\log_{10}$) (n = 422), median (IQR)	4.4 (2.6–5.3)	3.2 (2.6–4.9)	2.6 (2.6–4.9)	2.6 (2.6–4.4)	4.6 (2.6–5.3)	3.9 (2.6 5.0)
HIV1-RNA status at cancer diagnosis (cut point = 400 copies/mL), % (n)						
Undetectable	31% (16)	49% (80)	49% (41)	67% (6)	38% (43)	44% (186)
Detectable	69% (36)	51% (84)	51% (43)	33% (3)	62% (70)	56% (236)
Status at the end of follow-up (n = 783), % (n)						
Alive	81% (126)	61% (174)	67% (103)	61% (22)	84% (127)	70% (552)
Dead	19% (30)	39% (112)	33% (51)	39% (14)	16% (24)	30% (231)
Follow-up (years) (n = 783), median (IQR)	2.20 (0.55–6.13)	2.30 (0.66–4.91)	3.69 (0.62–8.87)	1.06 (0.59–5.42)	3.33 (0.92–5.84)	2.51 (0.69–6.13)
Type of cancer (n = 783), % (n)						
AIDS-defining cancers	82% (128)	66% (188)	70% (108)	72% (26)	75% (114)	72% (564)
Kaposi sarcoma	59% (92)	51% (147)	42% (65)	28% (10)	42% (64)	48% (378)
Non-Hodgkin lymphoma	20% (31)	13% (38)	27% (41)	19% (7)	22% (33)	19% (150)
Invasive cervical cancer	3% (5)	1% (3)	1% (2)	25% (9)	11% (17)	5% (36)
Non-AIDS-defining cancers	18% (28)	34% (98)	30% (46)	28% (10)	25% (37)	28% (219)
Anal	2% (3)	5% (15)	3% (4)	3% (1)	13% (19)	5% (42)
Breast	1% (2)	5% (15)	1% (1)	6% (2)	0% (0)	3% (20)
Colon	1% (2)	1% (3)	2% (3)	3% (1)	0% (0)	1% (9)
Hodgkin lymphoma	2% (3)	1% (4)	6% (9)	0% (0)	5% (7)	3% (23)
Lung	3% (4)	3% (8)	0% (0)	0% (0)	0% (0)	2% (12)
Prostate	0% (0)	2% (5)	1% (1)	3% (1)	3% (5)	2% (12)
Renal	1% (2)	2% (6)	0% (0)	0% (0)	0% (0)	1% (8)
Skin	4% (7)	7% (20)	5% (7)	6% (2)	1% (1)	5% (37)
Testicular	1% (1)	0% (0)	5% (7)	0% (0)	0% (0)	1% (8)
Other[a]	3% (4)	8% (22)	9% (14)	8% (3)	3% (5)	6% (48)

IQR interquartile range
[a]Other: acute leukemia (2–2%), bladder cancer (2–2%), brain cancer (5–6%), cancer with unknown primary (3–3%), chronic leukemia (1–1%), esophageal cancer (3–3%), eye cancer (1–1%), gall bladder (1–1%), gastric cancer (7–8%), laryngeal cancer (3–3%), not otherwise specified leukemia (3–3%), liver cancer (1–1%), multiple myeloma (2–2%), oral cancer (4–4%), ovarian cancer (2–2%), pancreatic cancer (1–1%), penile cancer (1–1%), sinus cancer (1–1%), soft tissue sarcoma (1–1%), thyroid cancer (4–4%)

Table 2 Patients' characteristics according to cancer type

	Non-AIDS-defining cancers (n = 219)	AIDS-defining cancers (n = 564)	Combined (n = 783)	P
Sex (n = 783), % (n)				< 0.001
Female	28% (61)	14% (79)	18% (140)	
Male	72% (158)	86% (485)	82% (643)	
Age at cancer diagnosis (n = 783), median (IQR)	45 (38–54)	37 (31–44)	39 (32–47)	< 0.001
Year of cancer diagnosis (n = 783), median (IQR)	2009 (2006–2012)	2008 (2004–2011)	2008 (2005–2011)	< 0.001
Years from HIV diagnosis to cancer diagnosis (n = 772), median (IQR)	5.26 (2.09–11.00)	0.82 (0.11–5.05)	1.67 (0.18–6.74)	< 0.001
Years from cART initiation to cancer diagnosis (n = 749), median (IQR)	3.08 (0.50–8.48)	0.02 (−0.08–0.86)	0.19 (−0.06–2.87)	< 0.001
Cancer diagnosis relative to cART initiation (n = 783), % (n)				< 0.001
Cancer diagnosis after cART initiation	79% (172)	50% (283)	58% (455)	
Cancer diagnosis before/at cART initiation/Did not start cART	21% (47)	50% (281)	42% (328)	
CD4 count (cells/µL) at cancer diagnosis (n = 537), median (IQR)	376 (229–573)	89 (29–230)	148 (44–364)	< 0.001
HIV-1 RNA at cancer diagnosis (log$_{10}$) (n = 422), median (IQR)	2.6 (2.6–3.7)	4.6 (2.6–5.2)	3.9 (2.6–5.0)	< 0.001
HIV-1 RNA status (cut point = 400 copies/mL), % (n)				< 0.001
Undetectable	70% (99)	31% (87)	44% (186)	
Detectable	30% (42)	69% (194)	56% (236)	
Status (n = 783), % (n)				0.20
Alive	67% (147)	72% (405)	70% (552)	
Dead	33% (72)	28% (159)	30% (231)	
Follow-up (yrs) (n = 783), median (IQR)	2.17 (0.66–5.13)	2.62 (0.69–6.34)	2.51 (0.69–6.13)	0.18

Numbers after percentages are frequencies. IQR: Interquartile range. Tests used: Pearson test for categorical variables; Wilcoxon Rank Sum test for continuous variables

adjusted hazard ratio [aHR] =1.08–2.47; p = 0.02). Similarly, age at cancer diagnosis and time from HIV diagnosis to cancer diagnosis were also significantly associated with mortality. Risk of mortality increased with age at cancer diagnosis (2% for each year; 95% CI 1.01–1.03; p = 0.002). From the time of HIV diagnosis, cancers diagnosed one year later were associated with a 3% higher hazard of mortality (95% CI 1.01–1.06; p = 0.01).

Results were fairly similar when ADC and NADC were considered separately (Table 4). Detectable viral load at diagnosis of an ADC was associated with an 83% increase in the adjusted hazard of mortality (95% CI 1.03–3.24; p = 0.04). In contrast, a detectable viral load at the time of NADC diagnosis was not associated with a higher hazard of mortality (aHR = 0.98; 95% CI 0.41–2.30; p = 0.96), although these hazard ratios did not statistically differ between ADC and NADC (p = 0.81, test for interaction). In general, there was little evidence that hazard ratios differed between ADC and NADC for any of the patient characteristics considered (p > 0.15 for all variables).

Discussion

In this multisite cohort study of HIV patients diagnosed with cancer across Latin America, we found that age, time since HIV diagnosis, and detectable viral load were predictive of mortality after accounting for cancer type, sex, cART use, and CD4 count. While ADC were the most prevalent cancers diagnosed, an increasing proportion of NADC were diagnosed in more recent years. Despite marked clinical differences in patient characteristics at cancer diagnosis, there was no meaningful difference in survival in the first year after cancer diagnosis for patients diagnosed with ADC versus those diagnosed with NADC, though there was a suggestion that NADC may be associated with increased mortality 3 and 5 years after diagnosis. In this region of low- and middle-income countries, these results reflect the dynamics of cancer epidemiology in HIV positive patients with increasingly available ART and longer life expectancy.

Site was also significantly associated with mortality. This might reflect varying prevalence of the different cancers and differences in access to treatment and care.

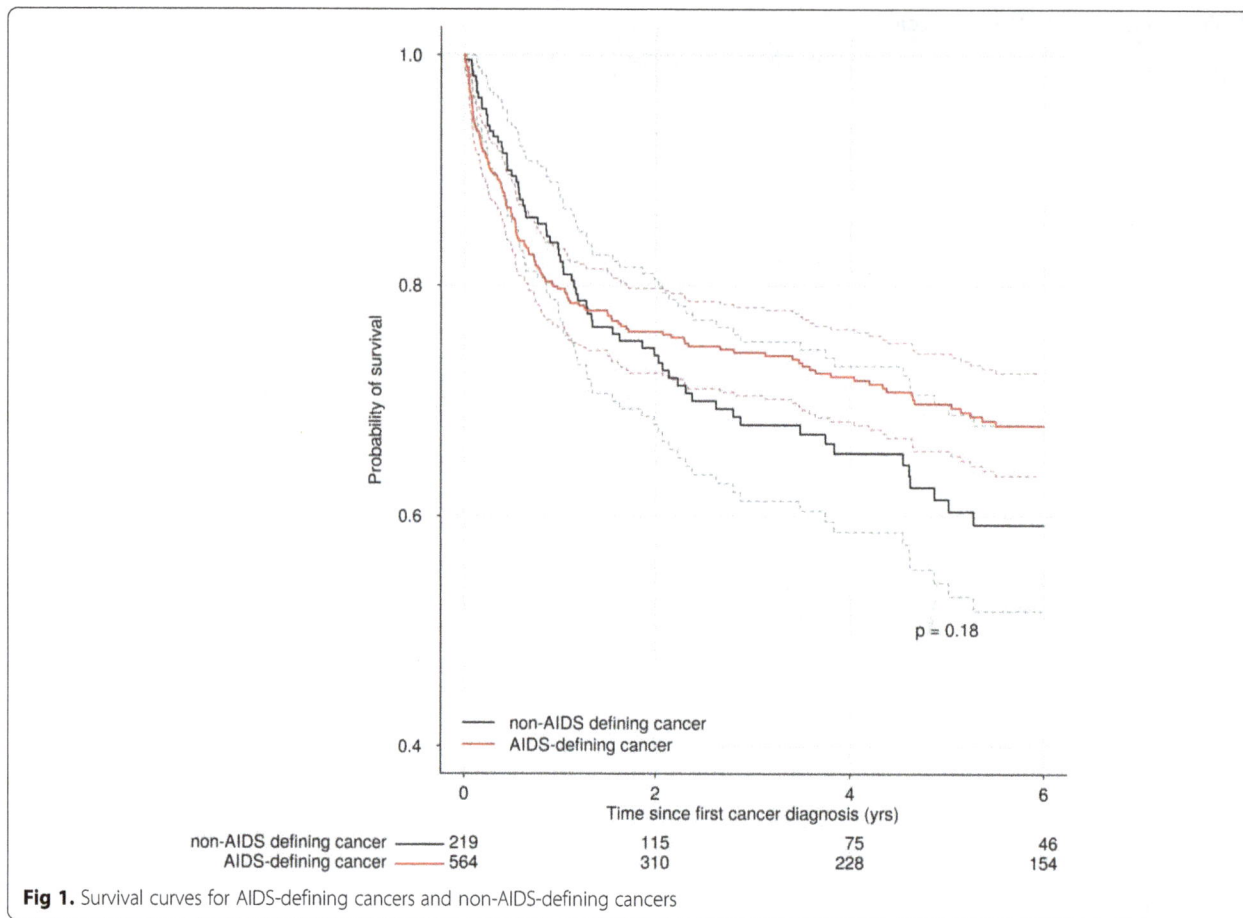

Fig 1. Survival curves for AIDS-defining cancers and non-AIDS-defining cancers

We observed an increased hazard of mortality following cancer diagnosis associated with detectable viral load (63% higher than patients with VL < 400 copies/ml); this hazard was particularly higher (83%) for those diagnosed with an ADC. HIV VL has been demonstrated in previous studies to predict mortality in patients diagnosed with ADC, particularly HIV-associated lymphomas [29–31]. Virologic suppression has also been associated with improved survival in studies of NADC [31, 32]. In our population, lack of virologic suppression was associated with mortality after cancer diagnosis and was independent of any observed immunologic association with mortality, suggesting that viral control may be a marker of other patient or clinical characteristics associated with improved cancer outcomes rather than the immunologic effect of HIV. In KS, the most frequent ADC in our study, HIV-1 has a direct role in disease pathogenesis, due to pro-oncogenic effects of HIV-1-encoded proteins such as the Tat protein. Tat, a regulatory protein released by HIV-infected cells, protects cells from apoptosis, promotes the growth of spindle cells in synergy with inflammatory cytokines, [33–35] and contributes to the intense neoangiogenesis found in KS lesions [36].

Our study did not find that CD4 at the time of cancer diagnosis was predictive of mortality following cancer diagnosis in any of the analyses performed, which differs from studies in high-income settings [32, 37]. Though median CD4 count at cancer diagnosis was significantly lower among patients diagnosed with an ADC versus those diagnosed with a NADC, CD4 count among all patients was very low in our cohort (median 148 cells/μl, IQR: 44–364) and 42% of all the patients were not on cART at cancer diagnosis, suggesting late HIV diagnosis or access to care. The very low CD4 counts among most patients and the fact that the majority had ADC may have limited our ability to detect a meaningful role of immunosuppression and mortality risk. Another possible explanation may be related to the high prevalence of KS, which if diagnosed in early stages and treated, generally has a good prognosis.

Although our study was focused on survival, it also describes cancer epidemiology of HIV-positive adults in the Latin America region. Five percent of patients overall were diagnosed with cancer during the study period; the majority of cases were ADC, and KS was the most frequent. KS incidence is geographically variable, and depends on the prevalence of human herpesvirus-8

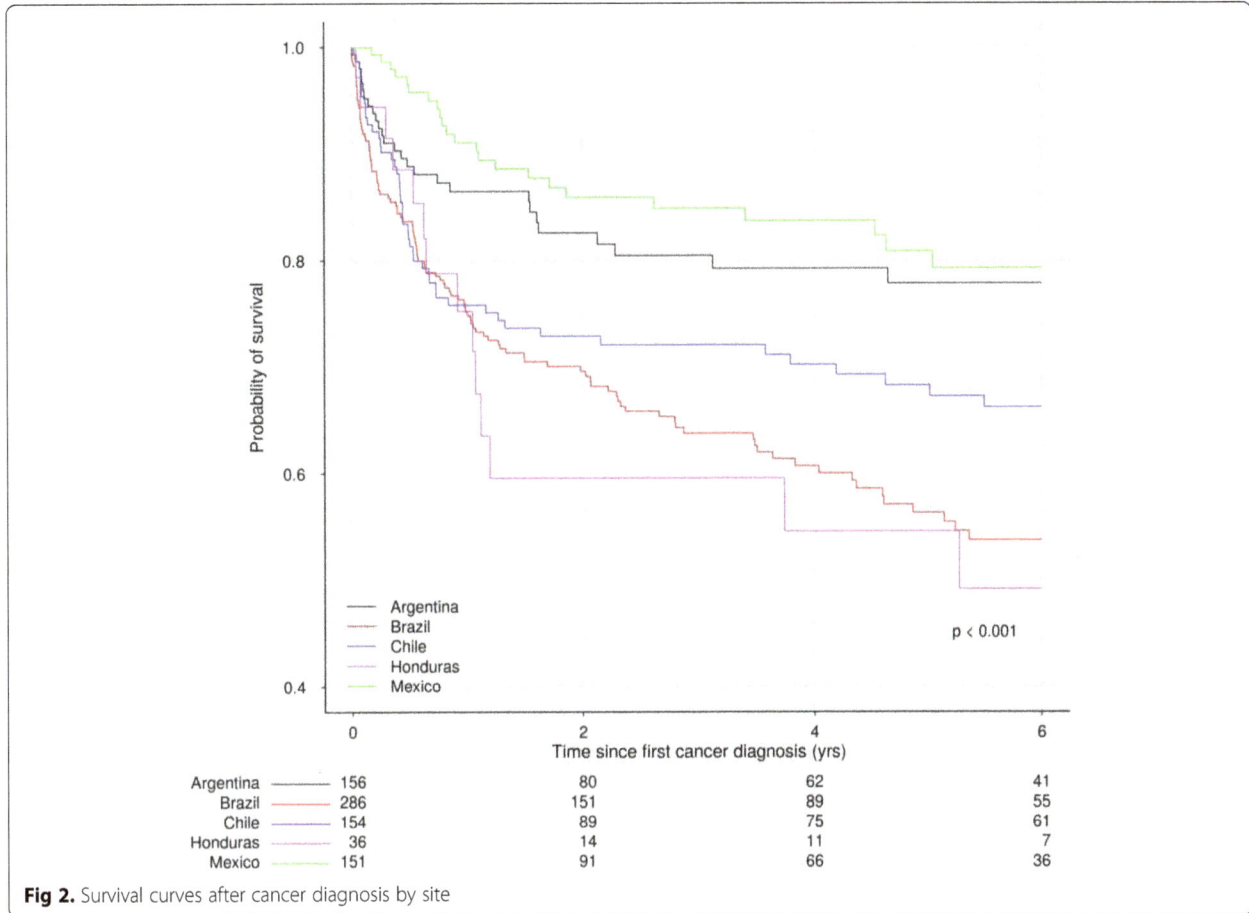

Fig 2. Survival curves after cancer diagnosis by site

Table 3 Unadjusted and adjusted results from the Cox proportional hazard models investigating the association between time from cancer diagnosis to death, dichotomizing HIV-1 viral load

Covariate	Unadjusted			Adjusted		
	HR	95% CI	P	HR	95% CI	P
Sex			0.41			0.22
Female (ref)	1.00			1.00		
Male	0.87	(0.61–1.22)		0.81	(0.57–1.14)	
Cancer diagnosis relative to cART initiation			0.61			0.41
Cancer diagnosis after cART initiation (ref)	1.00			1.00		
Cancer diagnosis before/at cART initiation/Did not start cART	0.93	(0.70–1.23)		0.87	(0.62–1.22)	
CD4 count (cells/μL) at cancer diagnosis			0.06			0.80
100	1.18	(0.96–1.44)		0.99	(0.82–1.21)	
200	1.03	(0.91–1.17)		0.98	(0.86–1.12)	
350 (ref)	1.00			1.00		
500	1.03	(0.89–1.19)		1.03	(0.90–1.17)	
HIV-1 RNA at cancer diagnosis			0.21			0.02
Undetectable (ref)	1.00			1.00		
Detectable (> 400 copies/mL)	1.28	(0.87–1.88)		1.63	(1.08–2.47)	
Years from HIV diagnosis to cancer diagnosis	1.03	(1.01–1.06)	0.01	1.03	(1.01–1.06)	0.01
Age at cancer diagnosis (per year)	1.02	(1.01–1.03)	0.003	1.02	(1.01–1.03)	0.002

Table 4 Adjusted analyses according to type of cancer (AIDS-defining cancer and non-AIDS-defining cancer)

Covariate	ADC			NADC			p (test for interaction)
	HR	95% CI	P	HR	95% CI	P	
Sex			0.08			0.86	0.18
Female (ref)	1.00			1.00			
Male	0.67	(0.43–1.05)		1.05	(0.61–1.80)		
Cancer diagnosis relative to cART initiation			0.59			0.94	0.81
Cancer diagnosis after cART (ref)	1.00			1.00			
Cancer diagnosis before/at cART initiation/Did not start cART	0.90	(0.60–1.33)		1.03	(0.42–2.52)		
CD4 count (cells/µL) at cancer diagnosis			0.87			0.66	0.23
100	1.08	(0.75–1.55)		1.09	(0.81–1.46)		
200	1.04	(0.83–1.32)		1.01	(0.89–1.15)		
350 (ref)	1.00			1.00			
500	0.96	(0.79–1.18)		1.05	(0.90–1.22)		
HIV-1 RNA at cancer diagnosis			0.04			0.96	0.81
Undetectable (ref)	1.00			1.00			
Detectable (400 copies/mL)	1.83	(1.03–3.24)		0.98	(0.41–2.30)		
Years from HIV diagnosis to cancer diagnosis	1.04	(1.00–1.07)	0.03	1.02	(0.98–1.07)	0.26	0.71
Age at cancer diagnosis (per year)	1.02	(1.01–1.04)	0.005	1.02	(1.00–1.04)	0.12	0.70

The last column provides p-values comparing hazard ratios for ADC vs. NADC using tests for interaction
AIDS-defining cancer (ADC); non-AIDS-defining cancer (NADC)
*= p-value from the model on the full cohort with the type of cancer interacted with the given variable. There were 219 subjects in the NADC cohort and 72 deaths. Similarly, there were 564 subjects in the ADC cohort and 159 deaths

infection, the prevalence of HIV, and access to HIV treatment [38, 39]. Our findings are consistent with other studies where ADC were still the most frequent malignancies observed, even in more recent years of the epidemic [20, 21, 40–42]. However, many recent reports describe an increasing proportion of cancers due to NADC, and occurring more frequently than ADC, among HIV cohorts [24, 43–48]. The most frequent NADC observed in our cohort were anal cancer, Hodgkin disease, and skin cancer, which likely are related to coinfection with oncogenic viruses such as HPV and EBV, and an aging population [24, 49–51]. Lung cancer was less frequently observed in our cohort compared to other reports, [24, 52] possibly due to differing patterns of tobacco use, diagnostic capabilities, or case ascertainment, which needs further exploration. Anal cancer was more frequent in FIOCRUZ-Brazil and INNSZ-Mexico; possibly related to more frequent anal cancer screening practices. These trends will probably continue to change as HIV-positive individuals live longer and antiretroviral therapy is started earlier. Of note, a high number of testis cancer was found in FA-Chile. Data from the general population show that Chile has a higher incidence of testis cancer (age-standardized rate 6.8 per 100,000 population) than the other countries participating in the study (ranging from 0.4 in Honduras to 5 per 100,000 population in Argentina) [53]. Further investigation will be needed

to determine whether there are particular associated factors in the HIV-positive population.

Across our region, cancer trends and mortality differed, likely reflecting differences in access to cART and HIV care historically. For example, FIOCRUZ-Brazil (which has had cART universally available since 1996) had the highest proportion of incident NADC diagnosed as well as high mortality following cancer diagnosis. Indeed, some studies from high-income settings with broad access to cART have also observed higher mortality for NADC than for ADC [22]. One important risk factor for incidence of and mortality after NADC is increasing age, an observation we also found in our study [32]. Older age alone has been associated with increased mortality in HIV and may be associated with poor response to HIV or cancer treatment or accumulation of other co-morbidities. Taken together, these findings underscore the epidemiologic changes observed in high-income settings of increased NADC incidence and mortality among an aging cohort of HIV patients that is also occurring in Latin America.

Lastly, our study is novel in its reporting of long term survival following cancer diagnosis in HIV patients in Latin America and showed important differences from what has been reported in high-income settings. Overall survival following cancer diagnosis in our study at one, three, and five years was 80%, 73%, and 68% respectively. In contrast, the five-year survival after cancer diagnosis was 54.5% following ADC diagnosis and approximately 65% following NADC diagnosis in the HIV Outpatient Study in the US [31]. Worm et al. reported five-year survival of 52.7% following NADC diagnosis in the D:A:D study [24]. These differences may be due to differences in specific types of cancers diagnosed (for instance, low rates of lung cancer observed in our cohort), patient characteristics (such as CD4 nadir or presence of co-infections, not included in our analysis), cancer treatment availability, or death ascertainment. Our study importantly adds to the understanding of cancer outcomes in HIV patients globally, including those from settings of limited resources and high prevalence of ADC.

There are limitations to our study to consider. First, though misclassification is a concern for any observational study, CCASAnet has gone to great lengths to maintain a high level of data quality including on-site audits of observational data collected [54]. It is possible that some cancer cases may be undiagnosed and therefore not included in this study due to differential rates of cancer screening or diagnosis. Second, our analysis was limited by high rates of missing laboratory data. This was addressed by multiple imputation in our analyses but is a common challenge for observational data in resource-limited settings. Third, other factors known to predict cancer outcomes were not included in this study, including cancer stage at diagnosis, cancer treatment, and smoking. Some studies from the US have suggested that HIV patients with cancer are less likely to receive appropriate cancer treatments compared to uninfected patients [55]. We did not have complete information available regarding cancer treatment received by patients and how this may differ by clinical site or patient characteristics such as cART use or immune status. Fourth, due to relatively low numbers of individual NADC diagnoses, we grouped the cancer diagnoses into ADC and NADC categories. Cancers are a heterogeneous mix of diseases and this approach, and the moderate numbers of events, may have limited our ability to detect clinical predictors of outcomes related to specific cancer diagnoses. Fifth, cancers diagnosed up to one year before the HIV diagnosis were included. It is probable that patients with ADC were more likely to be tested for HIV than patients with NADC, so there might be an under- representation of HIV patients with NADC in our cohort. Lastly, some studies have shown worse outcomes of NADC in HIV-positive people compared to the general population [1]. Our analysis lacks an HIV-uninfected population with which to compare survival outcomes following cancer diagnosis to evalu-ate the question of whether HIV patients in our region have comparably different outcomes than uninfected cancer patients.

Conclusions

As one of the first studies to describe survival after cancer diagnosis in HIV-positive individuals from Latin America, this study provides valuable information to be used at the local level and shows the need of continuing investigation of cancer epidemiology to establish effective prevention and screening policies in this region. Future work will be strengthened by increasing observation time as patients with HIV and cancer live longer, incorporating additional information about specific cancer therapies in the region, and utilizing regional national cancer registries that may improve ascertainment and allow for comparisons with the general populations.

Acknowledgements
We gratefully acknowledge all patients, caregivers, and data managers involved in the CCASAnet cohort. We also thank the Infectious Diseases Unit, Hospital Fernández, Buenos Aires, Argentina.

Fundings
This work was funded by the NIH-funded Caribbean, Central and South America network for HIV epidemiology (CCASAnet), a member cohort of the International Epidemiologic Databases to Evaluate AIDS (IeDEA) (U01AI069923). This award is funded by the following institutes: Eunice Kennedy Shriver National Institute Of Child Health & Human Development (NICHD), Office Of The Director, National Institutes Of Health (OD), National Institute Of Allergy And Infectious Diseases (NIAID), National Cancer Institute (NCI), and the National Institute Of Mental Health (NIMH).

Authors' contributions
VIF, CAJ, JC, BES, CMG and PC made substantial contributions to the conception and design of the study, VIF, AKP, BG, JN, BC, CC, DP, and PC acquired the data; VIF, CKJ, BES and KJ made substantial contribution to the interpretation of the data. CKJ and BES analyzed it. VIF, CKJ, JC, BES, CMG and PC drafted the article; all authors revised it critically for important intellectual content approved the final version for publishing.

Competing interests
The authors declare that they have no conflicts of interest.

Author details
[1]Fundación Huésped, Pasaje Gianantonio 3932, C1202ABB Buenos Aires, Argentina. [2]Vanderbilt University School of Medicine, 1161 21st Ave. S A2200 Medical Center North, Nashville, TN 37232, USA. [3]Instituto Nacional de Infectologia Evandro Chagas, Fundação Oswaldo Cruz, Av. Brasil, 4365 - Manguinhos, Rio de Janeiro, RJ 21040-900, Brasil. [4]Instituto Nacional de Ciencias Médicas y Nutrición Salvador Zubirán: Unidad del Paciente Ambulatorio (UPA), 5to piso Vasco de Quiroga # 15 Col. Sección XVI Delegación Tlalpan; C.P, 14000 Mexico City, Mexico. [5]Fundación Arriarán, Santa Elvira 629, Santiago, Chile. [6]Instituto Hondureño de Seguridad Social, Barrio la Granja, Tegucigalpa Honduras, Hospital Escuela Universitario: Av La Salud, Tegucigalpa, Honduras.

References

1. Coghill AE, Engels EA. Are cancer outcomes worse in the presence of HIV infection? Cancer Epidemiol Biomark Prev. 2015;24(8):1165–6.

2. Patel P, Hanson DL, Sullivan PS, et al. Incidence of types of cancer among HIV-infected persons compared with the general population in the United States, 1992-2003. Ann Intern Med. 2008;148(10):728–36.

3. Silverberg MJ, Chao C, Leyden WA, et al. HIV infection and the risk of cancers with and without a known infectious cause. AIDS. 2009;23(17):2337–45.

4. Bonnet F, Burty C, Lewden C, et al. Changes in cancer mortality among HIV-infected patients: the Mortalite 2005 survey. Clin Infect Dis. 2009; 48(5):633–9.

5. Franceschi S, Lise M, Clifford GM, et al. Changing patterns of cancer incidence in the early- and late-HAART periods: the Swiss HIV cohort study. Br J Cancer. 2010;103(3):416–22.

6. Powles T, Robinson D, Stebbing J, et al. Highly active antiretroviral therapy and the incidence of non-AIDS-defining cancers in people with HIV infection. J Clin Oncol. 2009;27(6):884–90.

7. Raffetti E, Albini L, Gotti D, et al. Cancer incidence and mortality for all causes in HIV-infected patients over a quarter century: a multicentre cohort study. BMC Public Health. 2015;15:235.

8. Shiels MS, Pfeiffer RM, Gail MH, et al. Cancer burden in the HIV-infected population in the United States. J Natl Cancer Inst. 2011;103(9):753–62.

9. Vandenhende MA, Roussillon C, Henard S, et al. Cancer-related causes of death among HIV-infected patients in France in 2010: evolution since 2000. PLoS One. 2015;10(6):e0129550.

10. Brickman C, Palefsky J. Cancer in the HIV-Infected Host: Epidemiology and Pathogenesis in the Antiretroviral Era. Curr HIV/AIDS Rep. 2015;12:388–96.

11. Lewden C, Salmon D, Morlat P, et al. Causes of death among human immunodeficiency virus (HIV)-infected adults in the era of potent antiretroviral therapy: emerging role of hepatitis and cancers, persistent role of AIDS. Int J Epidemiol. 2005;34(1):121–30.

12. Simard EP, Engels EA. Cancer as a cause of death among people with AIDS in the United States. Clin Infect Dis. 2010;51(8):957–62.

13. Sigel K, Crothers K, Dubrow R, et al. Prognosis in HIV-infected patients with non-small cell lung cancer. Br J Cancer. 2013;109(7):1974–80.

14. Spano JP, Massiani MA, Bentata M, et al. Lung cancer in patients with HIV infection and review of the literature. Med Oncol. 2004;21(2):109–15.

15. Pacheco AG, Tuboi SH, Faulhaber JC, et al. Increase in non-AIDS related conditions as causes of death among HIV-infected individuals in the HAART era in Brazil. PLoS One. 2008;3(1):e1531.

16. Grinsztejn B, Luz PM, Pacheco AG, et al. Changing mortality profile among HIV-infected patients in Rio de Janeiro, Brazil: shifting from AIDS to non-AIDS related conditions in the HAART era. PLoS One. 2013;8(4):e59768.

17. Luz PM, Bruyand M, Ribeiro S, et al. AIDS and non-AIDS severe morbidity associated with hospitalizations among HIV-infected patients in two regions with universal access to care and antiretroviral therapy, France and Brazil, 2000-2008: hospital-based cohort studies. BMC Infect Dis. 2014;14:278.

18. Cobucci RN, Lima PH, de Souza PC, et al. Assessing the impact of HAART on the incidence of defining and non-defining AIDS cancers among patients with HIV/AIDS: a systematic review. J Infect Public Health. 2015;8(1):1–10.

19. Fazito E, Vasconcelos AM, Pereira MG, et al. Trends in non-AIDS-related causes of death among adults with HIV/AIDS, Brazil, 1999 to 2010. Cad Saude Publica. 2013;29(8):1644–53.

20. Castilho JL, Luz PM, Shepherd BE, et al. HIV and cancer: a comparative retrospective study of Brazilian and U.S. clinical cohorts. Infect Agent Cancer. 2015;10:4.

21. Fink VI, Shepherd BE, Cesar C, et al. Cancer in HIV-infected persons from the Caribbean, central and South America. J Acquir Immune Defic Syndr. 2011; 56(5):467–73.

22. Gotti D, Raffetti E, Albini L, et al. Survival in HIV-infected patients after a cancer diagnosis in the cART era: results of an italian multicenter study. PLoS One. 2014;9(4):e94768.

23. Hleyhel M, Belot A, Bouvier AM, et al. Trends in survival after cancer diagnosis among HIV-infected individuals between 1992 and 2009. Results from the FHDH-ANRS CO4 cohort. Int J Cancer. 2015;137(10):2443–53.

24. Worm SW, Bower M, Reiss P, et al. Non-AIDS defining cancers in the D:a:D study–time trends and predictors of survival: a cohort study. BMC Infect Dis. 2013;13:471.

25. Narayan KM, Miotti PG, Anand NP, et al. HIV and noncommunicable disease comorbidities in the era of antiretroviral therapy: a vital agenda for research in low- and middle-income country settings. J Acquir Immune Defic Syndr. 2014;67(Suppl 1):S2–7.

26. McGowan CC, Cahn P, Gotuzzo E, et al. Cohort profile: Caribbean, central and South America network for HIV research (CCASAnet) collaboration within the international epidemiologic databases to evaluate AIDS (IeDEA) programme. Int J Epidemiol. 2007;36(5):969–76.

27. Selik RM, Mokotoff ED, Branson B, et al. Revised Surveillance Case Definition for HIV Infection — United States, 2014. Morb Mortal Wkly Rep. 2014;63(RR 03):1–10.

28. Carriquiry G, Fink V, Koethe JR, et al. Mortality and loss to follow-up among HIV-infected persons on long-term antiretroviral therapy in Latin America and the Caribbean. J Int AIDS Soc. 2015;18:20016.

29. Gopal S, Patel MR, Yanik EL, et al. Temporal trends in presentation and survival for HIV-associated lymphoma in the antiretroviral therapy era. J Natl Cancer Inst. 2013;105(16):1221–9.

30. Gopal S, Patel MR, Yanik EL, et al. Association of early HIV viremia with mortality after HIV-associated lymphoma. AIDS. 2013;27(15):2365–73.

31. Patel P, Armon C, Chmiel JS, et al. Factors associated with cancer incidence and with all-cause mortality after cancer diagnosis among human immunodeficiency virus-infected persons during the combination antiretroviral therapy era. Open Forum Infect Dis. 2014;1(1):ofu012.

32. Achenbach CJ, Cole SR, Kitahata MM, et al. Mortality after cancer diagnosis in HIV-infected individuals treated with antiretroviral therapy. AIDS. 2011; 25(5):691–700.

33. Barillari G, Sgadari C, Fiorelli V, et al. The tat protein of human immunodeficiency virus type-1 promotes vascular cell growth and locomotion by engaging the alpha5beta1 and alphavbeta3 integrins and by mobilizing sequestered basic fibroblast growth factor. Blood. 1999;94(2):663–72.

34. Cheung MC, Pantanowitz L, Dezube BJ. AIDS-related malignancies: emerging challenges in the era of highly active antiretroviral therapy. Oncologist. 2005; 10(6):412–26.

35. Ensoli B, Sturzl M, Monini P. Cytokine-mediated growth promotion of Kaposi's sarcoma and primary effusion lymphoma. Semin Cancer Biol. 2000;10(5):367–81.

36. Impola U, Cuccuru MA, Masala MV, et al. Preliminary communication: matrix metalloproteinases in Kaposi's sarcoma. Br J Dermatol. 2003;149(4):905–7.

37. Collaboration of Observational HIV Epidemiological Research Europe (COHERE) study group, Bohlius J, Schmidlin K, et al. Prognosis of HIV-associated non-Hodgkin lymphoma in patients starting combination antiretroviral therapy. AIDS. 2009;23(15):2029–37.

38. Bohlius J. AIDS-defining Cancer project working group for IeDEA and COHERE in EuroCoord; AIDS-defining Cancer project working group for IeDEA and COHERE in EuroCoord, Comparison of Kaposi sarcoma risk in HIV-positive adults across five continents: a multiregional multicohort study. Clin Infect Dis. 2017;65(8):1316-26.

39. Rohner E, Wyss N, Heg Z, et al. HIV and human herpesvirus 8 co-infection across the globe: systematic review and meta-analysis. Int J Cancer. 2016;138(1):45–54.

40. Laurido M, Uruena A, Vizzotti C, et al. Incidence variation in malignancies associated or not with AIDS at an outpatient care center, 1997-2005. Medicina (B Aires). 2007;67(3):243–6.

41. Zohar M, Micha B. Cancer incidence in people living with HIV/AIDS in Israel, 1981-2010. AIDS Res Hum Retrovir. 2015;31(9):873–81.

42. Sachdeva RK, Sharma A, Singh S, et al. Spectrum of AIDS defining & non-AIDS defining malignancies in North India. Indian J Med Res. 2016;143(Supplement): S129–35.

43. Dryden-Peterson S, Medhin H, Kebabonye-Pusoentsi M, et al. Cancer incidence following expansion of HIV treatment in Botswana. PLoS One. 2015;10(8):e0135602.

44. Chen N, Jen I, Chen YH, et al. Cancer incidence in a Nationwide HIV/AIDS patient cohort in Taiwan in 1998-2009. J Acquir Immune Defic Syndr. 2014; 65(4):463–72.

45. Chiu CG, Smith D, Salters KA, et al. Overview of cancer incidence and mortality among people living with HIV/AIDS in British Columbia, Canada: implications for HAART use and NADM development. BMC Cancer. 2017; 17(1):270.

46. Riedel DJ, Stafford KA, Vadlamani A, et al. Virologic and immunologic outcomes in HIV-infected patients with Cancer. AIDS Res Hum Retrovir. 2017;33(5):482–9.

47. Tanaka LF, Latorre MR, Gutierrez EB, et al. Risk for cancer among people living with AIDS, 1997-2012: the Sao Paulo AIDS-cancer linkage study. Eur J Cancer Prev.2017; 00:000 000.

48. Yang J, Su S, Zhao H, et al. Prevalence and mortality of cancer among HIV-infected inpatients in Beijing, China. BMC Infect Dis. 2016;16:82.

49. Clifford GM, Polesel J, Rickenbach M, et al. Cancer risk in the Swiss HIV cohort study: associations with immunodeficiency, smoking, and highly active antiretroviral therapy. J Natl Cancer Inst. 2005;97(6):425–32.

50. Crum-Cianflone N, Hullsiek KH, Marconi V, et al. Trends in the incidence of cancers among HIV-infected persons and the impact of antiretroviral therapy: a 20-year cohort study. AIDS. 2009;23(1):41–50.

51. Engels EA, Biggar RJ, Hall HI, et al. Cancer risk in people infected with human immunodeficiency virus in the United States. Int J Cancer. 2008; 123(1):187–94.

52. Silverberg MJ, Lau B, Achenbach CJ, et al. Cumulative incidence of Cancer among persons with HIV in North America: a cohort study. Ann Intern Med. 2015;163(7):507–18.

53. International Agency for Research in Cancer. Globocan 2012: Estimated Cancer Incidence, Mortality and Prevalence Worldwide in 2012. 2012 [Accessed 2018 06 Apr 2018]; Available from: http://globocan.iarc.fr/Pages/fact_sheets_cancer.aspx.

54. Duda SN, Shepherd BE, Gadd CS, et al. Measuring the quality of observational study data in an international HIV research network. PLoS One. 2012;7(4):e33908.

55. Suneja G, Boyer M, Yehia BR, et al. Cancer treatment in patients with HIV infection and non-AIDS-defining cancers: a survey of US oncologists. J Oncol Pract. 2015;11(3):e380–7.

22

Integration of human papillomavirus 16 in esophageal carcinoma samples

Shuying Li[1*], Haie Shen[1], Zhanjun Liu[1], Ning Li[1], Suxian Yang[1], Ke Zhang[1*] and Jintao Li[2*]

Abstract

Background: Esophageal carcinoma (EC) is one of the major cancers in China. In 1982, Syrjanen first hypothesized the relationship between human papillomavirus (HPV) infection and the development of esophageal cancer. Since then, many reports in the field have supported this viewpoint. This study investigated the etiological relationship between HPV infection and the occurrence of esophageal carcinoma at Tangshan City of the Hebei province in China.

Methods: 189 samples of esophageal carcinoma patients were collected. DNA and RNA were isolated from samples, HPV DNA was detected by polymerase chain reaction (PCR) using My09/11 for HPV L1, and HPV16 was determined using type-specific primer sets for HPV16 E6. The HPV16 integration site was verified by amplification of papillomavirus oncogene transcripts, and HPV16 oncogene transcript products were ligated to the pMD-18 T vector and sequenced to confirm the physical location of HPV16 integration.

Results: 168 HPV-positive samples were detected in 189 samples, and among them 76 specimens were HPV16 positive. Approximately 600 bp of the HPV16 oncogene transcript were detected in nine esophageal cancer samples. Sequence analysis revealed that HPV16 E7 integrated into human chromosome 2 in three samples, into human chromosome 5 in one sample, into human chromosome 6 in one sample, into human chromosome 8 in two samples, and into human chromosome 17 in two samples. The results verified that the integrated HPV16 E7 in five samples harbored one mutation of viral DNA compared with the HPV16 sequence provided in GenBank (K02718).

Conclusions: The high prevalence of HPV16 suggests that HPV16 may play an etiological role in the development of esophageal cancer. The integration of HPV16 into host cell chromosomes suggests that persistent HPV infection is key for esophageal epithelial cell malignant transformation and carcinogenesis.

Keywords: Esophageal carcinoma, Human papillomavirus, Infection, Integration, Etiology

Background

Esophageal carcinoma (EC) is one of the major cancers in China [1, 2]. Environmental factors and life styles of esophageal carcinoma patients have been widely researched [3–5], although the pathogeny of esophageal cancer has not yet been determined. In 1982, Syrjanen first hypothesized the relationship between human papillomaviruses (HPV) infection and the development of esophageal cancer [6]. Since then, many reports in the

field have supported this viewpoint [7–13]. Our previous work showed that high-risk HPV types 16 and 18 were detected in esophageal tumors [14], and HPV18 was localized in human chromosome 8 in the EC109 cell line [15], these results indicates that HPV infection is a pathogenic factor for esophageal cancer.

Few studies have described the HPV integration site, so the objective of the current work to discuss HPV16 infection and integration site in the human genome to better understand its role in esophageal cancer. HPV infection detected using My09/11 for HPV L1 (16), HPV16 was determined using type-specific primer sets for HPV16 E6, and integration site of HPV16 in esophageal cancer was analyzed by amplification of papillomavirus oncogene transcripts (APOT), which allowed the discrimination of

* Correspondence: lsy5001@sina.com; 877567295@qq.com; 511046476@qq.com
[1]North China University of Science and Technology (Hebei Key Laboratory for Chronic Diseases, Tangshan Key Laboratory for Preclinical and Basic Research on Chronic Diseases), No.21 Bohai Road, Caofeidian New Town, Tangshan City, Hebei Province 063210, People's Republic of China
[2]College of Life Science and Bio-engineering, Beijing University of Technology, Beijingcity, 100124, People's Republic of China

HPV mRNAs derived from integrated genomes [17]. The integration of HPV in the host chromosome integration site can be accurately located by detection of the transcription of poly (A) tail [18, 19]. Namely, first, cDNA was synthesized by reverse transcription using RNA as template, and $(dT)_{17}$-p3 as primer; second, PCR amplification was conducted using cDNA as template, p1-HPV16 E7 and p3 as primers; third, PCR was conducted using above PCR product as template, p2-HPV16 E7 and $(dT)_{17}$-p3 as primers; fourth, the PCR product was cloned into a pMD-18 T vector; fifth, sequencing analysis and blast in GenBank. The integration sites was determined by sequence alignment including both HPV and human chromosome sequence.

Materials

Sample collection and preparation

A total of 189 fresh surgically resected tissue samples and clinical information of patients were obtained in 2013.03 to 2015.12 after participants authorized and signed informed consent forms to participate in the study. All specimen donors were pathologically diagnosed with esophageal carcinoma, and treated at the pathology department of Tangshan people's hospital in Hebei province. The patients were from the Tangshan area, 136 cases were male, and 53 cases were female. The average age of subjects was 58 (range 40–76) years old. Subject were classified as follows according to clinical and pathological stages of esophagus carcinoma: 98 early-stage;, 63 middle -stage; and 28 late-stage. Tumor tissue differentiation was separated into 30 well-differentiated types, 104 moderately-differentiated types and 55 poorly-differentiated types. All fresh samples were stored at −80 °C prior to experiments.

HPV16/pBR322 and HPV18/pBR322 DNA plasmid containing the whole genome of HPV16 and HPV18, plasmid of beta-actin DNA containing part human housekeeping genes, and human embryonic kidney 293 (HEK293) cell line DNA were stored at −20 °C prior to experiments.

Methods

DNA extraction

DNA was extracted from each tissue specimen (approximately 25 mg) using a QIAamp DNA mini kit (QIAGEN, Hilden, Germany) according to the manufacturer's instructions, and each sample DNA was eluted with approximately 50 μl sterilized distilled water. The concentration of each extracted DNA was detected and diluted to 100 ng/μl. DNA was stored at −20 °C.

Detection of specimen quality and HPV DNA

The quality of each tissue sample DNA was analyzed by PCR amplification using housekeeping gene β-actin

primers [20], HEK293 cell line DNA was used as a positive control, sterile water was used as a negative control to ensure the quality of specimens.

HPV DNA of each specimen was detected by PCR amplification using My09/11 primers for HPV L1 (My09: 5′-CGTCCMARRGGAWACTGATC-3′, MY11: 5′-GCMCAGGGWCATAAYAATGG-3′, PCR products 450 bp) [16] and HPV16 E6-specific primers (forward: 5′- ACTGCGACGTGAGGTATATGAC-3′, reverse: 5′- TTGATGATCTGCAACAAGACATAC-3′, PCR products 320 bp), which were designed according to the GenBank-provided HPV16 gene sequences K02718.1 (http://www.ncbi.nlm.nih.gov/nuccore/K02718). Primers were synthezed by Sangon Biotech of Shanghai. The PCR products were resolved on a 1.0% agarose gel with Goldview I nuclear staining dye (BioTeke Corporation, Beijing, China) and observed with a UV transilluminator.

Total PCR reaction was performed using Ex Taq Polymerase kit (Takara Biotechnology Co., Ltd., Dalian, China) in a 25-μl volume containing 5 pmol each of the forward and reverse primers, 1 × Ex Buffer (MgCl$_2$ free), 0.2 mM mixture deoxynucleoside triphosphate (dNTPs), 2.5 mM MgCl$_2$, 1 U Ex Taq DNA polymerase, and 0.25 ng extracted DNA template and control template were added to the reaction system. The following cycling was used: 95 °C for 5 min, followed by 31 cycles of 95 °C for 30 s, 55 °C for 30 s, and 72 °C for 30 s. The final extension step was 72 °C for 5 min, and stored at 4 °C.

Reverse transcription (RT)

Every sample RNA was extracted using the RNeasy Mini kit (Qiagen GmbH, Hilden, Germany) according to manufacturer's instruction. Reverse transcription (RT) was performed using M-MLV Reverse Transcriptase kit (BioTeke Corporation, Beijing, China) according to the manufacturer's protocol in a total volume of 20 μl, consisting of 9.2 μl RNase-free H2O, 4 μl of 5× first-strand buffer, 1.0 μl RNase inhibitor (40 U), 50 ng total RNA, 1 μl (dT)17-p3 (10 pmol primer: GACTCGAGTCGACATCGATTTTTTTTTTTTTTTTT), 0.5 μl dNTPs (0.2 mM), and 1 μl super script reverse transcriptase (200 U). The RNA reverse transcription was performed at 42 °C for 50 min and deactivated at 70 °C for 15 min, and the resulting product was stored at 4 °C.

To ensure mRNA quality of each tissue sample, human housekeeping gene GAPDH was detected using RT-PCR for verification of viral-cell fusion transcripts. The RT reactions were performed according to above, and the cDNA was stored at 4 °C. The PCR was conducted using a Takara Ex Taq Polymerase kit in a 20 μl reaction mixture containing 1X Ex buffer (MgCl$_2$-free), 0.2 mM dNTPs, 2.5 mM MgCl$_2$, 1 unit Ex Taq DNA polymerase, 5 pmol each GAPDH primer (forward, 5′-CATCACCATCTTCCAGGA-3′ and reverse, 5′-GTC

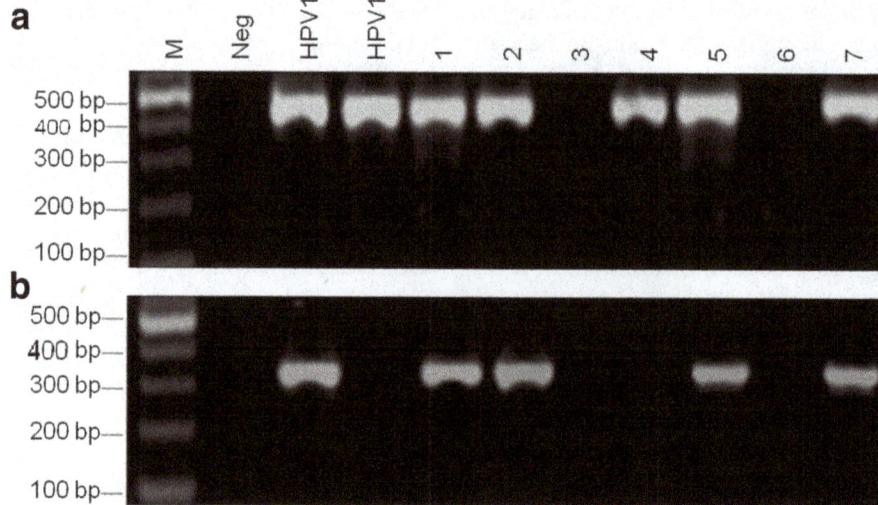

Fig. 1a Detection of HPV DNA using MY09/11 primers in esophageal carcinoma samples. M was 100 bp DNA ladder; Neg was a negative control; lanes 1–7 were detection of HPV DNA in different esophageal carcinoma samples. HPV16 and 18 were positive controls with the HPV16/pBR322 and HPV18/pBR322 templates. **b** Detection of HPV16 DNA using HPV16 E6 specific primers in esophageal carcinoma samples. M was 100 bp DNA ladder; Neg was a negative control; lanes 1–7 were detection of HPV16 DNA in different esophageal carcinoma samples. HPV16 was a positive control with HPV16/pBR322 template; HPV18 was a specific control using HPV18/pBR322

TACCACCCTATTGCA-3′) and 2 μl cDNA template. The PCR cycling profile was as follows: 95 °C for 5 min; followed by 31 cycles of 95 °C for 30 s, 52 °C for 30 s and 72 °C for 30 s; followed by a final extension at 72 °C for 5 min; and storage at 4 °C.

The viral-cell fusion transcripts analysis

The first PCR amplification was conducted according to Klaes et al. [17] in a 20 μl volume using HPV16 E7-specific forward primers for p1–16 (5′-CGGACAGA GCCCATTACAAT-3′) and reverse primers for p3 (5′-

```
                 104                                                           163
Query  1         TTCGGTTGTGCGTACAAAGCACACACGTAGACATTCGTACTTTGGAAGACCTGTTAATGG
Query  2         TTCGGTTGTGCGTACAAAGCACACACGTAGACAGTCGTACTTTGGAAGACCTGTTAATGG
Query  3         TTCGGTTGTGCGTACAAAGCACACACGTAGACAGTCGTACTTTGGAAGACCTGTTAATGG
Query  4         TTCGGTTGTGCGTACAAAGCACACACGTAGACAGTCGTACTTTGGAAGACCTGTTAATGG
Query  5         TTCGGTTGTGCGTACAAAGCACACACGTAGACAGTCGTACTTTGGAAGACCTGTTAATGG
Query  6         TTCGGTTGTGCGTACAAAGCACACACGTAGACAGTCGTACTTTGGAAGACCTGTTAATGG
Query  7         TTCGGTTGTGCGTACAAAGCACACACGTAGACATTCGTACTTTGGAAGACCTGTTAATGG
Query  8         TTCGGTTGTGCGTACAAAGCACACACGTAGACATTCGTACTTTGGAAGACCTGTTAATGG
Query  9         TTCGGTTGTGCGTACAAAGCACACACGTAGACATTCGTACTTTGGAAGACCTGTTAATGG
Sbjct  755       TTCGGTTGTGCGTACAAAGCACACACGTAGACATTCGTACTTTGGAAGACCTGTTAATGG  814
Consensus        TTCGGTTGTGCGTACAAAGCACACACGTAGACATTCGTACTTTGGAAGACCTGTTAATGG

                 164                                                      218
Query  1         GCACACTAGGAATTGTGTGCCCCATCTGTTCTCAGAAACCATAATCTACCATGGC
Query  2         GCACACTAGGAATTGTGTGCCCCATCTGTTCTCAGAAACCATAATCTACCATGGC
Query  3         GCACACTAGGAATTGTGTGCCCCATCTGTTCTCAGAAACCATAATCTACCATGGC
Query  4         GCACACTAGGAATTGTGTGCCCCATCTGTTCTCAGAAACCATAATCTACCATGGC
Query  5         GCACACTAGGAATTGTGTGCCCCATCTGTTCTCAGAAACCATAATCTACCATGGC
Query  6         GCACACTAGGAATTGTGTGCCCCATCTGTTCTCAGAAACCATAATCTACCATGGC
Query  7         GCACACTAGGAATTGTGTGCCCCATCTGTTCTCAGAAACCATAATCTACCATGGC
Query  8         GCACACTAGGAATTGTGTGCCCCATCTGTTCTCAGAAACCATAATCTACCATGGC
Query  9         GCACACTAGGAATTGTGTGCCCCATCTGTTCTCAGAAACCATAATCTACCATGGC
Sbjct  815       GCACACTAGGAATTGTGTGCCCCATCTGTTCTCAGAAACCATAATCTACCATGGC  869
Consensus        GCACACTAGGAATTGTGTGCCCCATCTGTTCTCAGAAACCATAATCTACCATGGC
```

Fig. 2 Alignment sequencing results compared with HPV16. Query 1–9: sequencing results for nine esophageal carcinoma specimens after PCR amplification with P2–16 E7-specific primers; Sbjct: part sequence of HPV 16E7-E1 in GenBank (K02718)

a

Query	253	CCGACCCCGCCGCCCCGGGCCTCGGCTCGCCCTCCGCACCCCCCCCTGCCCCCCCACCGT	312
		||||||||||||||||||||||||||||||||||||||||||||||||||||||||||||	
Sbjct	220441863	CCGACCCCGCCGCCCCGGGCCTCGGCTCGCCCTCCGCACCCCCCCCTGCCCCCCCACCGT	220441804
Query	313	TCGCCGCTGCAGGCGGTCGGCCGCCGCGATGAAGGCGAGCTCGGGGGGATCAGGGGAGCCC	372
		||||||||||||||||||||||||||||||||||||||||||||||||||||||||||||	
Sbjct	220441803	TCGCCGCTGCAGGCGGTCGGCCGCCGCGATGAAGGCGAGCTCGGGGGGATCAGGGGAGCCC	220441744
Query	373	CCCGTGCTTCCTGCGCTTCCCGCGGCCTGTGCGGGTGGTAAGTGGCGCCGAGGCCGAGCT	432
		||||||||||||||||||||||||||||||||||||||||||||||||||||||||||||	
Sbjct	220441743	CCCGTGCTTCCTGCGCTTCCCGCGGCCTGTGCGGGTGGTAAGTGGCGCCGAGGCCGAGCT	220441684

b

Query	263	TCCCACTCATCCTGTCACGTATATCATAGTGTTCTTGACTGGGCCATTCATCTAAGATGG	322
		||||||||||||||||||||||||||||||||||||||||||||||||||||||||||||	
Sbjct	62706962	TCCCACTCATCCTGTCACGTATATCATAGTGTTCTTGACTGGGCCATTCATCTAAGATGG	62707021
Query	323	GATTTACCCTGTGAAACAGGGAGAAGACTTATGGACCCCAAGCATCATTTCGAGTTGTAG	382
		||||||||||||||||||||||||||||||||||||||||||||||||||||||||||||	
Sbjct	62707022	GATTTACCCTGTGAAACAGGGAGAAGACTTATGGACCCCAAGCATCATTTCGAGTTGTAG	62707081
Query	383	TTGAGTTTTTAAAAGACATACATGCAAAGTTCCTTTGCTTTGGACCCTCTGCATTATTAA	442
		||||||||||||||||||||||||||||||||||||||||||||||||||||||||||||	
Sbjct	62707082	TTGAGTTTTTAAAAGACATACATGCAAAGTTCCTTTGCTTTGGACCCTCTGCATTATTAA	62707141

c

Query	262	CAGGATCTGATGACCCTGGAATATGTTCCAATACAGATTCAACCCAAGCACAGGTTTTGT	321
		||||||||||||||||||||||||||||||||||||||||||||||||||||||||||||	
Sbjct	63106224	CAGGATCTGATGACCCTGGAATATGTTCCAATACAGATTCAACCCAAGCACAGGTTTTGT	63106283
Query	322	TAGGCAAAAAGAGACTATTGAAAGCTGAGACTTTAGAATTGAGTGACTTATATGTTAGTG	381
		||||||||||||||||||||||||||||||||||||||||||||||||||||||||||||	
Sbjct	63106284	TAGGCAAAAAGAGACTATTGAAAGCTGAGACTTTAGAATTGAGTGACTTATATGTTAGTG	63106343
Query	382	ATAAGAAGAAGGATATGTCTCCACCCTTTATTTGTGAGGAGACAGATGAACAAAAGCTTC	441
		||||||||||||||||||||||||||||||||||||||||||||||||||||||||||||	
Sbjct	63106344	ATAAGAAGAAGGATATGTCTCCACCCTTTATTTGTGAGGAGACAGATGAACAAAAGCTTC	63106403

Fig. 3 Alignment sequencing results compared with human chromosome 2. **a-c**: Alignment sequencing results of three esophageal carcinoma specimens compared with human chromosome. Query: sequencing results for three esophageal carcinoma specimens after PCR amplification with P2–16 E7-specific primers; Sbjct: part sequence of human chromosome 2

Query	259	ATCAGTACTGTTTAAATGAAAACAAAATCATCGACACAATTAAAATGTATTTGCTGTGGG	318
		||||||||||||||||||||||||||||||||||||||||||||||||||||||||||||	
Sbjct	112664	ATCAGTACTGTTTAAATGAAAACAAAATCATCGACACAATTAAAATGTATTTGCTGTGGG	112723
Query	319	ATGAGCTTGTTTTCTGAGAACAAAGTGGCGCGTGGGCCAGCTTTGTCCTCCCCACAAGTG	378
		||||||||||||||||||||||||||||||||||||||||||||||||||||||||||||	
Sbjct	112724	ATGAGCTTGTTTTCTGAGAACAAAGTGGCGCGTGGGCCAGCTTTGTCCTCCCCACAAGTG	112783
Query	379	GTTGTCCCCTCCTCCCTGTACAAACCCAGGAGAGCCGGGAGGAGCAGCTCCCGCAGGACT	438
		||||||||||||||||||||||||||||||||||||||||||||||||||||||||||||	
Sbjct	112784	GTTGTCCCCTCCTCCCTGTACAAACCCAGGAGAGCCGGGAGGAGCAGCTCCCGCAGGACT	112843

Fig. 4 Alignment sequencing results compared with human chromosome 5. Alignment sequencing results of one esophageal carcinoma specimens compared with human chromosome. Query: sequencing results for one esophageal carcinoma specimens after PCR amplification with P2–16 E7-specific primers; Sbjct: part sequence of human chromosome 5

```
Query    260       TGTGTGTGTTTTCCAAGCCAACACACTCTACAGATTCTTTATTAAGTTAAGTTTCTCTAA    319
                   ||||||||||||||||||||||||||||||||||||||||||||||||||||||||||||
Sbjct    7885358   TGTGTGTGTTTTCCAAGCCAACACACTCTACAGATTCTTTATTAAGTTAAGTTTCTCTAA    7885299
Query    320       GTAAATGTGTAACTCATGGTCACTGTGTAAACATTTTCAGTGGCGATATATCCCCTTTGA    379
                   ||||||||||||||||||||||||||||||||||||||||||||||||||||||||||||
Sbjct    7885298   GTAAATGTGTAACTCATGGTCACTGTGTAAACATTTTCAGTGGCGATATATCCCCTTTGA    7885239
Query    380       CCTTCTCTTGATGAAATTTACATGGTTTCCTTTGAGACTAAAATAGCGTTGAGGGAAATG    439
                   ||||||||||||||||||||||||||||||||||||||||||||||||||||||||||||
Sbjct    7885238   CCTTCTCTTGATGAAATTTACATGGTTTCCTTTGAGACTAAAATAGCGTTGAGGGAAATG    7885179
```

Fig. 5 Alignment sequencing results compared with human chromosome 6. Alignment sequencing results of one esophageal carcinoma specimens compared with human chromosome. Query: sequencing results for one esophageal carcinoma specimens after PCR amplification with P2–16 E7-specific primers; Sbjct: part sequence of human chromosome 6

GACTCGAGTCGACATCG-3'); the reaction system included $1 \times$ Ex buffer, 2.5 mM $MgCl_2$, 0.2 mM dNTPs, 5 pM primers, 2 μl cDNA, and 1 U Ex Taq DNA polymerase. The PCR cycle was as follows: 95 °C for 5 min, followed by 30 cycles at 95 °C for 1 min, 56 °C for 1 min, 72 °C for 3 min, and a final extension at 72 °C for 5 min, and stored at 4 °C.

Nested PCR was performed with identical conditions except for the annealing temperature at 67 °C with the following primers: HPV16 E7-specific forward primer p2–16 (5'-CTTTTTGTTGCAAGTGTGACTCTACG-3') and reverse primer (dT)17-p3; 5 μl of the first round PCR product was used as template. To ensure specificity of these primers, HEK293 cell line DNA template was used as a negative control. The PCR products were resolved on a 1.0% agarose gel with Goldview I nuclear staining dye (Bio-Teke Corporation, Beijing, China) and observed with a UV transilluminator.

Cloning and sequence analysis for HPV16 integrated position in the human chromosome

The final nested PCR products were cloned into pMD-18 T vector according to reference [21], except the temperature of the target segment ligation to the pMD-18 T vector was changed to room temperature for 1 h. Then, commissioning Beijing Rui Bo Xing ke Biological Technology company to

```
a  Query    257       AATTCTAACATCTTAATTCTAAGTTAGCTTTGCAATAAAGATCAGTCCTCTTGAAGAAAT    316
                      ||||||||||||||||||||||||||||||||||||||||||||||||||||||||||||
   Sbjct    541129    AATTCTAACATCTTAATTCTAAGTTAGCTTTGCAATAAAGATCAGTCCTCTTGAAGAAAT    541188
   Query    317       TAACTAAATTTAGAATAAGACTAATCTGTCATAATTAACACAAATTTTCTCTATTTTTAT    376
                      ||||||||||||||||||||||||||||||||||||||||||||||||||||||||||||
   Sbjct    541189    TAACTAAATTTAGAATAAGACTAATCTGTCATAATTAACACAAATTTTCTCTATTTTTAT    541248
   Query    377       ATAGCAATGTTTTTCAACACAAACTTTGGATAACCTTAATAAAGTAACATAAAAACCACA    436
                      ||||||||||||||||||||||||||||||||||||||||||||||||||||||||||||
   Sbjct    541249    ATAGCAATGTTTTTCAACACAAACTTTGGATAACCTTAATAAAGTAACATAAAAACCACA    541308
b  Query    256       CATTTTTATATTCATTTCCTTTTAGGGTATGCATTTTTATACATCTGACTTTAACTGATA    315
                      ||||||||||||||||||||||||||||||||||||||||||||||||||||||||||||
   Sbjct    1512094   CATTTTTATATTCATTTCCTTTTAGGGTATGCATTTTTATACATCTGACTTTAACTGATA    1512153
   Query    316       AATGACTGTAAAGAGGTGTATCTTTATGGAATTGTAGAGGATTTGTTTCCAAAAAGGAGC    375
                      ||||||||||||||||||||||||||||||||||||||||||||||||||||||||||||
   Sbjct    1512154   AATGACTGTAAAGAGGTGTATCTTTATGGAATTGTAGAGGATTTGTTTCCAAAAAGGAGC    1512213
   Query    376       TGATGCTGCCGTTCTCAGTGACAAAGTTGATGCGTGTTTCATGTCTGTCTGCTCCCAGGT    435
                      ||||||||||||||||||||||||||||||||||||||||||||||||||||||||||||
   Sbjct    1512214   TGATGCTGCCGTTCTCAGTGACAAAGTTGATGCGTGTTTCATGTCTGTCTGCTCCCAGGT    1512273
```

Fig. 6 Alignment sequencing results compared with human chromosome 8. **a, b**: Alignment sequencing results of two esophageal carcinoma specimens compared with human chromosome. Query: sequencing results for two esophageal carcinoma specimens after PCR amplification with P2–16 E7-specific primers; Sbjct: part sequence of human chromosome 8

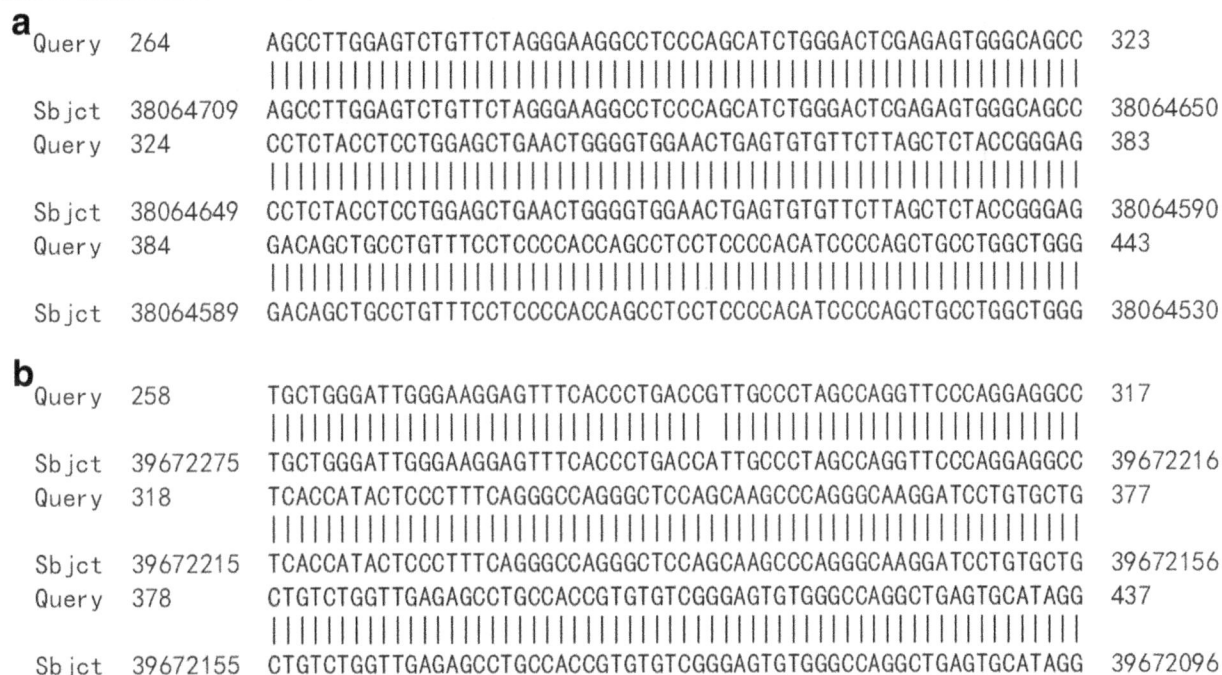

a

```
Query    264        AGCCTTGGAGTCTGTTCTAGGGAAGGCCTCCCAGCATCTGGGACTCGAGAGTGGGCAGCC    323
                    ||||||||||||||||||||||||||||||||||||||||||||||||||||||||||||
Sbjct    38064709   AGCCTTGGAGTCTGTTCTAGGGAAGGCCTCCCAGCATCTGGGACTCGAGAGTGGGCAGCC    38064650
Query    324        CCTCTACCTCCTGGAGCTGAACTGGGGTGGAACTGAGTGTGTTCTTAGCTCTACCGGGAG    383
                    ||||||||||||||||||||||||||||||||||||||||||||||||||||||||||||
Sbjct    38064649   CCTCTACCTCCTGGAGCTGAACTGGGGTGGAACTGAGTGTGTTCTTAGCTCTACCGGGAG    38064590
Query    384        GACAGCTGCCTGTTTCCTCCCCACCAGCCTCCTCCCCACATCCCCAGCTGCCTGGCTGGG    443
                    ||||||||||||||||||||||||||||||||||||||||||||||||||||||||||||
Sbjct    38064589   GACAGCTGCCTGTTTCCTCCCCACCAGCCTCCTCCCCACATCCCCAGCTGCCTGGCTGGG    38064530
```

b

```
Query    258        TGCTGGGATTGGGAAGGAGTTTCACCCTGACCGTTGCCCTAGCCAGGTTCCCAGGAGGCC    317
                    |||||||||||||||||||||||||||||||||||| |||||||||||||||||||||||
Sbjct    39672275   TGCTGGGATTGGGAAGGAGTTTCACCCTGACCATTGCCCTAGCCAGGTTCCCAGGAGGCC    39672216
Query    318        TCACCATACTCCCTTTCAGGGCCAGGGCTCCAGCAAGCCCAGGGCAAGGATCCTGTGCTG    377
                    ||||||||||||||||||||||||||||||||||||||||||||||||||||||||||||
Sbjct    39672215   TCACCATACTCCCTTTCAGGGCCAGGGCTCCAGCAAGCCCAGGGCAAGGATCCTGTGCTG    39672156
Query    378        CTGTCTGGTTGAGAGCCTGCCACCGTGTGTCGGGAGTGTGGGCCAGGCTGAGTGCATAGG    437
                    ||||||||||||||||||||||||||||||||||||||||||||||||||||||||||||
Sbjct    39672155   CTGTCTGGTTGAGAGCCTGCCACCGTGTGTCGGGAGTGTGGGCCAGGCTGAGTGCATAGG    39672096
```

Fig. 7 Alignment sequencing results compared with human chromosome 17. **a,b:** Alignment sequencing results of two esophageal carcinoma specimens compared with human chromosome. Query: sequencing results for two esophageal carcinoma specimens after PCR amplification with P2–16 E7-specific primers; Sbjct: part sequence of human chromosome 17

sequence. The sequencing results were blasted at NCBI (https://blast.ncbi.nlm.nih.gov/Blast.cgi?PROGRAM=-blastn&PAGE_TYPE=BlastSearch&LINK_LOC=blasthome), and HPV16 integration sites were determined in human chromosome for every integration specimen, severally.

Statistical analysis

Statistical analysis was performed using Statistical Package for the Social Sciences (SPSS) version 13.0 software. P –value of less than 0.05 was considered as statistically significant.

Results

Detection of specimen quality and HPV DNA

290-bp PCR products of β-actin were detected in 189 DNA samples, this result indicated that these DNA samples were in high quality and could meet the requirements for further experiments.

168 specimens were detected HPV positive among 189 samples using MY09 / 11 primers (Fig. 1a and b). All HPV-positive samples were amplified using HPV16 E6 specific primer sets, and among them 76 specimens were HPV16 positive (Fig. 1a and b).

HPV16 integration derived transcript in HPV16 E6 positive esophageal cancer samples

HPV16 integrated positions were confirmed in the HPV16 positive samples. Approximately 600 bp PCR

products were detected from nine HPV16 E6 positive samples by APOT. HPV16 E7 PCR products in nine samples were ligated into the pMD-18 T vector, and sequence analysis of HPV16 integration sites was performed. The sequence analysis showed that HPV16 E7 PCR products of nine samples were part of the HPV16 E7-E1 sequence, and compared with the HPV16 sequence provided in GenBank (K02718), the analysis results verified that integrated HPV16 E7 harbored one mutation from five samples of viral DNA (Fig. 2). Partial sequences from nine samples were similar to human chromosome sequences, as follows: three were similar to human chromosome 2 (Fig. 3a, b and c). One was similar to human chromosome 5 (Fig. 4), one was similar to human chromosome 6 (Fig. 5), two were similar to human chromosome 8 (Fig. 6a and b), and two were similar to human chromosome 17 (Fig. 7a and b).

The relationship between HPV16 integration and patient background

A total of fresh surgically resected tissue samples from 189 patients who were pathologically diagnosed with esophageal carcinoma were evaluated. The relationship between HPV16 integration and the patients' backgrounds are shown in Table 1. Statistical analysis showed that HPV16 integration was not significantly correlated with gender, age, histological differentiation and pathological stage.

Table 1 Background of esophageal cancer patients and HPV16 integration

Background	HPV16 positive ($n = 79$)	Samples ($n = 189$)	Integrated	Without integrated	X^2	P^a
sex					0.06	>0.05
male	55	136	7	48		
female	21	53	2	19		
age (year old)					1.38	>0.05
≤ 45	18	41	1	17		
46–64	28	70	3	25		
≥ 65	30	78	5	25		
differentiated type					0.09	>0.05
well differentiated	11	30	1	10		
moderately differentiated	49	104	6	43		
poorly differentiated	16	55	2	14		
pathological stages					2.99	>0.05
early stage	25	98	2	23		
middle stage	40	63	4	36		
late stage	11	28	3	8		
Total	76	189	9	67		

^{a}Notice: There were no statistically significant difference ($P>0.05$)

Discussion

High-risk HPV infection (such as HPV types16, HPV18, HPV31, HPV33, HPV35, HPV39, HPV45, HPV51, HPV52, HPV56, HPV58 and HPV59) have been identified as causative agents in cervix cancers [22, 23]. However, HPV has not been determined as to be a pathogenic factor for esophageal cancer occurrence thus far in highly prevalent regions [24, 25].

In the present study, HPV DNA from 189 patient tissue samples with pathologic diagnosis of esophageal carcinoma were examined, and a high prevalence was found (approximately 89% HPV DNA positive rate), and the HPV16 positive rate was 40.2%; Mehryar et al. [26] study showed that the prevalence of HPV types 16 and 18 was 40.40% and 47.47% in esophageal carcinoma for Tangshan, Hebei province, China, respectively, Dong et al. [7] study showed that Six HPV genotypes (HPV6, HPV16, HPV33, HPV39, HPV51, and HPV82) were present in at least 51.7% of the esophagealcarcinoma tissues, and combined with other studies [8–11], these findings indicate that HPV infection may be a pathogenic factor for esophageal cancers.

HPV16 integration was discovered in esophageal cancer cells from nine patient specimens, and HPV16 was found to be integrated into chromosomes 2, 5, 6, 8 and 17. With the integration of HPV18 in EC109 cells, these results indicate that HPV randomly integrates into the host chromosome and that the HPV viral genome is cleaved at the E1 and E2 ORFs for integration. Moreover, the E2 gene serves as a pivotal modulator for E6 and E7 gene expression in the viral life cycle. In many HPV-infected patients, HPV E2 restrains E6 and E7 gene transcription, which aids in the regulation of cellular proliferation [27]. Cleaving the E2 gene increased HPV E6 and E7 gene expression, which disrupts the cell cycle and leads to aberrant proliferation [28–30]. HPV E6 and E7 genes usually integrate into the host cell genome and require longer incubation periods for viral DNA replication and recombination to produce a variety of genetic changes in the viral and human genome. The expression levels of E6 and E7 simultaneously increased, which resulted in human chromosomal instability and the development of malignant tumors [18]. On the other hand, among nine integrated HPV16 specimens, three patient samples were in the late stage, including two females and one male, four patient samples from males were in the middle stage, and two patient samples from males were in the early stage; one was a well-differentiated sample, and six were moderately-differentiated samples, and two were poorly differentiated samples. Nine patient samples seem too small to be able to indicate that HPV16 integration is related to patient background (including gender, age, degree of differentiation, and pathological stages) and supports the assumption of preferred selective outgrowth of HPV-infected cells in preneoplastic lesions that express integrated viral oncogenes E6 and E7. The sequencing results showed one mutation for five DNA samples compared with the GenBank-provided HPV16 gene sequences of K02718.1 (http://www.ncbi.nlm.nih.gov/nuccore/K02718). This phenomenon may be different for local epidemic strains of HPV16. Next we will be to detect other HPV types infection and integration sites.

Conclusions

In this study, 76 specimens were HPV16 positive in 189 esophageal carcinoma samples, this result suggested that a high prevalence of HPV16 plays an etiological role in the development of esophageal cancer. The integration of HPV16 into host cell chromosomes suggests that persistent HPV infection is key for esophageal epithelial cell malignant transformation and carcinogenesis. However, HPV infection may be one of multiple risk factors of esophageal cancer. Further work is needed to elucidate the underlying mechanism, other types of HPV integration sites, the genetic changes associated with HPV infection, and the molecular mechanism of esophageal cancer occurrence.

Abbreviations

APOT: Amplification of papillomavirus oncogene transcripts.; EC: Esophageal carcinoma; HPV: Human papillomavirus; PCR: Polymerase chain reaction

Acknowledgements

Not applicable.

Funding

This study supported by the project of Science and technology for overseas scholars in Hebei Province (No.CY201620), the project of Hebei education department (No.ZD2016003), the Project of North China University Science and Technology (No. sp201506), Beijing Natural Science Foundation (No. 5162003).

Authors' contributions

Shuying Li, Ke Zhang, and Jintao Li, designed the study, performed the majority of the experiments, wrote the manuscript, and contributed equally to this work; Haie Shen, Ning Li, Suxian Yang, were samples collection, and performed some experiments; Zhanjun Liu, participated in the design of the study, and performed the statistical analysis. All authors read and approved the final manuscript.

Competing interests

The authors report no conflicts of interest.

References

1. He L, Fan J-H, Qiao Y-L. Epidemiology, etiology, and prevention of esophageal squamous cell carcinoma in China. Cancer Biol Med. 2017;14: 33–41.
2. Zhao J, He YT, Zheng RS, Zhang SW, Chen WQ: Analysis of esophageal cancer time trends in China, 1989–2008. Asian Pac J Cancer Prev 13:4613-4617, 2012.
3. Sun X, Chen W, Chen Z, Wen D, Zhao D, He Y. Population-based casecontrol study on risk factors for esophageal cancer in five high-risk areas in China. Asian Pac J Cancer Prev. 2010;11:1631–6.
4. Gholipour M, Islami F, Roshandel G, Khoshnia M, Badakhshan A, Moradi A, Malekzadeh R. Esophageal cancer in Golestan Province, Iran: a review of genetic susceptibility and environmental risk factors. Middle East J Dig Dis. 2016;8:249–66.
5. Zhang HZ, Jin GF, Shen HB. Epidemiologic differences in esophageal cancer between Asian and western populations. Chin J Cancer. 2012;31:281–6.
6. Syrjänen KJ. Histological changes identical to those of condylomatous lesions found in esophageal squamous cell carcinomas. Arch Geschwulstforsch. 1982;52:283–92.
7. Dong HC, Cui XB, Wang LH, Li M, Shen YY, Zhu JB, Li CF, Hu JM, Li SG, Yang L, et al. Type-specific detection of human papillomaviruses in Kazakh esophageal squamous cell carcinoma by genotyping both E6 and L1 genes with MALDI-TOF mass spectrometry. Int J Clin Exp Pathol. 2015;8:13156–65.
8. Türkay DÖ, Vural Ç, Sayan M, Gürbüz Y. Detection of human papillomavirus in esophageal and gastroesophageal junction tumors: a retrospective study by real-time polymerase chain reaction in an instutional experience from Turkey and review of literature. Pathol Res Pract. 2016;212:77–82.
9. Ludmir EB, Stephens SJ, Palta M, Willett CG, Czito BG. Human papillomavirus tumor infection in esophageal squamous cell carcinoma. J Gastrointest Oncol. 2015;6:287–95.
10. Georgantis G, Syrakos T, Agorastos T, Miliaras S, Gagalis A, Tsoulfas G, Spanos K, Marakis G. Detection of human papillomavirus DNA in esophageal carcinoma in Greece. World J Gastroenterol. 2015;21:2352–7.
11. Liu HY, Zhou SL, Ku JW, Zhang DY, Li B, Han XN, Fan ZM, Cui JL, Lin HL, Guo, et al. Prevalence of human papillomavirus infection in esophageal and cervical cancers in the high incidence area for the two diseases from 2007 to 2009 in Linzhou of Henan Province, northern China. Arch Virol. 2014;159: 1393–401.
12. Prakash Saxena PU, Fernandes DJ, Vidyasagar MS, Singh A, Sharan K. Detection of human papilloma virus in patients with squamous cell carcinoma of the esophagusplanned for definitive chemo-radiotherapy, and a study of their clinical characteristics. J Cancer Res Ther. 2016;12:871–5.
13. Pantham G, Ganesan S, Einstadter D, Jin G, Weinberg A, Fass R. Assessment of the incidence of squamous cell papilloma of the esophagus and the presence of high-risk human papilloma virus. Dis Esophagus. 2017;30(1):1–5.
14. Mehryar MM, Li SY, Liu HW, Li F, Zhang F, Zhou YB, Zeng Y, Li JT. Revalence of human papillomavirus in esophageal carcinoma in Tangshan, China. World J Gastroenterol. 2015;21(10):2905–11.
15. Zhang K, Li JT, Li SY, Zhu LH, Zhou L, Zeng Y. Integration of human papillomavirus 18 DNA in esophageal carcinoma 109 cells. World J Gastroenterol. 2011;17:4242–6.
16. Karlsen F, Kalantari M, Jenkins A, Pettersen E, Kristensen G, Holm R, Johansson B, Hagmar B. Use of multiple PCR sets for optimal detection of human papillomavirus. J Clin Microbiol. 1996;34:2095–100.
17. Klaes R, Woerner SM, Ridder R, Wentzensen N, Duerst M, Schneider A, Lotz B, Melsheimer P, von Knebel Doeberitz M. Detection of high-risk cervical intraepithelial neoplasia and cervical cancer by amplification of transcripts derived from integrated papillomavirus oncogenes. Cancer Res. 1999;59: 6132–6.
18. Hillemanns P, Wang XL. Integration of HPV16 and HPV18 DNA in vulvar intraepithelial neoplasia. Gynecol Oncol. 2006;100:276–82.
19. Klimov E, Vinokourova S, Moisjak E, Rakhmanaliev E, Kobseva V, Laimins L, Kisseljov F, Sulimova G. Human papilloma viruses and cervical tumours: mapping of integration sites and analysis of adjacent cellular sequences. BMC Cancer. 2002;2:1471–2407.
20. Lee DC, Cheung CY, Law AH, Mok CK, Peiris M, Lau AS. p38 Mitogen-activated protein Kinase-dependent Hyperinduction of tumor necrosis factor alpha expression in response to avian influenza virus H5N1. J Virol. 2005;79:10147–54.
21. Yuan B, Li XY, Zhu T, Yuan L, Hu JP, Chen J, Gao W, Ren WZ. Antibody study in canine distemper virus nucleocapsid protein gene-immunized mice. Genet Mol Res. 2015;14:3098–105.
22. Arbyn M, Tommasino M, Depuydt C, Dillner J. Are 20 human papillomavirus types causing cervical cancer? J Pathol. 2014;234:431–5.
23. Doorbar J, Egawa N, Griffin H, Kranjec C, Murakami I. Human papillomavirus molecular biology and disease association. Rev Med Virol. 2015;25:2–23.
24. Gao GF, Roth MJ, Wei WQ, Abnet CC, Chen F, Lu N, Zhao FH, Li XQ, Wang GQ, Taylor PR, Pan QJ, Chen W, Dawsey SM, Qiao YL. No association between HPV infection and the neoplastic progression of esophageal squamous cell carcinoma: result from a cross-sectional study in a high-risk region of China. Int J Cancer. 2006;119:1354–9.
25. Kamangar F, Qiao YL, Schiller JT, Dawsey SM, Fears T, Sun XD, Abnet CC, Zhao P, Taylor PR, Mark SD. Human papillomavirus serology and the risk of esophageal and gastric cancers: results from a cohort in a high-risk region in China. Int J Cancer. 2006;119:579–84.

26. Mehryar MM, Li SY, Liu HW, Li F, Zhang F, Zhou YB, Zeng Y, Li JT. Prevalence of human papillomavirus in esophageal carcinoma in Tangshan, China. World J Gastroenterol. 2015;21:2905–11.

27. Wells SI, Aronow BJ, Wise TM, Williams SS, Couget JA, Howley PM. Transcriptome signature of irreversible senescence in human papillomavirus-positive cervical cancer cells. Proc Natl Acad Sci U S A. 2003; 100:7093–8.

28. Bergner S, Halec G, Schmitt M, Aubin F, Alonso A, Auvinen E. Individual and complementary effects of human Papillomavirus Oncogenes on epithelial cell proliferation and differentiation. Cells Tissues Organs. 2016;201:97–108.

29. Ekalaksananan T, Jungpol W, Prasitthimay C, Wongjampa W, Kongyingyoes B, Pientong C. Polymorphisms and functional analysis of the intact human papillomavirus16 e2 gene. Asian Pac J Cancer Prev. 2014;15:10255–62.

30. Scheffner M, Romanczuk H, Münger K, Huibregtse JM, Mietz JA, Howley PM. Functions of human papillomavirus proteins. Curr Top Microbiol Immunol. 1994;186:83–99.

23

The current role and future prospectives of functional parameters by diffusion weighted imaging in the assessment of histologic grade of HCC

Vincenza Granata[1], Roberta Fusco[1,2*], Salvatore Filice[1], Orlando Catalano[1], Mauro Piccirillo[2], Raffaele Palaia[2], Francesco Izzo[2] and Antonella Petrillo[1]

Abstract

Hepatocellular carcinoma (HCC) is one of the most common human solid malignancies worldwide. Although the MRI is the technique that is best adapted to characterize HCC, there is not an agreement regarding the study protocol and even what the role of Diffusion-weighted imaging (DWI). The possibility that imaging study can correlate to histologic grade to selecting the therapeutic strategy would be valuable in helping to direct the proper management of HCC. Apparent Diffusion Coefficient (ADC) and IVIM-derived perfusion fraction (fp) and tissue diffusivity (Dt) values of HCC showed significantly better diagnostic performance in differentiating high-grade HCC from low-grade HCC, and significant correlation was observed between ADC, fp, Dt and histological grade.

Keywords: HCC, Magnetic resonance imaging, Diffusion weighted imaging, Histologic grade

Background

Hepatocellular carcinoma (HCC) is the most common primitive hepatic cancer [1, 2]. Imaging surveillance is a widely established tool that increases the probability of early detection of HCC, which is mandatory on patient at risk for this tumor since the treatment of HCC is different to other hepatic lesions [1]. According to the guidelines of National Comprehensive Cancer Network (NCCN) [3] and of European Association for the Study of the Liver (EASL) and American Association for the Study Liver Diseases National Comprehensive Cancer Network (AASLD), during the phase of HCC characterization, the diagnostic criteria should be used only for cirrhotic patients [4]. However, the up-to-date imaging-based criteria have several limits, counting the absence of recognized agreement concerning the precise descriptions of imaging features, binary classification (either definite or not definite HCC),

and disappointment to report non-HCC malignancies and vascular involvement [5]. Therefore, the American College of Radiology (ACR) has encouraged the use of Liver Imaging Reporting and Data System (LI-RADS) for the reading, recording and data collection of HCC nodules [6, 7]. Although imaging techniques allow identifying and characterizing of liver nodules with a higher diagnostic accuracy and Magnetic Resonance Imaging (MRI) is the diagnostic tool that should be chosen to survive HCC patients [8–10], however the gold standard to characterize liver lesions is still biopsy [11]. In fact, until now, histological analysis is the unique technique that allow to identify the histologic grade of HCC, that is one of the most predictive factors of survival for HCC patients [11]. During the last years, the possibility to obtain functional data by Diffusion-weighted imaging (DWI), it has seen born a great interest on this technique. DWI has been applied to liver imaging as an excellent tool for detection and characterization of focal liver lesions, increasing clinical confidence and decreasing false positives [11–14]. Oncology is a major field of application of DWI. The analysis of DW images can be done qualitatively and quantitatively, through the apparent diffusion coefficient (ADC) map.

* Correspondence: r.fusco@istitutotumori.na.it
[1]Radiology Division, Istituto Nazionale Tumori IRCCS Fondazione G. Pascale – IRCCS di Napoli, via Mariano Semmola, I-80131 Naples, Italy
[2]Hepatobiliary Surgical Oncology Division, Istituto Nazionale Tumori IRCCS Fondazione G. Pascale – IRCCS di Napoli, via Mariano Semmola, I-80131 Naples, Italy

Eco Planar Imaging (EPI) sequences are widely used for DWI, which are basically T2-W sequences, acquired with single shot technique and FS. Different series of DW images are acquired through modification of the gradient strength and magnitude, referred as b-value. One series should be obtained with a b-value of 0, meaning no gradient is applied and consequently no diffusion information is retrieved, giving similar information as T2 FS sequences. Another series should be obtained with a low b-value (b < 100), for lesion detection, while series obtained with a high b-value (such as b = 800) are important for liver lesion characterization [11–14]. DWI signal depends on the water mobility that is related to tissue characteristics [11]. Diffusion is quantified by a diffusion coefficient, the ADC. The ADC map is the graphical representation of the ratio of DW signal intensities and its measurements may discriminate between benign and malignant lesions. The ADC measurements are correlated to the sequence acquisition protocol and suffer from a lack of reproducibility, especially in respiratory triggering techniques, nodules of left liver lobe, smaller size and lesion heterogeneity [11]. Accurate estimation of ADC can be improved by acquiring a large number of b-values. ADC low values mean restricted diffusion, high ADC values mean free or unimpeded diffusion. Malignant tissue shows signal hyperintensity in DWI and signal hypointensity in the apparent diffusion coefficient (ADC) map [11]. Several researchers investigated, therefore, the values of ADC for lesion characterization. The ADC values for malignant lesions vary in literature widely and show a significant overlap with benign and other malignant lesions [11–14]. Le Bihan et al. as a first assessed the intravoxel incoherent motion (IVIM) and evaluated a more sophisticated method to define the relationship between signal attenuation and increasing b value that separately reproduce tissue diffusivity and tissue perfusion [12, 13]. IVIM data can be assessed qualitatively and quantitatively. The lesion characterization is done easier by quantitative data, while qualitatively method helped the detection of nodule [13]. In clinical practice DWI is widely employed after neoadjuvant therapy [14] or ablative techniques [15], to assess the efficacy of treatment. An emerging field of application of DWI is the evaluation of histological grade of the tumor [16]. Several researches have assessed the relationship between functional parameters obtained by DWI and histological grade of HCC [16–19]. Considering that the histologic grade of HCC is one of the most predictive factors of reappearance and survival after treatment and transplantation [16–19], the probability that imaging analysis could be associated to the histologic grade to selecting the therapeutic approach should guide the proper treatment of patient.

Our purpose is reporting an overview and update of the role of DWI in assessment of histologic grade of HCC.

Methods
This overview and update is the result of autonomous studies without protocol and registration number.

Search criterion
We evaluated several electronic databases, PubMed (US National Library of Medicine, http://www.ncbi.nlm.nih.-gov/pubmed), Scopus (Elsevier, http://www.scopus.com/), Web of Science (Thomson Reuters, http://apps.webofknowledge.com/) and Google Scholar (https://scholar.google.it/), using as search criteria the following key words: "hepatocellular carcinoma" AND "diffusion magnetic resonance imaging" AND "histologic grade", "hepatocellular carcinoma" AND "intravoxel incoherent motion" AND "histologic grade", "hepatocellular carcinoma" AND "multimodal imaging" AND "histologic grade". Our analysis enclosed the time between January 2000 and October 2017. Also, we evaluated the references of the searched studies for documents not indexed in the electronic databases. We retained solely the papers recording DWI results in the evaluation of histologic grade of HCC. Articles published in the English language from January 2000 to October 2017 were included. The absence of full text, overview analysis and conference papers were considered as exclusion criteria.

Histological grading assessment in HCC
The classical and most commonly adopted grading system for HCC is Edmondson–Steiner (ES) [20], published in the 1954 that organized the tumors in 4-tier histological grade distribution (Table 1). In contrast, and most likely due to differences from the ES classification, the World Health Organization (WHO) classification organized tumors in 3-tiers (Table 1) [21]. Usually the researches, when WHO classification is adopted, tend to assess each grade individually (G1 × G2 × G3), while when is adopted ES classification, they dichotomize them in low (G1 + G2) and high grades (G3 + G4).

Results
We collected 170 studies from the literature research from January 2000 to October 2017 considering the key words described above. However, 132 papers have different topic respect to correlation between HCC histologic grade and DWI and 24 studies corresponded to more than one excluded criteria. Therefore, fourteen articles were included at the end (Fig. 1).

Table 1 Histological features according to Edmondson and Steiner (ES) and WHO classification

Classification	Grades	Architecture	Cytology	Other features
Edmondson and Steiner	I	–	–	Areas of carcinoma where distinction from hyperplastic liver is difficult
	II	Trabecular, frequent acini (lumen varying from tiny canaliculi to large thyroid-like spaces)	Resemblance to normal hepatic cells; larger nuclei; abundant acidophilic cytoplasm	Cell borders sharp and clear cut; acini containing bile or protein precipitate
	III	Distortion of trabecular structure, acini less frequent than grade II	Larger, more hyperchromatic nuclei, granular but less acidophilic cytoplasm	Acini are less frequent; tumor giant cells may be numerous
	IV	Medullary, less trabeculae, rare acini	Highly hyperchromatic nuclei, scanty cytoplasm, with fewer granules	Loss of cell cohesiveness; giant, spindle or short-plump cells can be found
World Health Organization	Well differentiated	Thin trabecular, frequent acinar structures	Minimal atypia	Fatty change is frequent
	Moderately differentiated	Trabecular (3 or more cells in thickness) and acinar	Abundant eosinophilic cytoplasm, round nuclei with distinct nucleoli	Bile or proteinaceous fluid within acini
	Poorly differentiated	Solid	Moderate to marked pleomorphism	Absence of sinusoid-like blood spaces
	Undifferentiated	Solid	Little cytoplasm, spindle, or round-shaped cells	–

Discussion

The accurate detection of histologic grade of HCC is thought a main parameter in planning of the therapeutic approach [22]. Seeing that histological analysis of small doubtful nodule is often not feasible due to their location, the role of pre-operative imaging for the assessment of well, moderate and poorly differentiated HCCs is crucial [23]. DWI is a functional MRI technique that allows quantitative evaluation of water proton diffusion in tissues. HCC is characterized by increased cellularity and, thus, have restricted diffusion [11]. Intravoxel incoherent motion (IVIM) is a recently developed DWI-derived tool. IVIM can separate the effects of perfusion-related diffusion from pure molecular diffusion [11]. DWI and IVIM enable improved detection and characterization of HCC

[11]. According to Granata et al. [11] DWI and IVIM should be a role in predicting of the histological grade of HCC. In fact, they showed a good correlation between ADC, fp (perfusion fraction), and Dt (tissue diffusivity) and tumoral grading. ROC analyses showed that an ADC value of $2.11 \times 10-3$ mm2/sec, an fp value of 47,33% and an Dt value of $0.94 \times 10-3$ mm2/sec were the most accurate cut off levels to discriminate high grade versus low grade, with a sensitivity and specificity for ADC of 100 and 100%, for fp of 100 and 89%, for Dt of 100 and 74%, respectively. Guo et al. assessed the relationships of signal intensity (SI) and ADC with the histological grade in 27 resected HCC patients. They showed that there were no significant differences in ADC parameters or SI between higher or lower grade of HCC nodules. In fact the overall

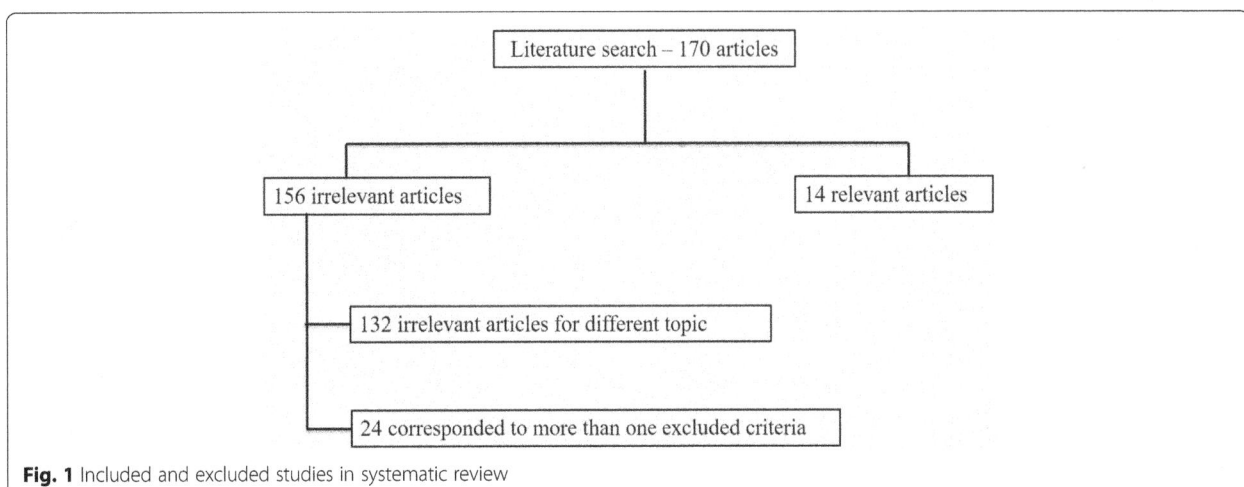

Fig. 1 Included and excluded studies in systematic review

ADC rate for all cases was $1.28 \pm 0.19 \times 10{-}3$ mm2/s. The ADC was $1.16 \pm 0.16 \times 10{-}3$ mm2/s for poorly differentiated nodules, lower than the well [$1.43 \pm 0.09 \times 10{-}3$ mm2/s] and moderately [$1.34 \pm 0.19 \times 10{-}3$ mm2/s] differentiated HCCs. The overall SI value was 75.66 ± 32.94. The mean SI value for the moderately differentiated HCCs was 54.37 ± 28.37, lower than the well (90.78 ± 27.49) and poorly (86.77 ± 31.51) differentiated [16]. Nakanishi et al. showed not only the utility of DWI for histological tumor grading, but also that ADC should be used as a preoperative prediction of early recurrence [22]. DWI is a valuable diagnostic tool, that allows not invasively characterizing biological tissues by measurement of properties of water diffusion, however there are results which are in contrast each one [12–19, 24–30]. Chen et al., in a meta-analysis, found that for differentiating well differentiated lesions from higher grades, DWI showed a low sensitivity (54%), high specificity (90%), and an excellent diagnostic performance (area under curve (AUC) = 0.9311). Conversely, in differentiating poorly differentiated lesion from lower grades, the sensitivity was 84%, the specificity 48%, showing a moderately high diagnostic performance [18]. Nasu et al. evaluated 125 resected HCCs showing no association between histological grade and ADC, while they found that SI of the HCC increased in higher grade [23]. Instead, Muhi et al. found significant changes in SI and ADC between different grades of 98 HCC nodules, although there was still considerable overlapping [24]. Nishie et al. found a relationship between ADC parameters and HCC histological data, but the difference was significant only between well-differentiated and poorly differentiated lesions [25]. Recent technique advance has endorsed the application of IVIM in predicting the histological grade of HCC [17]. By using the IVIM model diffusion features can be disconnected from pseudo diffusion caused by perfusion [12, 13]. According to Woo et al. IVIM-derived diffusion values (diffusion coefficient, Dt) had considerably higher diagnostic performance compared to ADC in discerning high grade (Fig. 2) from low grade HCC (Fig. 3) [17]. Conversely Granata et al. showed that the ADC had the best diagnostic performance, in comparison of fp and Dt [11].

However the mayor limit of DWI and IVIM parameters to discriminate the histological grade of HCC, as suggested by Ichikawa et al., is depending on the fitting methods used to obtained functional parameters, thus the fitting would be robust even though some errors might have occurred during image acquisition [29]. A prospective study with a larger cohort would be necessary to confirm the usefulness of the IVIM parameters for distinguishing poorly differentiated HCCs from other HCC grades and to establish the advantages of this method [29].

Several tumor features evaluated by imaging techniques can be associated with HCC prognosis after treatment [31]. Microvascular invasion (MVI), defined as microscopically detected tumor thrombi within small tumor or peritumoral vessels, to day, is considered a major risk factor of recurrence [31]. DWI and DWI-based approaches (IVIM and Kurtosis) play a pivotal role in assessment of MVI. Several researches have shown that higher tumor-to-liver signal intensity ratio and lower ADCs value can predict MVI [32–34]. This could be due to higher cellularity with restricted diffusion and decreased perfusion in MVI HCCs compared with no MVI HCC. Wang et al. assessed the role of kurtosis in HCC showing that mean kurtosis values increased in MVI positive patients so that those can be independent risk factors for MVI [35].

Another field of attention is the role of DWI in the assessment of immunotherapy. To date at the best of our knowledge there are not present in literature studies that describe the role of DWI in the assessment of HCC response after immunotherapy. However, Qin et al. [36] report the promising results of DWI in glioblastoma patients subjected to anti-PD1 therapy in order to differentiate patients who derive therapeutic benefit from those who do not. Preliminary data from advanced MRI assessment suggests that increase in volume of abnormal tissue with contrast enhancement, edema, and intermediate ADC occurs in most patients during the initial months of anti-PD1 ± anti-CTLA-4 immunotherapy. Among patients who appear to achieve therapeutic benefit, subsequent improvement in these MRI markers

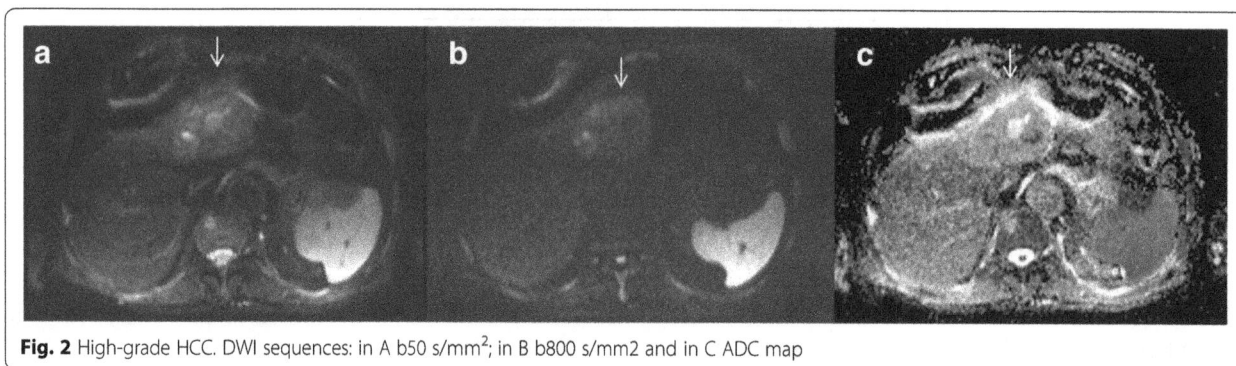

Fig. 2 High-grade HCC. DWI sequences: in A b50 s/mm^2; in B b800 s/mm2 and in C ADC map

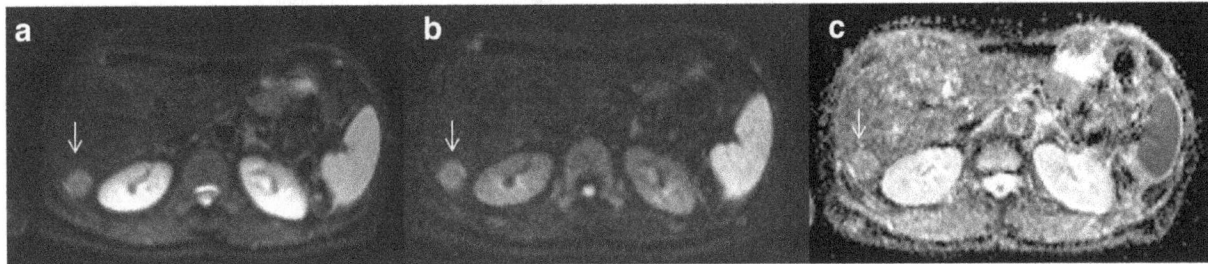

Fig. 3 Low-grade HCC. DWI sequences: in A b50 s/mm²; in B b800 s/mm2 and in C ADC map

was observed. Their findings suggest that volumetric change in ADC may correlate better with therapeutic benefit than RANO criteria measures. Therefore, future endpoint could be the evaluation of HCC tissue and in particular of immune cell infiltrate using DWI after immunotherapy [36].

Although there are the great advantages due to DWI and DWI-based approaches in detection and characterization of HCC, and DWI has been included in the Liver Imaging Reporting and Data System [9, 10], these approaches have several limitations. First, the performance of DWI for detection could be degraded due to the not standardized acquisition protocol, including the determination of optimal b values and breathing techniques across different modalities and medical centers. Therefore, universal thresholds for ADC and other quantitative parameters may not be acquirable. Second, DWI is sensitive to motion artifact; thus, detection and characterization of lesions can be mostly affected in the presence of motion artifacts [29].

Conclusion

The histologic grade of HCC is one of the most prognostic features of reappearance and survival after surgical treatment and transplantation. The probability that the imaging could identify the histologic grade of HCC should be a useful tool to guide the patient management. In this context, MRI study with the DWI sequences should be the method to choose because the ADC and IVIM-derived parameters are related to the histological grade of HCC. However, a larger study group would be necessary to confirm the usefulness of the IVIM parameters for distinguishing poorly differentiated HCCs from other HCC grades.

Abbreviations

AASLD: Association for the Study Liver Diseases National Comprehensive Cancer Network; ACR: American College of Radiology; ADC: Apparent diffusion Coefficient; AUC: Area under curve; Dt: Tissue diffusivity; DWI: Diffusion-weighted imaging; EASL: European Association for the Study of the Liver; fp: Perfusion fraction; HCC: Hepatocellular carcinoma; IVIM: Intravoxel incoherent motion; LI-RADS: Liver Imaging Reporting and Data System; MRI: Magnetic Resonance Imaging; NCCN: National Comprehensive Cancer Network

Acknowledgements
The authors are grateful to Alessandra Trocino, librarian at the National Cancer Institute of Naples, Italy. Additionally, authors are grateful to Assunta Zazzaro and Rita Guarino for collaboration.

Authors' contributions
VG conceived of the study, and participated in its design, coordination and drafting of the manuscript. RF participated in the studies collection and drafted the manuscript. SF, OC, MP, RP, FI, AP participated in the studies collection. All authors read and approved the final manuscript. Guarantor of the manuscript is Vincenza Granata. Each author have participated sufficiently in any submission to take public responsibility for its content.

Competing interests
The authors declare that they have no competing interests.

References
1. Bruix J, Sherman M. Management of hepatocellular carcinoma: an update. Hepatology. 2011;53:1020–2.
2. Piccirillo M, Granata V, Albino V, Palaia R, Setola SV, Petrillo A, Tatangelo F, Botti G, Foggia M, Izzo F. Can hepatocellular carcinoma (HCC) produce unconventional metastases? Four cases of extrahepatic HCC Tumori. 2013; 99(1):e19–23.
3. NCCN Clinical Practice Guidelines in Oncology on hepatobiliary Cancer Version 2016. http://www.nccn.org.
4. European Association for Study of Liver; European Organisation for Research and Treatment of Cancer. EASL-EORTC clinical practice guidelines: management of hepatocellular carcinoma. Eur J Cancer 2012;48(5):599–641. https://doi.org/10.1016/j.ejca.2011.12.021. Erratum in: Eur J Cancer 2012; 48(8):1255–1256.
5. An C, Rakhmonova G, Choi JY, et al. Liver imaging reporting and data system (LI-RADS) version 2014: understanding and application of the diagnostic algorithm. Clin Mol Hepatol. 2016;22(2):296–307.
6. American College of Radiology Liver Imaging Reporting and Data System Version 2014. ACR Web site http://www.acr.org/Quality-Safety/Resources/ LIRADS. Accessed 15 Apr 2016.
7. Santillan CS, Tang A, Cruite I, Shah A, Sirlin CB. Understanding LI-RADS. a primer for practical use Magn Reson Imaging Clin N Am. 2014;22:337–52.
8. Granata V, Petrillo M, Fusco R, Setola SV. de Lutio di Castelguidone E, Catalano O, Piccirillo M, albino V, Izzo F, Petrillo a. Surveillance of HCC patients after liver RFA: role of MRI with Hepatospecific contrast versus three-phase CT scan-experience of high volume oncologic institute. Gastroenterol Res Pract. 2013;2013:469097.
9. Granata V, Fusco R, Avallone A, Catalano O, Filice F, Leongito M, Palaia R, Izzo F, Petrillo A. Major and ancillary magnetic resonance features of LI-RADS to assess HCC: an overview and update. Infect Agent Cancer. 2017;12:23.
10. Granata V, Fusco R, Avallone A, Filice F, Tatangelo F, Piccirillo M, Grassi R, Izzo F, Petrillo A. Critical analysis of the major and ancillary imaging features of LI-RADS on 127 proven HCCs evaluated with functional and morphological MRI: lights and shadows. Oncotarget. 2017;8(31):51224–37.

11. Granata V, Fusco R, Catalano O, Guarino B, Granata F, Tatangelo F, Avallone A, Piccirillo M, Palaia R, Izzo F, Petrillo A. Intravoxel incoherent motion (IVIM) in diffusion-weighted imaging (DWI) for hepatocellular carcinoma: correlation with histologic grade. Oncotarget. 2016;7(48):79357–64.

12. Le Bihan D, Breton E, Lallemand D, Grenier P, Cabanis E, Laval-Jeantet M. MR imaging of intravoxel incoherent motions: application to diffusion and perfusion in neurologic disorders. Radiology. 1986;161:401–7.

13. Le Bihan D, Breton E, Lallemand D, Aubin ML, Vignaud J, Laval-Jeantet M. Separation of diffusion and perfusion in intravoxel incoherent motion MR imaging. Radiology. 1988;168:497–505.

14. Granata V, Fusco R, Catalano O, Filice S, Amato DM, Nasti G, Avallone A, Izzo F, Petrillo A. Early assessment of colorectal Cancer patients with liver metastases treated with Antiangiogenic drugs: the role of Intravoxel incoherent motion in diffusion-weighted imaging. PLoS One. 2015;10(11): e0142876.

15. Granata V, Fusco R, Catalano O, Piccirillo M, De Bellis M, Izzo F, Petrillo A. Percutaneous ablation therapy of hepatocellular carcinoma with irreversible electroporation: MRI findings. AJR Am J Roentgenol 2015;204(5):1000–7. d.

16. Guo W, Zhao S, Yang Y, Shao G. Histological grade of hepatocellular carcinoma predicted by quantitative diffusion-weighted imaging. Int J Clin Exp Med. 2015;8(3):4164–9.

17. Woo S, Lee JM, Yoon JH, Joo I, Han JK, Choi BI. Intravoxel incoherent motion diffusion-weighted MR imaging of hepatocellular carcinoma: correlation with enhancement degree and histologic grade. Radiology. 2014;270(3):758–67.

18. Chen J, Wu M, Liu R, Li S, Gao R, Song B. Preoperative evaluation of the histological grade of hepatocellular carcinoma with diffusion-weighted imaging: a meta-analysis. PLoS One. 2015;10(2):e0117661.

19. Li X, Li C, Wang R, Ren J, Yang J, Zhang Y. Combined application of Gadoxetic acid disodium-enhanced magnetic resonance imaging (MRI) and diffusion-weighted imaging (DWI) in the diagnosis of chronic liver disease-induced hepatocellular carcinoma: a meta-analysis. PLoS One. 2015;10(12):e0144247.

20. Edmondson HA, Steiner PE. Primary carcinoma of the liver: a study of 100 cases among 48,900 necropsies. Cancer. 1954;7:462–503.

21. World Health Organization Classification of Tumours by International Agency for Research on Cancer WHO classification of Tumours of the digestive system: volume 3. 4th revised ed. Lyon: International Agency for Research on Cancer; 2010.

22. Nakanishi M, Chuma M, Hige S, et al. Relationship between diffusion-weighted magnetic resonance imaging and histological tumor grading of hepatocellular carcinoma. Ann Surg Oncol. 2012;19(4):1302–9.

23. Nasu K, Kuroki Y, Tsukamoto T, et al. Diffusion-weighted imaging of surgically resected hepatocellular carcinoma: imaging characteristics and relationship among signal intensity, apparent diffusion coefficient, and histopathologic grade. AJR Am J Roentgenol. 2009;193:438–44.

24. Muhi A, Ichikawa T, Motosugi U, et al. High-b-value diffusion-weighted MR imaging of hepatocellular lesions: estimation of grade of malignancy of hepatocellular carcinoma. J Magn Reson Imaging. 2009;30:1005–11.

25. Nishie A, Tajima T, Asayama Y, et al. Diagnostic performance of apparent diffusion coefficient for predicting histological grade of hepatocellular carcinoma. Eur J Radiol. 2011;80:e29–33.

26. Zhou L, Rui JA, Wang SB, et al. Factors predictive for long-term survival of male patients with hepatocellular carcinoma after curative resection. J Surg Oncol. 2007;95(4):298–303.

27. Kim SH, Lim HK, Choi D, Lee WJ, Kim SH, Kim MJ, et al. Percutaneous radiofrequency ablation of hepatocellular carcinoma: effect of histologic grade on therapeutic results. AJR Am J Roentgenol. 2006;186:S327–33.

28. Ludwig JM, Juan C, Camacho JC, Nima Kokabi N, et al. The role of diffusion-weighted imaging (DWI) in Locoregional therapy outcome prediction and response assessment for hepatocellular carcinoma (HCC): the new era of functional imaging biomarkers. Diagnostics (Basel). 2015;5(4):546–63.

29. Ichikawa S, Motosugi U, Hernando D, Morisaka H, Enomoto N, Matsuda M, Onishi H. Histological grading of hepatocellular carcinomas with Intravoxel incoherent motion diffusion-weighted imaging: inconsistent results depending on the fitting method. Magn Reson Med Sci. 2017;

30. Shan Q, Chen J, Zhang T, Yan R, Wu J, Shu Y, Kang Z, He B, Zhang Z, Wang J. Evaluating histologic differentiation of hepatitis B virus-related hepatocellular carcinoma using intravoxel incoherent motion and AFP levels alone and in combination. Abdom Radiol (NY). 2017;42(8):2079–88.

31. Jiang HY, Chen J, Xia CC, Cao LK, Duan T, Song B. Noninvasive imaging of

32. hepatocellular carcinoma: From diagnosis to prognosis. World J Gastroenterol. 2018;24(22):2348–62.

32. Suh YJ, kim MJ, Jy C, Park MS, kim kW. Preoperative prediction of the microvascular invasion of hepatocellular carcinoma with diffusion-weighted imaging. Liver Transpl. 2012;18:1171–8.

33. Okamura S, Sumie S, Tonan T, Nakano M, Satani M, Shimose S, Shirono T, Iwamoto H, Aino H, Niizeki T, Tajiri N, Kuromatsu R, Okuda k NO, Torimura T. Diffusion-weighted magnetic resonance imaging predicts malignant potential in small hepatocellular carcinoma. Dig Liver Dis. 2016;48:945–52.

34. Xu P, Zeng M, Liu k S y, Xu C, Lin J. Microvascular invasion in small hepatocellular carcinoma: is it predictable with preoperative diffusion-weighted imaging? J Gastroenterol Hepatol. 2014;29:330–6.

35. Wang WT, yang L, yang ZX, Hu XX, Ding y y X, Fu CX, Grimm R, Zeng MS, Rao SX. Assessment of microvascular invasion of hepatocellular carcinoma with diffusion kurtosis imaging. Radiology. 2018;286:571–80.

36. Qin L, Li X, Stroiney A, Qu J, Helgager J, Reardon DA, Young GS. Advanced MRI assessment to predict benefit of anti-programmed cell death 1 protein immunotherapy response in patients with recurrent glioblastoma. Neuroradiology. 2017;59(2):135–45.

24

Extra-telomeric functions of telomerase in the pathogenesis of Epstein-Barr virus-driven B-cell malignancies and potential therapeutic implications

Silvia Giunco[1], Maria Raffaella Petrara[2], Manuela Zangrossi[2], Andrea Celeghin[2] and Anita De Rossi[1,2]* (iD)

Abstract

The Epstein-Barr virus (EBV) is a ubiquitous human γ-herpesvirus causally linked to a broad spectrum of both lymphoid and epithelial malignancies. In order to maintain its persistence in host cells and promote tumorigenesis, EBV must restrict its lytic cycle, which would ultimately lead to cell death, selectively express latent viral proteins, and establish an unlimited proliferative potential. The latter step depends on the maintenance of telomere length provided by telomerase. The viral oncoprotein LMP-1 activates TERT, the catalytic component of telomerase. In addition to its canonical role in stabilizing telomeres, TERT may promote EBV-driven tumorigenesis through extra-telomeric functions. TERT contributes toward preserving EBV latency; in fact, through the NOTCH2/BATF pathway, TERT negatively affects the expression of BZLF1, the master regulator of the EBV lytic cycle. In contrast, TERT inhibition triggers a complete EBV lytic cycle, leading to the death of EBV-infected cells. Interestingly, short-term TERT inhibition causes cell cycle arrest and apoptosis, partly by inducing telomere-independent activation of the ATM/ATR/TP53 pathway. Importantly, TERT inhibition also sensitizes EBV-positive tumor cells to antiviral therapy and enhances the pro-apoptotic effects of chemotherapeutic agents. We provide here an overview on how the extra-telomeric functions of TERT contribute to EBV-driven tumorigenesis. We also discuss the potential therapeutic approach of TERT inhibition in EBV-driven malignancies.

Keywords: Telomerase, TERT extra-telomeric functions, Epstein-Barr virus, Latent/lytic viral cycle, B-cell malignancies

Background

The Epstein-Barr virus (EBV) is a ubiquitous human γ-herpesvirus infecting more than 90% of the world's population. Primary infection with EBV is often asymptomatic, but it can also manifest as infectious mononucleosis. Although EBV may infect various cell types, such as epithelial cells and T or Natural Killer cells, it preferably infects B lymphocytes, in which it establishes a lifelong asymptomatic latent infection. In immunocompromised individuals, EBV may cause a wide range of cancers, of both hematopoietic and epithelial origin, including Burkitt's lymphoma (BL), Hodgkin's lymphoma (HL), post-transplant lymphoproliferative disorders (PTLD), AIDS-associated lymphomas, and nasopharyngeal and gastric carcinomas [1].

Like other γ-herpesviruses, EBV has both lytic and latent cycles. Primary EBV infection occurs in the oropharynx, leading to productive lytic infection of B lymphocytes. EBV antigens promote immune recognition, inducing an EBV-specific immune response which controls viral infection in the immunocompetent host, and the viral lytic cycle triggers the death of the infected cells [2]. In tumor cells, EBV expresses various sets of latency-associated proteins with transforming properties. The most restricted form of EBV latency ('latency I'), found in BL cells, is characterized by the selective expression of EBV nuclear antigen (EBNA)-1. A second latency program ('latency II'), in which EBV expresses EBNA-1 and the three latent membrane proteins (LMP-1, LMP-2A, LMP-2B), is found in tumor cells of HL and nasopharyngeal carcinomas. The full set of EBV-encoded

* Correspondence: anita.derossi@unipd.it
[1]Immunology and Molecular Oncology Unit, Istituto Oncologico Veneto (IOV)-IRCCS, Padova, Italy
[2]Department of Surgery, Oncology and Gastroenterology, Section of Oncology and Immunology, University of Padova, Padova, Italy

latency proteins ('latency III'), including the six EBNAs (EBNA-1, – 2, –3A, -3B, -3C, and -leader protein or LP) and the LMPs proteins, is usually present in PTLD and AIDS-associated lymphomas [1, 3]. In addition to its latent proteins, EBV encodes small non-polyadenylated, non-coding double-strand RNAs, called EBV-encoded RNAs (EBER), which are expressed in all forms of latency and may contribute to viral pathogenesis [4]. The oncogenic potential of EBV is highlighted by its ability to immortalize B cells in vitro, generating continuously proliferating lymphoblastoid cell lines (LCLs). LCLs may constitute an in vitro model of EBV-driven malignancies expressing the latency III program.

While latency programs predominate in EBV-driven tumors, lytic reactivation may occur in a small fraction of infected cells, favoring the spread of the virus [5, 6]. Lytic reactivation, induced by endogenous or exogenous stimuli, is orchestrated by up-regulation of two EBV immediate-early genes, *BZLF1* and *BRLF1* [7]. As lytic infection promotes the death of EBV-infected cells both in vitro and in vivo, the lytic induction strategy has been suggested as potential therapy to induce EBV-dependent tumor cell killing [8–10]. Triggering EBV lytic replication may be particularly effective and therapeutically important, as EBV lytic proteins can activate antiviral prodrugs, such as ganciclovir (GCV) or radiolabeled nucleoside analogs, which further promote the death of infected cells and also prevent the release of infectious viruses [11, 12]. Thus, the combination of antivirals with lytic cycle inducers is emerging as a promising strategy for treating EBV-driven tumors [13–15].

The establishment of EBV latency programs promotes cell proliferation, inhibits apoptosis, blocks viral lytic replication, and ensures accurate and equal partitioning of the episomal viral genome to daughter cells [16]. However, expression of latent EBV proteins is not sufficient to immortalize EBV-infected cells entirely. As in other oncogenic viruses, a critical step for EBV-driven transformation is to overcome cellular senescence and acquire unlimited proliferative potential. This step depends on activation of mechanisms for telomere maintenance [17, 18]. Although it has been suggested that in newly EBV-infected B lymphocytes telomere length can be maintained by alternative lengthening of telomeres (ALT) [19], only EBV-positive cells with sustained telomerase activity become truly immortalized, and it has been demonstrated that most EBV-driven tumors, as well as established LCLs, are telomerase-positive. By contrast, telomerase-negative EBV-infected cells, although exhibiting a prolonged lifespan, eventually undergo cellular senescence and terminate their lifespan through telomere shortening [17, 18]. In addition to its canonical role in stabilizing telomeres, current evidence shows that telomerase reverse transcriptase (TERT), the catalytic component of telomerase, can promote EBV-driven tumorigenesis through extra-telomeric functions [20–23]. Here we review the cross-talk between telomerase and EBV which is essential for the viral oncogenetic process and discuss potential therapeutic implications.

Telomere maintenance in EBV-infected cells: The canonical role of telomerase

Telomeres are specialized DNA structures located at the ends of chromosomes which are essential for stabilizing chromosomes by protecting them from end-to-end fusion and DNA degradation [24]. In human cells, telomeres are composed of (TTAGGG)n tandem repeats associated with telomere-binding proteins, the shelterin complex, which form a special T-loop-like structure, thus avoiding the ends of chromosomes being recognized as double-strand DNA damage [25]. The progressive loss of telomeric repeats, which occurs at each round of DNA replication due to the inability of DNA polymerase to replicate the 3′ end of chromosomes completely [26], reduces the length of telomeres to a critical size. Such critically short telomeres are no longer protected by the shelterin complex and are recognized as DNA double-strand breaks which trigger the DNA damage response (DDR), resulting in cellular senescence and apoptosis [25]. To circumvent replicative senescence and acquire the ability to sustain unlimited replicative potential, tumor cells must stabilize their telomeres.

Although EBV-infected B cells exhibit higher proliferative activity than resting primary B lymphocytes, very few EBV-carrying B cells eventually progress to immortalization: most of them reach a proliferative crisis and end their lifespan after about 150 population-doubling levels, according to genetic factors, including telomere length. Soon after EBV infection, B lymphocytes may exhibit multiple signs of telomere dysfunction and ALT markers, including highly heterogeneous telomeres, appearance of extra-chromosomal telomeric DNA, accumulation of telomere-associated promyelocytic leukemia nuclear bodies, and telomeric-sister chromatid exchange [19]. This phenotype seems to be associated with EBV-mediated displacement of shelterin proteins and uncapping problems at telomeres, which may favor the activation of the ALT mechanism. ALT is an inherently imprecise recombination-based mechanism which may fuel the chromosomal and genomic instability that characterize newly established LCLs [19, 27]. However, only LCLs developing strong telomerase activity overcome cellular crises and become stably immortalized [17, 18]. Established LCLs with sustained telomerase activity show minimal or no signs of telomere dysfunction [19], thus revealing the prominent role of telomerase activation in ensuring telomere integrity during EBV immortalization.

Telomerase is a ribonucleoprotein complex containing an internal RNA template (telomerase RNA component, TERC) and a catalytic protein, TERT, with telomere-specific reverse transcriptase activity. TERT, which synthesizes de novo telomere sequences using TERC as a template, is the rate-limiting component of the telomerase complex, and its expression is correlated with telomerase activity. Although TERC has broad tissue distribution and is constitutively present in normal and tumor cells, the expression of TERT is usually repressed in normal somatic cells and is essential for unlimited cell growth, thus playing a critical role in tumor formation and progression [28].

Regulation of telomerase operates at several levels: transcription, mRNA splicing, subcellular location of each component, and assembly of TERC and TERT in an active ribonucleoprotein. Transcription of the TERT gene is probably the key determinant in regulating telomerase activity, since TERT transcription is specifically up-regulated in cancer cells but silent in most normal ones. The TERT promoter reveals complex regulation dynamics, whereby multiple transcriptional regulatory elements play functional roles in different contexts, either individually or interactively. TERT contains recognition sequences for many important transcription factors such as TP53, P21, SP1, ETS, E2F, AP-1, HIF1A and MYC [29]. Regulation of TERT transcription may also involve DNA methylation, as the TERT promoter contains a cluster of CpG sites [29]. Somatic mutations in the promoter of the TERT gene, which increase gene expression by creating de novo binding sites for the ETS/TCF transcription factors, have also recently been described [30]. At post-transcriptional level, more than 20 different TERT variants have been reported, some of which probably play critical roles in regulating telomerase activity [31]. Telomerase activity is also controlled by post-translational modifications of the TERT protein. Phosphorylation of the protein at critical sites along the PI3K/AKT kinase pathway seems to be crucial for telomerase activity and nuclear localization. Active recruitment of telomerase to telomeres is a necessary regulatory step and involves telomere-associated shelterin proteins [32].

Studies aimed at defining the mechanism underlying EBV-induced telomerase activation have demonstrated that LMP-1, the major EBV oncoprotein, up-regulates telomerase activity both in epithelial cells [33, 34] and in B lymphocytes [35, 36]. In particular, it has been demonstrated that LMP-1 activates TERT in nasopharyngeal carcinoma cells through the AKT pathway [34]: in established LCLs, LMP-1 activates TERT at transcriptional level *via* the NF-κB and MAPK/ERK1/2 pathways [36]. Of interest, while in epithelial cells TERT expression is also MYC-dependent and the mutagenesis of MYC-

responsive E-box elements in the TERT promoter inhibits TERT transactivation by LMP-1 [33], in B cells TERT activation by LMP-1 is MYC-independent. In fact, mutagenesis in NF-κB binding sites, but not in MYC ones, inhibits LMP-1-transactivation of the TERT promoter [36]. This is of particular interest, since in most EBV-driven tumors, like the immunoblastic lymphomas occurring in AIDS patients and early PTLD lesions, *MYC* is in a germ-line configuration. In these malignancies, LMP-1 probably plays an essential role in TERT activation.

Role of TERT in switch of latent/lytic cycle of EBV

The canonical explanation for the tumor-promoting role of telomerase is that it allows cells to escape the barrier to unlimited replicative potential caused by telomere attrition. Accumulating evidence suggests that, besides its canonical role in stabilizing telomeres, TERT also has other biological functions, including enhancement of cell proliferation, resistance to apoptosis, and regulation of DDR, [37–39]. TERT can also alleviate levels of cellular reactive oxygen species (ROS) by enhancing cellular antioxidant defense systems, thus allowing cancer cells to evade death stimuli [40] and can stimulate the epithelial-mesenchymal transition and induce stemness [41, 42].

The extra-telomeric roles of TERT have also been described in EBV-driven lymphomagenesis. TERT plays a critical role in establishing EBV latency and preventing the EBV lytic cycle, thereby contributing to transformed phenotypes. In particular, high levels of endogenous TERT or ectopic TERT expression in TERT-negative EBV-infected B cells prevents the induction of the viral lytic cycle. By contrast, TERT silencing by specific siRNA or short-hairpin (sh)RNA induces the expression of BZLF1, EA-D and gp350 EBV lytic genes, and triggers a complete lytic cycle. This occurs in both EBV-immortalized and fully transformed B cells, thus supporting the concept that TERT is a critical regulator of the balance between viral latent and lytic cycles [20, 21]. The treatment of primary EBV-positive BL with zidovudine (AZT), a thymidine analog, has also been demonstrated to induce the EBV lytic cycle and cell death through the NF-κB pathway [43, 44]. As AZT may inhibit telomerase activity [45], this finding further supports the close relationship between TERT activity and the EBV latent/lytic cycle.

Studies aimed at defining the mechanism(s) by means of which TERT prevents the viral lytic cycle have demonstrated the involvement of the NOTCH2/BATF pathway. BATF is a transcription factor expressed in hematopoietic tissues and in B cells infected with EBV [46–48]. In LCL, BATF is a critically important survival factor being involved in the suppression of pro-apoptotic BIM and in the induction of MYC [48]. Notably, BATF has been shown to inhibit the expression of BZLF1, thus reducing EBV lytic replication in latently infected B cells [47]. Of interest, BATF is a target gene of the NOTCH signaling pathway in B cells [47]. High expression of TERT in LCLs has been shown to activate NOTCH2 at transcriptional level through the NF-kB pathway; in turn, NOTCH2 activates BATF, which negatively affects the expression of BZLF1, thus repressing the EBV lytic program [22]. Accordingly, pharmacological inhibition of NOTCH2 signaling by γ-secretase inhibitors decreases canonical NOTCH target genes expression, including BATF, with a concomitant increase in early and late EBV lytic genes, and thus triggers a complete lytic cycle in both LCL and EBV-positive BL cells [22].

More recently, the impact of TERT on EBV infection and viral gene expression has also been studied in epithelial cells [49]. Gastric carcinoma AGS cells with high telomerase activity show increased expression of latent EBV genes, indicating that telomerase directly contributes toward favoring the latency program in epithelial EBV-infected cells [49]. Thus, the ability of TERT to favor the latency program in both B lymphocytes and epithelial EBV-infected cells further supports the crucial role of telomerase in EBV-driven malignancies.

TERT inhibition as a therapeutic approach for EBV-driven malignancies

Telomerase inhibitors remain an attractive approach to target cancer cells, given the specificity of TERT expression in tumor cells. However, in theory, the time to antineoplastic effectiveness of telomerase inhibitors depends on the original length of the telomeres in cancer cells and, apparently, these agents are effective in halting tumor growth only after the cancer cells have shortened their telomeres. This aspect acquires particular importance in the context EBV-carrying malignancies as it has been demonstrated that EBV-positive BL cell lines show longer telomeres compared to EBV-negative BLs [50] and, during the early phases of EBV-induced growth of primary B cells, their telomeres length remain constant or even increase [19, 27, 51].

In this scenario, the evidence of extra-telomeric functions of TERT in cellular kinetics and resistance to apoptosis has recently opened the door to potential telomere length-independent therapeutic effects. In EBV-driven malignancies, besides sustaining the latency program required for the EBV-driven transformation, TERT may promote EBV tumor progression by enhancing the kinetics of cell proliferation. In fact, EBV-infected B cells with sustained telomerase activity grow faster than telomerase-negative cells [20]. Accordingly, TERT inhibition results in an anti-proliferative effect, inducing an accumulation of cells in the S phase, probably due to dephosphorylation of 4E-BP1, an AKT1-dependent substrate, which results in the decreased availability of proteins needed for cell cycle progression [21]. Thus, by slowing proliferation kinetics, TERT inhibition may represent an appealing suppressor strategy of EBV tumor growth.

As mentioned previously, the first mechanism by means of which short-term inhibition of TERT may induce cell death of EBV-transformed cells is induction of the EBV lytic cycle. Inhibition of TERT leads to down-regulation of BATF and up-regulation of BZLF1, the main regulator of the viral lytic cycle. Notably, cell death induced by TERT inhibition in EBV-positive cells does not depend only on the induction of the EBV lytic cycle: inhibition of TERT with short hairpin (sh)RNA in both EBV-positive and EBV-negative BL cell lines induces apoptosis via a AKT1/FOXO3/NOXA pathway [21]. In particular, TERT silencing induces inhibition of AKT1 kinase, which is associated with dephosphorylation/activation of the transcription factor FOXO3, an effector of AKT1 kinase functioning in several cell activities, including survival. In turn, FOXO3 induces up-regulation of NOXA, a pro-apoptotic protein, the expression of which is known to be blocked by latent EBV infection [52]. Thus, TERT inhibition can overcome the block of NOXA up-regulation induced by EBV, favoring cell apoptosis [21]. Notably, although pharmacological inhibition of AKT1 does not reveal any evidence of EBV lytic replication in EBV-positive B cells, thus indicating that the EBV lytic cycle induced by TERT inhibition occurs via an AKT1-independent pathway [21], the pharmacological inhibition of NOTCH2 triggers the EBV lytic cycle, thus confirming the critical involvement of the NOTCH2, BATF and BZLF1 pathways in the latent/lytic EBV cycle [22].

In EBV-positive tumor cells, the lytic cell cycle induced by TERT inhibition may be exploited to sensitize cells to antiviral drugs such as GCV. GCV is an antiviral prodrug activated by EBV lytic protein kinase [10, 11]. Phosphorylated/activate GCV competitively inhibits both viral and cellular DNA synthesis, thus resulting in both cell death of infected cells and reduction of viral replication [8]. Consequently, GCV markedly enhances the anti-proliferative and pro-apoptotic effects of TERT inhibition in both EBV-positive LCLs and BL [21]. Thus, the combination of antiviral drugs with strategies capable of inhibiting TERT expression/activity may result in therapeutically substantial effects in patients with EBV-related malignancies. Consistently, as EBV lytic reactivation after TERT inhibition is mediated by the NOTCH2/BATF pathway, GCV also enhances the apoptotic effect of γ-secretase inhibitors which, by blocking NOTCH2/BATF signaling, trigger viral lytic reactivation [22].

Most recent data show that LCLs and both EBV-positive and EBV-negative BL cells short-term treated with BIBR1532 (BIBR), a chemical compound which selectively inhibits the catalytic activity of TERT [53], undergo cell cycle arrest in S phase and apoptosis [23]. These effects are telomerase-specific and have not been observed in telomerase-negative cell lines. The cell cycle arrest and apoptosis subsequent to TERT inhibition are associated with and probably dependent on activation of the DDR pathway. TERT inhibition does induce DDR, highlighted by increased levels of γH2AX, activation of ATM and ATR and their downstream substrates CHK1, CHK2 and pro-apoptotic TP53. Notably, the DDR pathway activated after short-term exposure to BIBR is not related to telomere dysfunction, as BIBR treatment does not affect the mean and range of telomere lengths and γH2AX damage foci are randomly diffuse, rather than being specifically located on telomeres [23]. It has been demonstrated that the productive cycle of EBV elicits ATM-dependent DDR, and provides an S-phase-like cellular environment suitable for viral lytic replication [54]. Thus, it is reasonable that, in EBV-positive background, cell cycle arrest in S phase and DDR activation consequent upon TERT inhibition is partly orchestrated by the induction of the lytic cycle.

In addition, treatment of LCL with BIBR in combination with Fludarabine or Cyclophosphamide, two agents frequently employed to treat B-cell malignancies, induces a significant increase in specific cell death compared with results seen after treatment with chemotherapeutic agents alone. These results may

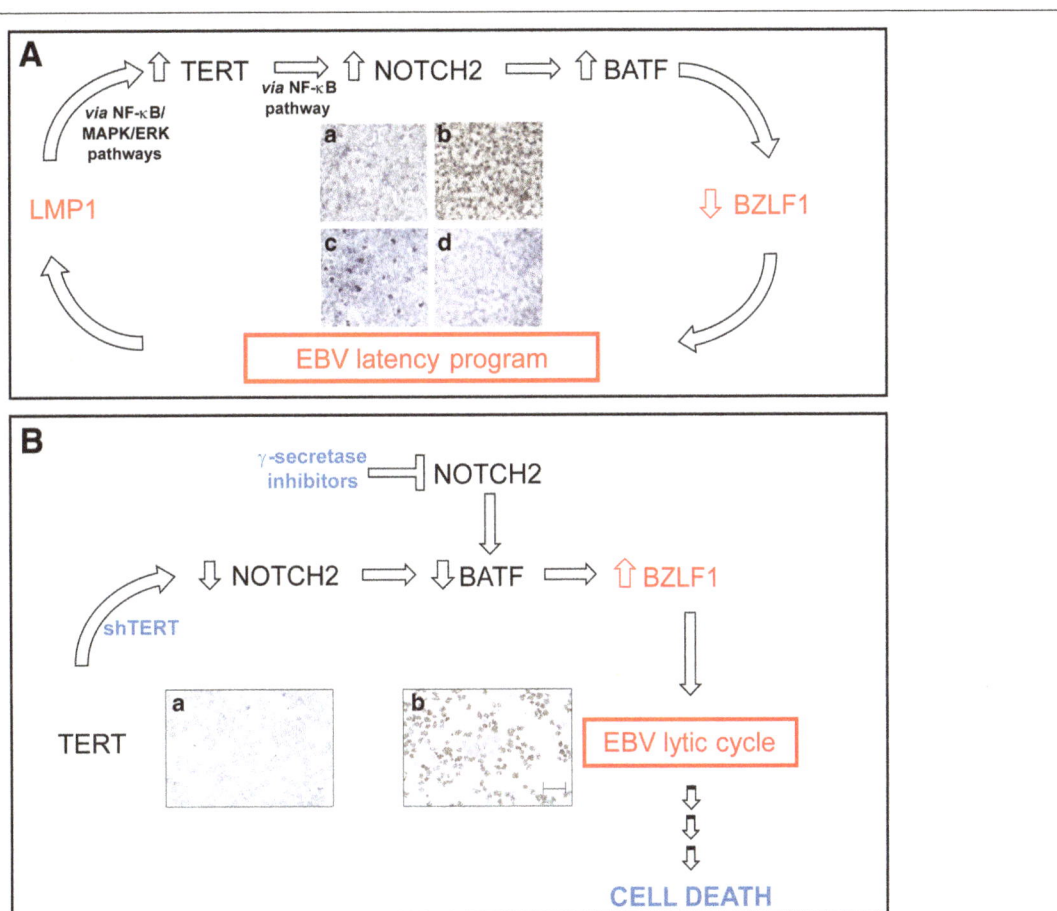

Fig. 1 TERT levels affect EBV latent/lytic status. **A**, cross-talk between EBV and TERT to sustain viral latency program: in EBV-infected primary **B** lymphocytes, activation of TERT occurs concomitantly with induction of latent EBV proteins and down-regulation of EBV lytic gene expression. EBV-encoded LMP-1 activates TERT at transcriptional level *via* NF-κB and MAPK/ERK1/2 pathways. In turn, TERT expression activates NOTCH2 at transcriptional level *via* NF-κB pathway. NOTCH2 activates BATF, which negatively affects the expression of BZLF1, a master regulator of viral lytic cycle, thus favouring induction and maintenance of EBV latency program, essential for EBV-driven transformation. Immunohistochemical image: TERT (*a, b*) and BZLF1 (*c, d*) protein expression in early- (*a, c*) and late- (*b, d*) infected B lymphocytes (X40). B, TERT or NOTCH inhibition triggers EBV lytic cycle: TERT silencing by shRNA (shTERT) or inhibition of NOTCH signaling by γ-secretase inhibitors lead to NOTCH2-dependent down-regulation of BATF and up-regulation of BZLF1, inducing a complete EBV lytic cycle. Immunohistochemical image: EBV lytic gp350 protein expression in EBV-positive BL cells untreated (*a*) and treated (*b*) for 72 h with shTERT (X20). Scale bar, 100 μm. See the text for details

lead to the substantial clinical application of TERT inhibitors in combination with standard chemotherapeutic protocols to treat EBV-positive B-cell malignancies [23].

Conclusions

Since a latent program is required to promote EBV tumorigenesis, whereas the lytic cycle induces cell death, the finding that TERT, besides maintaining telomere integrity, also plays a critical role in the establishment of EBV latency and in preventing the EBV lytic cycle (Fig. 1A), supports the view that TERT inhibition is an appealing therapeutic strategy against EBV-driven malignancies. By triggering the viral lytic cycle, TERT inhibition induces cell death (Fig. 1B) and sensitizes EBV-infected cells to antiviral drugs. Notably, besides triggering the viral lytic cycle *via* the NOTCH2/ BATF/BZLF1 pathway (Fig. 1B), short-term inhibition of TERT activates pro-apoptotic programs *via* the AKT1/ FOXO3/NOXA and ATM/ATR/TP53 pathways. Notably, cell cycle arrest and the pro-apoptotic effects of short-term TERT inhibition are independent of telomere length. Thus, in both EBV-driven and virus-unrelated B-cell malignancies inhibition of TERT seems to be an effective approach in inducing cell death, regardless of telomere length. In vitro experiments also demonstrate that the therapeutic approach based on inhibition of TERT enhances the pro-apoptotic and anti-proliferative effects of chemotherapeutic agents in EBV-transformed cells. Further studies of primary tumor cells from patients with EBV-driven malignancies and suitable animal models will pave the way for a solidly based pre-clinical rationale for including TERT inhibitors in chemotherapy protocols for treating these malignancies.

Abbreviations

ALT: Alternative length of telomeres; AZT: Zidovudine; BIBR: BIBR1532; BL: Burkitt's lymphoma; DDR: DNA damage response; EBER: EBV-encoded RNAs; EBNA: EBV nuclear antigen; EBV: Epstein-Barr virus; GCV: ganciclovir; HL: Hodgkin's lymphoma; LCL: Lymphoblastoid cell line; LMP: Latent membrane protein; PTLD: Post-transplant lymphoproliferative disorders; ROS: Reactive oxygen species; TERC: Telomerase RNA component; TERT: Telomerase reverse transcriptase

Acknowledgements

We would like to thank Dr. Marisa Zanchetta, Dr. Francesco Carmona and Dr. Silvia Sanavia from the Immunology and Molecular Oncology Unit, Istituto Oncologico Veneto (IOV)-IRCCS, Padova, Italy and Dr. Annalisa Dalzini from the Department of Surgery, Oncology and Gastroenterology, University of Padova, Italy, for their technical support.

Funding

This study was supported by funding from the Associazione Italiana per la Ricerca sul Cancro (Grant no. 14258 to ADR). SG received funds through a fellowship from the Istituto Oncologico Veneto IOV-IRCCS (Grant 5 × 1000).

Authors' contributions

All authors performed literature searches and contributed to writing this article. SG wrote the first draft of the manuscript. All authors contributed to its final version and approved its submission.

Competing interests

The authors declare that they have no competing interest.

References

1. Dolcetti R, Dal Col J, Martorelli D, Carbone A, Klein E. Interplay among viral antigens, cellular pathways and tumor microenvironment in the pathogenesis of EBV-driven lymphomas. Semin Cancer Biol. 2013;23:441–56.
2. Young LS, Rickinson AB. Epstein-Barr virus: 40 years on. Nat Rev Cancer. 2004;4:757–68.
3. Gloghini A, Dolcetti R, Carbone A. Lymphomas occurring specifically in HIV infected patients: from pathogenesis to pathology. Semin Cancer Biol. 2013; 23:457–67.
4. Yajima M, Kanda T, Takada K. Critical role of Epstein-Barr virus (EBV)-encoded RNA in efficient EBV-induced B-lymphocyte growth transformation. J Virol. 2005;79:4298–307.
5. Montone KT, Hodinka RL, Salhany KE, Lavi E, Rostami A, Tomaszewski JE. Identification of Epstein–Barr virus lytic activity in post-transplantation lymphoproliferative disease. Mod Pathol. 1996;9:621–30.
6. Xue SA, Labrecque LG, Lu QL, Ong SK, Lampert IA, Kazembe P, et al. Promiscuous expression of Epstein–Barr virus genes in Burkitt's lymphoma from the central African country Malawi. Int J Cancer. 2002;99:635–43.
7. Kenney SC, Mertz JE. Regulation of the latent-lytic switch in Epstein-Barr virus. Semin Cancer Biol. 2014;26:60–8.
8. Westphal EM, Mauser A, Swenson J, Davis MG, Talarico CL, Kenney SC. Induction of lytic Epstein-Barr virus (EBV) infection in EBV-associated malignancies using adenovirus vectors in vitro and in vivo. Cancer Res. 1999;59:1485–91.
9. Feng WH, Israel B, Raab-Traub N, Busson P, Kenney SC. Chemotherapy induces lytic EBV replication and confers ganciclovir susceptibility to EBV-positive epithelial cell tumors. Cancer Res. 2002;62:1920–6.
10. Feng WH, Cohen JI, Fischer S, Li L, Sneller M, Goldbach-Mansky R, et al. Reactivation of latent Epstein-Barr virus by methotrexate: a potential contributor to methotrexate-associated lymphomas. J Natl Cancer Inst. 2004; 96:1691–702.
11. Meng Q, Hagemeier SR, Fingeroth JD, Gershburg E, Pagano JS, Kenney SC. The Epstein-Barr virus (EBV)-encoded protein kinase, EBV-PK, but not the thymidine kinase (EBV-TK), is required for ganciclovir and acyclovir inhibition of lytic viral production. J Virol. 2010;84:4534–42.
12. Fu DX, Tanhehco Y, Chen J, Foss CA, Fox JJ, Chong JM, et al. Bortezomib-induced enzyme-targeted radiation therapy in herpesvirus-associated tumors. Nat Med. 2008;14:1118–22.
13. Perrine SP, Hermine O, Small T, Suarez F, O'Reilly R, Boulad F, et al. A phase 1/2 trial of arginine butyrate and ganciclovir in patients with Epstein-Barr virus-associated lymphoid malignancies. Blood. 2007;109:2571–8.
14. Wildeman MA, Novalic Z, Verkuijlen SA, Juwana H, Huitema AD, Tan IB, et al. Cytolytic virus activation therapy for Epstein-Barr virus-driven tumors. Clin Cancer Res. 2012;18:5061–70.
15. Stoker SD, Novalić Z, Wildeman MA, Huitema AD, Verkuijlen SA, Juwana H, et al. Epstein-Barr virus-targeted therapy in nasopharyngeal carcinoma. J Cancer Res Clin Oncol. 2015;141:1845–57.
16. Kang MS, Kieff E. Epstein-Barr virus latent genes. Exp Mol Med. 2015;47:e131.
17. Sugimoto M, Tahara H, Ide T, Furuichi Y. Steps involved in immortalization and tumorigenesis in human B-lymphoblastoid cell lines transformed by Epstein-Barr virus. Cancer Res. 2004;64:3361–4.
18. Jeon JP, Nam HY, Shim SM, Han BG. Sustained viral activity of epstein-Barr virus contributes to cellular immortalization of lymphoblastoid cell lines. Mol Cells. 2009;27:143–8.
19. Kamranvar SA, Chen X, Masucci MG. Telomere dysfunction and activation of alternative lengthening of telomeres in B-lymphocytes infected by Epstein-Barr virus. Oncogene. 2013;32:5522–30.
20. Terrin L, Dolcetti R, Corradini I, Indraccolo S, Dal Col J, Bertorelle R, et al. hTERT inhibits the Epstein-Barr virus lytic cycle and promotes the

proliferation of primary B lymphocytes: implications for EBV-driven lymphomagenesis. Int J Cancer. 2007;121:576–87.

21. Giunco S, Dolcetti R, Keppel S, Celeghin A, Indraccolo S, Dal Col J, et al. hTERT inhibition triggers Epstein-Barr virus lytic cycle and apoptosis in immortalized and transformed B cells: a basis for new therapies. Clin Cancer Res. 2013;19:2036–47.

22. Giunco S, Celeghin A, Gianesin K, Dolcetti R, Indraccolo S, De Rossi A. Cross talk between EBV and telomerase: the role of TERT and NOTCH2 in the switch of latent/lytic cycle of the virus. Cell Death Dis. 2015;6:e1774.

23. Celeghin A, Giunco S, Freguja R, Zangrossi M, Nalio S, Dolcetti R, et al. Short-term inhibition of TERT induces telomere length-independent cell cycle arrest and apoptotic response in EBV-immortalized and transformed B cells. Cell Death Dis. 2016;7:e2562.

24. Blackburn EH, Greider CW, Szostak JW. Telomeres and telomerase: the path from maize, Tetrahymena and yeast to human cancer and aging. Nat Med. 2006;12:1133–8.

25. Palm W, de Lange T. How shelterin protects mammalian telomeres. Annu Rev Genet. 2008;42:301–34.

26. Harley CB, Futcher AB, Greider CW. Telomeres shorten during ageing of human fibroblasts. Nature. 1990;345:458–60.

27. Kamranvar SA, Masucci MG. Regulation of Telomere Homeostasis during Epstein-Barr virus Infection and Immortalization. Viruses. 2017;9:pii: E217.

28. Hanahan D, Weinberg RA. Hallmarks of cancer: the next generation. Cell. 2011;144:646–74.

29. Akincilar SC, Unal B, Tergaonkar V. Reactivation of telomerase in cancer. Cell Mol Life Sci. 2016;73:1659–70.

30. Heidenreich B, Kumar R. TERT promoter mutations in telomere biology. Mutat Res. 2017;771:15–31.

31. Liu X, Wang Y, Chang G, Wang F, Wang F, Geng X. Alternative Splicing of hTERT Pre-mRNA: A Potential Strategy for the Regulation of Telomerase Activity. Int J Mol Sci. 2017;18:pii: E567.

32. Schmidt JC, Cech TR. Human telomerase: biogenesis, trafficking, recruitment, and activation. Genes Dev. 2015;29:1095–105.

33. Yang J, Deng X, Deng L, Gu H, Fan W, Cao Y. Telomerase activation by Epstein-Barr virus latent membrane protein 1 is associated with c-Myc expression in human nasopharyngeal epithelial cells. J Exp Clin Cancer Res. 2004;23:495–506.

34. Yang L, Xu Z, Liu L, Luo X, Lu J, sun L, et al. targeting EBV-LMP1 DNAzyme enhances radiosensitivity of nasopharyngeal carcinoma cells by inhibiting telomerase activity. Cancer Biol Ther. 2014;15:61–8.

35. Mei YP, Zhu XF, Zhou JM, Huang H, Deng R, Zeng YX. siRNA targeting LMP1-induced apoptosis in EBV-positive lymphoma cells is associated with inhibition of telomerase activity and expression. Cancer Lett. 2006; 232:189–98.

36. Terrin L, Dal Col J, Rampazzo E, Zancai P, Pedrotti M, Ammirabile G, et al. Latent membrane protein 1 of Epstein-Barr virus activates the hTERT promoter and enhances telomerase activity in B lymphocytes. J Virol. 2008; 82:10175–87.

37. Mukherjee S, Firpo EJ, Wang Y, Roberts JM. Separation of telomerase functions by reverse genetics. Proc Natl Acad Sci U S A. 2011;108:E1363–71.

38. Tátrai P, Szepesi Á, Matula Z, Szigeti A, Buchan G, Mádi A, et al. Combined introduction of Bmi-1 and hTERT immortalizes human adipose tissue-derived stromal cells with low risk of transformation. Biochem Biophys Res Commun. 2012;422:28–35.

39. Chen PC, Peng JR, Huang L, Li WX, Wang WZ, Cui ZQ, et al. Overexpression of human telomerase reverse transcriptase promotes the motility and invasiveness of HepG2 cells in vitro. Oncol Rep. 2013;30:1157–64.

40. Indran IR, Hande MP, Pervaiz S. hTERT overexpression alleviates intracellular ROS production, improves mitochondrial function, and inhibits ROS-mediated apoptosis in cancer cells. Cancer Res. 2011;71:266–76.

41. Liu Z, Li Q, Li K, Chen L, Li W, Hou M, et al. Telomerase reverse transcriptase promotes epithelial-mesenchymal transition and stem cell-like traits in cancer cells. Oncogene. 2013;32:4203–13.

42. Paranjape AN, Mandal T, Mukherjee G, Kumar MV, Sengupta K, Rangarajan A. Introduction of SV40ER and hTERT into mammospheres generates breast cancer cells with stem cell properties. Oncogene. 2012;31:1896–909.

43. Bayraktar UD, Diaz LA, Ashlock B, Toomey N, Cabral L, Bayraktar S, et al. Zidovudine-based lytic-inducing chemotherapy for Epstein-Barr virus-related lymphomas. Leuk Lymphoma. 2014;55:786–94.

44. Kurokawa M, Ghosh SK, Ramos JC, Mian AM, Toomey NL, Cabral L, et al.

45. Gomez DE, Armando RG, Alonso DF. AZT as a telomerase inhibitor. Front Oncol. 2012;2:113.

46. Echlin DR, Tae HJ, Mitin N, Taparowsky EJ. B-ATF functions as a negative regulator of AP-1 mediated transcription and blocks cellular transformation by Ras and Fos. Oncogene. 2000;19:1752–63.

47. Johansen LM, Deppmann CD, Erickson KD, Coffin WFI, Thornton TM, Humphrey SE, et al. EBNA2 and activated Notch induce expression of BATF. J Virol. 2003;77:6029–40.

48. Ma Y, Walsh MJ, Bernhardt K, Ashbaugh CW, Trudeau SJ, Ashbaugh IY, et al. CRISPR/Cas9 screens reveal Epstein-Barr virus-transformed B cell host dependency factors. Cell Host Microbe. 2017;21:580–91.

49. Rac J, Haas F, Schumacher A, Middeldorp JM, Delecluse HJ, Speck RF, et al. Telomerase activity impacts on Epstein-Barr virus infection of AGS cells. PLoS One. 2015;10:e0123645.

50. Mochida A, Gotoh E, Senpuku H, Harada S, Kitamura R, Takahashi T, et al. Telomere size and telomerase activity in Epstein-Barr virus (EBV)-positive and EBV-negative Burkitt's lymphoma cell lines. Arch Virol. 2005;150:2139–50.

51. Lacoste S, Wiechec E, Dos Santos Silva AG, Guffei A, Williams G, Lowbeer M, et al. Chromosomal rearrangements after ex vivo Epstein-Barr virus (EBV) infection of human B cells. Oncogene. 2010;29:503–15.

52. Yee J, White RE, Anderton E, Allday MJ. Latent Epstein-Barr virus can inhibit apoptosis in B cells by blocking the induction of NOXA expression. PLoS One. 2011;6:e28506.

53. Shirgahi Talari F, Bagherzadeh K, Golestanian S, Jarstfer M, Amanlou M. Potent human telomerase inhibitors: molecular dynamic simulations, multiple pharmacophore-based virtual screening, and biochemical assays. J Chem Inf Model. 2015;55:2596–610.

54. Kudoh A, Fujita M, Zhang L, Shirata N, Daikoku T, Sugaya Y, et al. Epstein-Barr virus lytic replication elicits ATM checkpoint signal transduction while providing an S-phase-like cellular environment. J Biol Chem. 2005;280:8156–63.

25

Glycogene expression profiles based on microarray data from cervical carcinoma HeLa cells with partially silenced E6 and E7 HPV oncogenes

Miguel Aco-Tlachi[1,2], Ricardo Carreño-López[2], Patricia L. Martínez-Morales[4], Paola Maycotte[4], Adriana Aguilar-Lemarroy[3], Luis Felipe Jave-Suárez[3], Gerardo Santos-López[1], Julio Reyes-Leyva[1] and Verónica Vallejo-Ruiz[1]* (iD)

Abstract

Background: Aberrant glycosylation is a characteristic of tumour cells. The expression of certain glycan structures has been associated with poor prognosis. In cervical carcinoma, changes in the expression levels of some glycogenes have been associated with lymph invasion. Human papillomavirus (HPV) infection is one of the most important factors underlying the development of cervical cancer. The HPV oncoproteins E6 and E7 have been implicated in cervical carcinogenesis and can modify the host gene expression profile. The roles of these oncoproteins in glycosylation changes have not been previously reported.

Methods: To determine the effect of the E6 and E7 oncoproteins on glycogene expression we partially silenced the E6 and E7 oncogenes in HeLa cells, we performed a microarray expression assay to identify altered glycogenes and quantified the mRNA levels of glycogenes by RT-qPCR. A protein-protein interaction network was constructed to identify potentially altered glycosylation pathways.

Results: The microarray analysis showed 9 glycogenes that were upregulated and 7 glycogenes that were downregulated in HeLa shE6/E7 cells. Some of these genes participate in glycosylation related to Notch proteins and O-glycans antigens.

Conclusions: Our results support that E6 and E7 oncoproteins could modify glycogene expression the products of which participate in the synthesis of structures implicated in proliferation, adhesion and apoptosis.

Keywords: Microarrays, Glycogene, Cervical cancer, HeLa cells, Human papillomavirus, E6 oncoprotein, E7 oncoprotein

Background

Glycosylation changes have been reported in cancer, and glycan structures are found in secreted proteins, membrane glycoproteins, and glycolipids. Glycans are involved in cellular adhesion, tumour proliferation, apoptosis, invasion, metastasis, angiogenesis and signal transduction [1].

In cervical cancer, the increased expression of some glycogenes such as *ST6GAL1* and *ST3GAL3*, has been correlated with deep stromal invasion and lymph node metastasis [2]. The increased expression of sialyltransferases genes could be related to an overexpression of sialylated antigens such as sialyl-T, sialyl-Le(a), and sialyl-Le(x), identified in cervical neoplasia [3–5].

Polylactosamine (polyLacNAc) is a glycan structure expressed during development and carcinogenesis, and β1,3-N-acetylglucosaminyl transferases (β3GnTs) participate in its synthesis. In cervical tissue, the increased expression of β3GnT2 has been detected in cervical intraepithelial neoplasia 3 (CIN3), and polyLacNAc expression is higher in cancer tissue [6]. The gene regulation of glycogenes is very complex, and little information exists about the factors that modify their expression during cervical transformation.

* Correspondence: veronica_vallejo@yahoo.com; vero.vallejoruiz@gmail.com
[1]Centro de Investigación Biomédica de Oriente, Instituto Mexicano del Seguro Social, Km. 4.5 Carretera Federal Atlixco-Metepec, Atlixco, C.P. 74360 Puebla, Mexico
Full list of author information is available at the end of the article

Cervical cancer tumours are associated with high-risk human papillomavirus infections. HPV-16 is the most prevalent high-risk HPV type, followed by HPV-18 and HPV-31 [7]. The HPV-18 type is the most prevalent genotype in cervical adenocarcinoma [8]. One of the key events of HPV-induced cervical cancer is the integration of the HPV genome into the host chromosome [9]. Expression of E6 and E7 genes is necessary for cell transformation induction and contributes to genome instability [10]. These viral oncoproteins have been implicated in the altered expression of different genes via different mechanisms. It has been reported that E6 can increase the expression of hTERT, the catalytic domain of telomerase, via transcription factor interactions, transcription repressor degradation, and chromatin structure modifications [11–13]. There are no reports about the roles of the E6 and E7 oncoproteins in glycosylation changes in the cervix.

The objective of this work was to identify glycogenes that modify their expression by partially silencing the HPV-18 E6 and E7 oncogenes in HeLa cells using microarray analysis.

Methods
Cell culture
HeLa cell line (VPH18+) from cervical cancer was used to perform the gene silencing. Cells were cultured and maintained in Dulbecco's Modified Eagle's Medium (DMEM) containing Earle's salts and L-glutamine (DMEM; Sigma, St. Louis, MO, USA), and supplemented with 10% foetal bovine serum, and 100 μg/ml streptomycin (Sigma). Cells were maintained at 37 °C in a 5% CO2 atmosphere. The culture medium was replaced every two days. Subconfluent adherent cells were harvested using a mixture of trypsin (0.025%) and EDTA (0.02%; Sigma) and washed with phosphate-buffered saline.

Gene silencing and clonal selection
Gene silencing in HeLa parental cells was achieved by cloning the shRNA sequence 5'-CTAACACTGGGTTA TACAA-3' into the pLVX-sh vector (pLVX-shE6/E7) (Clontech Laboratories, Mountain View, CA, USA). The 19-nucleotide sequence targets the E6 and E7 bicistronic mRNA [14]. As a control, the sequence 5'-GACTTCATA AGGCGCATGC-3' [15] was cloned into the pLVX-sh vector (pLVX-shControl). To obtain recombinant lentiviral particles carrying the respective constructs, Lenti-X 293 T cells were co-transfected with either pLVX-shControl or pLVX-shE6/E7 and Lenti-X HTX Packaging Mix (Clontech Laboratories, Mountain View, CA, USA). Lentiviruses were harvested from the supernatant and filtered. The presence of viral particles in the filtrate was confirmed using the LentiX-Gostik kit (Clontech Laboratories, Mountain View, CA, USA). Supernatants bearing lentivirus pLVX-shControl or pLVX-shE6/E7 were then used to transduce HeLa cells.

Transduced cells were selected with puromycin and when the culture reached 60% confluence, the cells were trypsinized and diluted to obtain monoclonal cultures. Screening of several HeLa clones carrying either shcontrol or shE6/E7 was performed by RT-qPCR to select clones with no change in the expression levels of E6/E7 or the best degree of gene silencing compare with parental HeLa cells (data not shown).

RT-qPCR
Total RNA from shcontrol and shE6/E7 HeLa monocultures was obtained using the NucleoSpin RNA II kit (Macherey-Nagel, Düren, Germany). In total, 500 ng of RNA was used to synthesize cDNA using random primers and the RevertAid First-Strand cDNA Synthesis kit (Thermo Fisher Scientific, USA).

To show that the amplification efficiencies of the E6, E7, *POFUT1*, *XXYLT1*, *DPY19L1*, *ALG14*, *UGT8*, *PIGV*, and *GALNT1* genes were optimal, standard curves were constructed with the following concentrations: 10, 1, 0.1, 0.01, and 0.001 ng/μL; HPRT was used as an endogenous gene. Each reaction was performed in a final volume of 10 μL comprising the following: 1 μL of cDNA template, 5 μL of 2X Maxima SYBER Green/Rox qPCR Master Mix (Thermo Fisher Scientific, USA), and 0.5 μL of 10 mM forward and reverse primers for the E6, E7, *POFUT1*, *XXYLT1*, *DPY19L1*, *ALG14*, *UGT8*, *PIGV*, *GALNT1* and HPRT genes (Table 1). The reactions were performed with a StepOne Real-Time PCR System (Applied Biosystems, Foster, CA), and the conditions were as follows: 95 °C for 10 min, followed by 40 cycles of 95 °C for 30 s, 60 °C 30 s, and 70 °C for 30 s.

To determine the mRNA levels the final reaction volume of 10 μL included 1 μL of cDNA template (0.5 ng/μL final concentration for the E6 and E7 genes and 0.1 ng/μL for the glycogenes), 5 μL of 2X Maxima SYBR Green/Rox qPCR Master Mix (Thermo Scientific, California, USA), 0.5 μL of forward and reverse primers (0.5 μM final concentration) and 3 μL of RNase free water. RT-qPCR was performed under the following conditions: 95 °C for 10 min, followed by 40 cycles of 95 °C for 30 s, 60 °C for 30 s and 70 °C for 30 s. The transcript levels of E6, E7 and the glycogenes were normalized to those of HPRT.

Relative quantification was performed using the comparative CT method with the formula $2^{-\Delta\Delta CT}$. The qPCR reaction was performed using the StepOneReal-Time PCR System (Applied Biosytems, Foster, CA).

Western blot
Protein extraction was performed by mechanical lysis from non-treated, shcontrol and shE6/E7 monocultures at 90% confluence. Next, 50 μg protein samples of each total cell extract were separated by 12% SDS-PAGE to analyze p53, whereas 70 μg protein samples were separated

Table 1 Sequences of the oligonucleotides used in the RT-qPCR assays to quantify E6, E7 and glycogenes expression level

Name	Sequence	PCR Product
E6 Forward	5'GCGACCCTACAAGCTACCTGAT 3'	295 bp
E6 Reverse	5'GCACCGCAGGCACCTTAT 3'	
E7 Forward	5' TGTCACGAGCAATTAAGCGACT 3'	215 bp
E7 Reverse	5' CACACAAAGGACAGGGTGTTC 3'	
POFUT1 Forward	5'CAGCCCAGTTCCCCGTCCTA3'	190 bp
POFUT1 Reverse	5'GAGCCTGCAGTCCCGTCCTTC3'	
UGT8 Forward	5'AAACCAGCCAGCCCACTACCAG3'	93 bp
UGT8 Reverse	5'GACACCAGCTCCAAAAGACACCAA3'	
XXLYLT1 Forward	5'GTGCTGGCTTGGGAACCTACTA3'	230 bp
XXLYLT1 Reverse	5'GCGGAACTGCCAGAATGTGT3'	
DPY19L1 Forward	5'GAGAGTGTACCCGTGTAATGTG3'	134 bp
DPY19L1 Reverse	5'GAGTGCAATCAAGCTTCCTCTA3'	
PIGV Forward	5' CCTGGGCAACTTGGACATA 3'	95 bp
PIGV Reverse	5' GGGCTTCTCTAGGGTCTTATTG 3'	
ALG14 Forward	5' CCGGGAGTCTCTCAGTATCTT 3'	100 bp
ALG14 Reverse	5' TCTAGGTGAGTAGGCATTGGA 3'	
GALNT1 Forward	5' GGATAAAGCCACAGAAGAGGATAG 3'	94 bp
GALNT1 Reverse	5' CAGGGTGACGTTTCGAAGAA 3'	
HPRT Forward	5'CCTGGCGTCGTGATTAGTGATGAT3'	136 bp
HPRT Reverse	5'CGAGCAAGACGTTCAGTCCTGTC3'	

by 15% SDS-PAGE to analyze E7. Samples were transferred to a polyvinylidene fluoride Immobilon-P membrane (Millipore, Darmstadt, Germany) and probed overnight at 4 °C with the antibodies anti-p53 (1:1000; Abcam ab1101), anti-E7 (1:1000; Abcam ab100953), and anti-β-actin (1:3000; Abcam ab8224). Signals were detected with an anti-HRP-conjugated secondary antibody (1:4000; Abcam ab97046) and developed with the ImmPACT™ DAB peroxidase substrate (Vector, Burlingame, CA. USA). Densitometric analysis was performed with ImageJ software.

Hybridization and microarray
Microarray analysis was performed at the Cellular Physiology Institute of UNAM as follows: total RNA from cell cultures was extracted with a Direct-zol™ RNA MiniPrep kit (Zymo Research, Irvine, CA, USA). Next, 10 μg of total RNA was used for cDNA synthesis incorporating dUTP-Alexa555 or dUTP-Alexa647 employing the First-Strand cDNA labelling kit (Invitrogen). Incorporation of the fluorophore was analyzed using the absorbance at 555 nm for Alexa555 (HeLa shE6/E7) and 650 nm for Alexa647 (HeLa shControl). Equal quantities of labelled cDNA were hybridized using UniHyb hybridization solution (TeleChem International INC) with a chip containing 35 K genes. Acquisition and

quantification of array images were performed using the ScanArray 4000 instrument with its accompanying software ScanArray 4000 from Packard BioChips, USA. For each spot, the Alexa555 and Alexa647 density and background mean values were calculated with ArrayPro Analyzer software from Media Cybernetics. Microarray data analysis was performed with GenArise (free) software, developed in the Computing Unit of the Cellular Physiology Institute of UNAM (http://www.ifc.unam.mx/genarise/). GenArise carries out several transformations: background correction, normalization, intensity filter, replicates analysis and selection of differentially expressed genes. Analyzed data were submitted to the NCBI-Gene Expression Omnibus database (accession number GSE90930).

Analysis of biological processes
Altered genes were analyzed using DAVID (Database for Annotation, Visualization, and Integrated Discovery) software (http://david.abcc.ncifcrf.gov/). Based on gene ontology (GO) [16], genes were classified according to their function in a biological process (BP), and a p-value < 0.05 was considered statistically significant.

Identification of glycogenes
We identified 336 glycogenes reported to date using the GlycoGene database (https://acgg.asia/ggdb2/index?doc), Consortium for Functional Glycomics-CAZy database (http://www.cazy.org/) and the published reports of glycogenes not included in the databases: *DPY19L1* gene, [17] and the *MANBAL* gene [18].

We selected genes with altered expression in the microarray corresponding to glycogenes.

Protein-protein interaction network
Predicted interaction network analysis was performed with Cytoscape 3.4.0 and the 'StringWSClient' plugin, considering a score of 0.4 as the confidence level.

Statistical analysis
Statistical analysis of the RT-qPCR results was performed using the Graph Pad programme. A One-way analysis of variance followed by Tukey's post-test was performed. A p-value < 0.05 was considered statistically significant.

Results
E6 and E7 oncogenes expression by RT-qPCR
RT-qPCR was performed to quantify and compare the E6 and E7 mRNA expression levels in HeLa-non-treated, HeLa shcontrol and HeLa-shE6/E7 cells. The E6 mRNA expression level in HeLa shcontrol cells was like that in HeLa-non-treated cells. By contrast, E6 mRNA was decreased by 60% in HeLa shE6/E7 cells compared to that in HeLa-non-treated and HeLa shcontrol cells ($p < 00.1$)

(Fig. 1). Similar results were obtained after analyzing E7 mRNA levels; its expression was decreased by 50% in HeLa shE6/E7 cells compared to that in HeLa-non-treated and HeLa shcontrol cells ($p < 00.1$).

E6 and E7 proteins expression by western blot analysis

We analyzed the p53 and E7 protein expression levels by Western blot. First, we indirectly analyzed the expression of the E6 protein by evaluating the quantity of the p53 protein, since the oncoprotein induces p53 degradation and can thus serve as a marker of E6 expression. The latter was analyzed due to reports that E6 detection is difficult using Western blot in the HeLa cell line [19]. The p53 protein level was increased in HeLa-shE6/E7 cells by 1.5- fold compared to that in HeLa-non-treated and HeLa shcontrol cells ($p < 0.001$) (Fig. 2), suggesting a decrease in E6 protein expression. By contrast, we analyzed E7 expression by detecting the protein directly. As expected, E7 protein expression was decreased by 0.5-fold in HeLa-shE6/E7 cells compared to that in HeLa-non-treated ($p < 0.001$) and HeLa shcontrol cells ($p < 0.05$) (Fig. 2). In summary, these results show that HeLa shE6/E7 cells display downregulated E6 and E7 mRNA and protein expression.

Cell organization, signalling and adhesion are the most affected biological processes under E6 and E7 downregulation

To analyze genes under E6 and E7 regulation, we performed a complete genome microarray comparing transcripts within HeLa shE6/E7 cells and HeLa shcontrol cells. Using GeneArise software, we identified 1157 genes exhibiting altered expression profiles in HeLa shE6/E7 cells compared with the control. The results showed altered genes with a Z-score > 2 for upregulated genes and a Z-score < 2 for downregulated genes. Thus, we identified 544 upregulated genes and 613 downregulated genes in E6 and E7 compared with the control (accession number GSE90930).

With the aim of been able to associate the 1157 altered genes according to their function, we performed an analysis with DAVID software and GO. The 1157 altered genes were related to differentiation, cell organization, signalling, translation, immune response, adhesion and cell cycle. Importantly, the results show that most of the expression changes in HeLa shE6/E7 cells correspond to genes associated with cell organization, signalling and cell adhesion (Fig. 3).

Glycogene expression is altered by the E6 and E7 oncoproteins

Next, to identify glycogenes among the altered genes in the microarray, we first identified all the glycogenes reported to date, by searching the GlycoGene database, Consortium for Functional Glycomics-CAZy database and published reports. Among the 336 glycogenes included in the database, 9 genes were upregulated in HeLa shE6/E7 cells (Z score > 2), including *ALG14*, *POFUT1*, *FUT4*, *MAN2A1*, *DPY19L1*, *C3orf21* (*XXYLT1*), *UGT2B17*, *IDUA* and *UGCGL1*. A total of 7 glycogenes were downregulated (Z score < 2), including *GALNT1*, *B4GALT2*, *UGT8*, *MANBAL*, *PIGV*, *FCMD* and *C1GALT1C1*.

Glycogene expression by qRT-PCR

Among the 16 glycogenes altered in the microarray assay, we evaluated 7 by RT-qPCR. The mRNA levels were evaluated for *POFUT1*, *DPY19L1*, *XXYLT1*, *ALG14*, *UGT8*, *PIGV*, and *GALNT1* in HeLa shcontrol and HeLa-shE6/E7 cells. The *POFUT1* and *ALG14* mRNA levels were increased on HeLa shE6/E7 cells compared to those in HeLa

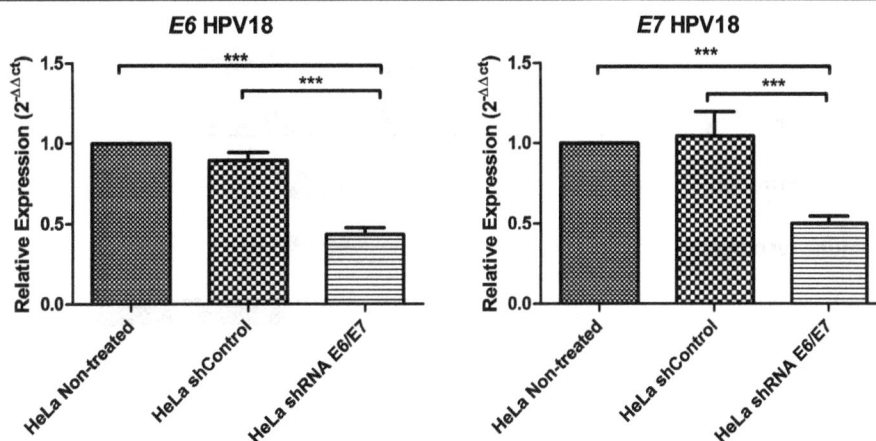

Fig. 1 Inhibition of HPV18 E6/E7 mRNA expression by shRNA E6/E7 in a HeLa cell line. HeLa cells were transfected with shRNA or shcontrol, and the relative expression of E6/E7 was determined by real-time PCR. The x-axis shows the different experiment groups; the y-axis shows the relative E6 and E7 mRNA expression, which was normalized to that in non-treated HeLa cells. Three independent experiments carried out in triplicate are shown, and the groups were analyzed by one-way analysis of variance (ANOVA) with the Tukey test. ***$p < 0.001$

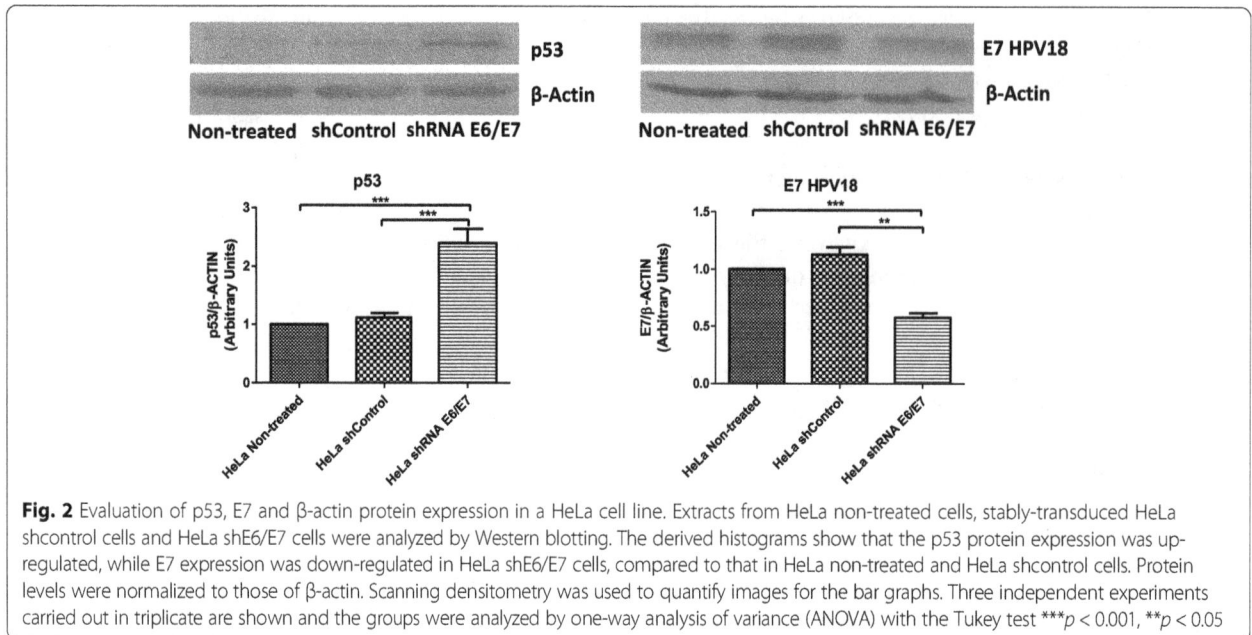

Fig. 2 Evaluation of p53, E7 and β-actin protein expression in a HeLa cell line. Extracts from HeLa non-treated cells, stably-transduced HeLa shcontrol cells and HeLa shE6/E7 cells were analyzed by Western blotting. The derived histograms show that the p53 protein expression was up-regulated, while E7 expression was down-regulated in HeLa shE6/E7 cells, compared to that in HeLa non-treated and HeLa shcontrol cells. Protein levels were normalized to those of β-actin. Scanning densitometry was used to quantify images for the bar graphs. Three independent experiments carried out in triplicate are shown and the groups were analyzed by one-way analysis of variance (ANOVA) with the Tukey test ***$p < 0.001$, **$p < 0.05$

shcontrol cells ($p < 0.05$) (Fig. 4). *DPY19L1* and *XXLT1* showed increased mRNA levels in HeLa shE6/E7 cells, but they were not statistically significant (Fig. 4).

The glycogenes downregulated in the microarray, *UGT8*, *PIGV*, and *GALNT1* were evaluated by RT-qPCR. Only *UGT8* showed statistically significant decreased expression in HeLa shE6/E7 cells; *PIGV* showed decreased expression but it was not statistically significant, and *GALNT1* did not showed expression changes (Fig. 5).

Next, we determined whether the glycogenes with altered expression in the microarray have been previously reported to have modified expression in cancerous tissues.

Among the 9 upregulated genes, only *POFUT1*, *FUT4*, *UGT2B17*, and *MAN2A1* have been reported to be altered in cancerous tissues. *FUT4* is increased in leukaemia, gastric, breast and colorectal cancer; *UGT2B17* is increased in endometrial cancer; *POFUT1* is increased in glioblastomas and oral squamous cell carcinoma, and *MAN2A1 is* decreased in glioblastoma (Table 2).

Next, we compared the downregulated glycogenes in HeLa shE6/E7 cells with those reported in cancerous tissues. Only 4 glycogenes have been reported in cancer. *GALNT1* is increased in bladder cancer, *C1GALT1C1* is increased in colorectal cancer and *UGT8* is increased in

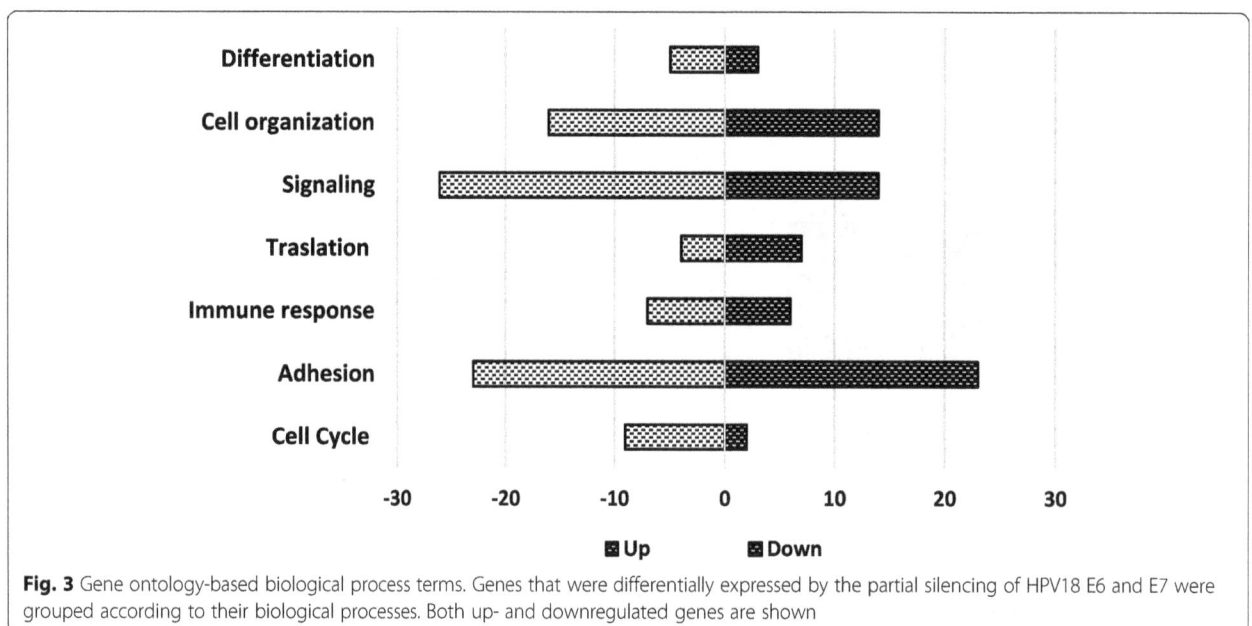

Fig. 3 Gene ontology-based biological process terms. Genes that were differentially expressed by the partial silencing of HPV18 E6 and E7 were grouped according to their biological processes. Both up- and downregulated genes are shown

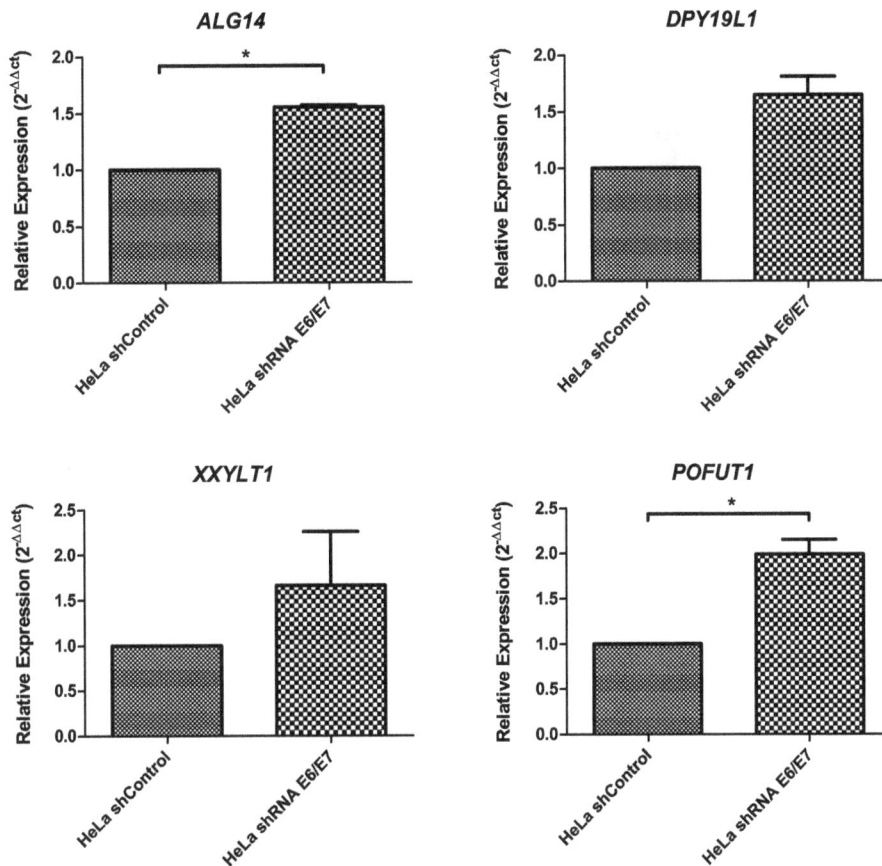

Fig. 4 Expression of *POFUT1*, *DPY19L1*, *XXYLT1*, and *ALG14* in shcontrol and shE6/E7 HeLa cells. The mRNA expression levels were determined by RT-qPCR. The mean ± SD of three independent experiments carried out in triplicate assays is shown; *P* < 0.05

breast cancer. For *B4GALT2* missense mutations, have been reported in colon cancer. The remaining glycogenes have not been reported to be altered in cancerous tissues (Table 3).

E6 and E7 activity may downregulate the notch glycosylation pathway and upregulate Tn and T antigens synthesis

To identify possible functional association among the enzymes coded by the altered glycogenes under E6 and E7 downregulation, we examined data with Cytoscape software to generate predicted protein-protein interactions. Analyses among all upregulated glycogenes revealed a network whithin 3 glycogenes: *FUT4, POFUT1, and XXYLT1* (Fig. 6a). By contrast, analyses among downregulated genes showed an interaction only between *GALNT1* and *C1GALT1C1* (Fig. 6b). These results suggest that *FUT4, POFUT1 and XXYLT1* as well as *GALNT1* and *C1GALT1C1* could be participating in the same glycosylation pathway.

Next, with the aim of investigating potential targets of the up- and downregulated glycogenes, an analysis was performed by text mining when considering 5 more proteins that could be interacting with the altered glycogenes. Thus, the network among upregulated glycogenes revealed a direct interaction between *NOTCH1* and *POFUT1* (Fig. 7).

Analysis among the downregulated genes revealed a direct interaction within *GALNT1*, *C1GALT1C1* and *MUC1* (Fig. 8), a protein that carries the Tn antigen, which is present in most of the cancers, including uterine cervical cancer cells [20–22].

Discussion

Glycosylation changes in cancer have been associated with immune modulation, cell-matrix interactions, cell invasion, metastasis, and angiogenesis [23], and some of these changes could be due to the dysregulation of glycogenes at the transcriptional level (25–28). In cervical neoplasia, an increased expression of the sialyltransferase genes *ST6GAL1* and *ST3GAL3* has been reported as well as increased sialic acid and the tumour antigens sLe(X), Tn

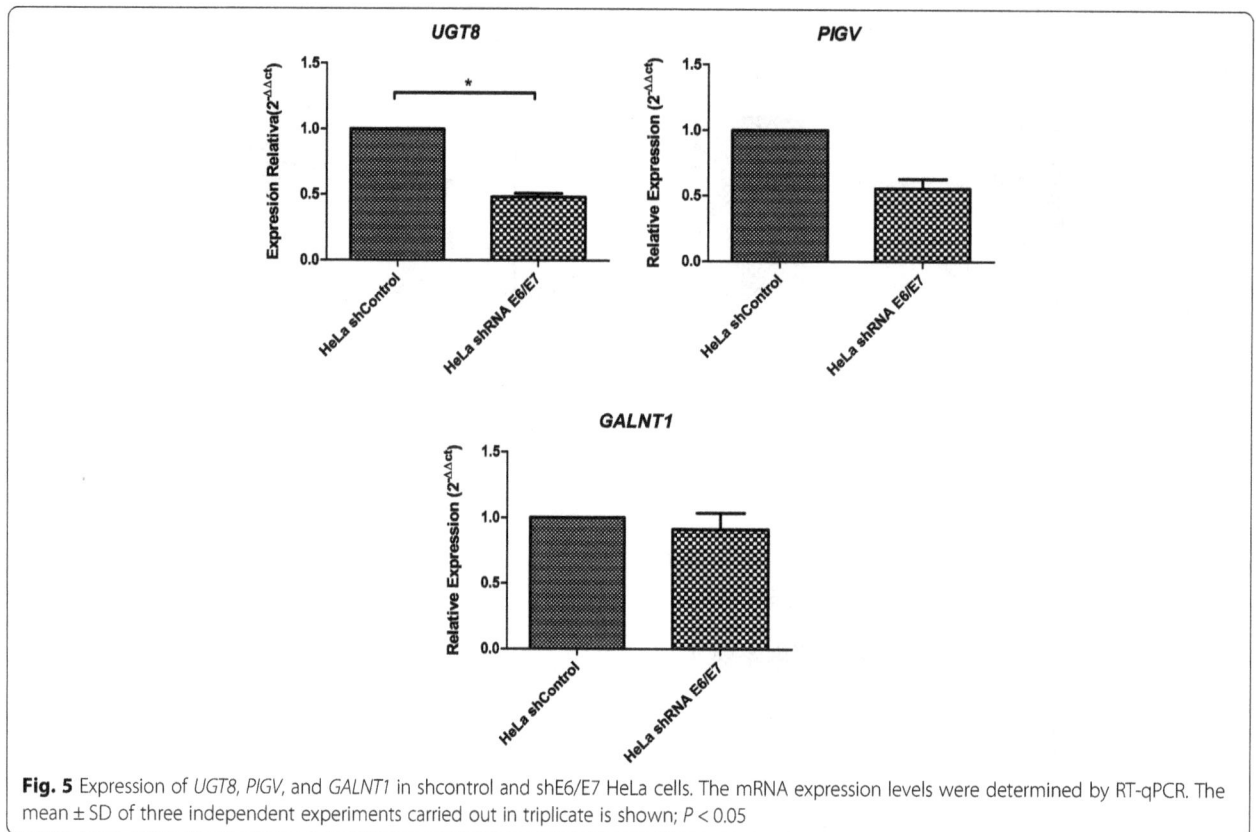

Fig. 5 Expression of *UGT8*, *PIGV*, and *GALNT1* in shcontrol and shE6/E7 HeLa cells. The mRNA expression levels were determined by RT-qPCR. The mean ± SD of three independent experiments carried out in triplicate is shown; $P < 0.05$

and sTn [2, 4, 5, 24, 25]. The role of HPV infection in the glycosylation changes in cervical neoplasia has not been studied. The viral oncoproteins E6 and E7 play a role in cellular transformation and have been implicated in the altered expression of several genes. Notably, the E6 and E7 oncoproteins can modulate gene expression by different mechanisms. It has been reported that E6 can increase the expression of hTERT via transcription factor interactions, transcription repressor degradation, and chromatin structure modifications [11–13]. The role of viral oncoproteins in the glycosylation changes detected in cervical cancer could be due to changes in glycogene expression.

In the present study, we report the potential effects of the E6 and E7 oncogenes in the expression changes of glycogenes. Analysis of the microarray assay results of HeLa cells with partially silenced E6 and E7 oncogenes showed that the cells displayed altered expression of the glycogenes *ALG14*, *POFUT1*, *FUT4*, *MAN2A1*, *DPY19L1*, *XXYLT1*, *UGT2B17*, *IDUA*, *UGCGL1*, *GALNT1*, *B4GALT2*, *UGT8*, *MANBAL*, *PIGV*, *FCMD*, and *C1GALT1C1*. Specifically,the results suggest that the E6 and E7 oncoproteins upregulate the expression of of *GALNT1*, *B4GALT2*, *UGT8*, *MAN BAL*, *PIGV*, *FCMD*, and *C1GALT1C1* whereas they downregulate *ALG14*, *POFUT1*, *FUT4*, *MAN2A1*, *DPY19L1*, *XXYLT1*, *UGT2B17*, *IDUA*, and *UGCGL1*. By RT-qPCR,

we confirmed the downregulation of UGT8 and the upregulation of *POFUT1* and *ALG14* in HeLa shE6/E7 cells. We observed that the mRNA level changes were not statistically significant for *XXYLT1*, *DPY19L1*, and *PIGV*. Although these glycogenes have not yet reported to be altered in cervical cancer, some have been reported to be aberrantly expressed in other cancer types, suggesting that they could be implicated in cervical transformation. In this manner, *MAN2A1* has been reported to be altered in glioblastoma [26], *GALNT1* is altered in bladder cancer, *C1GALT1C1* is altered in colorectal cancer [27], and *UGT8* is altered in breast cancer [28]. By contrast, our results indicate that *POFUT1*, *FUT4*, and *UGT2B17* are upregulated when E6 and E7 are knocked down, suggesting that the expression of these viral oncoproteins downregulates their expression. These results are contrary to reports on other cancer types, such as in leukaemia, glioblastoma, oral squamous cell carcinoma, gastric cancer, breast cancer, colorectal cancer, and endometrial cancer, wherein these genes are upregulated [26, 29–33]. These results indicate that the underlying mechanisms involved in their regulation are different depending on the type of cancer; for example, in human renal cell carcinoma, downregulation of *ST3GAL4* is associated with malignant progression, while in gastric cancer, upregulation is associated with malignant behaviour [34, 35].

Table 2 Glycogenes upregulated in HeLa shE6/E7 cells

Gene/enzyme	Enzyme function	Gene alteration in cancer and oncogenic associated-effects
ALG14 UDP-N-Acetylglucosaminyltransferase Subunit	Associates with ALG13 and transfers a GlcNAc on GlcNAc-PP-Dol (second step of N-linked glycosylation)	Not reported
FUT4 Fucosyltransferase 4	Catalyzes the transfer of fucose (Fuc) residues from GDP-Fuc to [Fucα1 → 2Galβ1 → 4GlcNAcβ1 → R] in α-1, 3 linkage	mRNA upregulated in acute myeloid leukaemia [54], gastric [30] and colorectal cancers [32]. Protein upregulated in breast cancer was associated with proliferation and metastasis [31]
MAN2A1 Mannosidase Alpha Class 2A Member 1	Hydrolyzes two peripheral mannosyl residues from Manα1--6(Manα1--3) Manα1--6(GlcNAcβ1--2Manα1--3) [Manβ1--4GlcNAcβ1--4GlcNAcβ1]- asparagine structure	MAN2A1– FER tyrosine kinase fusion gene is expressed in liver tumours, oesophageal adenocarcinoma, glioblastoma multiforme, prostate tumours, non-small cell lung tumours, and ovarian tumours [55].
DPY19L1 Dpy19 like 1 (C. elegans)	Participates in the C-mannosylation of tryptophan residues on target proteins.	Not reported
C3orf21 (XXYLT1) Xyloside Xylosyltransferase 1	Elongates the O-linked xylose-glucose disaccharide attached to EGF-like repeats (Notch proteins) by catalyzing the addition of the second xylose	Lower frequency of wild type genotype in the C3orf21 gene rs 2,131,877 locus in lung adenocarcinoma tissues [56]
IDUA Iduronidase, Alpha-L-	Cleaves α-linked iduronic acid residues from the nonreducing end of the glycosaminoglycans (GAGs), heparan sulfate, and dermatan sulfate	Not reported
UGT2B17 UDP Glucuronosyltransferase Family 2 Member B17	Catalyzes the glucuronidation of steroids (detoxification)	mRNA upregulated in endometrial cancer [33]
POFUT1 Protein O-Fucosyltransferase 1	Catalyzes the reaction that attaches fucose through an O-glycosidic linkage to a conserved serine or threonine of EGF domains	mRNA upregulated in glioblastomas [26] Protein upregulated in oral squamous cell carcinoma [29]
UGCGL1 UDP-Glucose Glycoprotein Glucosyltransferase 1	Reglucosylates single N-glycans near the misfolded part of the protein	Not reported

Table showing upregulated glycogenes, the names of the coded enzymes, their alteration in different cancer types and their oncogenic-associated-effects

Table 3 Glycogenes downregulated in HeLa shE6/E7 cells

Gene/enzyme	Enzyme function	Gene alteration in cancer and oncogenic- associated-effects
PIGV Phosphatidylinositol Glycan Anchor Biosynthesis Class V	Transfers the second mannose in the glycosylphosphatidylinositol (GPI) anchor	Not reported
GALNT1 Polypeptide N-Acetylgalactosaminyltransferase 1	Transfers N-acetylgalactosamine (GalNAc) to a serine or threonine residue O-glycosylation	mRNA upregulated in bladder cancer stem cells [57]
C1GALT1C1 C1GALT1 Specific Chaperone 1	Specific chaperone assisting the folding/stability of C1GALT1, for the generation of core 1 O-glycan T antigen	mRNA and protein upregulated in colorectal cancer [27]
FCMD Fukutin	Glycosyltransferase involved in the biosynthesis of α-dystroglycan (α-DG)	Not reported
MANBAL Mannosidase, beta A, lysosomal-like	Mannosidase beta-like	Not reported
B4GALT2 Beta-1,4-Galactosyltransferase 2	Transfers galactose to the terminal N-acetylglucosamine of complex-type N-glycans	Missense mutations in B4GALT2 gene in colon cancer with a predictive deleterious phenotype [58]
UGT8 Ceramide UDP-Galactosyltransferase	Catalyzes the transfer of galactose to ceramide (biosynthesis of GalCer)	mRNA and protein upregulated in breast [28] and increased protein expression in lung cancer [59]

Table showing downregulated glycogenes, the names of the coded enzymes and their alteration in different cancer types

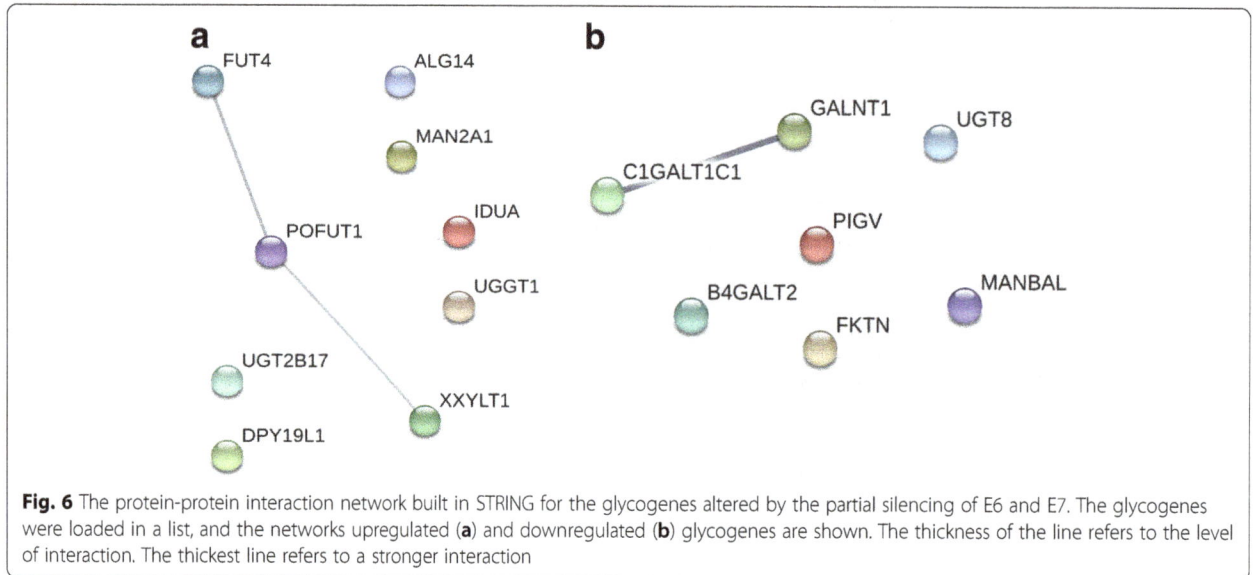

Fig. 6 The protein-protein interaction network built in STRING for the glycogenes altered by the partial silencing of E6 and E7. The glycogenes were loaded in a list, and the networks upregulated (**a**) and downregulated (**b**) glycogenes are shown. The thickness of the line refers to the level of interaction. The thickest line refers to a stronger interaction

The Human Protein Atlas database shows that the protein expression levels of Fut4, Man2A1 and Ugt2b17 are not increased in samples from patients with cervical cancer, and POFUT1 is detected at low and medium expression levels; these results agree with our results suggesting that the respective glycogenes are down-regulated in the presence of the E6/E7 oncoproteins. Moreover, *GALNT1*, and *C1CAGLT1C*, with higher expression in HeLa control cells, are reported to have medium and high expression levels in cervical cancer samples in this database, suggesting that viral oncoproteins could increase their expression in cervical cancer. Remarkably, in general, the data point to the same glycogene expression profile in cervical cancer.

In addition, functional bioinformatic analysis allowed us to elucidate the possible altered biosynthetic pathway considering the altered glycogenes and their potential targets. Thus, we identified that under higher E6 and E7 expression, the components of the Notch glycosylation pathway are downregulated, whereas the components of

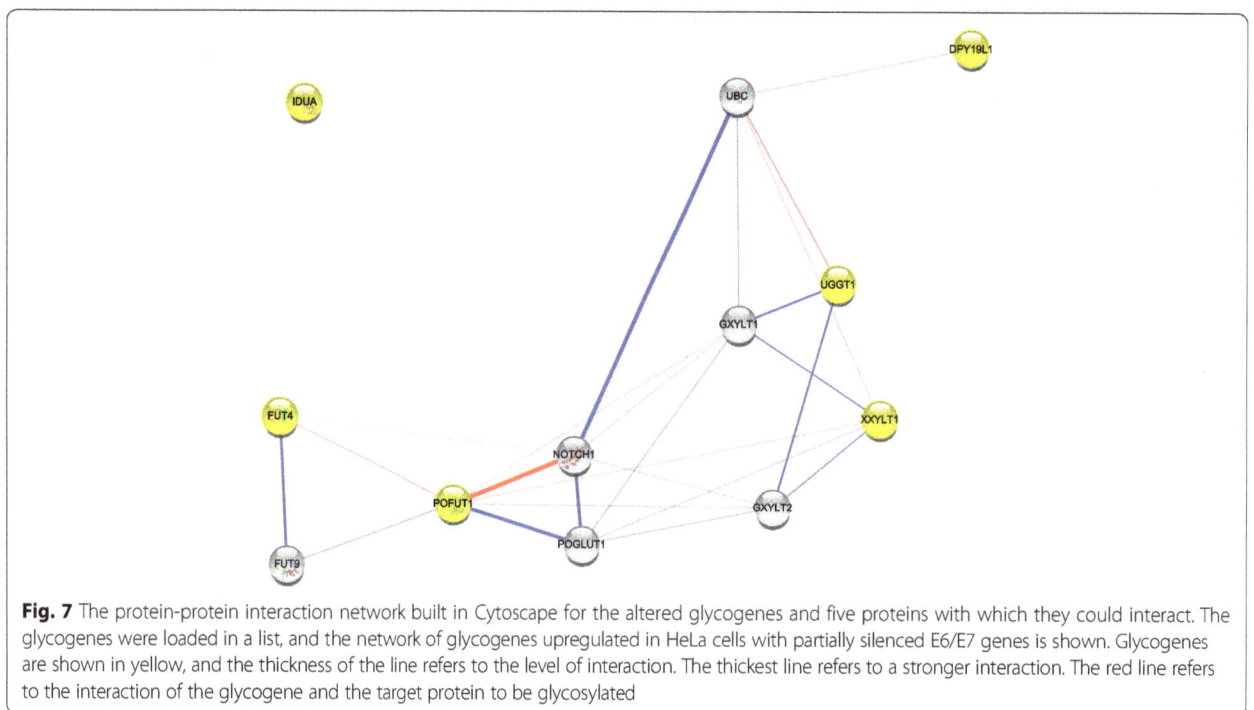

Fig. 7 The protein-protein interaction network built in Cytoscape for the altered glycogenes and five proteins with which they could interact. The glycogenes were loaded in a list, and the network of glycogenes upregulated in HeLa cells with partially silenced E6/E7 genes is shown. Glycogenes are shown in yellow, and the thickness of the line refers to the level of interaction. The thickest line refers to a stronger interaction. The red line refers to the interaction of the glycogene and the target protein to be glycosylated

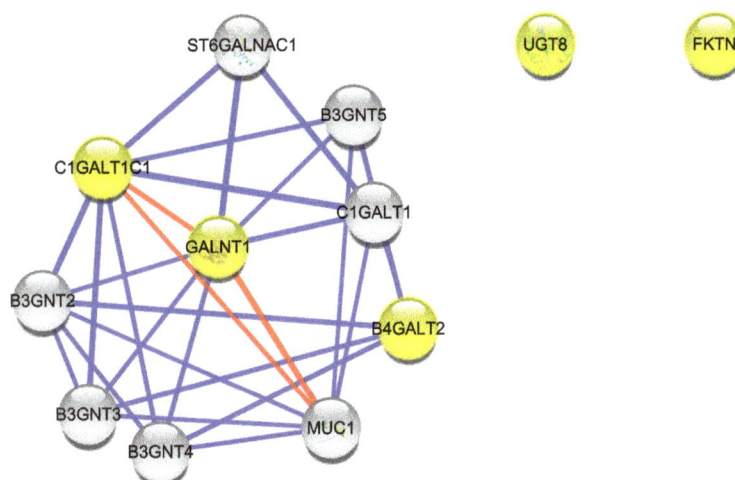

Fig. 8 The protein-protein interaction network built in Cytoscape for the altered glycogenes and five proteins with which they could interact. The glycogenes were loaded in a list, and the network of glycogenes downregulated in partially silenced HeLa cells is shown. Glycogenes are shown in yellow, and the thickness of the line refers to the level of interaction. The thickest line refers to a stronger interaction. The red line refers to the interaction of the glycogene and the target protein to be glycosylated

the synthesis of Tn and T antigens are upregulated. Interestingly, both mechanisms are aberrantly regulated in cancerous cell phenotypes [20, 36–38].

In the first case, analysis of the downregulated glycogenes under E6 and E7 activity and their potential targets showed a direct interaction within Pofut4 and Notch1. Pofut1 is an O-fucosyltranferase that modifies the extracellular EGF-like domains of Notch transmembrane proteins. The enzyme attaches a fucose via an O-glycosidic linkage to a conserved serine or threonine for proper protein folding [39]. Interestingly, defects in Notch receptor fucosylation by the deletion of POFUT1 have been implicated in the development of myeloid hyperplasia in adult mice. Moreover, POFUT1 deficiency provokes a slight decrease in Notch1 and Notch2 expression at the cell surface and abrogates the binding between Notch and its ligand Delta [40]. Additionally, evidence from *Drosophila* suggest that Pofut1 could exert a chaperone activity on the Notch protein. The absence of OFUT1 (Pofut1) leads to the decrease in Notch protein expression on the cell surface, whereas its overexpression increases the binding between Notch and its ligand [41]. Interestingly and consistent with this notion, the absence of OFUT1 leads to the retention of Notch in the endoplasmic reticulum [42]. In human cervical cancer, several reports indicate intracellular localization of the Notch1 protein [42–46]. Moreover, studies on cervical cancer showed that in a normal cervix, Notch-1 is more commonly membrane-localized than in a cancerous cervix [46]. Thus, our results could suggest that under downregulation of the enzyme Pofut1, the protein Notch1 could exhibit a decrease in its O-fucosylation pattern or in its presence at the cell membrane. Alteration of this particular glycogene could promote aberrant Notch signalling [47, 48].

In the second case, higher E6 and E7 expression, the glycogenes *GALNT1* and *C1GALT1C1* are upregulated. Since, GalNAc-T1 and C1GalT1 specific chaperone 1 participate in the Tn antigen O-glycosylation pathway [49, 50], the results suggest that E6 and E7 activity could promote Tn antigen biosynthesis by upregulating the expression of both enzymes. Mucin1 is a membrane-bound protein that participates in intracellular signalling and cell adhesion. The protein is O-glycosylated by several transferases, including GalNAc-T1 and the C1GalT1C1-C1GalT1 complex. Changes in this glycosylation process have been associated with different types of cancer [51]. Specifically, two tumour antigens expressed in carcinomas are Tn and sialyl-Tn; these structures are present in many mucin-type glycoproteins including Muc1 [49–51]. O-glycosylation that leads to Tn synthesis begins with the addition of an N-acetylgalactosamine to a Ser or Thr residue of the protein, catalyzed by GalNT1. Following Tn antigen formation, this new chain can serve as an acceptor for at least three other Golgi glycosyltransferases. The most common modification of the Tn antigen is the formation of the core 1 disaccharide (or T antigen) by the action of C1GalT1 (known as T-synthase), which requires the chaperone C1GalT1C1 (known as COSMC) for its activity. C1GalT1C1 resides in the endoplasmic reticulum and prevents the misfolding, aggregation, and proteasome-dependent degradation of newly synthesized T-synthase. In the absence of functional C1GalT1C1, the newly synthesized T-synthase is inactive and rapidly degraded. Loss of C1GalT1C1 function eliminates T-synthase activity and the consequential Tn antigen expression in several human tumours [50]. In summary, our results suggest an increase in Tn and T antigen synthesis in Mucin1 since the cells displayed an upregulation of both the GalNT1 and C1GalT1C1 proteins. In cervical cancer, Tn and sTn antigens are expressed in invasive squamous cell carcinomas, but not in a normal squamous epithelium [24].

By contrast, GalNT1 can exhibit a mucin-independent function in cancer and be implicated in other pathways, such as EGFR signaling, by increasing EGFR degradation via decreasing of EGFR O-glycosylation [52]. Moreover, GalNT1 can mediate the O-glycosylation of Sonic Hedgehog to promote signal activation in bladder cancer stem cells [53]. In the case of C1GalT1C1, forced expression of the chaperone in colon cancer cell lines increases T antigen expression and enhances cell growth, migration, and invasion, and this phenotype is associated with the increased phosphorylation of ERK and AKT. By contrast, knocking down C1GalT1C1 decreases malignant behaviours and the signalling pathways, suggesting that the chaperone can promote malignant phenotypes of colon cancer cells, mainly via activation of the MEK/ERK and PI3K/Akt signalling pathways [27].

These reports suggest that the glycogenes altered in the microarray assay of HeLa cells with partially silenced E6 and E7 oncogenes, could play important roles in cervical transformation that have not yet been explored.

Conclusions

Partially silencing of the E6 and E7 HPV oncogenes could be implicated in important glycosylation pathways altered in cervical cancer. In the present study, glycosylation of the Notch receptor and O-glycosylation type mucin were identified. The identified genes implicated in these pathways have not been reported in cervical cancer.

The analysis of glycogenes altered by the HPV oncoproteins E6 and E7 is a valuable tool to identify possible glycogenes implicated in the cervical transformation process and to understand the role of HPV infection in glycosylation changes detected in cervical cancer.

Abbreviations

CIN: Cervical intraepithelial neoplasia; HPV: Human papillomavirus; polyLacNAc: Polylactosamine; β3GnTs: β1,3-N-acetylglucosaminyl transferases

Acknowledgements

We thank to Lorena Chávez González, Simón Guzmán León, José Luis. Santillán Torres, and Jorge Ramírez for their technical assistance in the microarray determinations and Gerardo Coello, Gustavo Corral and Ana Patricia Gómez for their assistance with GenArise software.

Funding

This study was supported by the Instituto Mexicano del Seguro Social (grant no. FIS/IMSS/PROT/G14/1293). JRL has a fellowship from Fundación IMSS. MAT was supported by a Ph.D. fellowship from CONACYT (no. 242753), and from IMSS (98227565). Programa Cátedras CONACYT 2016 (no. 485) and Fondo Redes Temáticas de Investigación-CONACYT (253596).

Authors' contributions

MAT, GSL and JRL participated in the molecular biology experiments. MAT, RCL, PLMM, JRL and VVR participated in the in silico analysis. AAL and LJS participated in the gene silencing assay. MAT, PLMM and VVR participated in drafting the manuscript. All authors read and approved the final version of the manuscript.

Competing interests

The authors declare that they have no competing interests.

Author details

[1]Centro de Investigación Biomédica de Oriente, Instituto Mexicano del Seguro Social, Km. 4.5 Carretera Federal Atlixco-Metepec, Atlixco, C.P. 74360 Puebla, Mexico. [2]Posgrado en Ciencias Microbiológicas, Benemérita Universidad Autónoma de Puebla, Edificio 103-J Cd. Universitaria, Col. San Manuel, C.P. 72570 Puebla, Pue, Mexico. [3]Centro de Investigación Biomédica de Occidente, Instituto Mexicano del Seguro Social, Sierra Mojada 800, Col Independencia, C.P. 44340 Guadalajara, Jalisco, Mexico. [4]CONACYT- Centro de Investigación Biomédica de Oriente, Instituto Mexicano del Seguro Social, Km. 4.5 Carretera Federal Atlixco-Metepec, Atlixco, C.P. 74360 Puebla, Mexico.

References

1. Pinho S, Reis CA. Glycosylation in cancer: mechanisms and clinical implications. Nat Rev Cancer. 2015;15:540–55.
2. Wang PH, Li YF, Juang CM, Lee YR, Chao HT, Ng HT, et al. Expression of sialyltransferase family members in cervix squamous cell carcinoma correlates with lymph node metastasis. Gynecologyc Oncology. 2002;86:45–52.
3. Carrilho C, Cantel M, Gouveia P, David L. Simple mucin-type carbohydrate antigens (Tn, sialosyl-Tn and sialosyl-T) and gp 230 mucin-like glycoprotein are canddidate markers for neoplastic transformation of the human cervix. Virchows Arch. 2000;437:173–9.
4. Engelstaedter V, Fluegel B, Kunze S, Mayr D, Friese K, Jeschke U, et al. Expression of the carbohydrate tumour marker Sialyl Lewis a, Sialyl Lewis X, Lewis Y and Thomsen-Friedenreich antigen in normal squamous epithelium of the uterine cervix, cervical dysplasia and cervical cancer. Histol Histopathol. 2012;27:507–14.
5. Velázquez-Márquez N, Santos-López G, Jiménez-Aranda L, Reyes-Leyva J, Vallejo-Ruiz V. Sialyl Lewis x expression in cervical scrapes of premalignant lesions. J Biosci. 2012;37:999–1004.
6. Clark AT, Guimarães da Costa VM, Bandeira Costa L, Bezerra Cavalcanti CL, De Melo Rêgo MJ, Beltrão EI. Differential expression patterns of N-acetylglucosaminyl transferases and polylactosamines in uterine lesions. Eur J Histochem. 2014;58:2334.
7. zur Hausen H. Papillomavirus and cancer: from basic studies to clinical application. Nat Rev Cancer. 2002;2:342–50.
8. Dahlström LA, Ylitalo N, Sundström K, Palmgren J, Ploner A, Eloranta S, et al. Prospective study of human papillomavirus and risk of cervical adenocarcinoma. Int J Cancer. 2010;127:1923–30.
9. Zhao JW, Fang F, Guo Y, Zhu TL, Yu YY, Kong FF, et al. HPV16 integration probably contributes to cervical oncogenesis through interrupting tumor suppressor genes and inducing chromosome instability. J Exp Clin Cancer Res. 2016;35:180.
10. Korzeniewski N, Spardy N, Duensing A, Duensing S. Genomic instability and cancer: lessons learned from human papillomaviruses. Cancer Lett. 2011;305:113–22.
11. Gewin L, Myers H, Kiyono T, Galloway DA. Identification of a novel telomerase repressor that interacts with the human papillomavirus type-16 E6/E6-AP complex. Genes Dev. 2004;18:2269–82.
12. Wang S, Pang T, Gao M, Kang H, Ding W, Sun X, et al. HPV E6 induces eIF4E transcription to promote the proliferation and migration of cervical cancer. FEBS Lett. 2013;587:690–7.
13. Songock WK, Kim SM, Bodily JM. The human papillomavirus E7 oncoprotein as a regulator of transcription. Virus Res. 2017;231:56–75.
14. Butz K, Ristriani T, Hengstermann A, Denk C, Scheffner M, Hoppe-Seyler F. siRNA targeting of the viral E6 oncogene efficiently kills human papillomavirus-positive cancer cells. Oncogene. 2003;22:5938–45.

15. Qi Z, Xu X, Zhang B, Li Y, Liu J, Chen S, et al. Effect of simultaneous silencing of HPV-18 E6 and E7 on inducing apoptosis in HeLa cells. Biochem Cell Biol. 2010;88:697–704.

16. Huang DW, Sherman BT, Lempicki RA. Systematic and integrative analysis of large gene lists using DAVID bioinformatics resources. Nat Protoc. 2009;4:44–57.

17. Buettner FF, Ashikov A, Tiemann B, Lehle L, Bakker H. C. Elegans DPY-19 is a C-mannosyltransferase glycosylating thrombospondin repeats. Mol Cell. 2013;50:295–302.

18. Milde-Langosch K, Karn T, Schmidt M, zu Eulenburg C, Oliveira-Ferrer L, Wirtz RM, et al. Prognostic relevance of glycosylation-associated genes in breast cancer. Breast Cancer Res Treat. 2014;15:295–305.

19. Hall AHS, Alexander KA. RNA interference of human papillomavirus type 18 E6 and E7 induces senescence in HeLa cells. J Virol. 2003;77:6066–9.

20. Hirao T, Sakamoto Y, Kamada M, Hamada S, Aono T. Tn antigen, a marker of potential for metastasis of uterine cervix cancer cells. Cancer. 1993;72:154–9.

21. Kumar SR, Sauter ER, Quinn TP, Deutscher SL. Thomsen-Friedenreich and Tn antigens in nipple fluid: carbohydrate biomarkers for breast cancer detection. Clin Cancer Res. 2005;11:6868–71.

22. Danussi C, Coslovi A, Campa C, Mucignat MT, Spessotto P, Uggeri F, et al. A newly generated functional antibody identifies Tn antigen as a novel determinant in the cancer cell-lymphatic endothelium interaction. Glycobiology. 2009;19:1056–67.

23. Munkley J, Elliott DJ. Hallmarks of glycosylation in cancer. Oncotarget. 2016;7:35478–89.

24. Terasawa K, Furumoto H, Kamada M, Aono T. Expression of Tn and sialyl-Tn antigens in the neoplastic transformation of uterine cervical epithelial cells. Cancer Res. 1996;56:2229–32.

25. López-Morales D, Reyes-Leyva J, Santos-López G, Zenteno E, Vallejo-Ruiz V. Increased expression of sialic acid in cervical biopsies with squamous intraepithelial lesions. Diagn Pathol. 2010;4:74.

26. Kroes RA, Dawson G, Moskal JR. Focused microarray analysis of glyco-gene expression in human glioblastomas. J Neurochem. 2007;103:14–24.

27. Huang J, Che M, Lin N, Hung JS, Huang YT, Lin WC, et al. The molecular chaperone Cosmc enhances malignant behaviors of colon cancer cells via activation of Akt and ERK. Mol Carcinog. 2014;71:62–71.

28. P D, Owczarek T, Plazuk E, Gomułkiewicz A, Majchrzak M, Podhorska-Okołów M. Ceramide galactosyltransferase (UGT8) is a molecular marker of breast cancer malignancy and lung metastases. Br J Cancer. 2010;103:524–31.

29. Yokota S, Ogawara K, Kimura R, Shimizu F, Baba T, Minakawa Y, et al. Protein O-fucosyltransferase 1: a potential diagnostic marker and therapeutic target for human oral cancer. Int J Oncol. 2013;43:1864–70.

30. Petretti T, Schulze B, Schlag PM, Kemmner W. Altered mRNA expression of glycosyltransferases in human gastric carcinomas. Biochim Biophys Acta. 1999;1428:209–28.

31. Yan X, Lin Y, Liu S, Yan Q. Fucosyltransferase IV (FUT4) as an effective biomarker for the diagnosis of breast cancer. Biomed Pharmacother. 2015;70:299–304.

32. Petretti T, Kemmner W, Schulze B, Schlag PM. Altered mRNA expression of glycosyltransferases in human colorectal carcinomas and liver metastases. Gut. 2000;46:359–66.

33. Hirata H, Hinoda Y, Zaman MS, Chen Y, Ueno K, Majid S, et al. Function of UDP-glucuronosyltransferase 2B17 (UGT2B17) is involved in endometrial cancer. Carcinogenesis. 2010;31:1620–6.

34. Saito S, Yamashita S, Endoh M, Yamato T, Hoshi S, Ohyama C, et al. Clinical significance of ST3Gal IV expression in human renal cell carcinoma. Oncol Rep. 2002;9:1251–5.

35. Jun L, Yuanshu W, Yanying X, Zhongfa X, Jian Y, Fengling W, et al. Altered mRNA expressions of sialyltransferases in human gastric cancer tissues. Med Oncol. 2012;29:84–90.

36. Dang TP. Notch, apoptosis and Cancer. In: Reichrath J, Reichrath S, editors. Notch signaling in embryology and Cancer. US: Springer; 2012. p. 199–209.

37. Wei H, Cheng Z, Ouyang C, Zhang Y, Hu Y, Chen S, et al. Glycoprotein screening in colorectal cancer based on differentially expressed Tn antigen. Oncol Rep. 2016;36(3):1313–24.

38. Fu C, Zhao H, Wang Y, Cai H, Xiao Y, Zeng Y, et al. Tumor-associated antigens: Tn antigen, sTn antigen, and T antigen. HLA. 2016;88(6):275–86.

39. Stahl M, Uemura K, Ge C, Shi S, Tashima Y, Stanley P. Roles of Pofut1 and O-fucose in mammalian notch signaling. J Biol Chem. 2008;283:13638–51.

40. Yao D, Huang Y, Huang X, Wang W, Yan Q, Wei L, Xin W, et al. Protein O-fucosyltransferase 1 (Pofut1) regulates lymphoid and myeloid homeostasis through modulation of notch receptor ligand interactions. Blood. 2011;117:5652–62.

41. Okajima T, Reddy B, Matsuda T, Irvine KD. Contributions of chaperone and glycosyltransferase activities of O-fucosyltransferase 1 to notch signaling. BMC Biol. 2008;6(1).

42. Vodovar N, Schweisguth F. Functions of O-fucosyltransferase in notch trafficking and signaling: towards the end of a controversy? J Biol. 2008;7(2)

43. Zagouras P, Stifani S, Blaumueller CM, Carcangiu ML, Artavanis-Tsakonas S. Alterations in notch signaling in neoplastic lesions of the human cervix. Proc Natl Acad Sci. 1995;92:6414–8.

44. Daniel B, Rangarajan A, Mukherjee G, Vallikad E, Krishna S. The link between integration and expression of human papillomavirus type 16 genomes and cellular changes in the evolution of cervical intraepithelial neoplastic lesions. J Gen Virol. 1997;78:1095–101.

45. Ramdass B, Maliekal TT, Lakshmi S, Rehman M, Rema P, Nair P, et al. Coexpression of Notch1 and NF-kappaB signaling pathway components in human cervical cancer progression. Gynecolyc Oncology. 2007;104:352–61.

46. Song LL, Peng Y, Yun J, Rizzo P, Chaturvedi V, Weijzen S, et al. Notch-1 associates with IKKα and regulates IKK activity in cervical cancer cells. Oncogene. 2008;27:5833–44.

47. Maliekal TT, Bajaj J, Giri V, Subramanyam D, Krishna S. The role of notch signaling in human cervical cancer: implications for solid tumors. Oncogene. 2008;27:5110–4.

48. Sun L, Liu M, Sun GC, Yang X, Qian Q, Feng S, et al. Notch signaling activation in cervical Cancer cells induces cell growth arrest with the involvement of the nuclear receptor NR4A2. J Cancer. 2016;7:1388–95.

49. Ju T, Otto VI, Cummings RD. The Tn antigen-structural simplicity and biological complexity. Angew Chem Int Ed. 2011;50:1770–91.

50. Ju T, Aryal RP, Kudelka MR, Wang Y, Cummings RD. The Cosmc connection to the Tn antigen in cancer. Cancer Biomarkers. 2014;14:63–81.

51. Sousa AM, Grandgenett PM, David L, Almeida R, Hollingsworth MA, Santos-Silva F. Reflections on MUC1 glycoprotein: the hidden potential of isoforms in carcinogenesis. Acta Pathol Microbiol Immunol Scand. 2016;124:913–24.

52. Huang MJ, Hu RH, Chou CH, Hsu CL, Liu YW, Huang J, et al. Knockdown of GALNT1 suppresses malignant phenotype of hepatocellular carcinoma by suppressing EGFR signaling. Oncotarget. 2015;6:5650–65.

53. Li C, Du Y, Yang Z, He L, Wang Y, Hao L, et al. GALNT1-mediated glycosylation and activation of sonic hedgehog signaling maintains the self-renewal and tumor-initiating capacity of bladder cancer stem cells. Cancer Res. 2016;76:1273–83.

54. Stirewalt DL, Meshinchi S, Kopecky KJ, Fan W, Pogosova-Agadjanyan EL, Engel JH, et al. Identification of genes with abnormal expression changes in acute myeloid leukemia. Genes Chromosomes and Cancer. 2008;47:82–0.

55. Chen ZH, Yu YP, Tao J, Liu S, Tseng G, Nalesnik M, et al. MAN2A1-FER fusion gene is expressed by human liver and other tumor types and has oncogenic activity in mice. Gastroenterology. 2017;153:11203–2.

56. Yang L, Wang Y, Fang M, Deng D, Zhang Y. C3orf21 ablation promotes the proliferation of lung adenocarcinoma, and its mutation at the rs2131877 locus may serve as a susceptibility marker. Oncotarget. 2017;8:33422–31.

57. Ding M, Wang H, Wang J, Zhan H, Zuo YG, Yang DL, et al. ppGalNAc T1 as a potential novel marker for human bladder Cancer. Asian Pac J Cancer Prev. 2012;13:5653–72.

58. Venkitachalam S, Revoredo L, Varadan V, Fecteau RE, Ravi L, Lutterbaugh J, et al. Biochemical and functional characterization of glycosylation-associated mutational landscapes in colon cancer. Sci Rep. 2016;6:23642.

59. Rzechonek A, Cygan M, Blasiak P, Muszczynska-Bernhard B, Bobek V, Lubicz M, et al. Expression of Ceramide Galactosyltransferase (UGT8) in primary and metastatic lung tissues of non-small-cell lung Cancer. Adv Exp Med Biol. 2016;952:51–8.

26

Human papillomavirus genotype distribution in cervical cancer biopsies from Nepalese women

Sunil Kumar Sah[1†], Joaquin V. González[2,3†], Sadina Shrestha[1], Anurag Adhikari[4], Krishna Das Manandhar[6], Shyam Babu Yadav[5], David A. Stein[7], Birendra Prasad Gupta[6*] and María Alejandra Picconi[2,3]

Abstract

Background: Cervical cancer (CC) is the leading cause of morbidity and mortality from cancer in Nepalese women. Nearly all cases of CC are caused by infection with certain genotypes of human papillomavirus (HPV). Data on HPV genotype distribution in Nepalese CC patients is sparse. We aimed to determine the distribution of HPV genotypes in biopsies of CC tissue from Nepalese women.

Methods: This study examined 248 archived paraffin-embedded tissue specimens from CC cases from patients of B. P. Koirala Memorial Cancer Hospital, Bharatpur, Chitwan, Nepal. DNA was extracted from the biopsies and HPV detection performed by PCR. HPV genotyping was then carried out by a reverse line hybridization technique capable of identifying 36 distinct HPV genotypes.

Results: Most of the samples were from tumors that had been designated by hospital pathologists as squamous cell carcinoma (77.6%). 165 of the 248 samples contained DNA of sufficient quality for rigorous PCR testing. All the analyzable specimens were positive for HPV. The most common HPV genotypes, in decreasing order of frequency were 16, 18, 45, 33, 52, 56 and 31; most were found as single infections (94.5%). Together, HPV types 16, 18, and 45 were found in 92% of the tumor samples.

Conclusion: This study strengthens the knowledge-base of HPV genotype distribution in CC cases in Nepal. Hopefully, this information will be useful to the medical community and public health policy-makers in generating improved HPV-surveillance, −prevention and -treatment strategies in Nepal.

Keywords: Human papillomavirus, Cervical cancer, HPV genotyping, Nepal

Background

In 1983, Harald zur Hausen and colleagues isolated human papillomavirus (HPV)-16 and 18 from human cervical cancer (CC) tissues and helped define the central role of HPV in the development of CC [1]. HPV is now recognized as the etiologic agent causing almost all invasive CC and a major carcinogen causing other human malignancies as well, including vulvovaginal, oropharyngeal, penile, and anal cancers [2].

Currently, within the family *Papillomaviridae*, more than 200 HPV genotypes have been characterized [3]. Over 40 genotypes, all in the *Alphapapillomavirus* genus, can infect the female and male anogenital region. Infection with some of the genotypes can cause benign genital warts while others cause precursor cervical lesions, cervical intraepithelial neoplasia (CIN) and CC [4]. Of the 40, at least 12 HPV genotypes have been definitively associated with progression of CIN to CC and are considered carcinogenic to humans [5]. HPV genotypes 16, 18, 31, 33, 35, 39, 45, 51, 52, 56, 58, and 59 are classified as carcinogenic to humans (Group 1; often referred to as high-risk, HR), HPV-68 as probably carcinogenic to humans (Group 2A), HPV-types 26, 30, 34, 53, 66, 67, 69, 70, 73, 82, 85 and 97 (Group 2B) as possibly

* Correspondence: birendraphd@gmail.com
†Equal contributors
6Central Department of Biotechnology, Tribhuvan University, Kirtipur, Kathmandu, Nepal
Full list of author information is available at the end of the article

carcinogenic to humans, while HPV-6 and 11 (Group 3; often referred to as low-risk, LR) are not currently classifiable as to their carcinogenicity to humans [6]. Of the HR-HPV-genotypes, genotypes 31, 33, 35, 52 are phylogenetically related to HPV-16 while genotypes 39, 45, 59, and probably 68 are more closely related to HPV-18 [7].

Worldwide, CC is the fourth most common type of cancer among women, and causes over 40% mortality [8]. Currently, more than 80% of new CC cases are diagnosed in lower- and middle-income countries such as Nepal, India, Bangladesh and Sri Lanka [9]. Annually, in Nepal, over 2000 new cases of CC are diagnosed and over 1000 deaths are attributed to CC [10]. However, due to the lack of both a national screening program for CC and a reliable national database for cancer cases in general, the actual number of cases and deaths probably exceeds those reported estimates [11].

Nepal is located in Southern Asia, adjacent to both India and China, in the Himalayan region. Along with indigenous peoples, many of Nepal's inhabitants are descendants of migrants from India, southern China, Myanmar, Tibet and other areas of Central Asia, making Nepal a multiethnic and multicultural country. Nepal's population has been steadily rising in recent decades, currently reaching approximately 26 million (census 2011). As in most developing countries, a spectrum of sanitary and public health conditions are present, due at least in part to transportation limitations and reduced access to medical services in rural compared to urban areas.

Several studies have addressed the prevalence and genotypes of HPV circulating in Nepalese females having non-cancerous cytology, as well as in those having preneoplastic and neoplastic cervical lesions [9]. However, current and comprehensive data regarding HPV genotype distribution in Nepalese CC cases is scarce.

Although HPV-16 and 18 are the predominant HPV genotypes associated with CC worldwide, at least 25% of CC cases are associated with other HPV genotypes [12]. Differences in the relative prevalence of the various CC-associated HPV genotypes has been documented to occur both regionally and across more large-scale geographic areas [13].

Three prophylactic HPV vaccines are currently available worldwide: a quadrivalent vaccine was first licensed in 2006, a bivalent vaccine in 2007 and a nonavalent vaccine in 2014. All protect against infection with HPV-16 and 18; while the most recent also protects against five additional HR-HPV types (HPV-31, 33, 45, 52, and 58). Current evidence suggests the three vaccines offer comparable efficacy in prevention of CC. The choice of HPV-vaccine is typically based on data regarding a number of factors, including the type and scale of local HPV-associated pathologies, the target-populations for which the vaccine has been approved and product characteristics (e.g. cost, availability) [14].

The goal of this study was to determine the distribution of HPV-genotypes found in CC cases of Nepalese women. We are hopeful that this information will be useful to public-health officials for designing improved strategies for the prevention of HPV-infection and its related diseases.

Methods
Study design
A retrospective cross-sectional study was designed and coordinated by the BP Koirala Memorial Cancer Hospital (BPKMCH), Bharatpur, Chitwan, Nepal, in collaboration with the Central Department of Biotechnology, Tribhuvan University, Kritipur, Nepal, Kathmandu Research Institute for Biological Sciences, Lalitpur, Nepal, and the National Institute of Infectious Diseases (INEI) -ANLIS "Dr. Malbrán", Buenos Aires, Argentina. The study was approved by the Nepal Health Research Council.

Archived formalin-fixed paraffin-embedded sections of tumor tissue biopsies that had been excised from CC patients (30–99 year old women) during 2011 to 2014 at BPKMCH were examined. A random sampling method was used for tissue specimen selection and de-identification was done prior to specimen handling, to avoid any sampling-bias. Information regarding the age at collection, year of collection, and histological findings generated from the samples was obtained.

Fixed and paraffin embedded cervical tissue block processing
All cervical tumor tissue blocks were processed at INEI under stringent laboratory conditions to avoid contamination of or between samples. For each ten case-block of samples, a paraffin blank-block was also sectioned and included, as a control for contamination. One to five 10 μm sections of tissue from each sample were transferred to a 1.5 mL screw-cap tubes using a fresh tooth pick for each section, for use in downstream techniques described below. Fresh gloves were used for each case. After the sectioning of each case the scalpel used was cleaned with R-WAX (BioPack, Argentina). A blank-block was sectioned after each ten case-block.

DNA extraction
DNA was extracted from the sectioned blocks using a method developed at the United States Centers for Disease Control (US CDC) using the QIAamp DNA Blood MiniKit (QIAGEN) [15]. Briefly, 180 μl of ATL buffer was added to a microcentrifuge tube containing a single tissue section and heated at 120 °C for 20 min, which melted the paraffin. At approximately 5 min into the heating step, the tube contents were mixed by gentle

tapping. After heating, the samples were incubated at room temperature for 3 min, followed by quick centrifugation. Twenty microliters of proteinase K was added to the tube, followed by brief vortexing, then incubated at 65 °C for 16 h [15]. The tubes where then briefly centrifuged and 200 μl ATL buffer and 200 μl ethanol was added, yielding a final volume of around 400 μl. After a brief vortex the mixture was loaded into a QIAamp Mini spin column and centrifuged at 8000 rpm for 1 min. The elution steps were performed according to the manufacturer's protocol except the elution volume was 50 μl AE buffer pre-warmed to 55 °C.

HPV detection and genotyping

HPV detection was performed using PCR with biotinylated Broad-Spectrum General Primers (BSGP) 5+/6+ designed to amplify a highly conserved 140 bp fragment of the HPV-L1 gene [16]. Genotyping was carried out by a reverse hybridization line which identifies 36 HPV- genotypes (6,11,16,18,26,31,33,34,35,39,40,42,43,44,45,51,52,53,54,55, 56,57,58,59,61,66,68,70,71,72,73,81,82,83,84,89). Briefly, the denatured biotynilated amplicons, obtained from amplification of sample DNA with BSGP5+/GP6+ primers, were hybridized with genotype-specific oligonucleotide probes immobilized as parallel lines on membrane strips (Reverse Line Blot Hybridization, RLB). The hybrids were treated with alkaline phosphatase-streptavidin conjugate and substrate (ECL Detection Reagents) resulting in a chemiluminescent product subsequently detected by exposure to autoradiography film. The β-globin gene was co-amplified and its relative abundance detected in each sample, to serve as an internal control [17]. The INEI laboratory, which performed the HPV detection and genotyping in this work, is the HPV Regional Reference Laboratory for the Americas (within the Global HPV Laboratory Network (Global HPVLabNet)) and annually participates in an international Global HPV DNA typing proficiency study [18].

Data analysis

Data analysis was performed using Epi Info version 3.5.3 (US CDC). In determining the frequency of HPV genotypes, each sample was scored for the genotype detected and, if more than a single genotype was detected, for the combination of genotypes detected.

Results

Of the 248 paraffin embedded CC tissue blocks originally selected, the β-globin gene was amplifiable in only 165, thus our further analysis was restricted to this subset. Histological analysis of these samples revealed that 81 of the 165 blocks contained squamous cell carcinoma (Fig. 1).

All the 165 analyzed blocks were positive for HPV; among them, 156 (94.5%) were infected with a single genotype and 9 (5.5%) were infected with multiple genotypes. Almost all cases were positive for at least one HR-HPV genotype, and one sample harbored HPV-6 (Table 1). The HPV genotypes identified belong to one of five species of the fifteen total species of the α-papillomavirus genus: α5 (HPV-51; 0.5%), α6 (HPV-56; 2.3%), α7 (HPV-18, 39, 45 and 68; total: 20.7%), α9 (HPV-16, 31, 33, 35 and 52; total: 75.9%), and α10 (HPV-6; 0.5%).

The most common genotypes detected, in decreasing order of frequency, were HPV-16, 18, 45, 33, 52, 56, and 31. HPV-16, 18, and 45 were the three most prevalent types in all histological groups (squamous cell carcinoma, adenocarcinoma, and adenosquamous cell carcinoma). One or more of these three genotypes were detected in 152/165 (92%) of the tumor tissue samples.

Samples testing positive for HPV-18 or 45 were from women of a higher age than those infected with HPV-16 (Table 2). The mean ages of women with invasive CC associated with HPV-16, 18 and 45 were 45–57 years (95% CI 43.5–47.5), 55.4 years (50.3–60.6) and 52.3 years (44.1–60.5), respectively, while the average age of those with CC associated with any other HPV genotype was higher, at 56 years [53.9–58.1].

Discussion

This study defines the HPV-genotype distribution in the largest series of CC tissue samples from Nepal addressed to date. We analyzed archived biopsy specimens from the B.P. Koirala Memorial Cancer Hospital, one of the few hospitals in Nepal specializing in cancer diagnosis and treatment. Patients from throughout Nepal are referred to this hospital, thus the samples analyzed can be considered as representative of the Nepalese population overall.

In our study, HPV detection was performed by PCR using the BSGP5+/6 + multiplexed with-globin system, which is technically superior to the original GP5+/6+ PCR system [16], and suitable for large-scale epidemiological studies. The PCR system we used is designed to amplify fragmented DNA and thus the detection method of choice with archived formalin-fixed, paraffin-embedded tissues samples, which are prone to degradation from fixative-induced cross-linking [19].

In agreement with previously published studies on CC in local, regional and worldwide populations, we found that squamous cell carcinoma was the dominant CC histo-type (77.6%) [12].

Our results are consistent with previous studies documenting HPV-16 as the most common and HPV-18 as the second-most common genotypes associated with CC worldwide. We found HPV-16 and 18 to be associated

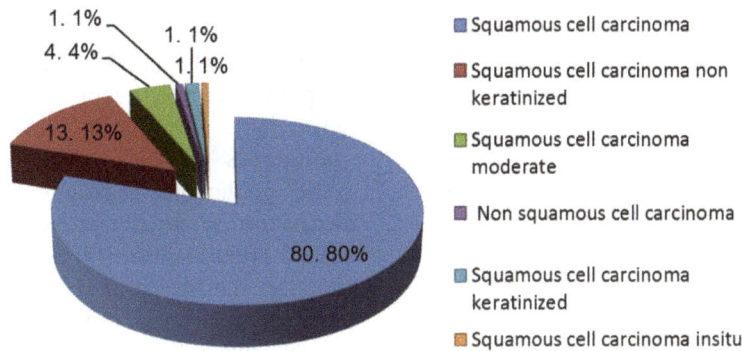

Fig. 1 Histological diagnosis of cervical cancer analyzed in the study

with 87% of the total CC tissue samples in our study, consistent with a previous study of 54 Nepalese cases detecting HPV-16/18 in 90% of samples [20] . Our study detected HPV-16/18 at a moderately higher rate than previously reported for Southern Asia (80%) [21], and the Asian region (71%) in a worldwide study [12], but a little smaller than those rates from Eastern India that exceeds 100%, considering multiple infections (HPV-16: 83.78%; HPV-18, 21.08%) [22].

HPV45 was the next most common genotype found in our study (4.8%), in agreement with previous publications on local and regional populations [12, 20]. Together the three most-common HPV genotypes (HPV-16, 18 and 45) were found in over 90% of our samples. Our results vary somewhat from a previous study which detected HPV-58 in 4.0% of Asia-wide samples [12] whereas here, with Nepal-only samples, HPV-58 was not detected at all. As well, HPV-56 was present in < 1% of samples in the Asia-wide data while in our study it was detected in 2.4% of samples.

The obtained results confirmed the inverse correlation between HPV genotype diversity and progressive disease [23]. Also in Nepal, the genotype distribution in normal cytology reveals a wide spectrum of HPV types, both low and high risk types, without marked predominance of none of them (HPV-70, 4.7%; HPV-16, 1.4%; HPV-58, 0.9%; HPV-56, 0.7%; HPV-18, 0.6%; HPV-52 y 39, 0.4%; HPV-35, 0.3%; HPV-33 y 45, 0.2%) [24–26]; as the severity of the cervical lesion increases, HR-HPV genotype become the most frequent types, being almost the only ones in CC, with a remarkable majority of HPV-16 and HPV-18, as it was shown in our study.

Most of the samples examined in this study were infected with only one HPV genotype, which is consistent with the previously observed inverse correlation between HPV diversity and neoplastic lesion [19]. Moreover, our findings are consistent with the ecological principles of competitive exclusion and carcinogenesis hallmarked by clonal expansion and evolution of transformed cells [27, 28].

Table 1 Distribution of HPV genotypes in cervical cancer from Nepalese women

HPV Genotype HR-HPV	Samples (n = 165) Frequency (%)	Single infection (a) Frequency (%)	Multiple infection (b) Frequency (%)
16	119 (72, 2)	111 (93.3)	8 (6.7)
18	25 (14,8)	22 (88.0)	3 (12.0)
31	3 (1.8)	2 (66.7)	1 (33.3)
33	4 (2,4)	4 (100)	0 (0)
35	2 (1,2)	2 (100)	0 (0)
39	2 (1,2)	1 (50)	1 (50)
45	8 (4,8)	6 (75)	2 (25)
51	1 (< 1)	0 (0)	1 (100)
52	4 (2,4)	2 (50)	2 (50)
56	4 (2,4)	4 (100)	0 (0)
68	1 (< 1)	1 (100)	0 (0)
LR-HPV			
6	1 (< 1)	1 (100)	0 (0)

Table 2 Distribution of HPV genotypes (single and multiple infections) in invasive cervical cancer according to age among Nepalese women

HPV genotype	Age (Years) Frequency (%)				Total Frequency (%)
	< 40	40–49	50–59	> 60	
6	0 (0%)	0 (0%)	1 (100.0%)	0 (0%)	1 (100%)
16	7 (6.3%)	27 (24.3%)	42 (37.9%)	35 (31.5%)	111 (100%)
18	1 (4.5%)	7 (31.8%)	6 (27.3%)	8 (36.4%)	22 (100%)
31	0 (0%)	1 (50.0%)	0 (0%)	1 (50.0%)	2 (100%)
33	0 (0%)	1 (25.0%)	0 (0%)	3 (75.0%)	4 (100%)
35	0 (0%)	1 (50.0%)	1 (50.0%)	0 (0%)	2 (100%)
39	0 (0%)	0 (0%)	0 (0%)	1 (100.0%)	1 (100%)
45	0 (0%)	2 (33.3%)	2 (33.3%)	2 (33.3%)	6 (100%)
52	1 (50.0%)	0 (0%)	0 (0%)	1 (50.0%)	2 (100%)
56	0 (0%)	0 (0%)	2 (50.0%)	2 (50.0%)	4 (100%)
68	0 (0%)	0 (0%)	1 (100.0%)	0 (0%)	1 (100%)
16 + 18	1 (33.3%)	0 (0%)	1 (33.3%)	1 (33.3%)	3 (100%)
16 + 39	0 (0%)	0 (0%)	0 (0%)	1 (100.0%)	1 (100%)
16 + 45	0 (0%)	0 (0%)	2 (100.0%)	0 (0%)	2 (100%)
16 + 51	0 (0%)	0 (0%)	1 (100.0%)	0 (0%)	1 (100%)
16 + 52	0 (0%)	1 (0%)	0 (0%)	0 (0%)	1 (100%)
31 + 52	0 (0%)	1 (0%)	0 (0%)	0 (0%)	1 (100%)

Our detection of HPV-6 in one CC biopsy containing no other HPV-genotypes is a rare and noteworthy event. According to the IARC-WHO Working Group Reports, the carcinogenic potential of HPV-6 and 11 is considered "not classifiable", a category which includes agents that are considered to have low carcinogenic potential, based on the available epidemiological and experimental data [28]. The rationale for this categorization of HPV-6 and 11, rather than the "probably not carcinogenic" classification, is the low but established probability of finding either genotype associated with a small percentage (0.45% [95% CI: 0.35–0.56]) of CC cases worldwide. It has been postulated that HPV-6 and other low-risk genotypes may in rare cases cause cancer as a result of unusual "virus-host circumstances" [29].

The results from this and previous studies documenting the presence of HPV-16 and 18 in a high percentage of CC tissue samples represent further evidence that implementation of an HPV vaccine program designed to address at least these two HPV genotypes could significantly lower the incidence of CC in Nepal. Fortunately, all three HPV vaccines provide considerable cross-protection against numerous disease-associated HPV types not specifically included as antigenic targets in the respective vaccine formulations. Based on evidence from clinical trials and post-introduction impact evaluations, the bivalent and quadrivalent HPV vaccines provide protection against HR-HPV genotypes other than HPV-16 and 18, such as HPV-31, 33 and 45, all of which have been implicated to cause preneoplastic lesions and subsequent cancer [30].

Numerous previous studies have made similar optimistic predictions regarding the potential of HPV-vaccination to greatly reduce the overall number of cervical abnormalities [14, 31]. Preceding studies in developing countries have documented that HPV vaccination supplemented with regular screening is a highly cost-effective strategy to reduce the incidence of and mortality from cervical cancer [32].

Conclusion

This study increases our knowledge of HPV genotype distribution in cervical cancer cases from Nepal. In anticipation that Nepal will soon implement more effective widespread public health measures to prevent HPV infections and their sequelas, particularly CC, it is important to have epidemiologic data regarding the prevalence of HPV genotypes. Considering the high prevalence of HPV-16 and 18 (83%) found in the CC from Nepalese women in this study, we expect that the widespread introduction of any of the approved HPV-vaccines will sharply decrease the incidence of CC in Nepal. Considering the cross-protection generated against most or all of the disease-associated HR-HPV genotypes by the currently-marketed vaccines, including the relatively inexpensive bivalent vaccine [30, 33], widespread vaccination with any of the current HPV vaccines is expected to have a multiplicity of benefits to Nepalese public health. It is our hope that this study will be useful to Nepalese public-health officials in generating improved strategies for prevention of HPV infection and its associated diseases, as well as pre- and post-vaccine surveillance.

Abbreviations

BPKMCH: B. P. Koirala memorial cancer hospital; BSGP: Broad-Spectrum General Primers; Ca: cancer; CC: cervical cancer; CDC: center for disease control; CI: confidence interval; CIN: cervical intraepithelial neoplasia; GHPVLN: Global HPV laboratory network; HPV: human papillomavirus; HR: high risk; ICC: invasive cervical cancer; LR: low risk; SCC: squamous cell carcinoma

Acknowledgements

We would like to thanks Dr. C. B. Pun, Dr. Sadina Shrestha, Keshav Prasad Paudel and the staff from BP Koirala memorial cancer hospital pathology department for their cooperation and expertise.

Funding

None

Authors' contributions

SKS, SS participated to archive the tissue blocks, provided the clinical, demographic information and histopathological report; JVG performed the genotyping assays, and participated in the analysis and interpretation of the results; BPG, AA, KDM, SBY participated to design the study and manuscript preparation; MAP and DAS participated in analysis and interpretation of the results, and writing of the manuscript. All authors read and approved the final manuscript.

Competing interest

The authors declare that they have no competing interests.

Author details

[1]B. P. Koirala Memorial Cancer Hospital, Bharatpur, Chitwan, Nepal.
[2]Oncogenic Viruses Laboratory, National Institute of Infectious Diseases-ANLIS "Dr. Malbrán", Av. Velez Sarsfield 563, C1282AFF Buenos Aires, Argentina.
[3]National and Regional HPV Reference Laboratory, National Institute of Infectious Diseases-ANLIS "Dr. Malbrán", Av. Velez Sarsfield 563, C1282AFF Buenos Aires, Argentina. [4]Kathmandu Research Institute for Biological Sciences, Lalitpur, Nepal. [5]Department of Health Service, Ministry of Health, Government of Nepal, Kathmandu, Nepal. [6]Central Department of Biotechnology, Tribhuvan University, Kirtipur, Kathmandu, Nepal. [7]Department of Biomedical Sciences, Oregon State University, Corvallis, Oregon, USA.

References

1. Dürst M, Gissmann L, Ikenberg H, Zur Hausen H. A papillomavirus DNA from a cervical carcinoma and its prevalence in cancer biopsy samples from different geographic regions. Proc Natl Acad Sci. 1983;80(12):3812–5.
2. MM wALBooMER J, Acos Mv, MANos° MM, xAvıER BosCH F, KUMMER JA: HUMAN PAPILLOMAVIRUS IS a NECESSARY CAUSE OF INVASIVE CERVICAL CANCER. WORLDWIDE. J Pathol 1999, 189:12–19.
3. Bzhalava D, Eklund C, Dillner J. International standardization and classification of human papillomavirus types. Virology. 2015;476:341–4.
4. De Villiers E-M, Fauquet C, Broker TR, Bernard H-U, zur Hausen H. Classification of papillomaviruses. Virology. 2004;324(1):17–27.
5. Muñoz N, Bosch FX, de Sanjosé S, Herrero R, Castellsagué X, Shah KV, Snijders PJ, Meijer CJ. Epidemiologic classification of human papillomavirus types associated with cervical cancer. N Engl J Med 2003. 2003;348:518–27.
6. Bouvard V, Baan R, Straif K, Grosse Y, Secretan B, El Ghissassi F, Benbrahim-Tallaa L, Guha N, Freeman C, Galichet L: A review of human carcinogens—part B: biological agents. In: Elsevier; 2009.
7. Harari A, Chen Z, Burk RD. Human papillomavirus genomics: past, present and future. In: Human Papillomavirus. Volume 45, edn.: Karger publishers; 2014. p. 1–18.
8. Jemal A, Bray F, Center MM, Ferlay J, Ward E, Forman D. Global cancer statistics. CA Cancer J Clin. 2011;61(2):69–90.
9. Sankaranarayanan R, Bhatla N, Gravitt PE, Basu P, Esmy PO, Ashrafunnessa K, Ariyaratne Y, Shah A, Nene BM. Human papillomavirus infection and cervical cancer prevention in India, Bangladesh, Sri Lanka and Nepal. Vaccine. 2008; 26:M43–52.
10. Denny L. Cervical cancer prevention and treatment in low-resource settings. A Textbook of Gynecology for Less-Resourced Locations London: Sapiens Pub. 2012:317–36.
11. Bruni L, Barrionuevo-Rosas L, Albero G: ICO information center on HPV and cancer (HPV Information Center). Human papilloma virus and related diseases in Bangladesh. In.: Summary report 2016–02-26 [Data Accessed]; 2015.
12. de Sanjose S, Quint WG, Alemany L, Geraets DT, Klaustermeier JE, Lloveras B, Tous S, Felix A, Bravo LE, Shin H-R. Human papillomavirus genotype attribution in invasive cervical cancer: a retrospective cross-sectional worldwide study. The lancet oncology. 2010;11(11):1048–56.
13. Schiffman M, Rodriguez AC, Chen Z, Wacholder S, Herrero R, Hildesheim A, Desalle R, Befano B, Yu K, Safaeian M. A population-based prospective study of carcinogenic human papillomavirus variant lineages, viral persistence, and cervical neoplasia. Cancer Res. 2010;70(8):3159–69.
14. Organization WH. Human papillomavirus vaccines: WHO position paper, may 2017–recommendations. Vaccine. 2017;
15. Steinau M, Patel SS, Unger ER. Efficient DNA extraction for HPV genotyping in formalin-fixed, paraffin-embedded tissues. The Journal of Molecular Diagnostics. 2011;13(4):377–81.
16. Schmitt M, Dondog B, Waterboer T, Pawlita M. Homogeneous amplification of genital human alpha papillomaviruses by PCR using novel broad-spectrum GP5+ and GP6+ primers. J Clin Microbiol. 2008;46(3):1050–9.
17. van den Brule AJ, Pol R, Fransen-Daalmeijer N, Schouls LM, Meijer CJ, Snijders PJ. GP5+/6+ PCR followed by reverse line blot analysis enables rapid and high-throughput identification of human papillomavirus genotypes. J Clin Microbiol. 2002;40(3):779–87.
18. Eklund C, Forslund O, Wallin K-L, Dillner J: Global improvement in genotyping of human papillomavirus DNA: the 2011 HPV LabNet International Proficiency Study. Journal of clinical microbiology 2013:JCM. 02453–02413.
19. Quint W, Jenkins D, Molijn A, Struijk L, van de Sandt M, Doorbar J, Mols J, Van Hoof C, Hardt K, Struyf F. One virus, one lesion—individual components of CIN lesions contain a specific HPV type. J Pathol. 2012;227(1):62–71.
20. Sherpa ATL, Clifford GM, Vaccarella S, Shrestha S, Nygård M, Karki BS, Snijders PJ, Meijer CJ, Franceschi S. Human papillomavirus infection in women with and without cervical cancer in Nepal. Cancer Causes Control. 2010;21(3):323–30.
21. Bruni L, BarrionuevoRosas L, Albero G, Aldea M, Serrano B, Valencia S: ICO Information Centre on HPV and Cancer (HPV Information Centre). Human Papillomavirus and Related Diseases in the World. Summary Report 2015. In.: HPV information center; 2014.
22. Senapati R, Nayak B, Kar SK, Dwibedi B. HPV genotypes distribution in Indian women with and without cervical carcinoma: implication for HPV vaccination program in Odisha, eastern India. BMC Infect Dis. 2017;17(1):30.
23. Stoler MH, Wright TC Jr, Sharma A, Apple R, Gutekunst K, Wright TL. High-risk human papillomavirus testing in women with ASC-US cytology: results from the ATHENA HPV study. Am J Clin Pathol. 2011;135(3):468–75.
24. Bruni L, Diaz M, Castellsagué M, Ferrer E, Bosch FX, de Sanjosé S. Cervical human papillomavirus prevalence in 5 continents: meta-analysis of 1 million women with normal cytological findings. J Infect Dis. 2010;202(12):1789–99.
25. De Sanjosé S, Diaz M, Castellsagué X, Clifford G, Bruni L, Muñoz N, Bosch FX. Worldwide prevalence and genotype distribution of cervical human papillomavirus DNA in women with normal cytology: a meta-analysis. Lancet Infect Dis. 2007;7(7):453–9.
26. Johnson DC, Bhatta MP, Smith JS, Kempf M-C, Broker TR, Vermund SH, Chamot E, Aryal S, Lhaki P, Shrestha S. Assessment of high-risk human papillomavirus infections using clinician-and self-collected cervical sampling methods in rural women from far western Nepal. PLoS One. 2014;9(6): e101255.
27. Depuydt CE, Thys S, Beert J, Jonckheere J, Salembier G, Bogers JJ. Linear viral load increase of a single HPV-type in women with multiple HPV infections predicts progression to cervical cancer. Int J Cancer. 2016;139(9):2021–32.
28. Shen-Gunther J, Wang C-M, Poage GM, Lin C-L, Perez L, Banks NA, Huang TH-M. Molecular pap smear: HPV genotype and DNA methylation of ADCY8, CDH8, and ZNF582 as an integrated biomarker for high-grade cervical cytology. Clin Epigenetics. 2016;8(1):96.
29. Schiffman M, Clifford G, Buonaguro FM. Classification of weakly carcinogenic human papillomavirus types: addressing the limits of epidemiology at the borderline. Infectious agents and cancer. 2009;4(1):8.
30. Malagón T, Drolet M, Boily M-C, Franco EL, Jit M, Brisson J, Brisson M. Cross-protective efficacy of two human papillomavirus vaccines: a systematic review and meta-analysis. Lancet Infect Dis. 2012;12(10):781–9.
31. Gertig DM, Brotherton JM, Budd AC, Drennan K, Chappell G, Saville AM. Impact of a population-based HPV vaccination program on cervical abnormalities: a data linkage study. BMC Med. 2013;11(1):227.

32. Gervais F, Dunton K, Jiang Y, Largeron N. Systematic review of cost-effectiveness analyses for combinations of prevention strategies against human papillomavirus (HPV) infection: a general trend. BMC Public Health. 2017;17(1):283.

33. Kavanagh K, Pollock KG, Cuschieri K, Palmer T, Cameron RL, Watt C, Bhatia R, Moore C, Cubie H, Cruickshank M. Changes in the prevalence of human papillomavirus following a national bivalent human papillomavirus vaccination programme in Scotland: a 7-year cross-sectional study. Lancet Infect Dis. 2017;17(12):1293–302.

HPV infection and p53 and p16 expression in esophageal cancer: are they prognostic factors?

Allini Mafra da Costa[1,2*], José Humberto Tavares Guerreiro Fregnani[1], Paula Roberta Aguiar Pastrez[1,3], Vânia Sammartino Mariano[1,3], Estela Maria Silva[1,3], Cristovam Scapulatempo Neto[1], Denise Peixoto Guimarães[3,4], Luisa Lina Villa[5,6], Laura Sichero[5], Kari Juhani Syrjanen[1,3,7] and Adhemar Longatto-Filho[1,3,8,9,10]

Abstract

Background: Esophageal squamous cell carcinoma (ESCC) is a highly lethal malignant tumor. Currently, Human papillomavirus (HPV) is suggested as a potential risk factor for esophageal cancer (EC) in addition to the classic risk factors, alcohol and tobacco, but this hypothesis still remains contradictory. We sought to investigate wether HPV and well-known biomarkers (p16 and p53) and patient-related factors that may have impact on survival of ESCC.

Methods: We conducted a prospective cohort study. By using multiplex PCR, we determined the prevalence of high risk HPV in ESCC, and evaluated the immunohistochemical expression of p16 and p53, molecular markers related to esophageal carcinogenesis in order to verify the potential influence of these variables in patients's survival. Survival rates were estimated using Kaplan-Meier methods. A multivariate confirmatory model was performed using Cox proportional hazards regression.

Results: Twelve (13.8%) of 87 patients were HPV-DNA positive. Positive reactions of p16 and p53 were 10.7% and 68.6%, respectively. Kaplan-Meier analysis indicated that men ($p = 0.025$) had poor specific-cancer survival and a shorter progression-free survival ($p = 0.050$) as compared to women; III or IV clinical stage ($p < 0.019$) had poor specific-cancer survival and a shorter progression-free survival ($p < 0.001$) compared to I and II clinical stage; not submitted to surgery (<0.001) and not submitted to chemoradiotherapy ($p = 0.039$) had a poor specific-cancer survival, as well. The multivariate analysis showed that HPV, p16 and p53 status are not predictive parameters of progression-free and specific-cancer survival.

Conclusion: HPV infection and p53 and p16 expression are not prognostic factors in ESCC.

Keywords: Human Papillomavirus, Esophageal cancer, Survival

Background

Presently, esophageal cancer (EC) is regarded as an important public health problem worldwide, being considered the eighth most common type of cancer and the sixth leading cause of cancer death according to estimates by GLOBOCAN 2012 [1].

Despite recent advances in multidisciplinary treatments, including radical surgical resection, chemotherapy and radiotherapy, the 5-year survival rate of patients with esophageal squamous cell carcinoma (ESCC) remains being less than 30%, and this is due mainly to atypical early symptoms, middle-to-late stage diagnosis, low treatment remission rates and high local recurrence rates, requiring the identification of a suitable biomarker to predict their long-term survival [2, 3].

Recently, evidence suggests that human papillomavirus (HPV) may play an important role in ESCC development; a number of studies in this area has increased steadily, as evidenced in several reviews [4–9]. First descriptions of

* Correspondence: mafra.allini@gmail.com
[1]Teaching and Research Institute, Barretos Cancer Hospital – Pius XII Foundation, Rua Antenor Duarte Vilela, 1331, Dr. Paulo Prata, Barretos, São Paulo 14784-400, Brazil
[2]Cancer Registry, Barretos Cancer Hospital – Pius XII Foundation, São Paulo, Brazil
Full list of author information is available at the end of the article

oral lesions associated with HPV were preceded by reports that suggested the involvement of viruses in the development of benign [10] and malignant [11] lesions of the squamous epithelium of the esophagus. These initial observations were based on the report of morphological similarities between HPV lesions in the genital tract (warts) and esophageal papillomas [10, 11].

The first report that demonstrated the presence of HPV in ESCC occurred more than 30 years [10]; however, its prevalence is significantly variable among different geographical regions, and its role in carcinogenesis is still a matter of debate. Although the number of studies and interest in the subject has increased in recent years, literature is still controversial [12]. Data accumulated reflects a trend linking HPV infection and EC in high risk areas, whereas in low-risk areas such association was not evident [13].

The molecular genetic background of ESCC, mainly researches on protein alterations, has been widely studied and may assist in the prognosis of patients [14]. Proteins such as p53, p16 and others have been considered as prognostic factors for ESCC [15].

The differential expression of the tumor suppressor protein p53 is one of the commonest abnormality in several cancer types, including EC, and its mutation is mainly related to cell invasion and metastasis, as well as being related to advanced stages of the disease [14]. These mutations can lead to an increase in expression of p53, which accumulates in the nuclei and can be detected by immunohistochemistry (IHC) methods [16, 17]. The p16 protein expression is frequently used as a surrogate marker for HPV infection, and was shown as a marker for responder and better prognosis among head and neck squamous cell carcinoma patients who underwent radiotherapy [18]. Similarly, high p16 expression supposedly correlates with favorable prognosis in esophageal squamous cell carcinoma as well [19, 20], although data are still limited and variable [16, 18–23].

A retrospective cohort study with 136 ESCC patients has showed that p53 overexpression was associated with poor prognosis in these patients and a significantly independent predictor of poor overall survival [16]. However, this prognostic role of p53 overexpression in ESCC remained unclear [16].

Necessary strategies to improve prognosis and survival rates in patients with EC require early diagnosis and treatment, which rely on studying and exploring factors that influence the prognosis of such neoplasia.

This study aimed to evaluate the correlation of HPV infection and the expression of p53 and p16 with clinicopathologic factors, and whether they are ESCC prognostic factors for cancer progression (survival).

Methods

This was a prospective cohort study. Briefly, the patients of both genders, aged above 18 years, admitted to the Barretos Cancer Hospital, with histopathological confirmation of ESCC, clinical indication for endoscopy and no previous treatment for cancer were included. Medical records were available to obtain clinical and follow-up data.

Sample collection, HPV detection and characterization

The procedure for conducting the Digestive Endoscopy followed the routine of the Department of Endoscopy at Barretos Cancer Hospital using sedation, flexible video endoscopes (Olympus 180, Japan; Fuginon 4400, Japan) and Single-Use Radial Jaw 4 Biopsy Forceps (Boston Scientific Corporation, Natick, MA). Biological samples were collected from tumors tissues, fixed in 10% buffered formalin and embedded in paraffin. Slides were routinely stained with Hematoxylin-Eosin.

HPV DNA, obtainened by organic extraction [24], was measured in all samples using type-specific PCR bead-based multiplex genotyping (TS-MPG) assays that combine multiplex polymerase chain reaction (PCR) and bead based Luminex technology (Luminex Corp., Austin, TX, USA), as described by Pastrez et al. and da Costa et al. [25, 26].

A primer set targeting the β-globin gene were included as a positive control for the quality of the template DNA and the mix without sample was a negative control. HPV multiplex PCR was performed with QIAGEN Multiplex PCR Kit (Qiagen, Dusseldorf, Germany), according to manufacturer's instructions, and the details of the reaction can be seen in Pastrez et al. [25] methodology.

For the hybridization assay, the mean fluorescence intensity (MFI) values were obtained when no PCR product was added to the mixture of hybridization was considered as background, for each probe, was performed according to Schmitt et al. (2006) [27]. The cutoff was calculated by adding 5 MFI for 1.1 X the value of median found, and values higher than 20 MFI was considered positive.

Immunohistochemistry

The immunohistochemistry expression of p16 and p53 proteins were analyzed in automated system (Ventana Benchmark ULTRA, CA, USA) using a primary antibody against p16 (monoclonal mouse anti-human p16INK4A protein, Clone E6H4TM, ready for use, Roche Brazil) and p53 (monoclonal mouse anti-human p53 protein, Clone DO-7, dilution 1:1200, Cell Marque, Rocklin, CA, USA). The scores for analysis oh the proteins and details can be seen in a former study recently published [25].

Statistical analysis

Survival rates were estimated in months, and survival was defined as the period from the date of diagnosis to the date of death or the date at which information was last obtained from the patient. For the analysis, the event of interest was death related to cancer to specific-cancer survival and the locoregional recurrence, progression or metastasis to progression-free survival. Cases that were alive or dead from other causes were censored to specific-cancer survival and without locoregional recurrence, progression or metastasis to progression-free survival. Such information was obtained through direct consultation to the death certificate or medical records. Multiple confirmatory models were used to check whether HPV, p53 and p16 status were related to prognosis of ESCC. Multivariable Cox proportional hazards regression models was used to estimate hazard ratios (HR) and 95% confidence intervals (CI) with adjustment for sex, clinical stage and treatment. Fisher exact test was used to association analysis. For tabulation and statistical analysis we used IBM® SPSS® Statistics 20.0.1 software for Windows (IBM Corporation, Route 100, Somers NY 10589). The level of statistical significance was set at 0.05 for all analysis.

Results

During the period between February 2013 and August 2014, 123 patients with ESCC were enrolled in this study. Age ranged from 41 to 92 years (mean = 60.9 years, SD = 10.3 years; median = 61 years). Patients characteristics are described in Table 1; HPV, p53 and p16 status versus patients characteristics are depicted in Table 2.

Kaplan-Meier analysis indicated that ESCC male patients had a poor specific-cancer survival ($p = 0.025$) and a shorter progression-free survival ($p = 0.050$); III or IV clinical stage ($p < 0.019$) had a poor specific-cancer survival and a shorter progression-free survival ($p < 0.001$); not submitted to surgery (<0.001) and not submitted to chemoradiotherapy (CTR) ($p = 0.039$) had a poor specific-cancer survival. Those patients with disease progression or metastasis (<0.001) had a poor specific-cancer survival (Table 3). The distribution of cases according to patients' characteristics and survival rates are shown with more details in Table 3 and the survival curves shown in Fig. 1.

In the multivariate analysis, using a confirmatory model, HPV, p16 and p53 did not show any prediction value related to the progression-free and specific-cancer survival. Results of the multivariable Cox regression analysis are shown in Table 4.

Discussion

Esophageal cancer is an extremely aggressive disease, which is usually diagnosed at an advanced stage, due mainly to the lack of specific initial symptoms. Consequently, EC infiltrates organs and metastasizes straightforwardly, resulting in poor prognosis and 5-year survival of 15–34% [28–30]. In cases of advanced

Table 1 Patients' characteristics

Variable	Category	n	%
Sex	Female	23	18.7
	Male	100	81.3
Age at diagnosis	≤ 60 years old	60	48.8
	> 60 years old	63	51.2
Alcohol consumption	≤ 20 years	24	19.5
	>20 years	99	80.5
Tobacco consumption	≤20 years	26	21.1
	>20 years	97	78.9
Clinical stage[a]	I	3	2.6
	II	26	22.8
	III	58	50.9
	IV	27	23.7
Histological grade *	Well differentiated	14	11.6
	Moderately differentiated	73	60.3
	Poorly differentiated	34	28.1
Surgery	No	102	82.9
	Yes	21	17.1
Radiotherapy	No	51	41.5
	Yes	72	58.5
Chemotherapy	No	45	36.6
	Yes	78	63.4
Progression	No	84	68.3
	Yes	39	31.7
Status	Death by cancer	93	75.6
	Alive	30	24.4
HPV[a]	Negative	75	86.2
	Positive	12	13.8
p16[a]	Negative	108	89.3
	Positive	13	10.7
p53[a]	Negative	37	31.4
	Positive	81	68.6

[a]There are missing values

disease, it is well established that standard treatment is CRT followed by surgery [31], which leads to downgrade the tumor stage and increase the complete resection rate [2]. However, the cure rate and survival of these patients is still low, requiring other methods which may assist in predicting survival and identification of potential responders to a given therapy.

Until now, published data demonstrate that clinic-histopathological factors, molecular biomarkers, and HPV infection are, possibly, predictive variables for neoadjuvant therapy [2, 31]. In head and neck cancer, HPV-positive patients have a better response to CRT

Table 2 HPV, p53 and p16 status versus patients' characteristics

Treatment	HPV[a]		p	p16[a]		p	p53[a]		p
	Negative	Positive		Negative	Positive		Negative	Positive	
Sex									
Female	16 (21.3)	3 (25.0)	0.720	18 (16.7)	5 (38.5)	0.071	6 (16.2)	17 (21.0)	0.624
Male	59 (78.7)	9 (75.0)		90 (83.3)	8 (61.5)		31 (83.8)	64 (79.0)	
Age at diagnosis									
≤ 60 years old	39 (52.0)	7 (58.3)	0.763	51 (47.2)	7 (53.8)	0.772	14 (37.8)	44 (54.3)	0.115
> 60 years old	36 (48.0)	5 (41.7)		57 (52.8)	6 (46.2)		23 (62.2)	37 (45.7)	
Alcohol consumption									
≤ 20 years	19 (25.3)	2 (16.7)	0.722	21 (19.4)	3 (23.1)	0.720	7 (18.9)	17 (21.0)	0.813
> 20 years	56 (74.7)	10 (83.3)		87 (80.6)	10 (76.9)		30 (81.1)	64 (79.0)	
Tobacco consumption									
≤ 20 years	14 (18.7)	5 (41.7)	0.125	25 (23.1)	1 (7.7)	0.295	8 (21.6)	18 (22.2)	0.572
> 20 years	61 (81.3)	7 (58.3)		83 (76.9)	12 (92.3)		29 (78.4)	63 (77.8)	
Clinical stage									
I or II	21 (29.2)	2 (16.7)	0.497	26 (26.0)	3 (23.1)	1.000	5 (14.3)	23 (30.3)	0.099
III or IV	51 (70.8)	10 (83.3)		74 (74.0)	10 (76.9)		30 (85.7)	53 (69.7)	
Histological grade									
Well differentiated	11 (15.1)	0 (0.0)	0.442	13 (12.3)	1 (7.7)	0.912	7 (18.9)	7 (8.9)	0.264
Moderately differentiated	42 (57.5)	9 (75.0)		62 (58.5)	9 (69.2)		19 (51.4)	49 (62.0)	
Poorly differentiated	20 (27.4)	3 (25.0)		31 (29.2)	3 (23.1)		11 (29.7)	23 (29.1)	
Surgery									
No	58 (77.3)	12 (100.0)	0.112	95 (88.0)	7 (53.8)	**0.006**	31 (83.8)	69 (85.2)	1.000
Yes	17 (22.7)	0 (0.0)		13 (12.0)	6 (46.2)		6 (16.2)	12 (14.8)	
Chemoradiotherapy									
No	18 (24.0)	0 (0.0)	0.140	24 (22.2)	2 (15.4)	0.803	7 (18.9)	17 (21.0)	0.871
Chemo or Radio	25 (33.3)	6 (50.0)		38 (35.2)	4 (30.8)		12 (32.4)	29 (35.8)	
Chemo and Radio	32 (42.7)	6 (50.0)		46 (42.6)	7 (53.8)		18 (48.6)	35 (43.2)	
HPV									
Negative	–	–	–	65 (85.5)	9 (90.0)	1.000	24 (88.9)	47 (83.9)	0.743
Positive	–	–		11 (14.5)	1 (10.0)		3 (11.1)	9 (16.1)	
p16[a]									
Negative	65 (87.8)	11 (91.7)	1.000	–	–	–	34 (91.9)	72 (88.9)	0.751
Positive	9 (12.2)	1 (8.3)		–	–		3 (8.1)	9 (11.1)	
p53[a]									
Negative	24 (33.8)	3 (25.0)	0.743	34 (91.9)	72 (88.9)	0.751	–	–	–
Positive	47 (66.2)	9 (75.0)		3 (8.1)	9 (11.1)		–	–	

[a]There are missing values
Entries in boldface are significantly different

and a higher survival rate in relation to HPV-negative cancers [32–34]. Due to the fact that the esophagus can also be infected with these viruses, a similar association and clinical characteristics [20] are supposed. However, the impact of HPV infection on the prognosis of ESCC is still uncertain [2, 35]. In addition, the recent advances in HPV vaccination can believed to improve the reduction of HPV-related tumors in non-gynecological cancers, which is a optimistic scenario to be proved in near future [36].

Previous work of our study group showed a rate of high-risk HPV infection in esophageal tumor samples (13.8%) [25, 26], which led us to investigate whether this event could influence the survival of our patients.

Table 3 Survival rates according to clinical and pathological data

Variable	Progression-free survival			Specific survival		
	Total events	One-year	p-value	Total events	One-year	p-value
Sex						
Female	4	86.7	**0.050**	14	72.3	**0.025**
Male	35	63.3		79	49.8	
Age at diagnosis						
≤ 60 years old	18	73.3	0.553	45	54.9	0.266
> 60 years old	21	63.0		48	53.2	
Alcohol consumption						
≤ 20 years	5	74.6	0.218	16	62.0	0.301
> 20 years	34	66.9		77	52.0	
Tobacco consumption						
≤ 20 years	11	51.3	0.158	19	49.0	0.796
> 20 years	28	73.1		74	55.3	
Clinical stage[a]						
I or II	6	91.2	**0.019**	13	78.6	**<0.001**
III or IV	32	57.9		73	44.2	
Histological grade[a]						
Well differentiated	4	76.2	0.170	10	63.5	0.426
Moderately differentiated	18	72.4		55	48.8	
Poorly differentiated	15	57.4		26	61.4	
Surgery						
No	32	65.8	0.486	84	47.5	**<0.001**
Yes	7	80.0		9	85.4	
Chemoradiotherapy						
No	8	72.4	0.731	24	34.6	**0.039**
Chemo or Radio	15	62.3		36	47.7	
Chemo and Radio	16	72.9		33	69.1	
HPV[a]						
Negative	23	69.3	0.885	56	52.6	0.093
Positive	3	71.4		11	31.3	
p16[a]						
Negative	35	66.9	0.956	84	52.4	0.739
Positive	4	75.2		9	60.6	
p53[a]						
Negative	12	66.3	0.892	27	51.4	0.584
Positive	26	67.0		63	54.9	

[a]There are missing values
Entries in boldface are significantly different

However, the current study demonstrated that HPV infection showed no impact on the survival of patients with ESCC and similar results were found in other studies [2, 35, 37, 38].

Hippelainen et al. (1993), e.g., detected HPV in 11% of the esophageal tumors analyzed but the infection was not associated with higher survival rate [38]. Dreilich et al. (2006) detected only HPV 16 in their esophageal samples and showed no influence of virus in survival or improvement of therapy response [35]. Liu et al. (2010) demonstrated that infection of HPV 16 and p53 protein expression were not correlated with survival during the 5-year follow-up period in ESCC [37]. Herbster et al. (2012) found mostly HPV 16 positive in esophageal

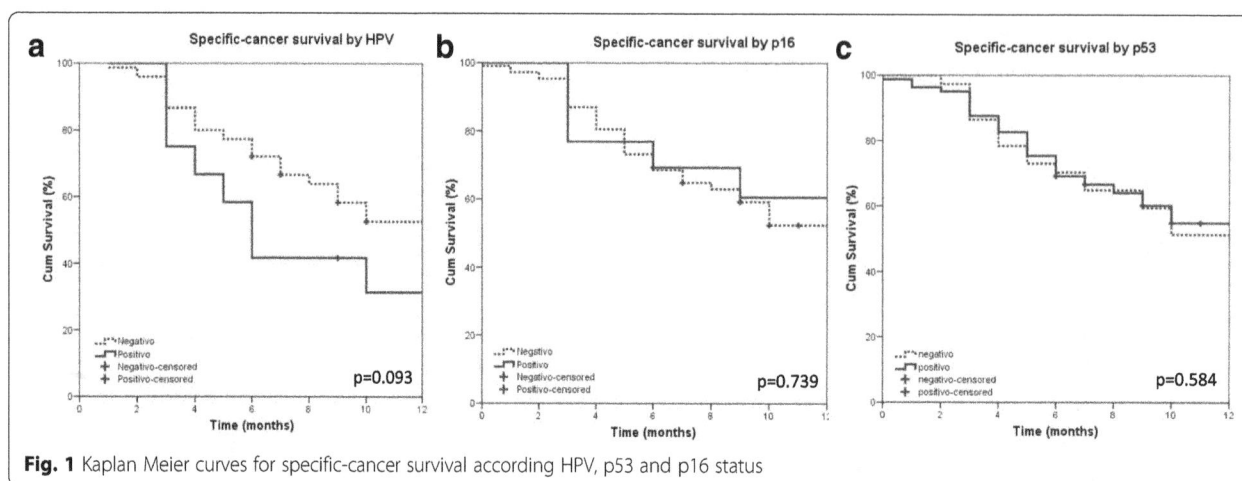

Fig. 1 Kaplan Meier curves for specific-cancer survival according HPV, p53 and p16 status

tumors, but this condition was not associated with overall survival [39]. Recently, Wang et al. (2015) demonstrated that the risk of developing multifocal ESCC was not significantly different between HPV-positive and HPV-negative groups. However, patients with HPV16 infection, specifically, had better response to CRT than those without HPV 16 infection [2].

Different results have also been reported in other studies. Cao et al. (2014) demonstrated that HPV infected patients had better 5-year rates of overall survival and reduction in the risk of death [22]. In contrast, Furihata et al. (1993) reported that HPV positive patients have worse survival than those HPV negative with overexpression of p53 in EC patients [40].

In addition to investigating HPV infection in EC, our group has also previously assessed the expression of molecular markers p53 and p16, considered to be essential G1 cell cycle regulatory genes whose loss of function is associated with ESCC carcinogenesis [41], and found that the expression of these proteins was significantly higher in tumor tissues compared to adjacent normal tissue to the tumor and also esophageal tissue from individuals without EC [25]. Based on this interesting result, we decided to evaluate the impact of increased expression of these proteins in EC as regards the survival of these patients. We find, through a multivariate analysis, that p53 and p16 expression showed no predictive value for progression-

free and specific-cancer survival. The results found in literature related to the expression of these markers and survival in ESCC are widely variable.

Currently, there are several studies trying to correlate the expression of p53 protein and mutations in the p53 gene with survival of patients carrying EC, and the results are widely variable. Bahnassy et al. (2005) and Huang et al. (2014) found that high p53 expression was associated with a poor survival rate in ESCC patients [42, 43]; and Han et al. (2007) showed that p53 expression was positively correlated with tumor stage and lymph node metastasis [44]. Ye et al. (2012) reported that p53 expression was not associated with the gender or age of the patient, but was associated with tumor differentiation degree and lymph node metastasis [45]. A retrospective cohort study of 136 ESCC patients, conducted to investigate the prognostic role of p53 in patients with ESCC suggested that overexpression of this protein was associated with poor prognosis in these patients, and it's a significantly independent predictor of poorer overall survival ($p = 0.04$) [16]. Furthermore, significant associations were also found between high expression of p53 and poor prognosis by Shang et al. (2014), Xu et al. (2014) and Chen et al. (2015), suggesting that this protein is an important biomarker candidate for the prognosis of patients with ESCC [3, 14, 23].

Similarly to our results, Chino et al. (2001) showed that p53 expression was not associated with tumor infiltration deepness, lymph node metastasis, or venous and/or lymphatic invasion [46]. Murata et al. (2013) examined the clinical and prognostic features of p53 immunohistochemical expression in 266 ESCC patients and found that the protein expression has no impact on the prognosis of ESCC, according to them, possibly due to their short follow-up time [47]. Furthermore, a p53 research group study demonstrated that, for EC, p53 immunohistochemistry does not correlate with response to chemotherapy, curative

Table 4 Risk of cancer progression or death according to HPV, p53 and p16 status

Model	Variable of interest[a]	Progression-free survival		Specific-cancer survival	
		HR	[CI$^{95\%}$]	HR	[CI$^{95\%}$]
1	HPV	1.042	[0.293: 3.709]	1.901	[0.926: 3.900]
2	p16	1.137	[0.383: 3.378]	1.268	[0.617: 2.604]
3	p53	1.318	[0.646: 2.689]	1.177	[0.726: 1.907]

[a]Model adjusted by sex. Clinical stage and treatment (surgery and chemoradiotherapy). HR: Hazard ratio

resection rate, or prognosis, whereas data from p53 mutation analyses are more consistent concerning the association of p53 mutation and poor survival [48]. These discrepancies may be related to several factors, including small sample sizes, patient selection bias, failure to take into account other prognostic parameters, differences in laboratory techniques (for example, the use of different monoclonal antibodies to screen for p53 expression) and a shorter time of follow-up [16, 47]. To date, the role of this protein in relation to EC patients' survival is not fully understood.

Unlike the large number of findings related to p53 overexpression and survival, studies seeking to correlate p16 expression with EC patient survival are scarce, since the vast majority uses this protein as an indirect marker for HPV infection.

Opposite to our findings, Cao et al. (2014) found that p16-positive patients had better 5-year rates of overall survival and progression free survival than p16-negative group [22] and similarly, Kumar et al. (2015) found that the p16 expression in ESCC correlates with a higher rate of pathologic complete remission in patients submitted to neo adjuvant chemotherapy, and could be considered as a predictive marker for response assessment. Furthermore, moderately differentiated histological grade, surgery, chemotherapy and progression or metastasis have shown their prediction value for specific-cancer survival [21]. However, no significant correlations were found between the proteins expression and clinical outcomes[1515], corroborating our findings.

Conclusions

HPV status did not statistically correlated to survival rates, despite the clear tendency of positive HPV cases to be more aggressive than the HPV negative, in opposition to HPV significance in oropharyngeal cancers.

Abbreviations

CI: Confidence Interval; CTR: Chemoradiotherapy; EC: Esophageal cancer; ESCC: Esophageal squamous cell carcinoma; HPV: Human papillomavirus; PCR: Polymerase chain reaction

Acknowledgements

The authors would like to thank the Barretos Cancer Hospital, HPV Teams at Barretos Cancer Hospital and Molecular Biology Laboratory, Center for Translational Research in Oncology, São Paulo Cancer Institute (ICESP), São Paulo, Brazil. CNPq Universal for providing supplies to the largest study, of which this study is a part of, entitled "The role of human papillomavirus (HPV) as the etiologic agent of esophageal cancer. A cross-sectional study, case-control and longitudinal at Barretos Cancer Hospital"(process: 482666 / 2012-9).

Funding

CNPq Universal for providing supplies to the largest study, of which this study is a part of, entitled "The role of human papillomavirus (HPV) as the etiologic agent of esophageal cancer. A cross-sectional study, case-control and longitudinal at Barretos Cancer Hospital"; (Grant number 482666/2012–9 to ALF); INCT HPV [Fundação de Amparo à Pesquisa do Estado de São Paulo (FAPESP) [Grant number 08/57889−1 to LLV]; Conselho Nacional de Desenvolvimento Científico e Tencnológico (CNPq) (Grant number 573799/ 2008–3 to LLV)].

Authors' contributions

AMC participated in the conception, design, development of methodology, acquisition of data, analysis and interpretation and writing of the manuscript; JHTGF participated in the conception, design, analysis and interpretation of data and review and revision of the manuscript; PRAP, VSM and EMS participated in the conception, design, development of methodology and acquisition of data; CSN, DPG developed the methodology and reviewed the manuscript; LS and LLV participated in the analysis and interpretation of data and review of the manuscript; KJS and ALF participated the conception, design, writing, review of the manuscript and study supervision. All authors read and approved the final manuscript.

Competing interests

The authors declare that they have no competing interests.

Author details

[1]Teaching and Research Institute, Barretos Cancer Hospital – Pius XII Foundation, Rua Antenor Duarte Vilela, 1331, Dr. Paulo Prata, Barretos, São Paulo 14784-400, Brazil. [2]Cancer Registry, Barretos Cancer Hospital – Pius XII Foundation, São Paulo, Brazil. [3]Molecular Oncology Research Center, Barretos Cancer Hospital – Pius XII Foundation, São Paulo, Brazil. [4]Department of Endoscopy, Barretos Cancer Hospital – Pious XII Foundation, Barretos, São Paulo, Brazil. [5]Molecular Biology Laboratory, Center for Translational Research in Oncology, Instituto do Câncer do Estado de São Paulo – ICESP, São Paulo, Brazil. [6]Department of Radiology and Oncology, School of Medicine, University of São Paulo, São Paulo, Brazil. [7]Department of Clinical Research - Biohit Oyj, Helsinki, Finland. [8]Medical Laboratory of Medical Investigation (LIM) 14, Department of Pathology, Faculty of Medicine, University of São Paulo, São Paulo, Brazil. [9]Research Institute of Life and Health Sciences (ICVS), University of Minho, Braga, Portugal. [10]ICVS / 3B's - Associated Laboratory to the Government of Portugal, Braga/Guimarães, Portugal.

References

1. GLOBOCAN 2012 v1.0, Cancer Incidence and Mortality Worldwide: IARC CancerBase No. 11 [Internet] [http://globocan.iarc.fr]. Accessed 27 Sept 2017.
2. Wang WL, Wang YC, Lee CT, Chang CY, Lo JL, Kuo YH, Hsu YC, Mo LR. The impact of human papillomavirus infection on the survival and treatment response of patients with esophageal cancers. J Dig Dis. 2015;16:256–63.
3. Chen J, Wu F, Pei HL, Gu WD, Ning ZH, Shao YJ, Huang J. Analysis of the correlation between P53 and Cox-2 expression and prognosis in esophageal cancer. Oncol Lett. 2015;10:2197–203.
4. Syrjanen K. HPV et tumeurs épidermoïdes bénignes et malignes de l'æsophag. In: PJ AF, Mougin C, editors. Papillomavirus Humains Biologie et pathologie tumorale. Paris: TEC & DOC; 2003.
5. Syrjanen KJ. HPV infections and oesophageal cancer. J Clin Pathol. 2002;55:721–8.
6. Syrjanen KJ. Human papillomavirus (HPV) infections and their associations with squamous cell neoplasia. Arch Geschwulstforsch. 1987;57:417–44.
7. Syrjänen K, Chang F, Syrjänen S. Infectious agents as etiological factors in esophageal carcinogenesis. In: Tahara E, Sugimachi K, Oohara T, editors.

Recent advances in gastroenterological carcinogenesis I. Bologna: Monduzzi Editore; 1996. p. 29–43.

8. Syrjanen K. HPV infections of the oesophagus. In: Papillomavirus infections in human pathology. New York: Wiley & Sons; 2000. p. 413–28.

9. Syrjanen K. HPV infections in etiology of benign and malignant sinonasal, bronchial and oesophageal squamous cell lesions. In: 4th International Multidisciplinary Congress EUROGIN (Monsonego J ed. Pp. 169–179). Bolongna: Monduzzi Editore; 2000. p. 169–79.

10. Syrjanen K, Pyrhonen S, Aukee S, Koskela E. Squamous cell papilloma of the esophagus: a tumour probably caused by human papilloma virus (HPV). Diagn Histopathol. 1982;5:291–6.

11. Syrjanen KJ. Histological changes identical to those of condylomatous lesions found in esophageal squamous cell carcinomas. Arch Geschwulstforsch. 1982;52:283–92.

12. Kamangar F, Chow WH, Abnet CC, Dawsey SM. Environmental causes of esophageal cancer. Gastroenterol Clin N Am. 2009;38:27–57. vii

13. Antunes LC, Prolla JC, de Barros LA, da Rocha MP, Fagundes RB. No evidence of HPV DNA in esophageal squamous cell carcinoma in a population of southern Brazil. World J Gastroenterol. 2013;19:6598–603.

14. Shang L, Liu HJ, Hao JJ, Jiang YY, Shi F, Zhang Y, Cai Y, Xu X, Jia XM, Zhan QM, Wang MR. A panel of overexpressed proteins for prognosis in esophageal squamous cell carcinoma. PLoS One. 2014;9:e111045.

15. Shibata-Kobayashi S, Yamashita H, Okuma K, Shiraishi K, Igaki H, Ohtomo K, Nakagawa K. Correlation among 16 biological factors [p53, p21(waf1), MIB-1 (Ki-67), p16(INK4A), cyclin D1, E-cadherin, Bcl-2, TNF-alpha, NF-kappaB, TGF-beta, MMP-7, COX-2, EGFR, HER2/neu, ER, and HIF-1alpha] and clinical outcomes following curative chemoradiation therapy in 10 patients with esophageal squamous cell carcinoma. Oncol Lett. 2013;5:903–10.

16. Yao W, Qin X, Qi B, Lu J, Guo L, Liu F, Liu S, Zhao B. Association of p53 expression with prognosis in patients with esophageal squamous cell carcinoma. Int J Clin Exp Pathol. 2014;7:7158–63.

17. Chang F, Syrjanen S, Syrjanen K. Implications of the p53 tumor-suppressor gene in clinical oncology. J Clin Oncol. 1995;13:1009–22.

18. Lassen P, Eriksen JG, Hamilton-Dutoit S, Tramm T, Alsner J, Overgaard J. Effect of HPV-associated p16INK4A expression on response to radiotherapy and survival in squamous cell carcinoma of the head and neck. J Clin Oncol. 2009;27:1992–8.

19. Sturm I, Petrowsky H, Volz R, Lorenz M, Radetzki S, Hillebrand T, Wolff G, Hauptmann S, Dorken B, Daniel PT. Analysis of p53/BAX/p16(ink4a/CDKN2) in esophageal squamous cell carcinoma: high BAX and p16(ink4a/CDKN2) identifies patients with good prognosis. J Clin Oncol. 2001;19:2272–81.

20. Cao F, Han H, Zhang F, Wang B, Ma W, Wang Y, Sun G, Shi M, Ren Y, Cheng Y. HPV infection in esophageal squamous cell carcinoma and its relationship to the prognosis of patients in northern China. ScientificWorldJournal. 2014;2014:804738.

21. Kumar R, Ghosh SK, Verma AK, Talukdar A, Deka MK, Wagh M, Bahar HM, Tapkire R, Chakraborty KP, Kannan RR. p16 expression as a surrogate marker for HPV infection in esophageal Squamous cell carcinoma can predict response to neo-adjuvant chemotherapy. Asian Pac J Cancer Prev. 2015;16:7161–5.

22. Cao F, Zhang W, Zhang F, Han H, Xu J, Cheng Y. Prognostic significance of high-risk human papillomavirus and p16(INK4A) in patients with esophageal squamous cell carcinoma. Int J Clin Exp Med. 2014;7:3430–8.

23. Xu XL. Zheng WH, Tao KY, Li XX, Xu WZ, Wang Y, Zhu SM, Mao WM: p53 is an independent prognostic factor in operable esophageal squamous cell carcinoma: a large-scale study with a long follow-up. Med Oncol. 2014;31:257.

24. Green MR, Sambrook J. Molecular Cloning: A Laboratory Manual, 4thed. New York: John Inglis N; 2012.

25. Pastrez PRA, Mariano VS, da Costa AM, Silva EM, Scapulatempo-Neto C, Guimaraes DP, Fava G, Neto SAZ, Nunes EM, Sichero L, et al. The relation of HPV infection and expression of p53 and p16 proteins in esophageal Squamous cells carcinoma. J Cancer. 2017;8:1062–70.

26. da Costa AM, Fregnani J, Pastrez PRA, Mariano VS, Neto CS, Guimaraes DP, de Oliveira KMG, Neto SAZ, Nunes EM, Ferreira S, et al. Prevalence of high risk HPV DNA in esophagus is high in Brazil but not related to esophageal squamous cell carcinoma. Histol Histopathol. 2017;11929

27. Schmitt M, Bravo IG, Snijders PJ, Gissmann L, Pawlita M, Waterboer T. Bead-based multiplex genotyping of human papillomaviruses. J Clin Microbiol. 2006;44:504–12.

28. World Health Organization. Genital human papillomavirus infections and cancer: memorandum from a WHO meeting. Bull World Health Organ. 1987; 65:817–27.

29. Shen ZY, Xu LY, Li EM, Shen J, Zheng RM, Cai WJ, Zeng Y. Immortal phenotype of the esophageal epithelial cells in the process of immortalization. Int J Mol Med. 2002;10:641–6.

30. Cervantes J. Update on the pathogenesis and immunotherapy of esophageal squamous cell carcinoma. Rev Gastroenterol Peru. 2004;24:165–70.

31. Tao CJ, Lin G, Xu YP, Mao WM. Predicting the response of Neoadjuvant therapy for patients with esophageal carcinoma: an in-depth literature review. J Cancer. 2015;6:1179–86.

32. Weinberger PM, Yu Z, Haffty BG, Kowalski D, Harigopal M, Brandsma J, Sasaki C, Joe J, Camp RL, Rimm DL, Psyrri A. Molecular classification identifies a subset of human papillomavirus–associated oropharyngeal cancers with favorable prognosis. J Clin Oncol. 2006;24:736–47.

33. Fakhry C, Westra WH, Li S, Cmelak A, Ridge JA, Pinto H, Forastiere A, Gillison ML. Improved survival of patients with human papillomavirus-positive head and neck squamous cell carcinoma in a prospective clinical trial. J Natl Cancer Inst. 2008;100:261–9.

34. Ang KK, Harris J, Wheeler R, Weber R, Rosenthal DI, Nguyen-Tan PF, Westra WH, Chung CH, Jordan RC, Lu C, et al. Human papillomavirus and survival of patients with oropharyngeal cancer. N Engl J Med. 2010;363:24–35.

35. Dreilich M, Bergqvist M, Moberg M, Brattstrom D, Gustavsson I, Bergstrom S, Wanders A, Hesselius P, Wagenius G, Gyllensten U. High-risk human papilloma virus (HPV) and survival in patients with esophageal carcinoma: a pilot study. BMC Cancer. 2006;6:94.

36. Skinner SR, Apter D, De Carvalho N, Harper DM, Konno R, Paavonen J, Romanowski B, Roteli-Martins C, Burlet N, Mihalyi A, Struyf F. Human papillomavirus (HPV)-16/18 AS04-adjuvanted vaccine for the prevention of cervical cancer and HPV-related diseases. Expert Rev Vaccines. 2016;15:367–87.

37. Liu WK, Jiang XY, Zhang MP, Zhang ZX. The relationship between HPV16 and expression of cyclooxygenase-2, P53 and their prognostic roles in esophageal squamous cell carcinoma. Eur J Gastroenterol Hepatol. 2010;22:67–74.

38. Hippelainen M, Eskelinen M, Lipponen P, Chang F, Syrjanen K. Mitotic activity index, volume corrected mitotic index and human papilloma-virus suggestive morphology are not prognostic factors in carcinoma of the oesophagus. Anticancer Res. 1993;13:677–81.

39. Herbster S, Ferraro CT, Koff NK, Rossini A, Kruel CD, Andreollo NA, Rapozo DC, Blanco TC, Faria PA, Santos PT, et al. HPV infection in Brazilian patients with esophageal squamous cell carcinoma: interpopulational differences, lack of correlation with surrogate markers and clinicopathological parameters. Cancer Lett. 2012;326:52–8.

40. Furihata M, Ohtsuki Y, Ogoshi S, Takahashi A, Tamiya T, Ogata T. Prognostic significance of human papillomavirus genomes (type-16, −18) and aberrant expression of p53 protein in human esophageal cancer. Int J Cancer. 1993;54:226–30.

41. Taghavi N, Biramijamal F, Sotoudeh M, Moaven O, Khademi H, Abbaszadegan MR, Malekzadeh R. Association of p53/p21 expression with cigarette smoking and prognosis in esophageal squamous cell carcinoma patients. World J Gastroenterol. 2010;16:4958–67.

42. Bahnassy AA, Zekri AR, Abdallah S, El-Shehaby AM, Sherif GM. Human papillomavirus infection in Egyptian esophageal carcinoma: correlation with p53, p21, mdm2, C-erbB2 and impact on survival. Pathol Int. 2005;55:53–62.

43. Huang K, Chen L, Zhang J, Wu Z, Lan L, Wang L, Lu B, Liu Y. Elevated p53 expression levels correlate with tumor progression and poor prognosis in patients exhibiting esophageal squamous cell carcinoma. Oncol Lett. 2014;8:1441–6.

44. Han U, Can OI, Han S, Kayhan B, Onal BU. Expressions of p53, VEGF C, p21: could they be used in preoperative evaluation of lymph node metastasis of esophageal squamous cell carcinoma? Dis Esophagus. 2007;20:379–85.

45. Ye B, Wang X, Yang Z, Sun Z, Zhang R, Hu Y, Lu Y, Du J. p53 and p73 expression in esophageal carcinoma correlate with clinicopathology of tumors. Hepato-Gastroenterology. 2012;59:2192–5.

HPV infection and p53 and p16 expression in esophageal cancer: are they prognostic...

227

46. Chino O, Kijima H, Shimada H, Nishi T, Tanaka H, Kise Y, Kenmochi T, Himeno S, Machimura T, Tanaka M, et al. Accumulation of p53 in esophageal squamous cell carcinoma. Int J Mol Med. 2001;8:359–63.

47. Murata A, Baba Y, Watanabe M, Shigaki H, Miyake K, Karashima R, Imamura Y, Ida S, Ishimoto T, Iwagami S, et al. p53 immunohistochemical expression and patient prognosis in esophageal squamous cell carcinoma. Med Oncol. 2013;30:728.

48. Kandioler D, Schoppmann SF, Zwrtek R, Kappel S, Wolf B, Mittlbock M, Kuhrer I, Hejna M, Pluschnig U, Ba-Ssalamah A, et al. The biomarker TP53 divides patients with neoadjuvantly treated esophageal cancer into 2 subgroups with markedly different outcomes. A p53 research group study. J Thorac Cardiovasc Surg. 2014;148:2280–6.

Reducing incidence of cervical cancer: knowledge and attitudes of caregivers in Nigerian city to human papilloma virus vaccination

Adaobi I. Bisi-Onyemaechi[1*], Ugo N. Chikani[1] and Obinna Nduagubam[2]

Abstract

Background: Despite the high prevalences of Human Papilloma Virus (HPV) infections and cervical cancer in Nigeria, utilization of the HPV vaccine as a highly effective preventive measure remains low. The aim of this study was to find out the awareness and attitudes of caregivers to HPV infections and the factors that determine acceptance of an HPV vaccine for their pre-adolescent girls.

Methods: This was a cross-sectional descriptive study of 508 caregivers of female children in Enugu Nigeria. A semi-structured questionnaire was used to collect information on knowledge of HPV, cervical cancer as well HPV vaccine and its acceptance for pre-adolescent female children. The data was analysed using descriptive statistics.

Results: Five hundred and eight (508) caregivers of female children were interviewed. Less than half, 221,(43.5%) of them knew about HPV, among these, 163 knew how HPV is transmitted. Only 12 (2.4%) of the caregivers know that an HPV infection is a major risk factor for cervical cancer. Among the 221 participants who knew the meaning of HPV, 132 (59.7%) were aware of an HPV vaccine. Only 26 (19.7%) of those aware of a vaccine agreed it can effectively prevent cervical cancer. Lack of awareness about the vaccine and accessibility were the major reasons given by parents on why the vaccine has not been received by their female children.

Conclusion: Despite high levels of education, awareness of HPV, HPV vaccine and the risks for cervical cancer remains low among caregivers in Enugu, south-east, Nigeria. Awareness and accessibility were the major determinants of HPV vaccine uptake among the caregivers. There is a need for massive and sustained awareness creation to increase HPV vaccination uptake in Nigeria.

Keywords: Awareness, Human papilloma virus, Cervical cancer, Vaccines, Nigeria

Background

Human Papilloma Virus (HPV) is the most common sexually transmitted virus and it is estimated that about 75% of sexually active women and men will acquire a genital HPV infection at some time [1]. HPV is known to affect adult and children alike and over 100 types of the HPV has been identified over the past few decades [2].

There has been an increasing interest in HPV because of their relationship with tumours particularly cervical. Epidemiological, molecular and clinical evidence has shown

that cervical cancer is caused by HPV. About 13genotypes are closely linked with cervical cancer especially genotypes 16 and 18 [3–11]. High risk Infections is usually persistent and should be the target of vaccination strategies [12].

Globally, cervical cancer is a major public health problem. Over 560,000 new cases and about 275,000 deaths are recorded each year, with more than 80% occurring in developing countries [13, 14]. It is the most common gynaecological cancer among women in sub-Saharan Africa [15]. It is estimated that 70,722 new cases of invasive cervical cancer occur annually in sub-Saharan Africa [16]. According to GLOBOCAN 2008, about14,089 new cervical cancer cases are diagnosed annually in Nigeria.

* Correspondence: adaobi.bisi-onyemaechi@unn.edu.ng
[1]College of Medicine, University of Nigeria Ituku-Ozalla, Enugu, Nigeria
Full list of author information is available at the end of the article

Cervical cancer is the second most common cancer in Nigeria and second to breast cancer among its female population [17–21]. In 2007, it was reported that 36.59 million women aged more than 15 years in Nigeria are at risk of developing cervical cancer. There are 9922 cases diagnosed annually with 8030 deaths. HPV prevalence is 24.8%. Incidence of cervical cancer in Nigeria is 250/100,000 women [22]. One of the preventive measures is the vaccination of pre-adolescents against oncogenic HPV. The vaccines are approved for administration to persons aged 9–26 years [9, 23, 24]. The target is to commence the vaccine among young children before they become sexually active. The cervical cancer control plan in Nigeria recommends visual inspection with acetic acid (VIA) or with Lugol's iodine, for screening, (secondary prevention strategy) of sexually-exposed women, and for primary prevention, HPV vaccination for girls aged 9 to 15 years. HPV vaccination has not been introduced in the vaccination schedule in Nigeria and is only available to people on personal arrangements. Programs are set up to vaccinate girls on adhoc, irregular and usually private basis.

A large number of European countries as well as United States, Australia and New Zealand have recommended including an HPV vaccine in the school vaccination program for young adolescent girls, often coupled with a catch-up program for older teenage girls [25, 26]. The vaccine has been found 70–100% effective in preventing cervical cancers [27–30]. The vaccines were licensed and introduced in Nigeria in 2009, uptake has ranged between 0 and 49% being utilized by only a few privileged population [30–32].

The knowledge of HPV infections and HPV vaccines, among the Nigeria population, are inadequate, and the cost of HPV vaccination per person is beyond what the average Nigerian can afford [33–36].

Awareness and knowledge of the infections and the vaccines would stimulate demand and uptake of the vaccines. Increasing demand may drive the introduction of the vaccine into the national immunization schedule thereby making the vaccine more affordable and accessible.

The aim of this study was to find out the knowledge and attitudes of parents to and the factors that determine the demand of HPV vaccine for their adolescent girls. This study was focused on the usefulness of HPV Vaccine as a preventive measure for the reduction of the incidence of cervical cancer hence the focus only on adolescent girls.

Methods
This was a cross-sectional descriptive study of 508 parents/caregivers of young children from primary schools in the three Local government councils of Enugu metropolis-Enugu-South, Enugu- North and Enugu-East. Fifteen primary schools were (five from each local council) were randomly selected for the study. The researchers attended the

Parents- Teachers forum of these schools. During the meeting, the researchers introduced themselves and the purpose of their research. They were then granted permission to administer the questionnaire to consenting parents of female children. Every eligible caregiver of a female child less than 18 years was recruited into the study. The data was collected consecutively from school to school. Data was collected between the months of January and July 2017. Data collection tool was semi-structured questionnaire reviewed by a panel of experts for validity. The questionnaire was either self-administered or interviewer-administered for study participants who were not literate. Items on the questionnaire include; socio-demographic variables; knowledge of cervical cancer; knowledge of HPV infections and HPV vaccines, their attitudes towards the effectiveness of the vaccines and reason (s) for uptake or otherwise of these vaccines for their adolescent girls. The data was analysed using descriptive statistics.

Results
A total of 508 caregivers were interviewed out of which 476 (93.7%) were below the age of 50 years. 385 (75.8%) were females and 123 (24.2%) males. Out of the 508 caregivers, 218 (42.9%) had more than one female child. The mean age of the children of the respondents was 7.3 years (SD + − 5.3) Three hundred and forty-seven (68.3%) had tertiary level of education while only 30 (5.9%) had no formal education. Three hundred and thirty (65%) caregivers were married (Table 1).

A total of 221 (43.5%) parents knew what HPV meant, among these, 163(74%) knew how it is transmitted (Tables 2 and 3).

Overall, only 21 (9.5%) of the parents who were aware of HPV knew the risk factors for genital HPV infections while a total of 66 (30%) of these knew that the risk of developing invasive cervical cancer is the major "sequale" following HPV infection (Tables 3 and 4).

Although 361(71%) of the respondents have heard about cancer of the cervix, 65% of them did not know what it means. Only 12 out of the 221(5.4%) participants that know about HPV are aware that it is risk factor for developing cervical cancer. These 12 were part of the 66 who identified that risk of developing cervical cancer as a sequale of genital HPV infections (Table 5).

Among the 221 participants who knew the meaning of HPV, 132 (59.7%) were aware of HPV vaccine. Furthermore, of the 132 participants who are aware of the HPV vaccine; only 26 (19.7%) agree that HPV vaccine can effectively prevent cervical cancer; 59(44.7%) didn't think so while 47(35.6%) had no idea.

Among those aware of the vaccine, 72 (54.5%) do not know what ages the HPV vaccine should be administered and only 6(2.75%) of the parents had given HPV vaccine to their eligible female children.

Table 1 Socio-demographic information of study participants

	Frequency	Percent
Age group		
< =25	116	22.8
26–30	86	16.9
31–35	94	18.5
36–40	87	17.1
41–45	62	12.2
46–50	31	6.1
> 50	32	6.3
Sex		
Male	123	24.2
Female	385	75.8
No of female children		
1	290	57.1
2	22	4.3
3	50	9.8
4	67	13.2
> 4	79	15.6
Level of education		
None	30	5.9
Primary	29	5.7
Secondary	102	20.1
Tertiary	347	68.3
Marital Status		
Single	154	30.3
Married	330	65.0
Divorced	7	1.4
Separated	17	3.3

Table 2 Knowledge about HPV

What is HPV	Frequency	Percent
Don't know	200	39.4
Human papilloma virus	221	43.5
It is a very bad disease	1	0.2
It is a virus and very deadly disease	1	0.2
Hepatisis vaccine	44	8.7
Human productivity virus	25	4.9
High power voltage	1	0.2
High productivity vaccine	8	1.6
Human power	1	0.2
A vaccine	1	0.2
Human positive virus	2	0.4
Hypertension	2	0.4
Human production value	1	0.2

Table 3 Knowledge about the risk factors for HPV infection

What are the risk factors for HPV infection?	Frequency	Percent
Don't know	89	40.3
Unprotected sex and multiple partners	20	9.0
Frequent cervical contact	1	0.5
Cancer and genital warts	15	6.8
Death	22	10.0
Promiscuity	58	26.2
Adolescence	2	0.9
Use of condom	1	0.5
Infection	2	0.9
In the womb	1	0.5
Early sex	1	0.5
Child birth	1	0.5
Stroke	1	0.5
Bleeding	1	0.5
Sickness	2	0.9
Vaginal discomfort	4	1.9
Total	221	100.0

The major reasons given by parents/caregivers for not giving HPV vaccine to their eligible children were that they were not aware of the vaccine (74.1%) and inability to access the vaccine among those aware of it. (72.5%) (Table 6).

Discussion

It was observed that many the study participants had formal education. The finding that 68.3% of the respondents had tertiary level of education signifies a high literacy level. However, despite this, awareness of cancer of cervix amongst them was low. This finding is similar to other studies in Nigeria, among women with similar social characteristics (age and educational attainment) where only a small proportion of respondents knew about the disease despite high levels of literacy [11, 36].

Table 4 Knowledge of the sequale of genital HPV infections

What is the hazard for HPV infection?	Frequency	Percent
Don't know	96	43.4
Risk of having cervical cancer	66	29.9
Death	51	23.1
Multiple sex partner	1	0.5
Infection	2	0.9
Yellow fever in fetus	1	0.5
Injury in the cervix	1	0.5
Bleeding	1	0.5
Chemical radiation	1	0.5
Genital warts	1	0.5
Total	221	100.0

Table 5 Knowledge about the risk factor for cervical cancer

What are the risk factors for cervical cancer?	Frequency n = 508	Percent
Don't know	265	52.2
Death	98	19.3
Sexual transmitted disease/unprotected sex	7	1.4
Early sex and multiple sex partners	4	.8
Multiple sexual partners	5	1.0
Sexual promiscuity	1	.2
Infection	62	12.2
Neck injury	1	.2
Cancer of the cervix	3	.6
Injury in the cervix	20	3.9
Pain in the cervix/womb	17	3.3
Affection	1	.2
Family planning inserts	2	.4
Vaginal Bleeding	3	.6
HPV infection	12	2.4
Instrumentation in female private part	2	.4
Sickness	1	.2
Low fertility	2	.4
Heredity	1	.2
Damage of the uterine wall	1	.2

However, in contrast, a similar study Ibadan that reported that awareness of cancer of cervix was up to 67% despite lower literacy level among the study participants [30, 35]. Another study in Lagos Nigeria reported an awareness level of up to 99% among nurses which is not unexpected as they were health workers with more access to health information [36].

Awareness about HPV infection was also low in this study; very few caregivers knew the risk factors for HPV infection as well as the relationship between HPV infection and cervical cancer. This may be because it is not part of routine health talks at ante-natal or immunization

Table 6 Reason (s) for not giving HPV vaccine by those aware of the vaccine

REASON	Frequency n = 132	Percent
I don't know how to access the vaccine	123	93.2
My daughter is too young to have risk of cervical cancer	94	71.2
I am worried about the safety of the vaccine	47	35.6
I am not sure of the effectiveness of the vaccine	26	19.7
The decision would be made by the child herself	108	81.8
The vaccine is expensive	25	18.9

sessions. These are the major places where most mothers get health information in this environment with limited access to internet and electricity. Similar finding of low awareness about HPV were also found in Lagos and Malaysia where only less than half of the mothers with similar educational attainment were aware of HPV disease [34]. However, in Ibadan Nigeria, awareness of HPV disease was found to be high [30]. This low level of awareness among the educated implies that a lot of information, communication and education strategies have tobe engaged to enlighten the public on a prevalent disease like cervical cancer. Health promotion strategies to educate the public about prevention of STIs of public health significance can be effective in preventing genital HPV infection and by extension cervical cancer [24].

Primary prevention of cervical cancer can be achieved through prevention and control of genital infection with oncogenic HPV types [24]. Oncogenic genital HPV infections can be prevented by vaccinating young female children with HPV vaccine. In Nigeria, mothers influence decision making particularly for their young female children; hence places with high concentration of mothers like antenatal classes, markets and parent-teachers forum meetings can be engaged to improve HPV awareness.

This study is similar to a number of other studies which have shown that awareness of the vaccine is also very low [11, 34, 35]. Also, more 90% of the respondents who were aware of the HPV vaccine cannot access it. This is worrisome because effective coverage of HPV vaccination requires both caregiver acceptance of the vaccines [5, 9] accessibility and affordability. Uptake rates cannot be improved when basic knowledge is lacking and vaccines inaccessible. This would result in underutilization of this preventive measure as was the case in this study.

As much as 45% of those aware of the vaccine do not agree that HPV vaccine can effectively prevent cervical cancer. Cost of the vaccine, concerns about the effectiveness and safety of the vaccine were reasonsgiven by the caregivers for poor uptake of HPV vaccines. Previous studies [33–36] have highlighted cost concerns as a major issue impeding the uptake of HPV vaccine, this study reveals knowledge gaps about the vaccine and accessibility as the more important factors than cost of the vaccine in our environment. Currently in Nigeria, HPV vaccine is optional, not included in the national immunization schedule and also not subsidized by government. Agida et al. [11] in their study observed that regardless of the current cost of the vaccine in Nigeria, acceptance was high among parents who were aware of the vaccine. Adequate information also needs to be provided to the parents and caregivers to dispel all wrong perceptions about HPV vaccine.

Awareness campaigns in places like ante-natal clinics, parents-teachers forums of schools etc., particularly amongst caregivers of young female children is pivotal to improving uptake of HPV vaccination and reducing incidence of cervical cancer in Nigeria. Governments should subsidize and include the HPV vaccine in National immunization schedules to encourage uptake and subsequently reduce the incidence of cervical cancer.

Conclusions

Despite high levels of education, the following, awareness of HPV infections and cervical cancer, and their related risk factors and HPV vaccines were low among caregivers of female children in Enugu, south-East, Nigeria.

Similarly history of HPV vaccination among the children of the respondents was low, accessibility and affordability was the most common challenge among those aware of the vaccine. There is a need for massive and sustained awareness creation to step up HPV vaccination in Nigeria.

Abbreviations

DNA: Deoxyribonucleic Acid; HPV: Human Papilloma Virus; LGA: Local government areas; STI: Sexually transmitted infection

Funding

The authors have no relevant financial relationship relevant to this article to disclose. This research did not receive any specific grant from funding agencies in the public, commercial, or not-for-profit sectors.

Authors' contributions

AB conceptualized the study, contributed to collection and analysis of data, reviewed the initial draft, wrote the final draft, and approved of the final manuscript to be submitted. UC contributed to initial conceptualization of the design, contributed in collection and analysis of data, and approved of the final draft to be submitted. ON contributed to initial conceptualization of the design, writing of the initial draft and approving of the final manuscript to be submitted.

Competing interests

The authors declare that they have no competing interests.

Author details

[1]College of Medicine, University of Nigeria Ituku-Ozalla, Enugu, Nigeria. [2]College of Medicine, Enugu State Teaching Hospital Parklane, Enugu, Nigeria.

References

1. Aral SO, Holmes KK. The epidemiology of STIs and their social and behavioural determinants: industrialized and developing countries. Sexually Transmitted Diseases. 4th 3ed ed. New York: McGraw-Hill; 2008. p. 53–92.
2. Syrjänen S, Puranen M. Human papilloma virus infections in children: the potential role of maternal transmission. Crit Rev Oral Biol Med. 2000;11(2): 259–74.
3. Prat J. Pathology of cancers of the female genital tract. Int J Gynecol Obstet. 2012;119:S137–50.
4. Stanley M. Human papilloma vaccines versus cervical cancer screening. Clin Oncol (R Coll Radiol). 2008;20:388–94.
5. Steller MA. Cervical cancer: A vaccine-preventable malignancy. Female Patient. 2006;31:9–10.
6. Erickson BK, Avarez RD, Huh WK. Human papilloma virus: what every provider should know. Am J Obstet Gynecol. 2013;208:169–75.
7. Haefner HK. Update on Human papilloma virus. Supplement to SRM. Nov 2008:15–6.
8. Paavonen J. Human papilloma virus infection and the development of cervical cancer and related genital neoplasia. Int J Infect Dis. 2007;11(Suppl 2):S3–9.
9. Escobar PF, Orr JW. The human papilloma virus vaccine: current status. Female Patient. 2008;33:18–22.
10. Patanwala IY, Bauer HM, Miyamoto J, Park IU, Huchko MJ, Smith-McCune KK. A systematic review of randomized trials assessing human papilloma virus testing in cervical screening. Am J Obstet Gynecol. 2013;208:343–53.
11. Agida TE, Akaba GO, Isah AY, Ekele B. Knowledge and perception of human papilloma virus vaccine among the antenatal women in a Nigerian tertiary hospital. Niger Med J. 2015;56:23–7.
12. Syrjänen S. Current concepts on human papilloma virus infections in children. APMIS. 2010;118(6–7):494–509.
13. Holland WW, Stewart S. Screening in adult women, screening in health care. Nuffield: Nuffield Provincial Trust; 1990. p. 155–72.
14. Ferlay J, Shin HR, Bray F, Forman D, Mathers C, Parkin DM. Estimates of worldwide burden of cancer in 2008. GLOBOCAN 2008. Int J Cancer. 2010; 127:2893–917.
15. Louie KS, de Sanjose S, Mayaud P. Epidemiology and prevention of human papilloma virus and cancer in sub-Saharan African: a comprehensive review. Tropical Med Int Health. 2009;14:1287–302.
16. Parkin DM, Sitas F, Chirenje M, Stein L, Abratt R, Wabinga H. Cancer in indigenous Africans-burden, distribution and trends. Lancet Oncol. 2008;9;683–92.
17. Morounke SG, Ayorinde JB, Benedict AO, Adedayo FF, Adewale FO, et al. Epidemiology and incidence of common cancers in Nigeria. J Cancer. Biol Res. 2017;5(3):1105.
18. Bruni L, Barrionuevo-Rosas L, Albero G, Serrano B, Mena M, Gómez D, Muñoz J, Bosch FX, De Sanjosé S.ICO/IARC Information Centre on HPV and Cancer (HPV Information Centre). Human Papilloma virus and Related Diseases in Nigeria. Summary Report 27 July 2017. [Accessed 5[th]aug 2018].
19. Awodele O, Adeyomoye AA, Awodele DF, Fayankinnu VB, Dolapo DC. Cancer distribution pattern in South-Western Nigeria. Tanzan J Health Res. 2011;13(2):125–31.
20. Rafindadi AH, Ahmed SA. Cancer in women and children in Zaria. Lagos: Proceedings of the association of pathologists in Nigeria Scientific Conference; 2005.
21. Ahmed SA, Sabitu K, Idris SH, Ahmed R. Knowledge, attitude and practice of cervical cancer screening among market women in Zaria, Nigeria. Niger Med J. 2013;54:316–9.
22. Pisani P, Parkin DM, Bray F, Ferley J. Estimates of the worldwide mortality from 25 cancers in 1990. Int J Cancer. 1999;83:870–3.
23. Erickson BK, Avarez RD, Huh WK. Human papilloma virus: what every provider should know. Am J ObstetGynecol. 2013;208:169–75.
24. Human papilloma virus vaccination. The American College of Obstetricians and Gynaecologists Committee Opinion no. 588. Obstet Gynecol. 2014;123: 712–8.
25. Markowitz LE, Dunne EF, Saraiya M, Lawson HW, Chesson H, Unger ER. Centers for Disease Control and Prevention (CDC); Advisory Committee on Immunization Practices (ACIP). Quadrivalent human papilloma virus vaccine: recommendations of the Advisory Committee on Immunization Practices (ACIP). MMWR Recomm Rep. 2007;56(RR-2):1–26.
26. Dahlström LA, Tran TN, Lundholm C, Young C, Sundström K, Sparén P.

Reducing incidence of cervical cancer: knowledge and attitudes of caregivers in Nigerian city to human...

233

Attitudes to HPV vaccination among parents of children aged 12-15 years—a population based survey in Sweden. Int J Cancer. 2010;126(2):500–7.

27. Harper DM, Franco EL, Wheeler C, Ferris DG, Jenkins D, Schuind A, et al; GlaxoSmithKline HPV Vaccine Study Group. Efficacy of bivalent L1 virus-like particle vaccine in prevention of infection with human papilloma virus types 16 and 18 in young women: a randomized control trial. Lancet 2004; 364:1757–1765.

28. Paavonen J, Naud P, Salmeron J, Wheeler CM, Chow SN, Apter D, et al. Efficacy of human papilloma virus (HPV)-16/18 ASO4-adjuvanted vaccine against cervical infection and pre-cancer caused by oncogenic HPV types (PATRICIA): final analysis of a double-blind, randomized study in young women. HPV PATRICIA Study Group Lancet. 2009;374:301–14.

29. Munaz N, Kjaer SK, Sigurdsson K, Iversen OE, Hermandez-Avila M, Wheeler CM, et al. Impact of human papilloma virus (HPV)-6/11/16/18 vaccine on all HPV-associated genital diseases in young women. J Natl Cancer Inst. 2010; 102:325–39.

30. Odetola TD, Ekpo K. Nigerian Women's perceptions about human papilloma virus immunizations. J Community Med Health Educ. 2012;2:191.

31. Olowookere SA, Abioye-KuteyiEA AEP, Fasure HA, Fayose O, Onakpoma F, Ibitoye A. Awareness and uptake of human papilloma virus vaccination and cervical Cancer screening among female undergraduate students in a tertiary institution in Nigeria. Nigerian Journal of Family Practice. 2012;3:27–32.

32. Ugwu EO, Obi SN, Ezechukwu PC, Okafor II, Ugwu AO. Acceptability of human papilloma virus vaccine and cervical cancer screening among female health-care workers in Enugu, Southeast Nigeria. Niger J Clin Pract. 2013;16:249–52.

33. Ezem BU. Awareness and uptake of cervical cancer screening in Owerri, south-eastern Nigeria. Ann Afr Med. 2007;6:94–8.

34. Ezenwa BN, Balogun MR, Okafor IP. Mothers' human papilloma virus knowledge and willingness to vaccinate their adolescent daughters in Lagos, Nigeria. Int J Women's Health. 2013;5:371–7.

35. Makwe CC, Anorlu RI. Knowledge of and attitude towards human papilloma virus infection and vaccines among female nurses at a tertiary hospital in Nigeria. Int J Womens Health. 2011;3:313–7.

36. Nnodu O, Erinosho L, Jamda M, Olaniyi O, Adelaiye R, Lawson L, et al. Knowledge and attitudes towards cervical cancer and human papilloma virus: a Nigerian pilot survey. Afr J Reprod Health. 2010;14:95–108.

Permissions

All chapters in this book were first published in IAC, by BioMed Central; hereby published with permission under the Creative Commons Attribution License or equivalent. Every chapter published in this book has been scrutinized by our experts. Their significance has been extensively debated. The topics covered herein carry significant findings which will fuel the growth of the discipline. They may even be implemented as practical applications or may be referred to as a beginning point for another development.

The contributors of this book come from diverse backgrounds, making this book a truly international effort. This book will bring forth new frontiers with its revolutionizing research information and detailed analysis of the nascent developments around the world.

We would like to thank all the contributing authors for lending their expertise to make the book truly unique. They have played a crucial role in the development of this book. Without their invaluable contributions this book wouldn't have been possible. They have made vital efforts to compile up to date information on the varied aspects of this subject to make this book a valuable addition to the collection of many professionals and students.

This book was conceptualized with the vision of imparting up-to-date information and advanced data in this field. To ensure the same, a matchless editorial board was set up. Every individual on the board went through rigorous rounds of assessment to prove their worth. After which they invested a large part of their time researching and compiling the most relevant data for our readers.

The editorial board has been involved in producing this book since its inception. They have spent rigorous hours researching and exploring the diverse topics which have resulted in the successful publishing of this book. They have passed on their knowledge of decades through this book. To expedite this challenging task, the publisher supported the team at every step. A small team of assistant editors was also appointed to further simplify the editing procedure and attain best results for the readers.

Apart from the editorial board, the designing team has also invested a significant amount of their time in understanding the subject and creating the most relevant covers. They scrutinized every image to scout for the most suitable representation of the subject and create an appropriate cover for the book.

The publishing team has been an ardent support to the editorial, designing and production team. Their endless efforts to recruit the best for this project, has resulted in the accomplishment of this book. They are a veteran in the field of academics and their pool of knowledge is as vast as their experience in printing. Their expertise and guidance has proved useful at every step. Their uncompromising quality standards have made this book an exceptional effort. Their encouragement from time to time has been an inspiration for everyone.

The publisher and the editorial board hope that this book will prove to be a valuable piece of knowledge for researchers, students, practitioners and scholars across the globe.

List of Contributors

Jin Zhao, Zhong Guo, Shuyan Pei, Chenjing Wang, Hongmei Qu, Jianbin Zhong, Ying Ma, Cong Nie and Dan Zhang
Medical College of Northwest University for Nationalities, Lanzhou 730030, People's Republic of China

Qiang Wang
Hospital of Longnan City, Longnan 746000, People's Republic of China

Tianbin Si
Gansu Provincial Cancer Hospital, Lanzhou 730050, People's Republic of China

M-N. Theodoraki, J. A. Veit, T. K. Hoffmann and J. Greve
Department of Oto-Rhino-Laryngology, Head and Neck Surgery, University Medical Center, Frauensteige 12, 89070 Ulm, Germany

Saad Saed Alghamdi
Laboratory Medicine, Faculty of Applied Medical Sciences, Umm Al-Qura University, Makkah 7607, Saudi Arabia

Amr Mohamed Mohamed
Laboratory Medicine, Faculty of Applied Medical Sciences, Umm Al-Qura University, Makkah 7607, Saudi Arabia
Clinical Laboratory Diagnosis, Department of Animal Medicine, Faculty of Veterinary Medicine, Assiut University, Assiut, Egypt

Mona Abdelfattah Ahmed
Medical Parasitology, King Abdullah Medical City, Makkah, Saudi Arabia
Parasitology Department, Faculty of Medicine, Ain-Shams University, Cairo, Egypt

Sabah Abdelghany Ahmed
Parasitology Department, Faculty of Medicine, Ain-Shams University, Cairo, Egypt

Sherif Ahmed Al-Semany
Oncology, King Abdullah Medical City, Makkah, Saudi Arabia
Department of Internal Medicine, Medical Oncology, Mansoura University, Mansoura, Egypt

Dina Abdulla Zaglool
Medical Parasitology, Al-Noor Specialist Hospital, Makkah, Saudi Arabia

Parasitology Department, Faculty of Medicine, Assiut University, Assiut, Egypt

Lawson JS, Ngan CC and Glenn WK
School of Biotechnology and Biomolecular Sciences, University of New South Wales, Sydney, Australia

Tran DD
School of Biotechnology and Biomolecular Sciences, University of New South Wales, Sydney, Australia
Douglass Hanly Moir Pathology, Sydney, Australia

Themba G. Ginindza, Joyce M. Tsoka-Gwegweni and Benn Sartorius
Discipline of Public Health, School of Nursing and Public Health, University of KwaZulu-Natal, 2nd Floor George Campbell Building, Mazisi Kunene Road, 4041 Durban, South Africa

Cristina D. Stefan
Walter Sisulu University, Umtata, South Africa

Xolisile Dlamini
Epidemiology Unit, Ministry of Health and Social Welfare, Mbabane, Swaziland

Pauline E. Jolly
Department of Epidemiology, University of Alabama, Birmingham, USA

Elisabete Weiderpass
Department of Medical Epidemiology and Biostatistics, Karolinska Institutet, Stockholm, Sweden
Department of Research, Cancer Registry of Norway, Institute of Population-Based Cancer Research, Oslo, Norway
Department of Community Medicine, Faculty of Health Sciences, University of Tromsø, The Arctic University of Norway, Tromsø, Norway
Genetic Epidemiology Group, Folkhälsan Research Center, Helsinki, Finland

Nathalie Broutet
World Health Organization; Department of Reproductive Health and Research, Geneva, Switzerland

Gary M. Clifford, Martyn Plummer and Silvia Franceschi
International Agency for Research on Cancer, 150 cours Albert Thomas, 69372 Lyon Cedex 08, France

Tim Waterboer, Bolormaa Dondog and Michael Pawlita
Infection, Inflammation and Cancer Program, German Cancer Research Center (DKFZ), Heidelberg, Germany

You Lin Qiao
Cancer Institute of the Chinese Academy of Medical Sciences, Beijing, China

Dimitri Kordzaia
Iv. Javakhishvili Tbilisi State University, Tbilisi, Georgia

Doudja Hammouda
Institut National de Sante Publique, Algiers, Algeria

Namory Keita
Department of Obstetrics and Gynaecology, Centre Hospitalier Universitaire de Donka, Conakry, Guinea

Nahid Khodakarami
Infertility and Reproductive Health Research Centre, Shahid Beheshti University of Medical Sciences, Tehran, Iran

Syed Ahsan Raza
Department of Surgery, The Aga Khan University, Karachi, Pakistan
Centre de Recherche du CHUM, Département de Médecine Sociale et Préventive Université de Montréal, Quebec, Canada

Ang Tshering Sherpa
Kist Medical College, Lalitpur, Nepal

Witold Zatonski
The Maria Sklodowska-Curie Memorial Cancer Center and Institute of Oncology, Warsaw, Poland

Balew Arega
College of Health Sciences, Debremarkos University, Debremarkos, Ethiopia
Department of Microbiology, Immunology andParasitology, School of Medicine, College of Health Sciences, Addis AbabaUniversity, Churchill Avenue, Addis Ababa, Ethiopia

Yimtubezinash Wolde-Amanuel and Daniel Asrat
Department of Microbiology, Immunology andParasitology, School of Medicine, College of Health Sciences, Addis AbabaUniversity, Churchill Avenue, Addis Ababa, Ethiopia

Kelemework Adane
Department of Microbiology and Immunology, College of Health Sciences, Mekelle University, Mekelle, Ethiopia

Ezra Belay
Department Medical Biochemistry, College of Health Sciences, Mekelle University, Mekelle, Ethiopia

Abdulaziz Abubeker
Department of Internal Medicine, School of Medicine, College of Health Sciences, Addis Ababa University, Churchill Avenue, Addis Ababa, Ethiopia

Lars Ivo Partecke, Felicitas Roetz, Claus-Dieter Heidecke and Wolfram von Bernstorff
Department of General, Visceral, Thoracic and Vascular Surgery, Universitätsmedizin Greifswald, Greifswald, Germany

Katharina Beyer
Department of General, Visceral, Thoracic and Vascular Surgery, Universitätsmedizin Greifswald, Greifswald, Germany
Department of General, Visceral and Vascular Surgery, Charité Universitätsmedizin Berlin, Campus Benjamin Franklin, Hindenburgdamm 30, 12203 Berlin, Germany

Frank Ulrich Weiss
Department of Obstetrics and Gynaecology, Universitätsklinikum Heidelberg, Heidelberg, Germany

Herbert Fluhr
Department of Medicine A, Universitätsmedizin Greifswald, Greifswald, Germany

Hugo Cruz
Microbiology, Faculty of Medicine of the University of Coimbra, 3004-504 Coimbra, Portugal

Célia Nogueira
Microbiology, Faculty of Medicine of the University of Coimbra, 3004-504 Coimbra, Portugal
CIMAGO, Faculty of Medicine of the University of Coimbra, 3001-301 Coimbra, Portugal
Medical Microbiology, Centre for Neuroscience and Cell Biology of the University of Coimbra, 3004-504 Coimbra, Portugal

Marta Mota
Microbiology, Faculty of Medicine of the University of Coimbra, 3004-504 Coimbra, Portugal
Medical Microbiology, Centre for Neuroscience and Cell Biology of the University of Coimbra, 3004-504 Coimbra, Portugal

Rui Gradiz
Physiopathology, Faculty of Medicine of the University of Coimbra, 3004-504 Coimbra, Portugal
Gastroenterology, University Hospitals of Coimbra, 3000-075 Coimbra, Portugal

Maximino Leitão
Gastroenterology, University Hospitals of Coimbra, 3000-075 Coimbra, Portugal

Maria Augusta Cipriano
Pathological Anatomy, University Hospitals of Coimbra, 3000-075 Coimbra, Portugal

Francisco Caramelo
Laboratory of Biostatistics and Medical Informatics, IBILI, Faculty of Medicine of the University of Coimbra, 3000-548 Coimbra, Portugal

Ana Alarcão
Pathology Institute, Faculty of Medicine of the University of Coimbra, 3004-504 Coimbra, Portugal

Francisco Castro e Sousa, Fernando Oliveira and Fernando Martinho
Department of Surgery, University Hospitals of Coimbra, 3000-075 Coimbra, Portugal

João Moura Pereira
Surgery, Regional Oncology Center of Coimbra, IPOFG, 3000-075 Coimbra, Portugal

Paulo Figueiredo
Histopathology, Regional Oncology Center of Coimbra, IPOFG, 3000-075 Coimbra, Portugal

Vincenza Granata, Roberta Fusco, Orlando Catalano, Francesco Filice and Antonella Petrillo
Radiology Division, "Istituto Nazionale Tumori - IRCCS - Fondazione G. Pascale", Via Mariano Semmola, Naples, Italy

Antonio Avallone
Abdominal Oncology Division, "Istituto Nazionale Tumori - IRCCS - Fondazione G. Pascale", Via Mariano Semmola, Naples, Italy

Maddalena Leongito, Raffaele Palaia and Francesco Izzo
Hepatobiliary Surgery Division, "Istituto Nazionale Tumori - IRCCS - Fondazione G. Pascale", Via Mariano Semmola, Naples, Italy

Li Qin, Lili Chen, Siting Zhao, Zhengxiang He and Xiaoping Chen
State Key Laboratory of Respiratory Disease, Guangzhou Institutes of Biomedicine and Health, Chinese Academy of Sciences, 190 Kaiyuan Avenue, Guangzhou Science Park, 510530 Guangzhou, China

Ming Ou-Yang, Chengzhi Zhou, Jianxing He and Nanshan Zhong
State Key Laboratory of Respiratory Disease, Guangzhou Institute of Respiratory Disease, First Affiliated Hospital, Guangzhou Medical University, 151 Yanjiang Road, 510120 Guangzhou, China

Changzhong Chen
Channing Laboratory, Brigham and Women's Hospital, 181 Longwood Ave, Boston, MA 02115, USA

Ran Xue and Pinghua Liu
Boston University, Boston, MA 02215, USA

Yu Xia
Department of Bioengineering, McGill University, Montreal, QC H3A 0C3, Canada

Hina Sarwath, Mahmoud Mohamed and Shahinaz Bedri
Department of Pathology and Laboratory Medicine, Weill Cornell Medicine – Qatar, Cornell University, Qatar Foundation - Education City, Doha, Qatar

Devendra Bansal and Ali A. Sultan
Department of Microbiology and Immunology, Weill Cornell Medicine – Qatar, Cornell University, Qatar Foundation - Education City, Doha, Qatar

Nazik Elmalaika Husain
Faculty of Medicine, Omdurman Islamic University, Omdurman, Sudan

Kasper Ingerslev and Jan Blaakaer
Department of Gynaecology and Obstetrics, Odense University Hospital, Denmark, Soendre Blvd. 29, 5000 Odense C, Denmark

Estrid Hogdall
Department of Pathology, Herlev and Gentofte Hospital, Denmark, Herlev Ringvej 75, 2730 Herlev, Denmark

Tine Henrichsen Schnack and Claus Hogdall
Gynaecologic Clinic, Copenhagen University Hospital, Denmark, Blegdamsvej 9, 2100 Copenhagen, Denmark

Wojciech Skovrider-Ruminski
Department of Pathology, Herlev Hospital, Denmark, Herlev Ringvej 75, 2730 Herlev, Denmark

Patrick W. Narkwa and Mohamed Mutocheluh
Department of Clinical Microbiology, School of Medical Sciences, Kwame Nkrumah University of Science and Technology, Kumasi, Ghana

David J. Blackbourn
Department of Microbial and Cellular Sciences, School of Biosciences and Medicine, University of Surrey, Surrey GU2 7XH, UK

Ruta Everatt and Irena Kuzmickiene
Laboratory of Cancer Epidemiology, National Cancer Institute, Baublio g. 3B, LT-08406 Vilnius, Lithuania

Edita Davidaviciene
Vilnius University Hospital Santaros Klinikos, P.Sirvio g. 5, LT-10214 Vilnius, Lithuania

Saulius Cicenas
Department of Thoracic Surgery and Oncology, National Cancer Institute, Santariskiu g. 1, LT-08660 Vilnius, Lithuania
Faculty of Medicine, Vilnius University, M.K.Ciurlionio g. 21, LT-03101 Vilnius, Lithuania

Susanne Hartwig and Géraldine Dominiak-Felden
Department of Epidemiology, Sanofi Pasteur MSD, 162 avenue Jean Jaurès, Lyon, France

Jean Lacau St Guily
Department of Otolaryngology-Head and Neck Surgery, Tenon Hospital – Assistance Publique-Hopitaux de Paris (AP-HP) and Sorbonne University-Paris 6, Pierre-et-Marie Curie University Cancerology Institute, 4 rue de la Chine, 75020 Paris, France

Laia Alemany
Cancer Epidemiology Research Program, Institut Català d'Oncologia (ICO)-IDIBELL, L'Hospitalet de Llobregat, Catalonia, Spain

Silvia de Sanjosé
Cancer Epidemiology Research Program, Institut Català d'Oncologia (ICO)-IDIBELL, L'Hospitalet de Llobregat, Catalonia, Spain
CIBER Epidemiologia y Salud Pública, Barcelona, Spain

Francesca Caccuri, Pietro Mazzuca, Cinzia Giagulli and Arnaldo Caruso
Section of Microbiology, Department of Molecular and Translational Medicine, University of Brescia, Brescia, Italy

Francesca Giordano, Ines Barone, Sebastiano Andò and Stefania Marsico
Department of Pharmacy, Health and Nutritional Sciences, University of Calabria, Arcavacata di Rende, Italy

Sook Ling Lai
Faculty of Dentistry, University of Malaya, Kuala Lumpur, Malaysia

Lee Fah Yap and Ian C. Paterson
Faculty of Dentistry, University of Malaya, Kuala Lumpur, Malaysia
Oral Cancer Research and Coordinating Centre, Faculty of Dentistry, University of Malaya, Kuala Lumpur, Malaysia

Anthony Rhodes
School of Medicine, Taylor's University, Subang Jaya, Selangor, Malaysia

Max Robinson
Centre for Oral Health Research, Newcastle University, Newcastle-upon-Tyne, UK

Hans Prakash Sathasivam
Centre for Oral Health Research, Newcastle University, Newcastle-upon-Tyne, UK
Ministry of Health, Kuala Lumpur, Malaysia

Maizaton Atmadini Abdullah
Faculty of Medicine and Health Sciences, University Putra Malaysia, Serdang, Malaysia

Kin-Choo Pua
Penang General Hospital, Penang, Malaysia

Pathmanathan Rajadurai
Subang Jaya Medical Centre, Subang Jaya, Selangor, Malaysia

Phaik-Leng Cheah
Faculty of Medicine, University of Malaya, Kuala Lumpur, Malaysia

Selvam Thavaraj
Head and Neck Pathology, Dental Institute, King's College London, London, UK

Ahmed M. Elhassan and Muntaser E. Ibrahim
Department of Molecular Biology, Institute of Endemic Diseases, University of Khartoum, Al-Qasr Street, , Khartoum, Sudan

Ghimja Fessahaye
Department of Molecular Biology, Institute of Endemic Diseases, University of Khartoum, Al-Qasr Street, , Khartoum, Sudan
Asmera College of Health Sciences, Asmara, Eritrea

Elwaleed M. Elamin
Faculty of Medical Laboratory Sciences, Alzaeim Alazhari University, Khartoum, Sudan

Ameera A. M. Adam
Faculty of Medical Laboratory Sciences, Department of Histopathology and Cytology, Al Neelain University, Khartoum, Sudan

Anghesom Ghebremedhin
Asmera College of Health Sciences, Asmara, Eritrea

Jean-Damien Combes
International Agency for Research on Cancer, 150 cours Albert Thomas, 69372 Cedex 08 Lyon, France

Silvia Franceschi
Cancer Epidemiology Unit, CRO Aviano National Cancer Institute IRCCS, Via Franco Gallini 2, 33081 Aviano, PN, Italy

Valeria I. Fink and Pedro Cahn
Fundación Huésped, Pasaje Gianantonio 3932, C1202ABB Buenos Aires, Argentina

Cathy A. Jenkins, Jessica L. Castilho, Anna K. Person, Bryan E. Shepherd, Karu Jayathilake and Catherine McGowan
Vanderbilt University School of Medicine, 1161 21st Ave. S A2200 Medical Center North, Nashville, TN 37232, USA

Beatriz Grinsztejn and Juliana Netto
Instituto Nacional de Infectologia Evandro Chagas, Fundação Oswaldo Cruz, Av. Brasil, 4365 - Manguinhos, Rio de Janeiro, RJ 21040-900, Brasil

Brenda Crabtree-Ramirez
Instituto Nacional de Ciencias Médicas y Nutrición Salvador Zubirán: Unidad del Paciente Ambulatorio (UPA), 5to piso Vasco de Quiroga # 15 Col. Sección XVI Delegación Tlalpan; C.P, 14000 Mexico City, Mexico

Claudia P. Cortés
Fundación Arriarán, Santa Elvira 629, Santiago, Chile

Denis Padgett
Instituto Hondureño de Seguridad Social, Barrio la Granja, Tegucigalpa Honduras, Hospital Escuela Universitario:Av La Salud, Tegucigalpa, Honduras

Shuying Li, Haie Shen, Zhanjun Liu, Ning Li, Suxian Yang and Ke Zhang
North China University of Science and Technology (Hebei Key Laboratory for Chronic Diseases, Tangshan Key Laboratory for Preclinical and Basic Research on Chronic Diseases), No.21 Bohai Road, Caofeidian New Town, Tangshan City, Hebei Province 063210, People's Republic of China

Jintao Li
College of Life Science and Bio-engineering, Beijing University of Technology, Beijingcity, 100124, People's Republic of China

Vincenza Granata, Salvatore Filice, Orlando Catalano and Antonella Petrillo
Radiology Division, Istituto Nazionale Tumori IRCCS Fondazione G. Pascale – IRCCS di Napoli, via Mariano Semmola, I-80131 Naples, Italy

Roberta Fusco
Radiology Division, Istituto Nazionale Tumori IRCCS Fondazione G. Pascale – IRCCS di Napoli, via Mariano Semmola, I-80131 Naples, Italy
Hepatobiliary Surgical Oncology Division, Istituto Nazionale Tumori IRCCS Fondazione G. Pascale – IRCCS di Napoli, via Mariano Semmola, I-80131 Naples, Italy

Mauro Piccirillo, Raffaele Palaia and Francesco Izzo
Hepatobiliary Surgical Oncology Division, Istituto Nazionale Tumori IRCCS Fondazione G. Pascale – IRCCS di Napoli, via Mariano Semmola, I-80131 Naples, Italy

Silvia Giunco
Immunology and Molecular Oncology Unit, Istituto Oncologico Veneto (IOV)-IRCCS, Padova, Italy

Anita De Rossi
Immunology and Molecular Oncology Unit, Istituto Oncologico Veneto (IOV)-IRCCS, Padova, Italy
Department of Surgery, Oncology and Gastro-enterology, Section of Oncology and Immunology, University of Padova, Padova, Italy

Maria Raffaella Petrara, Manuela Zangrossi and Andrea Celeghin
Department of Surgery, Oncology and Gastro-enterology, Section of Oncology and Immunology, University of Padova, Padova, Italy

Gerardo Santos-López, Julio Reyes-Leyva and Verónica Vallejo-Ruiz
Centro de Investigación Biomédica de Oriente, Instituto Mexicano del Seguro Social, Km. 4.5 Carretera Federal Atlixco-Metepec, Atlixco, C.P.74360 Puebla, Mexico

Miguel Aco-Tlachi
Centro de Investigación Biomédica de Oriente, Instituto Mexicano del Seguro Social, Km. 4.5 Carretera Federal Atlixco-Metepec, Atlixco, C.P.74360 Puebla, Mexico
Posgrado en Ciencias Microbiológicas, Benemérita Universidad Autónoma de Puebla, Edi icio 103-J Cd. Universitaria, Col. San Manuel, C. P. 72570 Puebla, Pue, Mexico

Ricardo Carreño-López
Posgrado en Ciencias Microbiológicas, Benemérita Universidad Autónoma de Puebla, Edi icio 103-J Cd. Universitaria, Col. San Manuel, C. P. 72570 Puebla, Pue, Mexico

Adriana Aguilar-Lemarroy and Luis Felipe Jave-Suárez
Centro de Investigación Biomédica de Occidente, Instituto Mexicano del Seguro Social, Sierra Mojada 800, Col Independencia, C. P. 44340 Guadalajara, Jalisco, Mexico

Patricia L. Martínez-Morales and Paola Maycotte
CONACYT- Centro de Investigación Biomédica de Oriente, Instituto Mexicano del Seguro Social, Km.4.5 Carretera Federal Atlixco-Metepec, Atlixco, C. P. 74360 Puebla, Mexico

Sunil Kumar Sah and Sadina Shrestha
B.P.Koirala Memorial Cancer Hospital, Bharatpur, Chitwan, Nepal

Joaquin V. González and María Alejandra Picconi
Oncogenic Viruses Laboratory, National Institute of Infectious Diseases-ANLIS "Dr. Malbrán", Av.Velez Sarsfield 563, C1282AFF Buenos Aires, Argentina
National and Regional HPV Reference Laboratory, National Institute of Infectious Diseases-ANLIS "Dr. Malbrán", Av.Velez Sarsfield 563, C1282AFF Buenos Aires, Argentina

Anurag Adhikari
Kathmandu Research Institute for Biological Sciences, Lalitpur, Nepal

Shyam Babu Yadav
Department of Health Service, Ministry of Health, Government of Nepal, Kathmandu, Nepal

Krishna Das Manandhar and Birendra Prasad Gupta
Central Department of Biotechnology, Tribhuvan University, Kirtipur, Kathmandu, Nepal

David A. Stein
Department of Biomedical Sciences, Oregon State University, Corvallis, Oregon, USA

José Humberto Tavares Guerreiro Fregnani and Cristovam Scapulatempo Neto
1Teaching and Research Institute, Barretos Cancer Hospital – Pius XII Foundation, Rua Antenor Duarte Vilela, 1331, Dr. Paulo Prata, Barretos, São Paulo 14784-400, Brazil

Allini Mafra da Costa
Teaching and Research Institute, Barretos Cancer Hospital – Pius XII Foundation, Rua Antenor Duarte Vilela, 1331, Dr. Paulo Prata, Barretos, São Paulo 14784-400, Brazil

Cancer Registry, Barretos Cancer Hospital – Pius XII Foundation, São Paulo, Brazil

Paula Roberta Aguiar Pastrez, Vânia Sammartino Mariano and Estela Maria Silva
Teaching and Research Institute, Barretos Cancer Hospital – Pius XII Foundation, Rua Antenor Duarte Vilela, 1331, Dr. Paulo Prata, Barretos, São Paulo 14784-400, Brazil
Molecular Oncology Research Center, Barretos Cancer Hospital – Pius XII Foundation, São Paulo, Brazil

Kari Juhani Syrjanen
Teaching and Research Institute, Barretos Cancer Hospital – Pius XII Foundation, Rua Antenor Duarte Vilela, 1331, Dr. Paulo Prata, Barretos, São Paulo 14784-400, Brazil
Molecular Oncology Research Center, Barretos Cancer Hospital – Pius XII Foundation, São Paulo, Brazil
Department of Clinical Research -Biohit Oyj, Helsinki, Finland

Adhemar Longatto-Filho
Teaching and Research Institute, Barretos Cancer Hospital – Pius XII Foundation, Rua Antenor Duarte Vilela, 1331, Dr. Paulo Prata, Barretos, São Paulo 14784-400, Brazil
Molecular Oncology Research Center, Barretos Cancer Hospital – Pius XII Foundation, São Paulo, Brazil
Medical Laboratory of Medical Investigation (LIM) 14, Department of Pathology, Faculty of Medicine, University of São Paulo, São Paulo, Brazil
Research Institute of Life and Health Sciences (ICVS), University of Minho, Braga, Portugal
ICVS / 3B's - Associated Laboratory to the Government of Portugal, Braga/Guimarães, Portugal

Denise Peixoto Guimarães
Molecular Oncology Research Center, Barretos Cancer Hospital – Pius XII Foundation, São Paulo, Brazil
Department of Endoscopy, Barretos Cancer Hospital – Pious XII Foundation, Barretos, São Paulo, Brazil

Laura Sichero
Molecular Biology Laboratory, Center for Translational Research in Oncology, Instituto do Câncer do Estado de São Paulo – ICESP, São Paulo, Brazil

Luisa Lina Villa
Molecular Biology Laboratory, Center for Translational Research in Oncology, Instituto do Câncer do Estado de São Paulo – ICESP, São Paulo, Brazil
Department of Radiology and Oncology, School of Medicine, University of São Paulo, São Paulo, Brazil

Adaobi I. Bisi-Onyemaechi and Ugo N. Chikani
College of Medicine, University of Nigeria Ituku Ozalla, Enugu, Nigeria

Obinna Nduagubam
College of Medicine, Enugu State Teaching Hospital Parklane, Enugu, Nigeria

Index

www.ingramcontent.com/pod-product-compliance
Lightning Source LLC
Chambersburg PA
CBHW080248230326
41458CB00097B/4160